WOMEN'S MENTAL HEALTH
A LIFE-CYCLE APPROACH

WOMEN'S MENTAL HEALTH

A LIFE-CYCLE APPROACH

Edited by

Sarah E. Romans, MB, ChB, MD

Shirley Brown Chair in Women's Mental Health Research,
Centre for Research in Women's Health
Consultant Psychiatrist, Sunnybrook and
Women's College Health Sciences Centre
Professor of Psychiatry, University of Toronto
Ontario, Canada

Mary V. Seeman, MD, DSc

Professor Emerita, University of Toronto
Centre for Addiction and Mental Health
Ontario, Canada

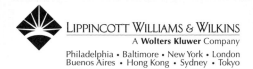

LIPPINCOTT WILLIAMS & WILKINS
A **Wolters Kluwer** Company

Philadelphia • Baltimore • New York • London
Buenos Aires • Hong Kong • Sydney • Tokyo

Executive Editor: Charles W. Mitchell
Managing Editor: Lisa R. Kairis
Project Manager: Bridgett Dougherty
Senior Manufacturing Manager: Benjamin Rivera
Marketing Manager: Adam Glazer
Design Coordinator: Terry Mallon
Production Services: Nesbitt Graphics, Inc.
Printer: Edwards Brothers

© 2006 by LIPPINCOTT WILLIAMS & WILKINS
530 Walnut Street
Philadelphia, PA 19106 USA
www.LWW.com

Library of Congress Cataloging-in-Publication Data

Women's mental health: a life-cycle approach / edited by Sarah Romans, Mary V. Seeman.
p. cm.
Includes bibliographical references and index.
ISBN 0-7817-5129-2
1. Women—Mental health. 2. Life cycle, Human. I. Romans, Sarah E. II. Seeman, M. V. (Mary Violette), 1935-
RC451.4.W6W65975 2006
362.2'082—dc22

2005003148

Care has been taken to confirm the accuracy of the information presented and to describe generally accepted practices. However, the authors, editors, and publisher are not responsible for errors or omissions or for any consequences from application of the information in this book and make no warranty, expressed or implied, with respect to the currency, completeness, or accuracy of the contents of the publication. Application of the information in a particular situation remains the professional responsibility of the practitioner.

The authors, editors, and publisher have exerted every effort to ensure that drug selection and dosage set forth in this text are in accordance with current recommendations and practice at the time of publication. However, in view of ongoing research, changes in government regulations, and the constant flow of information relating to drug therapy and drug reactions, the reader is urged to check the package insert for each drug for any change in indications and dosage and for added warnings and precautions. This is particularly important when the recommended agent is a new or infrequently employed drug.

Some drugs and medical devices presented in the publication have Food and Drug Administration (FDA) clearance for limited use in restricted research settings. It is the responsibility of the health care provider to ascertain the FDA status of each drug or device planned for use in their clinical practice.

10 9 8 7 6 5 4 3 2 1

To my mother, Francesca Sarah Chinnery Romans,
a powerful influence in my life

SARAH E. ROMANS

To the memory of my mother,
Sonia Brzezinska Szwarc

MARY V. SEEMAN

Contents

Contributors

Jean Addington, MD

Associate Professor, Psychiatry, University of Toronto; Director, PRIME Clinic, Centre for Addiction and Mental Health, Toronto, Ontario, Canada

Lisa Francesca Andermann, MPhil, MDCM, FRCPC

Assistant Professor, Culture, Community and Health Studies, Department of Psychiatry, University of Toronto, Toronto, Ontario; Psychiatrist, Department of Psychiatry, Mount Sinai Hospital, Toronto, Ontario, Canada

Leah K. Andrews, MB, ChB, FRANZCP

Senior Lecturer, Department of Psychological Medicine, University of Auckland, Auckland, New Zealand; Child and Adolescent Psychiatrist, Consultation Liaison Child Psychiatry, Starship Children's Health, Auckland District Health Board, Auckland, New Zealand

Jill A. Astbury, MEd, PhD

Research Professor, School of Psychology, Victoria University, Melbourne City, Victoria, Australia

Rosemary Basson, MD, FRCP (UK)

Clinical Professor, Director, Sexual Medicine Program, Department of Psychiatry, University of British Columbia, Vancouver, B.C.; Program Director, B.C, Center for Sexual Medicine, Vancouver General Hospital, Vancouver, B.C.

Robyn L. Bluhm, MA

PhD Candidate, Department of Philosophy, The University of Western Ontario, London, Ontario, Canada

Sheila B. Blume, MD

Clinical Professor of Psychiatry, School of Medicine, State University of New York at Stony Brook, Stony Brook, New York

Annie M. Bollini

Predoctoral Fellow, Department of Psychology, Emory University, Atlanta, Georgia

Elspeth A. Bradley, PhD, FRCPsych, FRCPC

Associate Professor, Department of Psychiatry, University of Toronto, Toronto; Surrey Place Centre, Psychiatrist-in-Chief, Biomedical Sciences and Research Division, Surrey Place Centre, Toronto, Ontario, Canada

Susan J. Bradley, MD

Professor, Psychiatry, University of Toronto, Toronto, Ontario; Psychiatrist, Psychiatry, Hospital for Sick Children, Toronto, Ontario, Canada

Anne E. Buist, MBBS, MMed, MD, FRANZCP

Associate Professor, Department of Psychiatry, University of Melbourne, West Heidelberg, Victoria, Australia; Deputy Director, Department of Psychiatry, Austin Health, West Heidelberg, Victoria, Australia

Cynthia M. Bulik

Distinguished Professor, Psychiatry/Nutrition, University of North Carolina, Chapel Hill, North Carolina

Joan Busfield, PhD

Professor, Department of Sociology, University of Essex, Colchester, Essex, United Kingdom

Helen F. K. Chiu, MBBS, FRCPsych

Professor, Department of Psychiatry, The Chinese University of Hong Kong, Tai Po, Hong Kong; Honorary Consultant, Department of Psychiatry, Shatin Hospital, Hong Kong

Marsha M. Cohen, MD, MHSc

Senior Research Scientist, Centre for Research in Women's Health; Professor, Department of Health Policy Management and Evaluation, University of Toronto, Toronto, Ontario, Canada

Judith H. Gold CM, MD, FRCPC, FRANZCP, DHumL (hc)
Private Practice of Psychiatry
Brisbane, Australia

Sophie Grigoriadis, PhD, MD, FRCRC
Assistant Professor, Department of Psychiatry, University of Toronto, Ontario, Canada; Psychiatrist, Department of Psychiatry, University Health Network and Sunnybrook and Women's College Health Sciences Centre, Toronto, Ontario, Canada

Sydney L. Hans, PhD
Associate Professor, School of Social Service Administration, The University of Chicago, Chicago, Illinois

Anne Hassett, MD, DGM, FRANZCP
Associate Professor, Psychiatry, University of Melbourne, Victoria, Australia; Clinical Director North West Aged Person's Mental Health Program, North West Mental Health, Melbourne Health Sunshine Hospital, Victoria, Australia

Judith V. Jordan, PhD
Assistant Professor, Department of Psychiatry, Harvard Medical School, Lexington, Massachusetts; Consulting Psychologist, Department of Psychology, McLean Hospital, Belmont, Massachusetts

Debra Kaminer
Lecturer, Department of Psychology, University of Cape Town, Rondebosch, Cape Town, South Africa

Javaria M. Khalid, BSc
Research Assistant, Women's Health Program, University Health Network, Toronto, Ontario, Canada

Marika Korossy, BA
Librarian and Resources Coordinator, The Joseph M. Berg Library and Biomedical Services and Research Division, Surrey Place Centre, Toronto, Ontario, Canada

Jayashri Kulkarni, MBBS, MPN, FRANZCP, PhD
Professor Department of Psychiatry and Psychological Medicine, Monash University, Clayton, Australia, Director, Alfred Psychiatry Research Centre, The Alfred Hospital, Melbourne, Australia

Ruth Lanius, MD
Assistant Professor, Department of Psychiatry, The University of Western Ontario, London, Ontario, Canada; Director, Traumatic Stress Service and WSIB Traumatic Stress Service Workplace Program, London Health Sciences Centre, London, Ontario, Canada

Florence Levy, MBBS, MD, FRANZCP
Conjoint Professor, School of Psychiatry, University of New South Wales, Sydney, Australia; Head, Child and Family East, Child and Adolescent Mental Health, Prince of Wales Hospital, Sydney, Australia

Ellen L. Lipman, MD, Msc
Associate Professor, Department of Psychiatry and Behavioural Neurosciences, McMaster University, Hamilton, Ontario, Canada; Child Psychiatrist, Department of Psychiatry and Behavioural Neurosciences, Faculty of Health Sciences, Hamilton Health Sciences, Chedoke Hospital, Hamilton, Ontario, Canada

Yona Lunsky, PhD, C.Psych
Assistant Professor, Department of Psychiatry, University of Toronto, Toronto, Ontario, Canada; Centre for Addiction and Mental Health, Psychologist, Dual Diagnosis, Centre for Addiction and Mental Health, Toronto, Ontario, Canada

Katharina Manassis, MD, FRCPC
Associate Professor, Department of Psychiatry, University of Toronto, Toronto, Ontario, Canada; Director, Anxiety Disorders Program, Department of Psychiatry, Hospital for Sick Children, Toronto, Ontario, Canada

Pamela Melding, MD
Department of Psychiatry
Faculty of Medical and Health Sciences The University of Auckland, Auckland, New Zealand

Carol Cooperman Nadelson, MD
Clinical Professor, Psychiatry, Harvard Medical School, Boston, Massachusetts; Director, Partners, Office for Women's Careers, Brigham and Women's Hospital, Boston, Massachusetts

Malkah Notman, MD
Clinical Professor, Department of Psychiatry, Harvard Medical School, Boston, Massachusetts; Director of Faculty Development, Department of Psychiatry, Cambridge Hospital, Cambridge, Massachusetts

David R. Offord*

Offord Centre for Child Studies and Department of Psychiatry and Behavioural Neuroscience, McMaster University, Hamilton, OH

Mary Kay O'Neil, PhD

Assistant Professor, Department of Psychiatry, University of Toronto; Visiting Scholar, Psychology Department, Concordia University, Montreal, Canada; Supervising and Training Analyst, Canadian Institute of Psychoanalysis, Montreal, Quebec, Canada

Clare Pain, MD, FRCPC

Assistant Professor Universities of Toronto and Western Ontario, Department of Psychiatry, Mount Sinai Hospital, Toronto, Ontario; Clinical Director of the Psychological Trauma Assessment Clinic in Toronto, and Director of Clinical Research for the Traumatic Stress Service in London, Department of Psychiatry, London Health Service Centre, Victoria Hospital, London, Ontario

Nalini Pandalangat, MA, M.Phil

Early Intervention Project Developer & Community Support Specialist, Community Support and Reserach Unit, Centre for Addiction and Mental Health, Toronto, Ontario, Canada

Mani N. Pavuluri, MD, PhD, FRANZCP

Associate Professor, Child Psychiatry, University of Illinois at Chicago, Chicago, Illinois; Director, Pediatric Mood Disorders Program, Institute for Juvenile Research

Chris Perkins, MB, ChB, FRANZCP

Mental Health Services for Older People, Tauranga Hospital, Tauranga, New Zealand

Lauren Reba

University of North Carolina, Chapel Hill, North Carolina

Gail Erlick Robinson, MD, D.Psych, FRCPC

Professor, Psychiatry and Obstetrics/Gynecology, University of Toronto, Toronto, Ontario, Canada; Director, Women's Mental Health Program, Psychiatry, University Health Network, Toronto, Ontario, Canada

Anne E. Rhodes, PhD

Assistant Professor, Department of Psychiatry and Public Health Sciences, University of Toronto; Research Scientist, Mental Health Department, St. Michael's Hospital, Toronto, Canada

Sarah E. Romans, MB, ChB, MD

Shirley Brown Chair in Women's Mental Health Research, Centre for Research in Women's Health; Consultant Psychiatrist, Sunnybrook and Women's College Health Sciences Centre; Professor of Psychiatry, University of Toronto, Ontario, Canada

Zainab Sabuwalla, BS

Department of Psychology, Emory University, Atlanta, Georgia

Soraya Seedat, MBChB, FC Psych, MMed (Psych)

Associate Professor, Department of Psychiatry, University of Stellenbosch, Cape Town, South Africa

Berit Schei

Professor, Department of Public Health, Norwegian University of Science and Technology, Trondheim, Norway; Consultant, Department of Obstetrics and Gynecology, St. Olavs Hospital, Trondheim, Norway

Frauke T. K. Schultze-Lutter, M. Psych., PhD

Scientific-psychological Head of FETZ; Early Recognition and Intervention Centre for Mental Crises, FETZ, Department of Psychiatry and Psychotherapy, University of Cologne, Cologne, Germany

Mary V. Seeman, MDCM, FRCPC, DSc

Professor Emerita, Psychiatry, University of Toronto, Ontario, Toronto, Canada; Staff Psychiatrist, Schizophrenia and Continuing Care, Centre for Addiction and Mental Health, Toronto, Ontario, Canada

Donna E. Stewart, MD, FRCPC

University Professor and Chair, Psychiatry, OB-GYN, University of Toronto, Toronto, Ontario, Canada; Director and Chair of Women's Health, Women's Health, University Health Network, Toronto, Ontario, Canada

Hermano Tavares, MD PhD

Institute of Psychiatry, University of Sao Paulo, Brazil

*Deceased

Deborah J. Walder, PhD
Department of Psychiatry, Massachusetts General Hospital, Charlestown, Massachusetts

Elaine Walker, PhD
Instructor of Psychology, Department of Psychiatry, Harvard Medical School; Staff Psychologist, Department of Psychiatry, Massachusetts General Hospital, Charlestown, Massachusetts

M. Louise Webster MBChB, FRACP, FRANZCP
Senior Lecturer, Department of Psychological Medicine, University of Auckland, Auckland, New Zealand; Child and Adolescent Psychiatrist, Consultation Liaison Child Psychiatry, Starship Children's Health, Auckland District Health Board, Auckland, New Zealand

Charmaine C. Williams, PhD, RSW
Assistant Professor
Faculty of Social Work, University of Toronto, Toronto, Canada

Monica L. Zilberman, MD, PhD
Post-doctoral Fellow, Faculty of Medicine, University of Sao Paulo, Sao Paulo, Brazil; Psychiatrist, Institute of Psychiatry, Hospital das Clinicas, Sao Paulo, Brazil

Kenneth J. Zucker, PhD
Professor, Departments of Psychology and Psychiatry, University of Toronto, Ontario, Canada; Centre for Addiction and Mental Health; Head, Child and Adolescent Gender Identity Clinic, Child, Youth, and Family Program, Toronto, Ontario, Canada

Preface

Women's mental health is receiving increased attention from scholars, practitioners, the media, and the public at large. There is now a widespread appreciation that biologically determined gender and socially determined gender play major roles in the way health, including mental health, is conceptualized. This heightened awareness is seen at all levels of scientific understanding, from the sociocultural through to the hormonal, cellular, and DNA levels—areas of increased biomedical investigation and activity. Simultaneous advances in knowledge have been occurring at each of these levels, and the time is now ripe to integrate gender-relevant findings across these levels.

An acceptable definition of women's mental health has not yet been clearly delineated (Weisman, 1997). Some have suggested that this field should be defined as the study of disorders that occur only in women, mainly in women, or that take a more serious course in women than in men. However, as chapters in this book (e.g., ADHD, conduct disorder) clearly show, it is also important to study gender differences in conditions that occur less frequently in women or that take a relatively less serious course in women and girls. Such a "gender lens" can inform ideas of etiology, phenotype (the boundaries of a disorder), and intervention.

It is now recognized that the origins, expression, and course and outcome, as well as responses to treatment of all psychiatric illnesses, differ in women and men. Traditionally, researchers and research funders were male, and women were excluded from participation in research trials. There were two cogent reasons advanced at the time for the exclusion of women. In the aftermath of the thalidomide and diethylstilbestrol crises, the health of the developing fetus was an important consideration; women (later modified to women without reliable contraception) were seen as risky participants in research studies because they could be or could become pregnant. Improved surveillance methods have minimized these concerns. The second area of concern arose from a naive awareness of the importance of the menstrual cycle and its interrelationship with physiologic processes. In the past, the menstrual cycle was primarily viewed as a confounding factor, which could upset the clear interpretation of research results. By contrast, now most researchers see that the periodicity of the menstrual cycle makes it an ideal focus for research, being neither too rapid, as are many ultradian rhythms, nor too protracted as are seasonal cycles, for ready study. This view that detailed investigation of the menstrual cycle itself can shed light on other chronobiological processes shows how far our concepts about gender and health have advanced in the last twenty years.

The entry of women into the echelons of research has also spurred our appreciation of gender and gender determinants of health and illness. It appears that women researchers may ask different questions and use different methodologies. Women's research is characterized by the inclusion of both quantitative and qualitative methods, a focus on the context of disorder, a reduction of the hierarchical relationship between researchers and their participants, and the embrace rather than the avoidance of complexity (Campbell & Wasco, 2000; Hoffman, 2000). We celebrate the burgeoning contributions being made by women researchers by commissioning these chapters written almost entirely by women. This volume firmly takes a woman's point of view. Of course, there are major overlaps between research conducted by women and men. Discoveries made by men about men usually apply to women too. But it is important, we think, to publicize work done by women that applies to women. Such insights will also, in large measure, apply to men.

The editors of this book had three guiding principles in mind that determined the structure and content of the volume: development, culture, and stress.

The concept of development, the process of becoming bigger, fuller, more active or more visible, and subsequently older and more involuted, the evolution from simpler to more complex and then, perhaps, back to simpler again, underpins our ideas about mental health. Many psychiatric theorists have addressed the development of the individual over time (the Freuds, Sigmund and Anna, Klein, Homey, Piaget, Erickson, Winnicott, Beck, Vaillant, Miller, Maslow, Gilligan). There are several threads to the development of the human being: physical, cognitive-intellectual, emotional, interpersonal, reproductive, and occupational, each with its own path. These threads are usually assumed to be developing synchronously. However, chapters in this volume (such as those on body image and eating disorders in adolescent girls, Chapter 8, and intellectual disability, Chapter 17) discuss the confusion in thinking that arises when one thread lags behind the others.

The link between developmental processes and mental disorders is a two-way street. Some disorders appear to be preordained from the start but await a certain level of development before they surface. The unfolding processes of schizophrenia (Chapters 9 and 14 on psychosis), substance abuse (Chapters 10 and 13), and gender difference in the rates of depression becoming manifest at puberty (Chapters 4 and 12) show how the developmental stage determines the phenotype of disorders. These are complex concepts whose sex and gender implications are as yet poorly analyzed. The other direction, more clearly described, documents how a mental disorder often delays a normal developmental sequence. This probably affects all developmental threads, but is most clearly documented for the interpersonal–social. Many chapters in this volume allude to this; it is clearly articulated in Chapter 8, where the impact of an eating disorder on psychosocial development in adolescence is discussed and illustrated in a memorable case history. The development of aging women is usually conceptualized as a loss of previously attained skills; the chapters in the section on aging identify new areas of mastery that challenge the mature woman. The psychogeriatric literature has traditionally been very attuned to developmental considerations. There is a problem in the psychiatric literature arising from the epidemiologic custom of separating studies of adults under 65 from those aged 65 and over. This custom has imposed an artificial disconnection in what is a continuous process of evolution and involution.

There is an additional way in which the dynamic model of development is relevant to women's mental health. The history of ideas about women's mental health itself has evolved and now draws on a diverse base of research in biomedicine, psychology, philosophy, anthropology, sociology, and women's and gender studies. Efforts of integration across disciplinary boundaries, bringing together current and complementary discourses, will advance the field's evolution.

The influence of culture is seen in all manifestations of mental health and psychiatric disorders. The editors sought a main introductory chapter on the cultural aspects of development and also received an arresting commentary on it. We aimed to include the perspectives of women from around the English-speaking world. We did not wish to narrow the scope of this volume only to insights from the developed world and strove not to present them as universal conclusions based only on the experience of one cultural group. In this, we and our contributors were limited by the global politics of health research funding; our contributors, mainly, have drawn on the available published research data that emanate from developed economies. The generalizability of these findings is suspect, as several contributors point out. Although the editors asked contributors to consider the developmental and cultural underpinnings of their topic, this was, of course, not always possible.

A third underlying focus was the effect of stress in general and stressors specific to women in particular on the course of individual disorders. This has been more fully developed in some chapters than in others (Chapters 3, 11, and 16) and is important because women's health is more adversely affected by stressors than is men's health (Sandanger and colleagues, 2004).

Structure of the book

In accord with the predesignated focus on development, culture, and stress, the book has a developmental structure and a cultural/stress focus within each section.

First, an introductory section summarizes the three key areas. This section sets the framework for thinking about women's mental health. The chapters address women's development, cultural effects on women, and stress as it affects women. These are not sharply demarcated topics, and the editors were pleased to find considerable overlap in the concepts outlined in each. We arranged for commentaries for each of these introductory chapters in order to include a diversity of ideas, to limit Eurocentrism, and to broaden the debate. Each chapter stands alone as a thoughtful and well-informed general essay but is enriched by reading it together with the specific commentaries, as well as the linked chapters.

Then follow four sections on mental health issues that present at different stages of a woman's life: childhood, adolescence, adulthood, and aging. Each section has a reflective commentary on its content from experts, selected for their appreciation of the global implications of both the research evidence and their clinical expertise. In addition, we have included a section on reproductive health, traditionally the essence of women's health, and how it remains a key concern for researchers and service planners. There are unique mental health aspects to female reproductive health, as our contributors outline. Its commentary alerts the reader to high-grade research which may be published regionally, for example, in Scandinavia; this may be particularly valuable because its cultural context may differ.

The book ends with a section on services for women, again with thoughtful commentary. The topic of services for women is a vexed discussion arena requiring more information and discussion. Many key questions appear difficult to study directly. We would like to know how gender determines help-seeking around the world, which health delivery systems work best for women or men in different contexts, and the cost-benefit ratios for each type of delivery system in each cultural setting, to determine the optimal delivery system for each region. Our contributors have deftly summarized the current state of awareness and outlined the gross deficits in evidence-based knowledge.

The book is directed at mental health professionals in practice and in training and general health students of the many mental health disciplines. The editors expect that different readers will learn different lessons from this volume. We trust that it will prove useful to many. This volume builds on the fine work of many predecessors who have written books, chapters, and research articles; designed conferences; and established journals to further the understanding of women's mental health. We have not covered all psychiatric disorders in a comprehensive manner. We focused on those matters that seemed most germane between 2002 and 2004. We hope to create a culture that will inspire others to fill the gaps evident in this volume; such is the process of development.

The editors sincerely thank Alexandra Romic, at the Centre for Research in Women's Health, Toronto, for her intelligent commitment to the production of this book; we owe her a great debt.

References

Campbell R, Wasco SM. Feminist approaches to social science: epistemological and methodological tenets. Am J Community Psychol. 2000;28:773–791.

Hoffman E. Women's health and complexity science. Acad Med. 2000;75:1102–1106.

Sandanger I, Nygard JF, Sorensen T, Moum T. Is women's mental health more susceptible than men's to the influence of surrounding stress? Soc Psychiatry Psychiatr Epidemiol. 2004;39:177–184.

Weisman CS. Changing definitions of women's health: Implications for health care and policy. Matern Child Health J. 1997;1:179–189.

Introduction

A Relational-Cultural Theory of Human Development: The Power of Connection

Judith V. Jordan

Traditional psychological theories have tended to focus on the individual as the unit of study, and there has been an undue emphasis on the separate self. The dominant Western psychological research paradigm has focused on individual differences in personality and trait psychology. These research models have emphasized the development of "the separate self," autonomy, and self-sufficiency. Logical, abstract functioning has been privileged as a sign of "maturity." The dominant culture (White, middle class, male, heterosexual) of the twenty-first century United States celebrates the importance of separation, "going it alone," individual competition, and achievement.

Feminist scholars, however, have questioned the construction of norms of healthy "human" development based on studies of men and theories propounded largely by men (1,2). These models of human development have typically pathologized those aspects of development that have to do with emotional expression, acknowledgment of vulnerability and dependence, and desire for connection with others. The achievement of personal autonomy, independence, and strength, measured by the capacity to resist the influence of others, has been celebrated as signifying personal health. These qualities have been delegated by gender, with boys and men seen as carrying the qualities of independence, self-sufficiency, and an instrumental orientation while girls and women have been seen as the "carriers" (2) of the nurturing and caring, relational tendencies in humans.

RELATIONAL-CULTURAL MODEL

A new model of development, based on listening to women's experience (3,4) and on research on women's lives (1) has arisen in response to the limitations of the more traditional theories. This relational-cultural theory of development and clinical practice (RCT) has been developed over the past 25 years at the Stone Center at Wellesley College (3–5). It is rooted in the groundbreaking work of Jean Baker Miller (2). Its core tenets postulate that women (all people) grow through and toward connection; mutual empowerment characterizes healthy relationships; mutual empathy is the process through which growth occurs. Growth-fostering relationships generate what Jean Baker Miller called "the five good things": a sense of zest, increasing clarity, productivity/creativity, a sense of worth, and desire for more connection. Disconnections occur in all relationships when there is empathic failure, hurt, misunderstanding, and unresponsiveness; they are inevitable and ubiquitous. When acute disconnections are reworked, connections are strengthened. When a person is hurt (let's say a person with less power, like a child or therapy patient) and is able to represent the experience to the more powerful person, who responds in a caring way, the injured person actually experiences a sense of "mattering" to the other person and of being effective in relationship. This is relational competence; it produces a sense of well-being, hope, and growing connection. If, however, the more powerful person who has participated in the hurt does not acknowledge the other's pain and does not respond as if the other's pain matters to him or her, the less powerful and hurt person is left feeling alone, scared, and vulnerable. In this case, the injured person will withdraw, disconnect, keep those aspects of herself out of relationship. She will use strategies of disconnection or survival to stay safe. In the process, however, she brings less and less of herself into relationship, thus limiting the potential for mutual growth. She will become less authentic, less fully representing her experience in that relationship. These places of disconnection become the source of what we call chronic disconnection. Jean Baker Miller (4) has used the term "condemned isolation" to characterize these places of painful disconnection; in condemned isolation, a person feels outside the human community, unable to move into relationships to reestablish connection, and often feels enormous shame and self-blame. The person feels she has caused the isolation and is, in some essential way, "bad" or unlovable. The path of human development is through movement to increasingly differentiated and growth-fostering connection; chronic disconnections are most destructive when they result from the unresponsiveness of or violations by important and powerful people in our lives.

Although acute disconnections can be reworked and thereby strengthen and transform connections, when disconnections are not repaired or responded to empathically they lead to significant pain. The original injury, not responded to in a caring way and repeated many times in the course of a child's development, becomes the core of the protective disconnection. This injury can result from a traumatic violation of the child's sense of safety (physical or sexual abuse, either acute or chronic), an ongoing context of humiliation or violation, or more chronic neglect and general unresponsiveness. All of these situations lead to chronic disconnection and the development of relational images unfavorable to the movement into new relationships. Thus, for a child who is treated abusively, an organizing and central relational image might be: "Whenever I allow myself to be vulnerable, I am treated in a hurtful and frightening way. There is no empathy in those who are here to care for me." Or another child might develop the relational expectation: "Whenever I represent my real experience of anger, I am attacked or abused." In a less traumatic picture, the child might develop the following relational image that contributes to chronic disconnection: "I am responded to more positively when I suppress my real feelings and act cheerful for my parents." These kinds of relational images take people out of connection. To the extent that the relational images are very central, generalized to new situations, and characterized by both pervasiveness and inflexibility, they will keep people locked into certain patterns of disconnection. While these images are importantly formed in early parent–child relationships, they are subject to change throughout the life span.

Since isolation is viewed as the primary source of suffering for human beings, those forces that take us out of connection become especially relevant. Shame arises when we feel unworthy of connection, when empathic responsiveness seems beyond our grasp (6). Shame interferes with moving into relationships where old, maladaptive relational images can be shifted. There is a sense of loss of empathic possibility or the belief that someone could respond empathically to us. Shame leads to isolation and often involves an experience of immobility; in shame, one is aware of wanting to feel connected but one feels unable to reach out or to move into the necessary vulnerability to participate in an authentic relationship with others. Shame is an intrinsically interpersonal affect. Experientially, it is about our whole sense of ourselves; our very being feels unworthy of connection.

Shame drives people into isolation and silence. While it arises spontaneously and is seen as one of the original affects in infants (7), shaming is also done to people to exercise social and political control. If those at the center (8) shame those at the margin or those who are outside the dominant value structure, very often they can disempower and silence them. The dominant group tells the nondominant group that its way of being is insufficient, not as "good" as the dominant group's (you're too needy, you value the wrong things, your sexuality is sick, your hair is too kinky). Shaming becomes a major psychological and political force in controlling people. Shaming, isolation, and silencing go hand in hand. They are often used by the powerful to disempower those with less power. As Karen Laing noted, "Isolation is the glue that holds oppression in place" (9).

THE ROLE OF CULTURE

The relational-cultural model is an evolving theory. Initially labeled "self-in-relation," then "relational development," it is currently referred to as 'relational-cultural" theory, or RCT. This latest designation best captures the fact that this is a model that fully embraces the power of context and sociocultural forces in individual development. It furthermore attempts to include an analysis of the role of power imbalances. Rather than "the self," connection and context are placed at the center of this new understanding of human beings. Proponents of the Stone Center model care about suffering incurred at the individual level, but we also care about the effects of disconnection at a societal level, the ways that power differentials, forces of stratification, privilege, and marginalization can disconnect and disempower individuals and groups of people. It is essential that we look at context and not assume that the person (or group) presenting with pain *is* the problem.

While many theories arising in the dominant culture would have us believe that psychological theory is value-neutral and scientifically "objective," RCT emphasizes instead the importance of making the biases visible rather than invisible and looking at difference in terms of power differentials and stratifications imposed by the culture. Thus Jordan and Walker (10) write that listening to the voices of historically marginalized women will "challenge our assumption of a powerful mythic norm that would define 'woman' as a white, economically privileged, able-bodied, and heterosexual female. Unchallenged, this norm becomes a standard against which all women's experience is interpreted and evaluated. Therefore, the extent to which any individual woman conforms to this norm becomes almost by default the measure by which she is deemed worthy of notice or fit for connection."

Just as theories do not exist outside of culture, relationships do not exist outside of culture. To the extent that a culture devalues certain qualities and even disavows them, those people who tend to represent these qualities will be devalued. These discredited qualities will be used as a rationalization to demonstrate the basic inferiority of the people who express them; ultimately this inferiority will be invoked as a reason why "these people" should not be allowed access to power or political equality. Ignoring the range of cultural influences on people's development ensues from a psychology that overemphasizes internal traits and individual difference. It makes what is intrinsically political and cultural appear to be a result of personal pathology. In this quest to explain all pathology as personal, mothers are blamed (11) and individuals are "healed" back into adhering to the dominant narratives. The power imbalances in patriarchal nuclear families are rarely examined nor are the effects on people of racism, sexism, heterosexism, classicism, and overemphasis on being able-bodied.

MUTUALITY

RCT is not a stage or step model of development and certainly does not espouse a linear picture of growth. Rather, movement toward mutuality in relationship is at the core. *Movement toward,* not *attainment of* mutuality is to be emphasized. Mutuality involves profound mutual respect and mutual openness to change and responsiveness. It does not necessarily mean equality, although an understanding of the forces of power is very important. There is an emphasis on movement and change and mutual responsiveness. Jean Baker Miller once said, "In order for one person to grow in a relationship, both people must grow" (personal communication).

Mutual empathy is the pathway of growth. Empathy involves a movement of understanding and "joining with" another person; it is a complex process of affective and cognitive responsiveness. In the movement of empathy, people feel connected, joined, understood. Mutual empathy suggests that in order for empathy to lead to a sense of being with another, being understood and "mattering," each person must allow the other to see his or her influence or impact. In a therapy situation, the client must be able to see that she has "moved" the therapist, had an impact. The therapist must allow his or her responsiveness to show. I, client, can see, feel, and know that I have touched you, therapist. This provides the way out of the chronic disconnection and isolation that brings people into therapy. In therapy and in life, this movement of mutual openness to influence, of letting someone else participate in changing us as we also affect them, is at the core of relational growth.

DEVELOPMENTAL ASPECTS OF RCT

As a developmental theory, RCT poses questions and suggests a shift in focus. It does not yet, and may never, present a sequential picture of growth or stages of development. In fact, a model of linear, stepwise path of development may violate the essential complex and contextual nature of growth that RCT espouses. RCT emphasizes the centrality of growth toward relational mutuality and expanding capacity for connection. Just as the neurobiologists stress the plasticity of brain function, RCT points to the ways people continue to grow in relationship throughout the life span. While early relationships lay down certain relational schema, images, or expectations, these are not immutable. Given a mutual and reparative relational context, people can rework the relational expectations both psychologically and neurologically. In that sense, this is an optimistic model of potential relational and neurobiologic flexibility.

RCT points to the development of relational *competence* and also to the forces that interfere with the experience of competence both in relationships and in instrumental arenas.

Relational competence involves movement toward mutuality and mutual empathy; the development of anticipatory empathy; noticing and caring about our impact on others; being open to being influenced; enjoying relational curiosity; experiencing vulnerability as inevitable and a place of potential growth rather than danger; creating good connection rather than exercising power over others as the path of growth (6). Relational competence evolves in the process of having an impact on another human being and caring about that impact. When one is not responded to, one feels ineffective; there is a drop in energy, loss of clarity and sense of worth, and often a deadening or withdrawal.

The development of mutual empathy is crucial to this movement of relational competence. There is abundant emphasis that we are hardwired for empathy (12). Babies cry in response to the distress cries of other infants (13). There is likely a neurological basis for the development of empathy. But modern Western cultures tend to support the development of empathy in girls and discourage it in boys. Girls are encouraged to be empathic, "tuned in," and relational. Boys are supported for being agentic and for being engaged in instrumental competence. The "boy code" (14) indicates that boys and men should be tough, autonomous, abstract, and linear rather than emotive and intuitive in their thinking; most important, they should not show vulnerability or a need for connection. In Western culture, little girls are encouraged to learn and elaborate empathic skills. They are supported in their expressions of care for others and allowed a wide range of emotional expression. They are also allowed to be aware of their vulnerability.

Girls are typically seen to put a great deal of energy into building relationships in which sharing, self-disclosure, and mutual support constitute the main "activity." Maccoby has shown (15) that in same-sex peer groups, boys tend to become preoccupied with power and hierarchy and are directed toward action rather than relationship. Boys tend to attribute success to personal effort and failure to chance whereas girls do the opposite (16), but girls typically excel in school in the early years and show fewer behavioral problems than boys do.

Adolescence

Carol Gilligan (1) has traced a path of strong development and clear voices from early childhood until early adolescence when girls begin to "lose their voice." As

Gilligan addresses it (17), girls begin to doubt their own knowledge, lose their clarity, and keep aspects of themselves out of relationship in order to stay in relationship. This paradox is about the loss of authentic representation of experience in early adolescence as girls begin to see relationships with boys as primary; they learn to suppress their anger, their assertiveness, and their sexuality in order to accommodate to the experiences of boys.

As gender issues exert more force in girls' lives and as they see themselves more as objects than subjects, there is a loss of clarity, and the ability to represent themselves fully in relationships is increasingly diminished. We see an increase in "symptoms" and pathology as girls get disconnected from themselves and each other. In adolescence, girls begin to experience an increase in depression, eating disorders, and substance abuse; they suffer violence at the hands of partners they have chosen. Many begin to retrieve memories of childhood sexual and physical abuse and suffer with severe dissociative and traumatic symptoms. There is a drop in self-esteem for many, particularly White girls. This is the time of entry into adult status, a status importantly informed by heterosexual attachments and patriarchal norms. Girls are increasingly disconnected from their inner experience and from each other, as they are encouraged to seek their primary affectional attachments with boys. In the heterosexual pairing, girls often feel a drop in competence. The rules that may have applied to their same-sex friendships suddenly seem useless. There is a sense of being relationally incompetent.

Until recently, the psychology of adolescence was often written as if what happened for boys and girls had parallel antecedents and was experienced in similar fashion. An individualistic bias in most traditional developmental theories suggested that the teen years were the time for separation, for becoming "one's own man" (18). Recently, psychologists working on the development of girls have suggested that for girls the "crisis of adolescence" is not so much caused by hormones, body change, and the push to separate from family as by the social context and disempowering messages girls begin to receive as they move into the adolescent world of heterosexual pairing, where socialization includes learning to be an object to another's subject. During this time of transition, the hardiness, robustness, zest, and confidence of the prepubescent girl are often replaced by accommodating to others, pretending not to know things, and keeping large aspects of themselves out of relationship. Girls learn in adolescence that the rules of success are made by men and that females are to play a subordinate role. They fear being too bright, too assertive, and too strong. In adolescence the paths of gender socialization begin to collide. Boys, socialized to be in control, instrumental, unemotional, rational, and independent, begin to come into more intimate relationship with girls who have been taught to be loving, caring, and empathic. The culture encourages girls to objectify their own bodies. It is in adolescence that girls experience a dramatic decline in self-esteem. Tracy Robinson and Janie Ward have suggested that African American girls face particular challenges in adolescence that threaten their belief in themselves. These authors suggest several pathways for the "development of a belief in self far greater than anyone's disbelief" (19). Importantly, this includes the capacity for critical thinking vis-à-vis the values of the dominant culture. In order to be resilient and maintain authenticity and a sense of empowerment, all girls must develop the capacity for resistance that Robinson and Ward delineated for African American girls. Girls and women from the dominant White middle-class culture have much to learn from girls and women who are marginalized about the development of courage, resistance, and resilience.

Adulthood

In adulthood, RCT suggests we continue to bring relational images into new relationships. To the extent that these images prevent our engagement in growth-fostering relationships, they will limit our development. But with the right context, these images can be reworked in such a way that *relational possibility* is created. In a safe enough context, one can begin to relinquish the more limiting strategies of disconnection and begin to trust that another person will be truly and safely responsive and that both people will be working toward mutual respect and mutual empathy. As a person begins to see the real responsiveness and respect in the other person, she will feel safer in moving into the necessary vulnerability to build an authentic relationship. In mutual relationship both parties will use anticipatory empathy to engage with awareness of the possible impact on others of their feelings and actions. The yearning for connection is a constant in life and will reemerge as the person begins to relinquish her conviction that relationships cannot be responsive or growth fostering.

WORKING WITH TRAUMA: AN EXAMPLE OF MOVEMENT FROM DISCONNECTION TO CONNECTION

Working with traumatized people provides a clear picture of the dynamics of chronic disconnection and the healing movement of connection. Let us look at chronic childhood sexual abuse. In chronic sexual abuse of a child, there is a profound violation of the child's well-being and a profound absence of empathy on the part of the perpetrator. In the abusive aspects of the relationship, the adult fails to take into account the impact of the abuse on the child or fails to care about the impact. The child is psychologically, physically, and neurobiologically injured by the adult's preoccupation with his or her needs and failure to notice the needs of the child. While the child may initially seek to protest or reestablish safety, the message from the abusing adult will inevitably be one of not caring or refuting the child's experience. In our model, the child attempts to represent her real experience of being hurt and is told in many different ways that her protest is not respected. She may even be punished further. The child quickly learns both helplessness and "not mattering." She also learns to take large chunks of her experience out of relationship. She no longer represents her true feelings, and she attempts to protect her vulnerability by withdrawing, moving into chronic disconnection and protective inauthenticity. She unfortunately learns the lesson: "I do not matter, I cannot have an impact on this other person, I am relationally incompetent, and I am to blame." She moves into the trauma pattern of isolation, immobility, helplessness, self-blame, and shame. Thus relational violation at its extreme creates severe, traumatic disconnections. Her neurobiology is affected by this pattern of learned helplessness (20), and it also makes it more difficult for her to reenter possibly growth-fostering relationships. For the abuse survivor, connection does not equal safety. To sit in a therapist's office is often triggering and terrifying: the patient with post-traumatic stress disorder (PTSD) is in a heightened sense of vulnerability, often flooded with the fear of being in the presence of a powerful other who is supposed to be trustworthy, and behind closed doors. This situation alone often triggers large traumatic disconnects. As treatment begins and the client begins to relinquish certain protective strategies of disconnection, she may move into more terror. The healing is often characterized by big, chaotic shifts in the movement of relationship. But it is in working with trauma that therapists often see the most touching and profound movement from isolation to reconnection. Connections heal. The challenge in working with trauma is to help the survivor stay safe enough through the disconnections so that therapy is not jeopardized. For the therapist, the challenge is to stay in authentic responsiveness in such a way that the client can see that she is having an impact, is being responded to in a caring way, and is relationally effective. As the highly reactive neurochemistry begins to reequilibrate and the relational images modify, the client will begin to be able to establish more trust and engagement in growth-fostering relationship.

RESEARCH SUPPORTING THE POWER OF CONNECTION

Increasingly, research is providing the data that connection is central to human development. A longitudinal study conducted by Resnick (21) found that a good relationship with an adult (either a parent or someone in the school system) was the single best protection against the high-risk behaviors of adolescence (suicide, violence, and substance abuse). Shelly Taylor and associates (22), reviewing the studies of stress and the "fight-or-flight" response, found that these early studies were done on male organisms (rats, monkeys, humans, etc.). In replicating the studies with females, these researchers found that females tend to move toward connection when stressed. They named this the "tend-and-befriend" tendency. It is interesting that one of the core pieces of "knowledge" in Western psychology, that animals flee or fight when stressed, has now been seen as clearly gender skewed.

Researchers studying the pathways of pain have discovered recently that social pain and physical pain share parts of the same underlying brain processing system (the anterior cingulate cortex). They note that we are actually hard-wired to experience distress upon separation and comfort upon reunion, and they conclude "social connection is a need as basic as air, water or food and that like the more traditional needs the absence of social connection causes pain" (23).

Allan Schore (12), exploring the psychobiology of attachment in the mother–infant dyad, notes that mutuality enhances the development of the right prefrontal context in both mother and child. This is the part of the brain that mediates empathic cognition and perception of emotional states and modulates amygdala functions. Mutual responsiveness actually creates growth in this essential part of the brain. Interruption of mutuality interferes with its development; repair has to be interactive, through mutual influences. The exciting and relatively burgeoning field of neurobiology and functional MRIs is beginning to name and trace the centrality of mutuality and connection in brain development and functioning (12,24,25). Thus, at a neuronal level, we are beginning to see the ways in which we as human beings are hard-wired to connect. These data cast doubt on many of the old "Separate Self" models of psychological growth.

Another line of research that increasingly supports the primacy of connection and mutuality is the work being done on resilience. Although many studies of resilience examine factors within the individual such as temperament, hardiness, and intelligence (26), there is also a large body of research supporting the importance of relationships in the development of psychological resilience (27). RCT points to the importance of relational contexts and the power of mutual support and mutual engagement in the development of resilience (27). It is not simply receiving support that facilitates resilience; it is also providing support. Or as RCT describes this phenomenon, participating in growth-fostering relationships where all people are growing and changing.

NEW DIRECTIONS IN RELATIONAL-CULTURAL THEORY

Relational-cultural theory originated in response to a perceived misunderstanding of the psychology of women in traditional Western psychological theories. By listening to the voices of women, new visions of women's strengths, vulnerabilities, and patterns of growth were discovered. The crucial shift in this model was to place connection and context or culture at the core of the work. As the model has been elaborated over the last quarter century, it has expanded to include a revision in understanding of the psychology of boys and men (14,28). It has also been used to better understand group and institutional dynamics (29,30). While the application has been largely in the world of clinical practice, Jean Baker Miller's original book (2) presented data regarding social dynamics and change that have been central to this work. Increasingly, we are using the understanding of individual dynamics to explore better societal and group dynamics. The original work of Jean Baker Miller, revolutionary in message, continues to be used to understand social change and social action. The model has been used to better explicate the role of connections in business and organizations (30), therapy groups (29), the mother–son relationship (31), couples dynamics (28), the neurobiology of trauma (20), and racism (32). A relational practice manual has been written to guide the formation and use of relational practice groups (33). These relational practice groups have been used in prisons, housing projects for formerly homeless women and children, staff groups in psychiatric facilities, groups of chronically mentally ill people, with mothers and sons, and among supervisors in hospitals. A scale measuring mutual psychological development (34) and a relational health indices scale have been constructed (35); a scale to measure "organizational relational health" is under construction (36).

RCT began with listening to women's experience in order to more accurately describe women's psychological development. Increasingly, it is focused on correcting the misrepresentations of human experience that are brought about by an overemphasis on separation, individualism, and denial of vulnerability. RCT seeks to embrace the complexity of human life and relationships. Its practitioners value connection and the capacity for mutuality. RCT is a work in progress. As such, we who practice RCT struggle to dwell in a place of openness and uncertainty. We believe in the ultimate human responsibility of being responsive to one another and believe that when mutual empathy is operating, relationships become the sustaining force in people's lives.

REFERENCES

1. Gilligan C. In a Different Voice. Cambridge, MA: Harvard University Press, 1982.
2. Miller J. Toward a New Psychology of Women. Boston: Beacon, 1976.
3. Jordan J, Kaplan A, Miller JB, et al. Women's Growth in Connection. New York: Guilford, 1991.
4. Miller JB, Stiver I. The Healing Connection. Boston: Beacon, 1997.
5. Jordan JV, ed. Women's Growth in Diversity. New York: Guilford, 1997.
6. Jordan J. Toward connection and competence. Work in Progress no 83. Wellesley, MA: Stone Center Working Paper Series, 1997.
7. Tomkins S. Shame. In: Nathanson D, ed. The Many Faces of Shame. New York: Guilford, 1987.
8. hooks b. Feminist Theory from Margin to Center. Boston: South End, 1984.
9. Laing K. In pursuit of parity: teachers as liberators. Katalyst Leadership Workshop, World Trade Center, Boston, 1998.
10. Jordan JV, Walker M, Hartling L. The Complexity of Connection. New York: Guilford, 2004.
11. Caplan P. Don't Blame Mother: Mending the Mother–Daughter Relationship. New York: Harper and Row, 1989.
12. Schore A. Affect Dysregulation and Disorders of the Self. New York: Norton, 2003.

13. Hoffman M. Sex differences in empathy and related behaviors. Psychol Bull 1997;84:712–722.
14. Pollack W. Real Boys. New York: Owl, 1999.
15. Maccoby, E. Gender and relationships: a developmental account. Am Psychol 1990;45:513–520.
16. Dweck C, Reppucci N. Learned helplessness and reinforcement responsibility in children. J Pers Soc Psychol 1973;25:1090–1116.
17. Gilligan C, Lyons NP, Hanmer T, eds. Making Connections: The Relational Worlds of Adolescent Girls at Emma Willard School. Cambridge, MA: Harvard University Press, 1990.
18. Levinson D. The Seasons of a Man's Life. New York: Alfred Knopf, 1978.
19. Robinson T, Ward J. A belief in self far greater than anyone's disbelief: cultivating resistance among African American females adolescence. Women Therapy 1991;2:81–103.
20. Banks A. PTSD: Brain chemistry and relationships. Project Report no 8. Wellesley, MA: Stone Center Working Paper Series, 2001.
21. Resnick M, Bearman P, Blum R, et al. Protecting adolescents from harm: findings from the National Longitudinal Study on adolescent health. JAMA 1997;278:823–832.
22. Taylor SE, Klein L, Lewis BP, et al. Biobehavioral responses to stress in females: tend-and-befriend, not fight-or-flight. Psychol Rev 2000;107:411–429.
23. Eisenberger N, Lieberman M. Why It Hurts to Be Left Out: The Neurocognitive Overlap Between Physical and Social Pain (in press).
24. Amen D. Healing Anxiety and Depression. New York: Putnam, 2003.
25. Siegel DJ. The Developing Mind: Toward a Neurobiology of Interpersonal Experience. New York: Guilford, 1999.
26. Kobasa SC, Puccetti MC. Personality and social resources in stress resistance. J Pers Soc Psychol 1983;4594:839–850.
27. Jordan JV. Relational resilience. Work in Progress no 57. Wellesley, MA: Stone Center Working Paper Series, 1992.
28. Bergman SJ. Men's psychological development: a relational perspective. Work in Progress no 48. Wellesley, MA: Stone Center Working Paper Series, 1991.
29. Fedele N. Relationships in groups: connection, resonance and paradox. Work in Progress no 69. Wellesley, MA: Stone Center Working Paper Series, 1994.
30. Fletcher J. Disappearing Acts: Gender, Power and Relational Practice at Work. Cambridge, MA: MIT Press, 1999.
31. Dooley C, Fedele N. Mothers and sons: raising relational boys. Work in Progress no 84. Wellesley, MA: Stone Center Working Paper Series, 1999.
32. Walker M. When racism gets personal. Work in Progress no 93. Wellesley, MA: Stone Center Working Paper Series, 2001.
33. Jordan JV, Dooley C. Relational practice in action: a group manual. Progress Report no 6. Wellesley, MA: Stone Center Working Paper Series, 2000.
34. Genero N, Miller JB, Surrey J. The mutual psychological development questionnaire. Project Report no 1. Wellesley, MA: Stone Center Working Paper Series, 1992.
35. Liang B, Taylor SE, Williams LM, et al. The relational health indices. Work in Progress no 92. Wellesley, MA: Stone Center Working Paper Series, 1998.
36. Banks A, Hartling L. Organizational health indices. Stone Center Project Report. Wellesley, MA: Stone Center Working Paper Series (in press).

SUGGESTED READINGS

Jordan JV, Kaplan A, Miller JB, et al. Women's Growth in Connection. New York: Guilford, 1991.
Jordan JV, ed. Women's Growth in Diversity. New York: Guilford, 1997.
Jordan JV, Walker M, Hartling L. The Complexity of Connection. New York: Guilford, 2004.
Miller JB, Stiver I. The Healing Connection. Boston: Beacon, 1997.
Walker M, Rosen W. How Relationships Heal: Stories from Relational-Cultural Therapy. New York: Guilford, 2004.

Chapter 1 Commentary
Psychoanalytic Perspectives
Malkah Notman, Carol Nadelson

Chapter 1 by Judith V. Jordan represents one model of conceptualizing development, based on the work of Jean Baker Miller. This theory has served a worthwhile purpose in emphasizing the critical role of relationships and a relational approach for women. It is also useful in emphasizing the role of values and culture in development and the limitations of seeing the individual as the sole focus of theoretical understanding and treatment.

It is important to place this work in the context of other theories and scholarship in psychoanalysis and development that have preceded it, such as object relations theory, psychology of the self, and relational theory and also to integrate it with current knowledge about biologic factors in development. The description of "traditional" psychoanalysis as emphasizing individual development and separation as a goal can be modified to recognize this pluralism and the "connection" with other theories.

An interesting addition would be a discussion of harmful or problematic connections, such as aggressive, sadistic, or ambivalent ones and the affects involved, in women as well as men, children, and parents. Self-in-relation is thus a complex subject, highlighted by the Jordan chapter. It is an excellent way to open a volume addressing the many complex issues involved in women's mental health.

Mary Kay O'Neil

The introductory chapter to this volume on women's mental health describes the relational-cultural theory (RCT) of human development, a valuable addition to developmental theory and the psychotherapeutic repertoire. As Drs. Notman and Nadelson have already noted, RCT is based on the pioneering work of Jean Baker Miller and the Stone Center's 25 years of study focused primarily on women's mental health and well-being. RCT underlines the intrinsic role of relationship and cultural values in either fostering or impeding psychosocial development. Concomitant contemporary research in the areas of social support and neurobiology substantiates the Stone Center's emphasis on the power of relational connection in psychological well-being.

The author asserts that traditional psychological theories have tended to focus on the individual as the unit of study and have placed undue emphasis on the separate self. Other models of development, based on studies of men, inaccurately pathologized normal emotionality, vulnerability, dependence, and relational needs and promoted personal autonomy, independence, and power. These assertions were true until 30 to 40 years ago, until the loud voice of feminism and the emergence of a biopsychosocial frame of reference brought about a major revolution in psychoanalytic thinking about womanhood. It was also necessary because, prior to the emergence of psychoanalytic, psychodynamic theories, the inner workings of the human mind and self-development were scarcely understood. That traditional theory has changed to include the relational, social, and biologic aspects of women's self-development is documented, for example, in the Journal of the American Psychoanalytic Association's 1976 and 1996 supplements on women's psychology (1,2). Other contemporary psychoanalytic writers such as Jessica Benjamin (3,4) and Ethel Person (5) have further contributed to the understanding of self-development, gender, and relationship within a sociocultural context. The burgeoning development of attachment theory based on the work of Bowlby et al. (6) and the more recent work of Fonagy et al. (7) lends further support to the relevance of RCT as a theory of women's development. Clinically, RCT emphasizes growth-fostering relationships based on mutual empathy and empowerment and the deleterious effects of shame and isolation fostered by disconnection. This emphasis mirrors the shift in the traditional psychotherapeutic approach from a one-person to a two-person psychology. That is, it is now well recognized that the therapist is emotionally engaged with the patient(s) in the therapeutic enterprise. Advances in the understanding of failures of empathy in the vicissitudes of development are ongoing (8).

The relational-cultural model was initially "self-in-relation." The "self" was deleted to "fully embrace the power of context and sociocultural forces in individual development." Leaving out the self was probably necessary to emphasize and more fully understand the impact of the relational-cultural context on women's development. To make RCT a well-rounded model of women's development and more potent in its clinical effectiveness, the self now needs to be reinstated. Self-development occurs within relationships; growth-fostering relationships cannot be established without an intact self. Just as RCT has made major advances in the last 25 years, so too have the traditional psychological theories. The integration of theories of self-development and theories of relational-cultural development can only be mutually enriching and beneficial to the understanding of women and their mental health.

REFERENCES

1. J Am Psychoanal Assoc. Female Psychol: 1976 (Suppl); 24(5).
2. J Am Psychoanal Assoc. 1996 (Suppl); 44/s.
3. Benjamin J. The Bonds of Love. New York: Pantheon, 1988.
4. Benjamin J. Like Subjects, Love Objects. New Haven: Yale University Press, 1995.
5. Person ES. Feeling Strong: The Achievement of Authentic Power. New York: William Morrow, 2002.
6. Goldberg S, Muir R, Kerr J. (eds.). Attachment Theory: Social Development and Clinical Perspectives. Hillsdale, NJ: Analytic, 1995.
7. Fonagy P. et al. Affect Regulation, Mentalization, and the Development of the Self. New York: Other Press, 2002.
8. Maroda KJ. Seduction, Surrender, and Transformation: Emotional Engagement in the Analytic Process. Relational Perspectives Book Series. Vol. 13. Hillsdale NJ: Analytic, 1999.

CHAPTER 2

Women, Culture, and Development

Lisa Francesca Andermann

This chapter explores the relationships between the mental health of women and their social worlds by examining the areas of culture and development. The term "development" is used to denote the growth of an individual across the life span and also in the sense of social and economic development. As this topic presents an unlimited area of study, the chapter will be organized around several important foci, using an anthropologic perspective: women's roles and the social position of women in different cultures, access to education, literacy levels, the effects of poverty, the value of women's work, violence, sexism, and women's access to health services, in particular mental health services. In short, this chapter addresses how women's environments, geographic, economic, and social (including society, culture, community, and family), intersect with women's health and well being.

Using a developmental approach to follow these topics through the various life stages helps to delineate the influence of society and culture on women's mental health. Learning from exceptions to the rule, where these occur, is also valuable. The chapter begins with a look at socialization into gendered roles, a process that begins at birth. A childhood lens puts the focus on education and literacy, puberty rituals, and female circumcision. An adult perspective looks at women's work, marriage, and childbearing; the focus in aging is menopause and senescence. At each stage, examples from different cultural groups in both the developed and developing world are presented.

CULTURAL COMPETENCE AND WOMEN'S MENTAL HEALTH

In this era of globalization, migration, and social complexity, the ability to work comfortably in situations of cultural diversity has become an important part of current practice for mental health professionals. This begins with some familiarity with cultural differences, but the development of true cultural competence involves four main categories: knowledge, attitudes, skills, and experience.

In terms of women's mental health, this means that knowing general details about a particular culture is not enough. One must take into account women's roles, status in society, educational and vocational opportunities, and religious beliefs and practices. While these may vary within cultures across social class or other divisions, the important point is that, if not approached from a gender perspective, this information may not always be obtained from the usual sources. In a culturally complex clinical situation, the clearest form of communication is between clinician and client, where questions can be asked directly. When language issues are present, working with professional interpreters avoids situations where husbands or other family members are asked to translate, a situation which may obscure the woman's voice. Cultural consultants who have insider knowledge of a particular culture can also provide useful collateral information.

The inclusion of gender and mental health issues and the promotion of women's mental health in books such as *Where There Is No Psychiatrist,* a mental health-care manual for developing countries, send an important message to all health-care workers (1). Patel states that "the promotion of gender equality, by empowering women to make decisions that influence their lives and educating men about the need for equal rights, is the most important way of promoting women's mental health" (p. 229). The book then offers practical suggestions on asking about stress in the domestic situation, how to ensure regular follow-up for women, asking permission to speak to husbands or family members for collateral history, as well as larger advocacy issues such as how to begin psychoeducational or support groups for women in the community.

BIRTH

As universal as the origin of species, the process of childbirth and the rituals, regulations, and social influences that surround it have developed into a collection of beliefs and behaviors as diverse as the cultures in which they are found. Describing these in detail would be far beyond the scope of this chapter; however, several themes emerge in which commonalities can be examined.

The first theme pertains to the strong preference, in some cultures, for male children. This is because of the importance of heredity and the maintenance of the male line in patrilineal societies, a guarantee of the continuity of the family. This will have a bearing on inheritance, including land ownership, and sometimes position and rank in society. Added to this are other financial considerations: in many places, the families of girl children bear the added burden of having to provide a dowry at the time of marriage, which presents a heavy load for many who are at the brink of poverty.

While developments in medical technology have allowed for screening and improving fetal outcomes, this has had the unintended effect of allowing parents to screen for the sex of the fetus. This possibility of choice has resulted in situations where healthy pregnancies may be terminated if the sex is not desirable.

In China, which instituted a one-child policy in the late 1970s to combat overpopulation, pressures on couples to have a male child have greatly increased. As well as "quantity," China has been interested in "quality" of births, instituting a law in 1995 restricting "imperfect" births, part of a greater government scheme intimately tied to interventions in reproductive health. Dikotter (2) examines these eugenic developments in detail within the historical, political, and economic context of Chinese society, describing the impact of current legislation on the personal lives of both men and women. When women in China are found to have "unauthorized" pregnancies not in compliance with the one-child policy, involuntary abortions or forced sterilization may occur or they risk high fines or the destruction of home or possessions (3).

Around the world, demographers have documented "missing women"—male:female sex ratios that favor men—in India 920 women for every 1,000 men, in China 100 women for every 113.8 men (3). They also cite the Indian government statistic that, out of 8,000 abortions at a clinic in Bombay, India, 7,999 were of female fetuses. Whether due to female infanticide or prenatal screening, the results are the same. This pattern has also been reported in the Middle East, with dramatic ratios as low as 48 women to 100 men in the United Arab Emirates. Economist Amartya Sen has calculated that there are over 100 million "missing" women in the world (3). In an attempt to explain this phenomenon, Sen links the interaction between economic reforms and cultural values that produce situations of gender subordination for women. In this way, development policies such as agricultural reforms, also known as structural adjustment policies, may actually (inadvertently) have a negative impact on women's health in terms of their nutritional status, levels of stress, and worsening poverty, leading to decreased access to health care.

At the other end of the reproductive spectrum, Hmong immigrants from Laos to the United States are reported to have one of the highest birthrates in the world, 9.5 children per couple, compared to the rate of White Americans, 1.9 children, and Black Americans, 2.2 children (4). This rate is thought to be a result of a combination of early marriage and a suspicious attitude toward Western medicine, including contraception, and is likely to decrease as young Hmong became more acculturated to life in America. In her insightful study of cultural misunderstandings between a Hmong family and the American medical establishment, Fadiman explains that

> the Hmong have many reasons for prizing fecundity. The most important is that they love children. In addition, they traditionally value large families because many children were needed to till the fields in Laos and to perform certain religious rites, especially funerals; because the childhood mortality rate in Laos was so high; because so many Hmong died during the war and its aftermath; and because so many Hmong still hope that their people will someday return to Laos and defeat the communist regime. In the refugee camps, Hmong newborns were often referred to as "soldiers" and "nurses." (4, p. 72)

The last sentence alludes to the concept of early socialization into gendered roles, beginning in the cradle.

There are also numerous traditions and taboos concerning the birth process itself. For example, the Hmong believe that it is important to bury the placenta in the dirt floor of the house, so that after death it can be found by the soul and worn as a "jacket" on a journey to the land of the ancestors, where one day the soul is reborn as a new baby (4). How this belief, along with so many others, has been transformed in an era of migration, hospital births, and modernized accommodations that lack dirt floors has been a process of ongoing negotiation.

Beliefs about pollution and taboo as means of regulating women's sexuality before, during, and after childbirth are commonly found around the world. Women are often kept in confinement for a specific period of time, usually weeks, after childbirth before being allowed to reintegrate into marital life and the wider society. Lewis's study of ritual among the Gnau people of New Guinea describes in intricate detail the ways in which men and women's lives in this traditional culture are bound by their beliefs. This is demonstrated by their performance of rituals that link them to others in the community, the local environment, and the supernatural world (5).

Another area of study has been the effects of poverty on childbearing and maternal and child health. In a moving and well-researched ethnography on women's lives in a Brazilian shantytown, anthropologist Nancy Scheper-Hughes (6) studies the links between social class and reproduction and finds that "poverty interacts in many different ways to produce child mortality and to shape reproductive thinking and practice" (p. 326). She describes the ways that scarcity affects maternal thinking, particularly difficulties in coping with extremely high rates of infant mortality, to the extent of bringing about a situation she describes as "the social production of indifference to child death." This does not imply that women do not experience the loss of their infants, but rather that they have come to differentiate the greater grief associated with the loss of an older child, who is already formed and with whom there is greater attachment, from the infant, in whom little has thus far been invested. Women in this environment have been demoralized to the point of seeing their breast milk as no good, spoiled, or sour and feeling that they have nothing left to give to their children. However, in order to reach their preferred family size, they must often bear two or three times that number of pregnancies, with the physical and psychological burdens this entails, in order to ensure a few surviving offspring. All of this is occurring in an environment of oppression with minimal government support for the very poor and with strong Catholic beliefs, which, among other things, forbid the use of contraception. Despite all the hardships, Scheper-Hughes is able to document survival skills and resilience among these women that provide hope for the future.

CHILDHOOD

Childhood is a time of rapid growth and learning in many spheres: physical, psychological, and cognitive, including mastery of language and a wide variety of interactions with the wider world. Culture is woven into the consciousness of a child during family activities—including daily chores, play, games, food, social occasions, religion and festivals, and contact with siblings, parents, grandparents, and the extended family and beyond. While the psychiatric and psychological literature offers many theories of child development, less has been written about the impact of culture on this critical period or how culture is learned.

In a chapter on gender, development, and psychopathology, Notman and Nadelson (7) write that "the role of particular cultural practices, including gender differences in child rearing, are manifest from infancy. Differences in parental behavior, especially those related to concepts of male and female roles, are powerful forces contributing to differences in male and female development" (p. 2). Examples of these differences—the ways that culturally constructed gender roles are passed from one generation to the next—taken from a variety of ethnographic studies and other sources are presented below.

In the memoir *Wild Swans* (8), which describes the lives of four generations of Chinese women during decades of massive political upheaval and social change during the nineteenth and twentieth centuries, Jung Chang describes how her great-grandmother, typical of millions of her era, was born to a working-class family without intellectual background or official post, and because she was a girl, was not given a proper name. She was simply called "Number Two Girl" (*er-ya-tou*). She had been promised by her family, at age 6, to the newborn son of a friend when he became of age, and the wedding took place when he turned 14 years old. Chang explains that, in this time of arranged marriages, it was considered one of the duties of a wife "to help bring up her husband." Girls were taught that "a virtuous woman should suppress her emotions and not desire anything beyond her duty to her husband" (p. 34). Notably, when Number Two Girl had a daughter of her own, the baby was given a real name. However, despite this nod to encouragement of her own identity, the baby girl (Chang's grandmother) was not able to escape the practice of binding feet. At age 2, her feet were tightly bound with cloth, breaking the bones in her arches and causing lifelong excruciating pain, all done to satisfy men's idea of feminine beauty.

Psychological anthropologist Jean Briggs's description of the emotional education of a 3-year-old Inuit girl in Canada's Arctic brings us to how culture is learned, the process of creating children "who think and feel like Inuit" (9). Through detailed ethnographic analysis of family "dramas" or social interactions, she outlines the process of Inuit education, whose goal of "increasing thought" in children is hidden in playful questions asked by adults. These repeated interactions, as encapsulated in the case study of one child's development, make visible the wider processes of socialization. However, because each of these interactions and new understandings is negotiated and renegotiated on an individual level, Briggs concludes that children cannot acquire a "fixed set of understandings" or a "total culture" through this very active learning process.

In another Inuit example, the ethnography of the Netsilik Eskimo of the central Canadian Arctic describes another important feature of the socialization of children, the learning of male and female roles (10). This traditional hunting society had a clear division of labor between the sexes, with a focus on husband and wife as collaborative partners in the subsistence of the nuclear family, although the husband held a superior position as head of the household. While the men hunted and fished, the women worked at home preparing food and animal skin clothing, which were equally essential to the survival of the family. Learning occurred through observation and imitation, with boys and girls each following their same-sex parents from a very young age. Balikci describes how spending almost all their time in the company of their parents within the confines of the igloo and its surroundings, and growing up in close association with the adult world, children quickly adopted the roles of the same-sex parent. This closeness is true of many traditional societies, where families live at much closer quarters, both spatially and psychologically, than in more modernized societies.

In the mainstream North American setting, *In a Different Voice,* Gilligan's influential psychological study of women's development begins in childhood and goes on through various stages of development through interviews with different age groups (11). Written in the early 1970s, this study was one of the first to explore differences between the sexes in terms of conceptions of self and morality and tries to understand the roots of women's position in society, what Gilligan terms "woman's place in man's life cycle." One of the well-known findings from this study is that even from a very young age, female children value interpersonal relationships and begin to order their worldview according to this principle of human connectedness. In contrast, boys often take a more logical and hierarchical approach to solving dilemmas. This leads to a tension between women and men, based on their use of different models of human relations: connectedness versus hierarchy. Both connectedness and hierarchy co-exist in the parent–child relationship and continue to be negotiated from that point onward as the child makes his or her way out into the world.

Formal learning—school-based education and literacy—is another of the tasks of childhood. Much has been written about the link between lack of education and the disparities in the economic, political, and health status of women around the world (3). When resources are scarce, girls in many countries often stay home while school fees are dedicated for their brothers. Families may not be aware of the importance of this decision to their daughters' futures.

ADOLESCENCE

Sexual maturation occurs in several steps, beginning as a girl approaches the age of puberty. Hormonal and physical changes, the development of secondary sexual characteristics, and finally, the onset of menarche, signal a shift in psychological identity that may take several years to fully integrate. The understanding that menarche has a potential for pregnancy and thus leads to the next stage in the life cycle of an adult woman is often viewed as a source of anxiety and risk (7). Peer groups generally become more important at this time, as girls begin to move beyond the immediate family as a source of role modeling and support, and issues of self-esteem, self-confidence, and physical attractiveness come to the forefront.

Puberty rites are common in many cultures to mark this time of change. These may be in the form of public rites, religious ceremonies, or social gatherings. Lewis (5) presents a detailed analysis of the intricate puberty rituals performed among the Gnau of New Guinea. For both female and male initiates, this is a major event of public recognition, involving elaborate decoration, feasting on ritual foods, and the reinforcement of social linkages within the family. For boys, the ritual includes a form of "symbolic menstruation" as they are made to bleed from their penises. Although, when asked by Lewis whether this male bloodletting was meant to resemble menstruation, the Gnau denied this idea, the behavior also occurs among other groups in New Guinea, and is described in this way in other anthropologic literature.

Female circumcision, also known as female genital mutilation (FGM), is another cultural tradition that occurs in many parts of the world, particularly in Africa and the Middle East, at the time of puberty or before, often in girls as young as 6–10 years of age. This procedure, the aim of which is to guarantee women's virginity and diminish their sexual pleasure, has an enormous impact on the development of female and sexual identity in the countries where it is practiced. In addition to these psychological effects, medical morbidity, infection, and chronic pain, occurring both at the time of the circumcision and possibly for years after, at the time of first sexual contact or childbirth, may have long-standing, even life-threatening, repercussions. The women are at greater risk of HIV transmission because damage to the urinary tract and vagina may lead to fistulas and other possibilities of infection (3).

A firsthand account of this difficult and painful experience is provided by Aman, a Somali woman, in her memoirs (12). To place this experience in perspective, anthropologist Janice Boddy describes female circumcision in the social context of Somali culture, a Muslim, male-dominated, pastoralist society. Although Islam does not specifically sanction this practice, or gender inequality in general, it is customary in Somalia to view women's status as inferior to that of men and for women to be bound by male authority. Concepts of honor, reputation, and independence are the foundations of Somali social organization. However, it is precisely these values, which are seen by Somalis to be unachievable by women because of their sexuality, that keep them in a morally inferior position. Boddy writes:

> Female fertility is highly prized; it is associated with plenty, prosperity, and life, with the continuation of the lineage through the birth of sons, and with the virtues of pity, mercy and compassion. Nevertheless, women are considered socially less developed than men. They regularly and involuntarily menstruate; they give birth and lactate; when pregnant they publicly display their sexuality, their ties, that is, to other humans. All these natural conditions that women cannot control are seen to represent weakness and a lack of independence, the antithesis of the social ideal. (12, p. 318)

Boddy cautions for the need to understand this practice in context, as it is generally older women and mothers who ensure its continuation. Peer pressure and a fear that, without it, marriage might be difficult or impossible keep it going. There are some changes currently being made among more educated women, with less radical operations being performed; some have been reduced to a symbolic pinprick.

Immigration has led to greater awareness of this issue because FGM procedures are being performed or requested in Europe and North America. Groups such as Amnesty International have brought this issue to world attention in calling for an annual "International Zero Tolerance to FGM Day" and lobbying African governments to sign a declaration "to protect African women from cultural and traditional belief systems that are inimical to the sexual and reproductive rights of women in the continent" (13). However, many women still see this practice as central to their social identity. Aman herself describes her infibulated body as "clean, closed and smooth" with its own aesthetic value (12). Desjarlais et al. (3, p. 139) present the case example of West African immigrant women in France, who face a difficult bind between risking legal charges and public trials (to have their daughters circumcised) and risking ostracism from the West African community. Without more local support to negotiate these cultural conflicts, it will be difficult to find meaningful solutions that will allow for a fuller inclusion of these young women in a changing society.

Body image and reproduction are intimately linked as attention to physical attractiveness grows more important during adolescent years (7). Eating disorders have been particularly studied in this regard, and comparisons made across cultures where physical preferences vary considerably. Anorexia is generally thought to be a particularly Western disorder, perhaps even considered as a culture-bound syndrome of Western Europe and North America (14). Much has been written about the impact and immediacy of Western media favoring thinner and thinner models and actresses, who predominate as role models for generations of impressionable young women. But how is this related to the development of an eating disorder? Eating disorders, including anorexia and bulimia, have been described in many places around the world. However, prevalence rates vary considerably, and they may be quite rare outside of a Westernized context. A careful analysis of questionnaires is needed to avoid misinterpreting culturally consistent responses. For example, in India answering positively about "engaging in dieting behavior" could mean observing religious Hindu fasts, or in China "cutting food into small pieces" is appropriate for eating with chopsticks (14). In these countries, eating disorders are rarely found. In other parts of Asia, some atypical eating disorders are described that do not include the phobia of fatness, central to the definition of the disorder given in the American Psychiatric Association's *Diagnostic and Statistical Manual of Mental Disorders.*

Anne Becker (15) was in the fortunate position of being able to conduct a study of eating disorders among adolescent girls in Fiji, a remote group of islands in the South Pacific, just as television was making its first appearance. There had been no previously published studies on the effects of the introduction of television on the eating habits of a media-naive population. The study began in 1995, just as television went on the air in Fiji, and a follow-up was done three years later. Becker's group found a significant increase in scores, indicating disordered eating, following television exposure. Although no subjects met criteria for anorexia, self-induced vomiting to control weight had gone from 0% in 1995 before television to 11.3% only three years later (15). There was an increase in body dissatisfaction during this time as girls expressed wanting to emulate characters they saw on television. Most interestingly, this rapid change took place in a setting where traditional Fijian culture saw a more robust physique as the ideal body shape and encouraged large appetites at feasts and family gatherings. Thus, the introduction of Western media imagery can be directly linked to the internalization of a new cultural ideal of thinness and the development of body dissatisfaction, leading in some cases to disordered eating.

Regardless of cultural differences, there is a major difference in ratios between males and females with eating disorders ranging from 1:10 to 1:20 (16). Dysfunctional eating behaviors are a complex combination of sociocultural, psychological, and biologic factors. The illness and its related behaviors often gives individuals a way to focus their attention away from stressful life problems and can result in delays in their dealing with developmental issues, including sexual function, because they maintain a prepubertal physique long into adolescence and beyond.

ADULTHOOD

Women's work and motherhood are the major roles in the adult lives of many women around the world. It is well known that work is related to mental health in that it increases self-esteem and financial independence. However, the reverse is also true, and the burden of overwork, both inside and outside the home, and often both simultaneously, can contribute to a situation of fatigue, anxiety, and worry. Women's work is often undervalued and underpaid. They may also spend more hours working than men from the same social class. In studies tracking time allocation of housework and child care, women in Africa worked on average 67 hours per week compared to 54 hours for men (3). This level of productivity may be affected by several other factors, including nutritional deficits and hunger. A study by the World Health Organization (WHO) estimated that 60% of women in developing countries were undernourished and nearly two thirds of women clinically anemic (3).

To get an idea of these difficulties firsthand, the narrative of a Dalit woman named Viramma, marginalized in her village as an untouchable, is instructive (17). The narrative, told to two French researchers over a period of 10 years, traces Viramma's life story from her childhood, beginning with marriage at age 11, soon followed by childbirth and the rituals around the births of her 12 children, through years of heavy agricultural work, punctuated by the annual cycle of festivals and religious life. Viramma says, ". . . we mothers always have a fire in our belly for our children: we must feed them, keep them from all sickness, raise them to become men or women who are going to work" (17, p. 96). This is especially important as an insurance policy for aging parents in her culture as in many places where there is no social assistance or old age pension. Viramma continues to describe her role as a mother: "what's more important for us women than children? If we don't draw anything out of our womb, what's the use of being a woman?" (p. 104). However, it is more often men that determine a woman's role in the family. Tseng writes that "in many societies women are considered significant only for bearing children, particularly sons" (14, p. 383). If this expectation is not fulfilled, then the husband can cast the woman out of the home, or have her replaced by another wife.

Level of education has a direct correlation with women's status in the family, ability to gain financial independence, access to better health care, and achievement of better mental health. When this opportunity is not available, because of scarce resources, or is lost because of political changes, the mental health of women suffers. In some parts of rural India, the literacy rate for village women may be as low as 12.3%, one of the lowest in the world (18). Even where opportunities for schooling do exist, many more boys attend than girls, and fathers are said to keep their daughters out of classes "because they fear she will start saying 'No' . . . and start having her own opinions" (p. 28).

Under the Taliban rule in Afghanistan, education for women was one of the first things to be outlawed. A study comparing the mental health of women in Afghanistan living in areas under Taliban control and other areas with that of women in a refugee camp in Pakistan found that major depression was much more prevalent under the Taliban (73%–78% versus 28%) and suicidal ideation in Taliban-controlled areas was much higher (73%) than in non-Taliban areas (18%) (19). In contrast to the minority party in power, a majority of the population, both men and women, believed that the protection of women's rights and equal opportunities for women in education and the workplace would be needed as a basic step to rebuild the community.

Deprivation of educational opportunities occurs in subtler ways as well. In the novel *Brick Lane* (20), which tells the story of a Bangladeshi immigrant woman who joins her husband in London, Nazneen, the main character, asks her husband if she can attend English classes at a local college. His answer is "What for? . . . You're going to be a mother. Will that not keep you busy enough?" (p. 62). This brings up the issue of acculturation and the difficulties that women may experience when forced to adjust to a new environment without language skills or family support. Immigration can bring a sudden loss of role for women, as whatever authority they may have had within their households is eroded by their new situation, and their children, who learn new languages more quickly, may step in to act as their intermediaries at doctors' appointments and at the bank. In her description of South East Asian immigrants in California, Fadiman writes that "of all the stresses in the Hmong community, role loss—the constellation of apparent incompetencies that convinced Lia's mother she was stupid—may be the most corrosive to the ego" (4, p. 206). While the psychological implications of this are not known, it can be imagined that this would have far-reaching effects on self-confidence and a woman's sense of agency.

The experience of succumbing to a medical illness can also have an impact on a woman's marital and family life. Jilek-Aall (21) presents the narrative of a young woman with epilepsy in Tanzania who relates that she had a seizure, upon which her "husband was furious. He gave my baby to his brother's wife, returned me to my parents, and demanded back the bridal price he had paid them to marry me. My parents had to comply for it is our custom that a man can do this if he is not satisfied with his wife" (p. 49). It was only after months of shame and stigmatization, given that epilepsy is feared as being a contagious disease in many parts of Africa, that this woman found treatment in a local clinic and, once stabilized on medication, was finally accepted back by her husband and reunited with her children.

Violence also adds to the difficulty of women's lives and their burden of mental distress. Domestic violence has a range of intensities. Female infanticide is described as an extreme form of domestic violence (14). More organized forms of violence, such as involuntary prostitution or female sexual slavery, also carry mental health risks, as well as risks for physical health and HIV infection in particular (3). During times of a breakdown of social order such as war or rebellion, rape is all too common, and may lead to long term psychological sequelae, particularly if children are born from these unions.

Violence is not always interpersonal but can occur on a larger scale. In *Women, Poverty and AIDS,* Farmer (22) defines "structural violence" as a set of historically and economically driven processes and forces that conspire to constrain individual agency, where neither nature nor individual will is at fault. He examines the interrelationships between women, poverty, and AIDS in an attempt to make explicit that, as a group, poor women, precisely because of the economic injustices they face, deal with higher rates of HIV infection than if they were grouped according to any other cultural, national, or occupational classification. The three case studies of women that he presents from Haiti, Harlem, and rural India illustrate this point; the women are each HIV positive and linked by poverty. He broadens his analysis in *Infections and Inequalities* (23) to include the global plague of tuberculosis, again making the argument that social inequality—poverty and lack of health resources—and disease are intimately linked: "In South Africa, say, these forces include poverty and racism; in other settings, gender inequality conspires with poverty to lead to higher incidence of tuberculosis in poor women" (p. 259).

Situations of extreme stress may lead to changes in the usual patterns of distribution of mental illness and related behaviors. It is generally known that, while women might attempt suicide more frequently, men more often complete suicide (16). However, in certain environments such as rural China, the suicide rate is higher for women, particularly young women. Tseng (14) postulates that the role of young females "as unmarried women, young wives, or daughters-in-law" contains more distress and is less favorable relative to the role of men, leaving them with fewer options with which to cope and foresee a future for themselves. (See the Section VI summary on Aging by Chiu, pp. 321–322, where the issue of suicide rates in Chinese women is developed as an example of the way culture impacts mental health in the aging women.)

An interesting epidemiologic finding in Ethiopia, which has not been shown elsewhere, pertains to age of onset of schizophrenia. Positive symptoms generally occur at younger ages in men (17–27 years) than in women (17–37 years) (16). Despite this difference, rates of schizophrenia are similar in women and men. The best-known cross-cultural studies of schizophrenia are a series conducted by the World Health Organization in the 1970s and 1980s that demonstrate better outcome of schizophrenia in developing countries than in the developed world (14). A more recent WHO report (24) comments on three types of biases that may influence age of onset of schizophrenia. First, male patients may require earlier hospitalization because of maladaptive or antisocial behavior. Second, traditional societies may "protect" young women from hospitalization for a stigmatizing illness, and, third, the availability of psychiatric services (leading to diagnosis and case identification) varies considerably in many parts of the world. They believe that higher expectations for young men to succeed at work and support a family may lead to earlier age of onset of schizophrenia in vulnerable males because of increased stress and that "differences in social roles and cultural norms . . . influence, at least partially, gender differences in risk, onset, course and outcome in schizophrenia" (24).

A recent community-based study from Ethiopia showed a reversal in age of onset between males and females, with younger age of onset of psychotic symptoms in females, 21 years versus 23.8 years in males (25). There was also a male:female ratio of almost 5:1. The authors suggest two possibilities for earlier age of onset in females. The first is that is it not uncommon in Ethiopia to report women as being younger than they actually are. They give more weight to the second possibility, which is that in rural Ethiopia, females have significantly higher scores for stressful life events, such as arranged marriages at a young age, abductions, and gynecologic difficulties, including multiple pregnancies, abortions, and childbirth, in areas without adequate medical services. Also, females in this study population experienced many of these adverse life events earlier than males. In a review article, Leung and Chue (26) discuss issues of sex differences in schizophrenia, giving details about age of onset in different settings. They report that marriage is sometimes found to delay onset, especially for males, while a positive family history tends to equalize age of onset in both sexes.

A WHO report entitled *Mental Health of Indigenous Peoples* (27) refers to Goldschmidt's concept of the "human career" as a means for individuals to achieve a sense of accomplishment in their lives, whether physical, social, or reproductive, ensuring the continuation of the society. Cohen writes:

> Whatever its size, complexity or environment, a central task of any culture is to provide its members with a sense of meaning and purpose in the world. What happens then, when a people's way of life is destroyed through disease, genocide, loss of territory, and repression of language and culture, when pathways to meaning are no longer available? (p. 12).

When a breakdown of the social fabric occurs, psychopathology, demoralization, and mortality may result. What role does gender play in this? In a study by the Baffin Psychiatric Consultation Service of the University of Toronto among the Inuit of the Canadian Arctic, women outnumbered men 3:2 for psychiatric consultations. However, reasons for consultation differed greatly between women and men, with more than twice as many women referred for depression (37.8% versus 16.4%), while more men were referred for suicidal attempts or ideation (32.8% versus 20.6%) and conflicts with the law (29.9% versus 4.4%) (28). In order to treat these populations, one must go beyond a simple biomedical approach, taking a broad historical, cultural, and community view, because "efforts to rebuild supportive environments for children, youth and their families must be an integral component of any mental health program for indigenous peoples" (27, p. 27).

Another important determinant of family structure is the system of kinship or descent, which determines how individuals are connected through family ties and obligations. In patrilineal societies, which are most common, the family name is passed down from the father to male children and grandchildren, and children are seen to belong to the kinship group of the father. In matrilineal societies, which comprise about 14% of family systems, such as those found in Micronesia, titles are passed down from mother to daughter and granddaughter (14). However, although descent follows the female line, authority is held by the woman's husband and brothers, so that authority and descent do not converge as they do in patrilineal societies.

AGING: MENOPAUSE, WIDOWHOOD, AND END-OF-LIFE ISSUES

Menopause marks the transition to postreproductive life for women. Although a universal biologic event, it brings with it a variety of cultural factors that influence reactions to this change (14). Much has been written about the symptoms attributed to menopause in various cultures, as reviewed by Charney (29), who explores the psychiatric, gynecologic, and transcultural literature on this topic. Lock (30) has written at length about this area and has studied menopause in Japan and North America to see whether the differences in its presentation were due to culture, biology, or a combination. In her overview, Charney, citing Lock, concludes that "not only can cultural beliefs influence the construction, nature and interpretation of menopause, but subtle biologic differences can also shape the subjective experience of individuals, and may ultimately mold cultural interpretations of this stage of the reproductive life cycle" (29, p. 429). Differences in diet, lifestyle, health status, childbearing, and social roles are some of the factors that must be taken into account in studies of this kind.

Retirement is described by Tseng (14) as a "product of industrialized society." In many parts of the world and most of history until recently, people continued to work and contribute as long as they were physically able. However, when people are made to retire involuntarily or are financially unprepared, retirement can become a very stressful time rather than one of leisure. Because of women's status in many societies, with lower incomes and perhaps dependence on a husband or male relatives, a woman can suddenly be placed in a precarious position late in life.

Ramphele (31) examines political widowhood in South Africa, exploring the position of woman as shifting from a representation of personal to public loss. She describes widowhood as a liminal state where local customs, from black clothing to certain eating rituals, are followed, as in many cultures, to indicate the particular social position of being a wife without a husband. She writes that "a woman's body, as the embodiment of the generative and reproductive power that knits generations together, holds the secret of her ability to concomitantly embody ritual danger and ritual power" (31, p. 115). Despite this power, the female body "usually requires a male body to render it whole and acceptable." The example of *sati* in India, a Hindu practice where widows join their husbands in death on the funeral pyre, is given as the ultimate joining of women and men's bodies. However, a lot of controversy exists concerning this rare illegal practice, which can be seen as a cultural form of suicide. On the one hand, it is the embodiment of a religious ideal, showing the devotion of a spouse honoring her husband's lineage. But it may be the result of social pressures to express grief in a particular way, a result of coercion on the part of the husband's family, and not all the woman's free choice (3). In cultures with a patrilineal system where women have no property rights, widows are dependent on their male relatives to support them and may choose *sati* as a way out, not to remain at their mercy (32). Whereas widowed men are encouraged to do so, widows in India are not allowed to remarry and so are excluded from most ceremonies and the chance to participate fully in life (14).

With changing times, the status of being a grandmother may no longer mean that childrearing days are over. When parents divorce, migrate to seek employment, or become ill and die of diseases such as AIDS, grandparents are often called out of "retirement" to help raise their grandchildren (32). In societies like India where the extended family is of primary importance, grandparents have close contact with the younger generations when the joint family structure is maintained, although this is changing rapidly as more nuclear family households move out on their own.

As women of a certain age are freed from their traditional roles, they may gain a certain authority. Elders are often accorded great respect and direct the activities of the kinship group. This is especially important in the case of hunter-gatherer cultures or groups with an oral tradition, where knowledge of the environment has been critical for survival. Among the Netsilik of northern Canada, elderly women often adopted a grandson or granddaughter, whom they referred to as their "walking stick," implying that they would provide for them through hunting and family support as they got older (10).

In his overview of mental health and well-being, which explores the factors contributing to fulfillment in life and longevity, Vaillant (33) makes reference to a longitudinal study of nuns by Snowdon (2001), who asked 180 nuns to write a brief autobiography of a few pages and then classified these according to the expression of positive emotion. Vaillant reports that only 24% of the nuns with the most positive emotion in their statements died by age 80 years, while 54% of those with the least positive emotion died by the same age. With this evidence, Vaillant proposes that subjective well-being can be linked to good health and longevity, that "subjective well-being makes available personal resources that can be directed toward innovation and creativity in thought and action . . . [and] becomes an antidote to learned helplessness" (p. 1380), the latter term being one of the factors associated with depression and unhappiness.

There is an enormous amount of variation in rituals of death and mourning, with a wide variety of meanings, beliefs, and expectations. In many parts of Africa, elders take on important new status through death, as they are believed to join the ancestors whose role it is to watch over the generations and protect the village (14). Funerals are therefore an opportunity for people to link the past and present and celebrate their collectivity. Sometimes mourning customs are used to reinforce social systems. In matrilineal Micronesian society, Ifaluk women do not openly grieve for their husbands but are culturally expected to grieve for their fathers and brothers, their blood relatives (14). Given these gender differences, one can only say that the representations of women in society continue even after death and form part of the larger cosmology, which in turn guides the beliefs and influences the status of women in future generations.

FUTURE DIRECTIONS

The *World Mental Health Report* (3), which has been cited several times in this chapter, devotes a chapter to issues of women's mental health and presents a review of the literature analyzing the social origins of distress. The authors compare ethnographic, epidemiologic, and clinical studies from around the world, examining the multiple social forces that contribute to increased rates of psychological and psychiatric distress in women. Their conclusions are that "poverty, domestic isolation, powerlessness (resulting, for example, from low levels of education and economic dependence), and patriarchal oppression, are all associated with higher prevalence of psychiatric morbidity (exclusive of substance disorder) in women" (3, p. 183). Other issues of importance include hunger, work, and violence in various forms—sexual, reproductive, and domestic violence. Examples include findings of higher rates of depression, anxiety disorders, and unspecified nonpsychotic disorders in women in India, Brazil, and several African countries. WHO takes the analysis further and reviews hypothesized explanations for these gender differences. For example, WHO cites the well-known early study of depression in a London suburb by Brown and Harris (1978), who found that four vulnerability factors explained class differences in depression among working-class and middle-class women: loss of parent, three or more children at home, lack of a confiding intimate relationship, and unemployment. Similar findings around gender differences have been noted since in many other settings, in both the developed and the developing world (Table 2.1). Many researchers have also reported on hypothesized social origins of gender differences in psychiatric disorders (Table 2.2).

New research is also looking at the evolutionary roles of women of different generations; an example is a recent study of the fitness benefits of prolonged postreproductive lifespan in women (42). The "grandmother hypothesis" poses the question: Unlike other animal species, why do women survive so long after their reproductive capacity has ceased? A comparative multigenerational study of Finland and Canada using premodern demographic records has now shown that postreproductive mothers enhance the success of their offspring to produce children of their own, contributing to earlier and more numerous grandchildren. In other words, the presence of a grandmother leads to more grandchildren, and more "genetic success" in evolutionary terms. How this will apply to modern times, and to different family structures, remains to be seen but will lead to interesting research questions.

Further studies looking for correlations between improvements in women's lives, such as reduction in poverty or more secure social positions, and improvements in mental health outcomes, would provide more hopeful evidence, since, unfortunately, most of the research in this area has done the important initial

TABLE 2.1

International Research Findings Showing Higher Prevalence of Psychiatric Disorder and Psychological Distress in Women

Research Study	Location	Psychiatric Disorder	Methods	Results
Chakraborty (34)	India	Psychological distress	Community survey (n = 13,335)	Higher frequency in women
Gureje et al. (35)	Nigeria	Major depression	CIDI interview (n = 187)	1. Major depression is three times higher in women than men 2. Dysthymia is more than twice as high
Jablensky (36)	China, India, Sri Lanka	Schizophrenia	Literature review	Higher prevalence for women in three of four studies
Almeida-Filho (37)	Brazil	Psychiatric disorders	Community survey (n = 6,741)	Higher prevalence of nonpsychotic disorders in women
Mari et al. (38)	Brazil	Psychotropic drug use	—	Women use more tranquilizers than men
Amowitz et al. (19)	Afghanistan	Major depression	—	Depression and suicidal ideation more prevalent in Taliban-controlled areas

Modified from Desjarlais et al., *World Mental Health Report* (3, p. 182).

TABLE 2.2

Hypothesized Social Origins of Gender Differences in Psychiatric Disorders

Research Study	Location	Psychiatric Disorder	Hypothesized Social Origins
Mari (39)	Brazil	Minor psychiatric morbidity	Housing issues and sharing living with nonfamily is associated with distress
WHO (40)	International survey	Substance abuse	Unequal social distress, marital stress, isolation of domesticity
Naeem (41)	Pakistan	Major depression	Lack of intimate, confiding relationship with husband
Almeida-Filho (37)	Brazil	Nonpsychotic disorders	Housewife role as risk factor for psychiatric morbidity linked to marital status, education, occupation
Becker et al. (15)	Fiji	Eating disorders	Introduction of Western media and television

Modified from Desjarlais et al., *World Mental Health Report* (3, p. 184).

work of linking negative impacts of social factors with mental health, and has shown that there is much room for improvement.

It is only by taking a view that includes a combination of local knowledge and global relevance that more progress will be made in understanding the social determinants of women's mental health.

REFERENCES

1. Patel V. Where There Is No Psychiatrist: A Mental Health Care Manual. London: Gaskell, 2003.
2. Dikotter F. Imperfect Conceptions: Medical Knowledge, Birth Defects and Eugenics in China. New York: Columbia University Press, 1998.
3. Desjarlais R, Eisenberg L, Good B. et al. World Mental Health: Problems and Priorities in Low-Income Countries. New York: Oxford University Press, 1995.
4. Fadiman A. The Spirit Catches You and You Fall Down: A Hmong Child, Her American Doctors and the Collision of Two Cultures. New York: Farrar, Strauss and Giroux, 1997.
5. Lewis G. Day of Shining Red: An Essay on Understanding Ritual. Cambridge: Cambridge University Press, 1980.
6. Scheper-Hughes N. Death Without Weeping: The Violence of Everyday Life in Brazil. Berkeley and Los Angeles: University of California Press, 1992.
7. Notman M, Nadelson C. Gender, development and psychopathology: a revised psychodynamic view. In: Seeman M, ed. Gender and Psychopathology. Washington: American Psychiatric Association Press, 1995.
8. Chang J. Wild Swans. New York: Anchor, 1992.
9. Briggs J. Inuit Morality Play: The Emotional Education of a Three-Year-Old. New Haven, CT: Yale University Press, 1998.
10. Balikci A. The Netsilik Eskimo. New York: Natural History Press, 1970.
11. Gilligan C. In A Different Voice: Psychological Theory and Women's Development. Cambridge, MA: Harvard University Press, 1998.
12. Barnes VL, Boddy J. Aman: The Story of a Somali Girl. Toronto: Vintage Canada: 1995.
13. Amnesty International, International Zero Tolerance to FGM Day: Effective measures needed to protect girls from female genital mutilation. Press Release, February 6, 2004.
14. Tseng W-S. Clinician's Guide to Cultural Psychiatry. San Diego: Academic, 2003.
15. Becker AE, Burwell RA, Gilman SE, et al. Eating behaviours and attitudes following prolonged exposure to television among ethnic Fijian adolescent girls. Br J Psychiatry 2002;180:509–514.
16. Sadock BJ, Sadock VA, eds. Kaplan and Sadock's Comprehensive Textbook of Psychiatry. Philadelphia: Lippincott Williams & Wilkins, 2000.
17. Racine J, Racine J-L. Viramma: Life of an Untouchable. New York: Verso, 1997.
18. Stackhouse J. Out of Poverty and into Something More Comfortable. Toronto: Random House Canada, 2000.
19. Amowitz L, Heisler M, Iacopino V. A population-based assessment of women's mental health and attitudes towards women's rights in Afghanistan. J Women's Health 2003;12:577–587.
20. Ali M. Brick Lane. London: Doubleday, 2003.
21. Jilek-Aall L. Forty years of experience with epilepsy in Africa. In: Schachter S, Andermann L. eds. The Brainstorms Village: Epilepsy in our World. Philadelphia: Lippincott Williams & Wilkins, 2003:37–52.
22. Farmer P. Women, poverty and AIDS. In: Farmer P, Connors, M, Simmons J, eds. Women, Poverty and AIDS: Sex, Drugs and Structural Violence. Monroe: Common Courage, 1996:3–38.
23. Farmer P. Infections and Inequalities: The Modern Plague. Berkeley: University of California Press, 1999.
24. Piccinelli M, Gomez Homen F. Gender Differences in the Epidemiology of Affective Disorders and Schizophrenia. Geneva: World Health Organization, 1997.
25. Kebede D, Alem A, Shibre T, et al. Onset and clinical course of schizophrenia in Butajira-Ethiopia. Soc Psychiatry Psychiatr Epidemiol 2003;38:625–631.
26. Leung A, Chue P. Sex differences in schizophrenia, a review of the literature. Acta Psychiatr Scand 2000;101:3–38.
27. Cohen A. The Mental Health of Indigenous Peoples: An International Overview. Geneva: World Health Organization, 1999.
28. Abbey SE, Hood E, Young LT, et al. Psychiatric consultation in the eastern Canadian Arctic: III. Mental health issues in Inuit women in the eastern Arctic. Can J Psychiatry 1993;38:32–35.
29. Charney DA. The psychoendocrinology of menopause in cross-cultural perspective. Transcultural Psychiatr Res Rev 1996;33:413–429.
30. Lock M. Encounters with Aging: Mythologies of Menopause in Japan and North America. Berkeley and Los Angeles: University of California Press, 1993.

31. Ramphele M. Political widowhood in South Africa: the embodiment of ambiguity. In: Kleinman A, Das V, Lock M, eds. Social Suffering. Berkeley and Los Angeles: University of California Press, 1997.

32. Dennerstein L, Kane P. Introduction: gender, health and societies. Transcultural Psychiatr Res Rev 1996;33:377–390.

33. Vaillant GE. Mental Health. Am J Psychiatry 2003;160:1373–1384.

34. Chakraborty A. Social Stress and Mental Health: A Social-Psychiatric Field Study of Calcutta. Sage, 1990.

35. Gureje O, Obikoya B, Ikuesan BA. Prevalence of specific psychiatric disorders in an urban primary care setting. E African Med J 1992;69:282–287.

36. Jablensky A. Schizophrenia in the third world: an epidemiological perspective. Working paper, International Mental and Behavioral Health Project, Center for the Study of Culture and Medicine, Harvard Medical School, Boston, MA, 1993.

37. Almeida-Filho N. Becoming modern after all these years: social change and mental health in Latin America. Working paper, International Mental and Behavioral Health Project, Center for the Study of Culture and Medicine, Harvard Medical School, Boston, MA, 1993.

38. Mari J, Almeida-Filho N, Coutinho E, et al. The epidemiology of psychotropic use in the City of Sao Paulo. Psychol Med 1993;23:467–474.

39. Mari J. Psychiatric morbidity in three primary medical care clinics in the city of Sao Paulo. Soc Psychiatry 1987;22:129–138.

40. World Health Organization. Women and substance abuse, 1992 Interim Report. Geneva: WHO Programme on Substance Abuse.

41. Naeem S. Vulnerability factors for depression in Pakistani women. J Pak Med Assoc June 1992;137–138.

42. Lahdenpera M, Lummaa V, Helle S, et al. Fitness benefits of prolonged post-reproductive lifespan in women. Nature 2004;428(6979):178–181.

Chapter 2 Commentary
A Feminist Perspective
Charmaine C. Williams

Lisa Andermann's anthropologic perspective reminds us that in many contexts the social determinants of mental health are not under the control of women. Whether living in conditions of national prosperity or national deprivation, women and girls are constrained in their efforts to achieve health and gain access to safe, effective health care. Too commonly, women and female children are the most deprived members of any nation-state.

Dr. Andermann deftly directs us to a critical view of the female development process. She challenges decontextualized biologic narratives of birth, maturation, and death by presenting the sociopolitical, cultural, and economic context of women's experiences of mental health. The prenatal and childbirth periods are revealed as stages for establishing the value of mothers and their daughters. Childhood is represented as a period for intense socialization into approved adult female roles. Adolescence becomes a time for regulating women's sexual behavior and disciplining their sexual attractions. Adulthood brings years devoted to productivity but in a context that devalues and diminishes female productivity. Finally, women's elder years are identified as a time when they are no longer defined by the presence of men in their lives, but in the absence of men, they are both socially and materially impoverished. Dr. Andermann makes it clear that each stage of individual development brings new threats to the mental health of women throughout the world. Yet, I appreciate that her chapter does not dwell exclusively on the negative. She also presents indicators of hope and alternate possibilities. Both theory and practice point the way toward restructuring of social and material arrangements to reduce female disadvantage.

Still, I believe that the chapter reveals a deficiency of the anthropologic gaze. Too often, this gaze is revealed as not only Western, but also racist, sexist, heterosexist, and otherwise oppressive. The Western gaze is present in the exotification of practices in the so-called developing world, presenting them as failures to attain our own idealized cultural arrangements. The racism of the gaze is revealed in presenting post-partum "confinement" in "other" cultures as punitive, omitting other information that would clarify its role in assuring sufficient tranquility for mother–child bonding and rest. The sexism of the gaze is revealed in the focus on women as prereproductive, reproductive, or postreproductive, implying they have few functions beyond the production of subsequent generations. Finally, the heterosexism of the gaze is revealed in the emphasis on sexuality as expressed exclusively through male–female pairings, rendering invisible the other possibilities for love and intimacy. The narrowing of our view to this particular gaze suggests the world should be judged against Western, white, reproductive, heterosexual functioning in order to gauge the desirability of patterns of individual and social development. I do not, however, hold Dr. Andermann responsible for fashioning this gaze; by drawing on the literature that exists, she inevitably reproduces its oppressive undertones.

One possibility for moving beyond the problematic gaze that has influenced work conducted under the rubric of anthropologic cross-cultural or transcultural study is to focus less on what "other" cultures practice in female development. We can shift the gaze to a broader focus on the elements that seem to persist as threats to women's mental health and well-being in all contexts. Violence is a universal threat to women's mental health. Whether that violence emerges in war, family violence, sexual exploitation, or some other form, we recognize its damage and its relevance across contexts. Hegemonic ideals of femininity are a universal threat to women's mental health. Rigid expectations for female presentation contribute to eating disorders, the self-destructive pursuit of cosmetic surgeries, genital mutilations, and other practices that we recognize as damaging and relevant across contexts. Patriarchal capitalism is a universal threat to women's mental health. Lack of control over resources, the commodification of women's bodies, devaluing women's work inside and outside of the home, and other economic abuses are practices that we recognize as damaging to women's capacities to maintain mental health across contexts. We should be working with researchers in other contexts to reframe a gaze that includes scrutiny of our own practices and their continuity with other methods of gender-based mental abuse that have local and international implications. The benefits and challenges of such collaborations are being explored in a growing literature on international research collaborations (1–4). The task is demanding, but the potential reward is compelling. With all of us sharing a reframed gaze, we can work toward the improved mental health of women all over the world.

REFERENCES

1. Bowes A. Evaluating an empowering research strategy: reflections on action-research with South Asian Women. Sociological Research Online 1996;1(1). http//www.socresonline.org.uk/1/1/1 .html#top
2. Byron J, Thorburn D. Gender and international relations: a global perspective and issues for the Caribbean. Feminist Review 1998;59: 211–232.
3. Gaskell J, Eichler M. White women as burden: on playing the role of feminist "experts" in China. Womens Stud Int Forum 2001;24(6):647–651.
4. Maina-Ahlberg B, Nordberg E, Tomson G. North–South health research collaboration: challenges in institutional interaction. Soc Sci Med 1997;44(8):1229–1238.

Women and Stress

Elaine Walker, Zainab Sabuwalla,
Annie M. Bollini, Deborah J. Walder

The issue of sex differences in the response to stress has both health and social implications. Conventional wisdom has been of two minds on the issue. One perspective, shared by some in the scientific community, views women as being more reactive to stressful events than men (1), but another, more recent popular conception is that women cope better with stress (2). Empirical research findings indicate that the situation is more complex than either of these perspectives.

Research on the biobehavioral impact of psychosocial stress has burgeoned in the past two decades. We know that stress can adversely affect both physical and mental health and that these effects are mediated by changes in biologic systems that govern the stress response (3). There is no doubt that, among mammals, both sexes manifest biologic and behavioral reactions when exposed to stress. However, recent evidence indicates that the nature of these responses varies for men and women. Thus, it is not simply a matter of greater or lesser stress reactivity in females. Instead, it appears that the sexes differ in a constellation of factors that determines the nature of their measured responses to stressful events.

In this chapter, we discuss the empirical research findings on the nature of the stress response in males and females. The objective is to answer three questions: (1) Do the sexes differ in their psychological and behavioral responses to stress? (2) Do the sexes differ in their biologic responses to stress? and (3) What are the mental health implications of these differences for men and women?

HISTORICAL BACKGROUND

Past theoretical models of the human stress response were dominated by theories that did not distinguish between the responses manifested by males and females. Further, until the mid-1990s, laboratory studies examining physiologic stress responses in human beings were predominantly focused on men; women comprised a minority of research participants (4). The reason for excluding women from such studies was partly that scientists believed the greater neuroendocrine variability in women, attributable to the menstrual cycle, had the potential to obscure the findings. The past decade has witnessed greater inclusion of women in scientific investigations, and there is now a more substantive body of theory and empirical findings addressing gender differences.

In reviewing the historical antecedents to contemporary research on stress, it is apparent that one of the most influential theoretical frameworks in the field has been the notion of the "fight-or-flight" response to stress (5). Stress-induced activation of the sympathetic nervous system is assumed to mediate this response via its innervation of the adrenal medulla, which triggers a hormonal cascade and the secretion of catecholamines (e.g., norepinephrine and epinephrine), both of which affect the brain and other organs. The nature of the stressor determines whether the organism fights or flees in response to sympathetic activation. When the stressor is appraised as one that can be overcome, then "fight," or aggressive behavior, is the response, but when the stress is produced by a more formidable threat, "flight" is more likely. Thus the response to stress is presumably aimed at enhancing survival.

Other researchers elaborated on this approach and hypothesized biobehavioral interactions in the stress response. In 1936 Helen Flanders Dunbar, a medical doctor, suggested a relationship between psychosomatic diseases and certain types of personality. Around the same time, Hans Selye proposed a model of the "stages" of the stress response, which he subsequently revised (6). The model posits that the mammalian response to stress or threat entails a "General Adaptation Syndrome" (GAS) and is characterized by a set of resistance and adjustment reactions. The first of the three stages is the *alert* or *alarm* phase, in which the organism experiences homeostatic disruption. The second phase is *resistance*, in which the organism attempts, both biologically and behaviorally, to adapt to or eliminate the stressor. The third phase, which occurs if the organism is unsuccessful in coping with the stressor, involves *exhaustion* or *decompensation*. The issue of gender has rarely been raised as a relevant factor in determining the qualitative or quantitative aspects of these stages. But subsequent research findings provide reason to believe that gender may indeed moderate the stress response, especially the nature of the individual's reaction in the alarm and resistance stages.

In a recent paper, Shelley Taylor and her colleagues (4) proposed a new model of the stress response that posits an important gender difference. Based on their review of the empirical literature as well as evolutionary theories about biobehavioral sex differences, Taylor et al. proposed that the notion of "fight or flight" does not aptly describe the response to stress in females. Instead, the female stress response is better described as a pattern of "tend-and-befriend." They propose that "Tending involves nurturant activities designed to protect the self and offspring that promote safety and reduce distress; befriending is the creation and maintenance of social networks that may aid in this process" (p. 411). Further, they suggest that the mechanisms that subserve the tend-and-befriend pattern emanate from the neural systems that subserve the "attachment-caregiving" system. We will examine some evidence for this in our discussion of biologic sex differences in stress.

Of course, as Taylor et al. (4) point out: "Biology is not so much destiny as it is a central tendency, but a central tendency that influences and interacts with social, cultural, cognitive, and emotional factors." Indeed, empirical research on gender and stress indicates that gender moderates the biobehavioral response to stress exposure. Human males and females conceptualize and respond to stress in different ways.

GENDER DIFFERENCES IN MENTAL DISORDERS

There are sexually differentiated rates of many medical conditions. For example, women are more likely to acquire an autoimmune disease and are more susceptible to Alzheimer's and epilepsy, whereas men are more susceptible to cardiovascular disorders (7–9). Cardiac arrest is much more common in men; however, women have lower recovery and survival rates from heart attack, which is the leading cause of death among American women. Given these differences in susceptibility to physical health problems, it is not surprising that there are sex differences in patterns of mental disorders.

In a seminal paper, Carolyn Zahn-Waxler reviewed sex differences in psychopathology and proposed that they have their basis in biologically determined sex differences in temperament (10). The other chapters in this volume discuss research findings that are consistent with this assumption. Across cultures, there is a preponderance of men with antisocial and other externalizing disorders, and significantly more women with internalizing disorders, especially those that are presumed to be linked with stress. Thus, more women than men meet diagnostic criteria for depression and post-traumatic stress disorder (PTSD), especially following exposure to stress (4,10,11). The predominance of females with depression and PTSD also holds for children. It is of interest to note, however, that among subgroups expected to encounter high levels of stress, such as police officers, there are no gender differences in rates of PTSD or its symptoms, a finding that suggests that women may self-select for such occupations (11). These and related findings have raised pivotal questions about possible sex differences in exposure or response to stress.

THE BEHAVIORAL RESPONSE TO STRESS

SELF-REPORTED STRESS

When males and females are asked to report on the stresses they experience in everyday life, females tend to report more stressors (12). In fact, a recent meta-analysis revealed developmental continuity in this trend; compared to males, females of all ages report more stressful events than males (13).

The gender difference in self-reported stress escalates following puberty. Compared to younger and older individuals, adolescents generally report a greater number of stressful events (13). But the postpubertal rise in self-reported stress is greater for girls than boys, although there is little developmental change during adolescence in the number of stress events reported by females (14). With advanced age, there is a decline in self-reported stress for both sexes, but elderly women continue to report more stress than elderly men.

The nature of the stressful events also differs by gender. Males report more physical conflicts, accidents, and negative work and school events. In contrast, females report more stressful interpersonal events, especially stressful experiences that involve significant others. For example, Hagedoorn et al. (15) examined levels of psychological stress in geriatric couples and found that women's stress was determined by both their own and their spouse's health status. For males, in contrast, only their own health status was related to their psychological stress. Thus women seem to be more emotionally distressed by health problems in significant others. Consistent with this, female elderly caregivers reported experiencing more stressors than their male counterparts despite apparent uniform caregiving experiences across the sexes (16).

There are also differences in the emotional responses to stressors described by men and women (17). Women are more likely to endorse feelings of emotional vulnerability and sensitivity, whereas men are more likely to endorse items describing tension, irritability, and being easily upset.

There is a dearth of literature examining gender differences in self-reported stress across cultures, although the data available indicate that females report more stress than males across cultures (18). This conclusion is tentative, given the limited research available. Yet consistency across cultures, despite differences in social customs, suggests that gender differences in self-reported stress have biologic underpinnings.

When considering the sex difference in self-reported stress, it is important to keep in mind that there are also sex differences in the likelihood of recalling and reporting stressful events. One likely reason for this is that females engage in more cognitive rumination about adverse events (19). In other words, they direct attention inwardly, on negative feelings and thoughts. Similarly, there is evidence that compared to males, females recall more details of negative life events (20). Thus the higher rate of self-reported everyday stressors among females may reflect a cognitive style that makes it easier for them to recall past adverse events.

Another important consideration is the evidence that the gender difference is reversed for more serious stressors, or *traumatic* events, and this also appears to hold across cultures (21). The preponderance of self-reported traumatic events for males is most pronounced in the categories of physical attacks and accidents. In striking contrast, females are much more likely than males to experience one of the chief traumas linked with distress and PTSD, namely, sexual abuse and assault (20,22). Females are about three times more likely than males to be victims of sexual abuse or assault, and this may contribute to the higher rate of PTSD observed in women.

CYCLIC CHANGES IN FEMALES' SUBJECTIVE STRESS

Temporal variations in subjective stress parallel hormonal variations during the menstrual cycle. In the premenstrual phase, when estrogen is low, women report feeling more stress than during the postmenstrual phase (i.e., 4 to 5 days after menstruation) (23). Further, women with more severe premenstrual symptoms report more stress overall (23). They also rate events as more stressful than do women without premenstrual symptoms, women using oral contraceptives, and males, despite equal ratings among the groups on the frequency of stressful events (24). Thus premenstrual symptoms appear to heighten sensitivity to stress, perhaps because monthly hormonal variations affect mood, which in turn influences how events are perceived.

REACTIONS TO THE STRESS OF TRAUMA AND LOSS

Given that females report more stress than males, we turn to the question of whether this indicates that females are exhibiting a stronger response to stressors when they occur, rather than simply being exposed to more frequent or severe stressors. The limited available research findings indicate that when confronted with the same stressor, females have a greater subjective response and more behavioral sequelae than males. As noted previously, females of all ages are more likely to exhibit PTSD following exposure to significant stressors. Further, this differential susceptibility has its origins in childhood. For example, Ronen, Rahav, and Rosenbaum (25) assessed Middle Eastern children's reactions to the 1991 Gulf War. Although boys and girls reported comparable levels of anxiety and behavioral problems before the war, girls felt more anxious during the war and manifested greater increases in the frequency of certain behavior problems, such as stuttering, sleep disturbances, and fear of sleeping alone. Yet, it is noteworthy that sex differences in behavioral reaction to the war were only observed for the adolescent cohort, and younger children did not differ in war-related symptoms based on gender. This mirrors the findings on developmental changes in gender differences in self-reported stress in community samples and suggests that pubertal changes can amplify sensitivity to stress in females.

There is some evidence that there are cultural differences in the consequences of stress for males and females. In a study of work-related stress in the United States, United Kingdom, Taiwan, and South Africa, there were few gender differences for the type of stressors experienced; however, gender groups differed in how job stress was related to their overall mental health (26). Based on self-report of mental well-being, American males showed the strongest relation between stress and health, but the association was weakest for British and South African females. These findings suggest that the way occupational stressors influence mental health may vary by sex and culture.

Despite the evidence that females show a more pronounced psychological response to stress, their physical health reactions may not be as strong as those shown by males. The most informative research on this issue comes from studies of partner loss. After loss of a spouse, both men and women suffer higher rates of physical illnesses than their married counterparts (2). However, compared to women, men who lose a spouse are significantly more vulnerable to health problems and have higher rates of mortality. Males who experience loss show higher rates of suicide, heart disease, liver disease, and accidents. Recent studies have shown that the increased mortality risks of widowhood among men extend for years after partner loss, suggesting that loss of a spouse constitutes a chronic stress for men. As discussed below, it is likely that these sex differences are partially mediated by differences in the neurohormonal and cardiovascular responses to stress. But they may also be a result of gender differences in coping strategies.

There is a substantial body of research on gender differences in behavioral coping reactions to loss and separation, particularly partner loss (2). Although feelings of distress are normative after partner loss, males and females exhibit very different coping strategies. The differences parallel those described by Taylor and colleagues (4), with women seeking more social contact and men being more likely to engage in avoidance coping, which sometimes involves dysfunctional distracting behaviors like heavy drinking. For example, in a study of partner loss, widowed men who refused to participate in interviews but completed questionnaires by mail were more depressed than those who agreed to the interview (2). The opposite pattern was observed among widows, with the more depressed agreeing to the interview.

Men employ avoidant or withdrawal strategies when dealing with other types of major life stressors as well. For example, most men with prostate cancer avoid disclosure about the illness when possible, but the majority of women with breast cancer seek opportunities to discuss their illness with others (27). Women are also more likely to attend support groups and share their emotional reactions (28). Again, gender differences in cognitive and coping styles may contribute to the observed gender differences in the diagnosis of stress-related psychiatric disorders.

Other empirical research shows that women generally tend to cope with stress by focusing on and sharing their emotional reactions. Garnefski and colleagues measured individuals' strategies for regulating their emotions following stressful life events and found that women were much more likely than men to engage in cognitive strategies involving rumination and elaborating on the emotional aspects of the event (29). Women also used more active social coping, like seeking social support and engaging in positive reappraisal, and positive self-talk. In fact, women report greater use of the majority of coping behaviors when compared to men (27).

Similar gender differences are observed in the behavior of parents who have been exposed to stressful, conflictual interactions in the course of the workday (30). Repetti found that fathers who had experienced a stressful workday were more likely to be interpersonally conflictual or to withdraw from their families at home that evening. Women, on the other hand, were more nurturant and caring toward their children on their stressful workdays.

THE BIOLOGIC RESPONSE TO STRESS

Given the evidence that women express more subjective distress in response to stress, we now turn to the biologic level of analysis. As mentioned earlier, exposure to stress activates the body to respond. This is reflected in multiple neural systems, including the hypothalamic-pituitary-adrenal (HPA) axis, the cardiovascular system, the immunologic system, and various neurotransmitter systems, especially the catecholamines. Published reports on gender differences in the biologic indicators of the stress response have primarily focused on the steroid hormones governed by the HPA axis.

GENDER DIFFERENCES IN THE HPA RESPONSE TO STRESS

The hypothalamic-pituitary-adrenal (HPA) axis is one of the key neural systems mediating the effects of stress on behavioral maladjustment and psychiatric illnesses (3,31). The HPA axis involves three chemical messengers: corticotropin-releasing hormone (CRH), adrenocorticotropic hormone (ACTH), and glucocorticoids. In response to stress, cells in the periventricular nucleus of the hypothalamus release CRH. The pituitary contains receptors for CRH, and when these are stimulated, the pituitary releases ACTH. ACTH then signals the adrenal cortex to release glucocorticoids, including cortisol in primates and corticosterone in rats. Glucocorticoids have effects throughout the body, and they are critical to the physiologic changes that constitute the adaptation to stress. Glucocorticoid receptors, located in various regions throughout the brain, serve to regulate the activity of the HPA axis through neural feedback systems.

Research on rodents has been consistent in revealing sex differences in HPA activity, with female rats showing greater basal corticosterone levels than males (32). Similarly, female rats manifest greater increases in ACTH and corticosterone in response to both acute and chronic stressors (32). In rodents, sex is also linked with the expression of corticosteroid receptors and the morphology of the hippocampal pyramidal neurons. But research on human subjects does not parallel the results observed in rodents. This points to important limitations on generalization across species.

In humans, the research on baseline cortisol and ACTH generally reveals minimal or no sex differences. Some tests of adults' basal levels of HPA functioning show that men have greater ACTH secretion than women, but there appear to be no sex differences in basal cortisol secretion (33). Several studies of adolescents have also shown no gender difference in levels of cortisol (34), although a few indicate that boys have higher levels of ACTH than girls (35).

Data from a recent study of adolescents conducted in our laboratory are consistent with previous reports in showing no significant sex difference in baseline cortisol. Participants range in age from 12 to 17 years, and include both normal adolescents (n = 26) and a group (n = 54) of adolescents who met diagnostic criteria of the *Diagnostic and Statistical Manual of Mental Disorders* (DSM-IV) for an Axis II personality disorder. During the laboratory assessment of this sample, saliva cortisol was measured five times. Figure 3.1 shows cortisol values, by

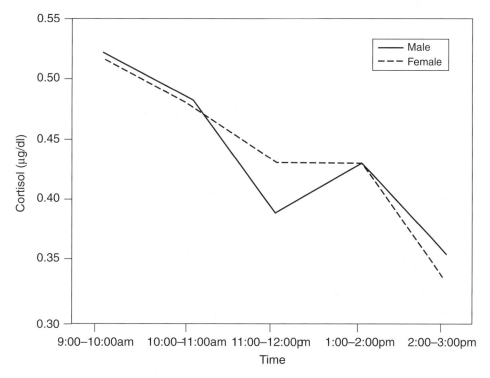

FIGURE 3.1 ● Cortisol levels for male and female adolescents.

time, for males and females. As can be seen, the temporal trends are similar. Thus, during this critical developmental period, when females report significantly more stress than males, baseline stress hormone secretion shows no sex difference.

More consistent evidence of gender differences does emerge, however, from studies of stress-induced cortisol secretion. In response to laboratory challenges, including psychosocial stress and "real-world" examination stress, adult male subjects generally show greater cortisol and ACTH responses than female subjects. In a series of studies by Kirschbaum and colleagues (33,36), participants engaged in a brief public speaking task combined with a mental arithmetic task in front of an audience. There was a twofold to fourfold increase in cortisol above baseline for both sexes when exposed to this stressor, but males had a larger mean cortisol increase. Similar results have been reported for sex differences in response to a laboratory stress that involved social aggression (7). Males had the largest reactivity on cortisol, although women showed a more self-reported hostility. No sex differences have been reported in the cortisol response to a physical challenge (bicycle ergometry test) or a CRH challenge (injection of corticotropin-releasing hormone) (36).

It is relevant to note that Kirschbaum et al. (33) have proposed that gender differences may be obscured in total plasma cortisol stress responses, while gender differences emerge for ACTH and free salivary cortisol. These researchers showed that ACTH responses to stress were elevated in men compared to women, independent of menstrual cycle phase or contraceptives use (33). For saliva cortisol, women in the luteal phase had a stress response comparable to that of men, whereas women in the follicular phase and those on oral contraceptives showed lower cortisol responses. These observations highlight the need to distinguish between the total cortisol *secretion* and the bioavailable cortisol *levels*.

While research on young and middle-aged adults suggests that stress-induced activation of the HPA axis is more pronounced for males, studies of elderly subjects do not yield this pattern. Instead, it appears that the sex difference in the cortisol response to stress may be reversed with advanced age. Seeman et al. (37) found higher cortisol reactivity in elderly women compared to elderly men in response to a driving simulation challenge. These observations were corroborated using a 30-minute cognitive challenge paradigm; among older subjects, females exhibited a greater response than males, but among younger subjects, males exhibited a greater salivary cortisol response (37). Similar results were reported by Laughlin and Barret-Connor (38). This developmental shift in gender differences suggests that gonadal hormones may play a role in the cortisol response to stress.

Given the evidence that males and females differ in the intensity of their concern with socioemotional issues, we might also expect them to differ in their biologic response to stressors that vary in social salience. Consistent with this notion, there are gender differences in the nature of the stressors that elicit more pronounced cortisol responses. Stroud, Salovey, and Epel (39) randomly assigned adult subjects to achievement or rejection stress conditions. The achievement condition involved challenging cognitive tasks, and the social rejection condition involved challenging social interactions. There were no sex differences in mood ratings following the stressors; however, men showed significantly greater cortisol responses to the cognitive challenges, whereas women showed greater responses to the social rejection. These findings are consistent with the notion that women are more invested in social relations, whereas men are more concerned with achievement.

In biologic challenges to the HPA axis, the findings on gender differences are mixed. Gallucci et al. (40) found that women exhibited a greater and more prolonged ACTH response to a CRH challenge than men, but there was no significant sex difference in cortisol secretion. In contrast, Dorn et al. (35) found greater secretion of ACTH in male than female adolescents following a CRH challenge. Again, these findings may indicate a reversal in sex differences with age, although further studies are needed before such conclusions are drawn.

OTHER ASPECTS OF THE NEUROCHEMICAL RESPONSE TO STRESS

Sex differences in other neurochemical indices of stress have received relatively little attention compared to hormones secreted by the HPA axis. Some studies have shown that epinephrine increases in response to cognitive challenges (mirror tracing and mental arithmetic) are greater in males than females (41). Similarly, adolescent boys, compared with girls, show significantly higher levels of norepinephrine.

Oxytocin is a pituitary hormone secreted in response to a variety of events, including stressors, in both males and females. It appears to serve as a counter-regulator of other neural systems that are activated by stress, including the HPA axis, and its release is linked with enhanced sedation, relaxation, and maternal and other affiliative behavior. A review by Taylor et al. (4) of research on both animals and humans indicates that oxytocin release in response to stress is significantly greater in females. As described below, this is consistent with evidence that androgens inhibit oxytocin release, while estrogen enhances it. In addition, endogenous opioid peptides serve to augment affiliative behaviors, especially in females. Taylor et al. (4) discuss findings from a variety of sources to show female responses of the sympathetic nervous system and HPA axis are down regulated by oxytocin, which in combination with endogenous opioid mechanisms and estrogen, fosters maternal and affiliative behavior in response to stress. In contrast, stress appears to enhance the "fight-or-flight" stress response in males.

PHYSIOLOGIC MANIFESTATIONS OF THE RESPONSE TO STRESS

There are documented sex differences in the cardiovascular response to stress, with males typically showing more pronounced responses. Reviews of the literature have revealed that males have higher heart rate and blood pressure at rest and greater challenge-induced increases in heart rate and especially blood pressure (38). Among the stressors that have been found to induce a greater cardiovascular response in males are thermal stress (cold air/water), physical exertion stress, social hassles, and orthostatic stress. Further, males show more protracted cardiovascular responses to acute stress than women (7,8). Taken together, these findings are generally consistent with the higher rate of cardiovascular disease in men. Of note, however, some studies show no sex differences in cardiac and/or blood pressure responses following psychosocial or physical challenges (7,42).

As with self-reported stress, studies of women at different phases of the menstrual cycle reveal temporal variations in women's vascular response to stress. For example, Hastrup and Light (43) found sex differences in blood pressure during the follicular (but not the luteal) phase of the menstrual cycle. Jern et al. (44) found more pronounced hemostatic response to mental stress during the luteal phase than during the follicular phase.

There has been a paucity of research on sex differences on skin conductance indicators of the stress response. The limited data that are available indicate no sex difference in baseline skin conductance; however, males show greater skin conductance than do females in response to video clips depicting fearful and angry interactions, whereas females were more physiologically reactive to sad themes (45).

GONADAL HORMONES AND THE BIOLOGIC STRESS RESPONSE

Sex hormones are one likely source of sex differences in the response to stress. Gonadal hormones influence the neural systems involved in the stress response beginning in the fetal period via organizational effects on the brain (4). During the postnatal period, gonadal hormones have both activational and organizational effects on the function of the nervous system. Yet the mechanisms through which these hormones alter the stress response in humans are not fully understood.

There is an abundance of research suggesting a complex bidirectional relationship between the HPA axis and hypothalamic-pituitary-gonadal (HPG) axis (46,47). One complicating factor in extrapolating from this body of literature is the fact that it is primarily based on animal research. As noted, it now appears that sex differences in the stress response vary across species.

The limited data available indicate that, in postmenopausal women, there are significant inhibitory effects of estrogen treatment on both the HPA axis and catecholamine response to stress. Further, data from human studies suggest that progesterone influences the HPA axis response to stress by modulating sensitivity to negative feedback (32). The research findings we have reviewed here indicate that there are changes in the pattern of sex differences in the stress response across the life span. This suggests that hormonal changes associated with maturational processes can differentially alter the nature of stress responses in males and females.

Despite our increasing knowledge of the stress response at the behavioral and biologic level, the precise nature of the interaction between the HPA and HPG axes, and the underlying mechanisms at various points throughout development, remain unclear. Increasing evidence that 1) abnormalities in both of these systems may play a critical role in the development of psychiatric and medical disorders and 2) that the systems are sexually differentiated, highlight the need for future studies aimed at clarifying the potential role of this hormonal milieu in mediating (or moderating) the biologic response to stress.

CONCLUSIONS

The research literature on sex differences in stress indicates that males and females differ in their responses to stress at multiple levels of analysis: subjective psychological reactions, biologic responses, behavioral responses, and mental and physical health consequences. Yet, the direction of the sex difference is not consistent across these levels of analyses. On some levels women appear to be more vulnerable than men, but on others they are more resilient.

The empirical findings are consistent in showing that women are more likely than men to identify events as stressors and to describe a stronger subjective emotional response to them. In large part, this seems to be one facet of a more generalized tendency for females to recall and share information about negative experiences and emotions. This gender difference in "social-cognitive style" is also reflected more broadly in the tendency for females to express both positive and negative emotion with greater frequency and intensity than males (45).

Yet, the data on various facets of the biologic response to stressors indicate that males often show a more pronounced reaction. Studies of ACTH and cortisol secretion generally suggest that there are no gender differences in baseline levels. But there is support for a sex difference in activation of the HPA axis in response to stress in adults; when a difference is detected, it is more likely to involve greater cortisol or ACTH responses in males. Similarly, with respect to the cardiovascular response to stress, the data tend to indicate that males manifest a stronger response than females. The greater biologic response to stress in males, especially stress-induced by performance demands, may contribute to the higher risk for cardiovascular disorder in men as well as the higher rate of morbidity and mortality following loss. However, there is also some evidence that the gender difference in the magnitude of the neurohormonal stress response reverses with advanced age. These maturational changes should be examined further because they may hold clues to underlying hormonal mechanisms.

Another salient gender difference in the response to stress is observed at the level of behavioral coping. In response to stressful events, females of all primate species, including humans, are more inclined than males to seek social proximity to others (4). Most often females seek social contact with other females with whom they have established relationships. It may be this propensity that provides women with an advantage over men in coping with significant personal losses. In contrast, the "fight-or-flight" pattern is more characteristic of males, who are more likely to act aggressively in response to stress. This behavioral tendency may account for the higher rate of self-reported traumatic experiences among males, especially those involving injury or interpersonal aggression.

Finally, at the level of psychiatric symptoms, we see a more pronounced link with stress among women. Women are more likely to manifest psychiatric symptoms and to meet criteria for psychiatric syndromes, especially PTSD, following exposure to stress. It is important to keep in mind, however, that the diagnosis of such symptoms and syndromes is based on self-report. Thus the higher prevalence in women may simply reflect the tendency for females to more readily recall and verbalize negative experiences and emotions. This should be taken into consideration when formulating and applying diagnostic criteria. At the biologic level, the stress response may be as strong or stronger in males, yet females will more often meet clinical criteria for stress-related disorders.

Conclusions about gender differences in the stress response should also take developmental level into consideration. As noted, the stress sensitivity of females may change across the life span and with the menstrual cycle. The developmental trend entails changes during adolescence and with advanced age. This pattern could be interpreted as a reflection of hormonal influences. To date, however, our understanding of the relation between sex hormones and the stress response is limited (32).

As mentioned previously, most of the published research on the relation between gonadal hormones and the stress response is based on animal models, typically rodents. It appears that there are species differences in the biologic mechanisms subserving the stress response that limit the generalizability of the animal findings to human gender differences. As a consequence, there is a need for more systematic, empirical research aimed at elucidating the effects of sex hormones on the stress response in males and females. The field of stress research has evolved over the past few decades, and we now have excellent paradigms and reliable biologic assays for exploring multiple aspects of the human response to stress. Thus the stage is set for conducting informative research about the psychobiologic underpinning of sex differences.

Finally, the links between psychological and biologic manifestations of stress should be subjected to further exploration. At the present time, the diagnostic approach to stress-related disorders is based almost exclusively on patient self-report. Yet, we know that the adverse physical consequences of stress exposure are mediated by the biologic factors. In the future, the accuracy of diagnosis of stress-related disorders might be enhanced by incorporating biologic measures that index the neurohormonal and physiologic indicators. The combination of psychological and biologic measures might also lead to a better understanding of the nature of sex differences in the clinical manifestations of stress-related disorders.

REFERENCES

1. Bonner CA. Psychogenic factors as causative agents in manic-depressive psychoses. In: Lewis NDC, ed. Manic-Depressive Psychosis. New York: Friedman, 1932:121–130.
2. Stroebe M, Stroebe W, Schut H. Gender differences in adjustment to bereavement: an empirical and theoretical review. Rev Gen Psychol 2001;5:62–83.
3. Sapolsky RM. Why Zebras Don't Get Ulcers. New York: Friedman, 1994.
4. Taylor SE, Klein LC, Lewis BP, et al. Biobehavioral responses to stress in females: tend-and-befriend, not fight-or-flight. Psychol Rev 2000;107:411–429.
5. Cannon WB. The Wisdom of the Body. New York: Norton, 1932.
6. Selye H. History of the stress concept. In: Goldberger L, Breznitz S, eds. Handbook of Stress: Theoretical and Clinical Aspects. 2nd Ed. New York: Free Press, 1993:7–17.
7. Earle TL, Linden W, Weinberg J. Differential effects of harassment on cardiovascular and salivary cortisol stress reactivity and recovery in women and men. J Psychosom Res 1996;46:125–141.
8. Matthews KA, Gump BB, Owens JF. Chronic stress influences cardiovascular and neuroendocrine responses during acute stress and recovery, especially in men. Health Psychol 2001;20:403–410.
9. Jacobson DL, Gange SJ, Rose NR, et al. Epidemiology and estimated population burden of selected autoimmune disease in the United States. Clin Immunol Immunopathol 1997;84:223–242.
10. Zahn-Waxler C. Warriors and worriers: gender and psychopathology. Dev Psychopathol 1993;5:79–89.
11. Pole N, Best SR, Weiss DS, et al. Effects of gender and ethnicity on duty-related posttraumatic stress symptoms among urban police officers. J Nerv Ment Dis 2001;189:442–448.
12. Turner RJ, Avison WR. Status variations in stress exposure: implications for the interpretation of research on race, socioeconomic status, and gender. J Health Soc Behav 2003;44:488–505.
13. Davis MC, Matthews KA, Twamley EW. Is life more difficult on Mars or Venus? A meta-analytic review of sex differences in major and minor life events. Ann Behav Med 1999;21:83–97.
14. Allgood-Merten B, Lewinsohn PM, Hops H. Sex differences and adolescent depression. J Abnorm Psychol 1990;99:55–63.
15. Hagedoorn M, Sanderman R, Ranchor AV, et al. Chronic disease in elderly couples: are women more responsive to their spouses' health condition than men? J Psychosom Res 2001;51:693–696.
16. Bookwala J, Schulz R. A comparison of primary stressors, secondary stressors, and depressive symptoms between elderly caregiving husbands and wives: the caregiver health effects study. Psychol Aging 2000;15:607–616.
17. Smith LL, Reise SP. Gender differences on negative affectivity: an IRT study of differential item functioning on the Multidimensional Personality Questionnaire Stress Reaction scale. J Pers Soc Psychol 1998;75:1350–1362.
18. Caballo VE, Cardena E. Sex differences in the perception of stressful life events in a Spanish sample: some implications for the Axis IV of the DSM-IV. Pers Indiv Diff 1997;23:353–359.
19. Nolen-Hoeksema S. Responses to depression and their effects on the duration of depressive episodes. J Abnorm Psychol 1991;100:569–582.
20. Hankin BL, Abramson LY, Siler M. A prospective test of the hopelessness theory of depression in adolescence. Cog Therap Res 2001;25:607–632.
21. Gavranidou M, Rosner R. The weaker sex? Gender and post-traumatic stress disorder. Depress Anxiety 2003;17:130–139.

22. Kaplan SJ, Pelcovitz D, Labruna V. Child and adolescent abuse and neglect research: a review of the past 10 years. Part I: Physical and emotional abuse and neglect. J Am Acad Child Adolesc Psychiatry 1999;38:1214–1222.
23. Woods NF, Lentz MJ, Mitchell ES, et al. Perceived stress, physiologic stress arousal, and premenstrual symptoms: group differences and intra-individual patterns. Res Nurs Health 1998; 21:511–523.
24. Gallant SJ, Popiel DA, Hoffman DM, et al. Using daily ratings to confirm premenstrual syndrome/late luteal phase dysphoric disorder: I. Effects of demand characteristics and expectations. Psychosom Med 1992;54:149–166.
25. Ronen T, Rahav G, Rosenbaum M. Children's reactions to a war situation as a function of age and sex. Anxiety Stress Coping 2003;16:59–69.
26. Miller K, Greyling M, Cooper C, et al. Occupational stress and gender: a cross-cultural study. Stress Med 2000;16:271–278.
27. Tamres LK, Janicki D, Helgeson VS. Sex differences in coping behavior: a meta-analytic review and examination of relative coping. Pers Soc Psychol Rev 2002;6:2–30.
28. Kiss A, Meryn S. Effect of sex and gender on psychosocial aspects of prostate and breast cancer. Br Med J 2001;323:1055–1058.
29. Garnefski N, Teerds J, Kraaij V, et al. Cognitive emotion regulation strategies and depressive symptoms: differences between males and females. Pers Indiv Diff 2004;36:267–276.
30. Repetti RL, Wood J. Effects of daily stress at work on mothers' interactions with preschoolers. J Fam Psychol 1997;11:90–108.
31. Walker EF, Diforio D. Schizophrenia: a neural diathesis-stress model. Psychol Rev 1997;104: 667–685.
32. Young EA, Altemus M. Puberty, ovarian steroids, and stress. Ann NY Acad Sci 2004;1021: 124–133.
33. Kirschbaum BM, Kudielka J, Gaab NC, et al. Impact of gender, menstrual cycle phase and oral contraceptives on the activity of the hypothalamic-pituitary-adrenal axis. Psychosom Med 1999;61:154–162.
34. Susman EJ, Granger DA, Murowchick E, et al. Gonadal and adrenal hormones: developmental transitions and aggressive behavior. Ann NY Acad Sci 1996;794:18–30.
35. Dorn LD, Burgess ES, Susman EJ, et al. Response to CRH in depressed and nondepressed adolescents: does gender make a difference? J Am Acad Child Adolesc Psychiatry 1996;35:764–773.
36. Kirschbaum C, Klauer T, Flipp SH, et al. Sex-specific effects of social support on cortisol and subjective responses to acute psychological stress. Psychosom Med 1995;57:23–31.
37. Seeman TE, Singer B, Wilkinson CW, et al. Gender differences in age-related changes in HPA axis reactivity. Psychoneuroendocrinology 2001;26:225–240.
38. Laughlin GA, Barret-Connor E. Sexual dimorphism in the influence of advanced aging in adrenal hormone levels: the Rancho Bernardo Study. J Clin Endocrinol Metab 2000;85:3561–3568.
39. Stroud LR, Salovey P, Epel ES. Sex differences in stress responses: social rejection versus achievement stress. Biol Psychiatry 2002;52:318–327.
40. Gallucci W, Baum A, Laue L, et al. Sex differences in sensitivity of the hypothalamic-pituitary-adrenal axis. Health Psychol 1993;12:420–425.
41. Stoney CM, Davis MC, Matthews KA. Sex differences in physiological response to stress and in coronary heart disease: a causal link? Psychophysiology 1987;24:127–131.
42. Sgoifo A, Braglia F, Costoli T, et al. Cardiac autonomic reactivity and salivary cortisol in men and women exposed to social stressors: relationship with individual ethological profile. Neurosci Biobehav Rev 2003;27:179–188.
43. Hastrup JL, Light KC. Sex differences in cardiovascular stress responses: modulation as a function of menstrual cycle phases. J Psychosom Res 1984;28:475–483.
44. Jern C, Manhem K, Eriksson E, et al. Hemostatic responses to mental stress during the menstrual cycle. Thromb Haemost 1991;66:614–618.
45. Kring AM, Gordon AH. Sex differences in emotion: expression, experience, and physiology. J Pers Soc Psychol 1998;74:686–703.
46. Tilbrook AJ, Turner AI, Clarke IJ. Effects of stress on reproduction in non-rodent mammals: the role of glucocorticoids and sex differences. Rev Reprod 2000;5:105–113.
47. Viau V. Functional cross-talk between the hypothalamic-pituitary-gonadal and -adrenal axes. J Neuroendocrinol 2003;14:506–513.

Chapter 3 Commentary
A Perspective from South Africa

Soraya Seedat, Debra Kaminer

Findings of a female predominance of stress-related disorders (such as post-traumatic stress disorder and major depression) have been robustly documented over time and across cultural settings. Yet the critical issue in stress research is trying to establish why women are more likely than men to develop these disorders. From an evolutionary perspective, it has been suggested that differences in the stress response can be explained not only in terms of personality and cultural differences within a population but also in terms of *gender differences* in the pursuit of life goals. For example, it has been suggested that women's greater investment in developing social support networks and nurturing relationships as compared with men may, in fact, translate to greater vulnerability when faced with stressors that have negative interpersonal consequences (1).

In conceptualizing and responding to stress, men and women arguably utilize different cognitive and emotional strategies. In contrast to men, who are more likely to employ avoidance strategies (characteristic "fight–flight" pattern) and to focus on personal autonomy, women are more likely to display coping strategies that are characteristically affiliative or prosocial. But it can also be argued that these gender-differential responses cannot be considered outside of a biobehavioral framework. In Chapter 3, Walker, Sabuwalla, Bollini, and Walder provide an insightful review of gender differences in biologic responses to stress, with reference to the hypothalamic-pituitary-adrenal-gonadal, catecholamine, and autonomic nervous systems. Two points are worth noting: First, gender differences are neither *universal* nor *fixed* across the age spectrum. Second, across neuroendocrine, physiologic, and behavioral parameters of measurement, male-female differences have shown wide variation.

At a biologic level, men show stronger neuroendocrine and cardiovascular responses when exposed to stress. Women, on the other hand, manifest more pronounced emotional responses. This is an interesting paradox. On one level women appear to be more vulnerable than men to stress; at another level they appear to be more resilient. Other trends are worth noting. When exposed to a psychological stress, men have a larger mean cortisol and ACTH response than women, but in response to a biologic stress, gender findings are mixed and some studies demonstrate no significant differences in cortisol levels. Even within the same sex, there is some indication that certain personality traits may buffer the glucocorticoid response to stress. For example, one study has demonstrated that healthy males who characterized themselves as less attractive, somewhat introverted, socially inept, slightly distrusting of others, and with lower self-esteem had greater cortisol responses than males without these characteristics (2). In addition, "high-stressed" females (those who scored high on a chronic workload scale) had higher cortisol levels than high-stressed males or low-stressed males and females. Clearly, the link between biologic indicators of stress and psychological manifestations warrants further exploration.

To inform the developmental underpinnings of gender differences in the stress response, Lanius, Bluhm, and Pain explore the impact of early traumatic experience on brain development and emotional regulation (see Chapter 11 of this book). To support their hypothesis that abnormal neural functioning is at the core of emotional dysregulation seen in trauma-related disorders [namely, PTSD and borderline personality disorder (BPD)], they draw on the neuroimaging literature of emotional states in healthy subjects, patients with PTSD, and patients with BPD.

While gender, in itself, can influence the nature of early adverse experience, studies have also shown that at the level of neurodevelopment, significant gender differences exist in brain laterality and hormonal milieu. For example, one theory posits that exposure to significant stressors during a sensitive developmental period in an infant can cause the brain to develop along a stress-responsive pathway through a cascade of neurobiologic effects (3). Teicher et al. (3) have also hypothesized that exposure to corticosteroids in infancy may be a crucial factor in organizing the brain to develop in this manner. When stress comes along (for example in the form of postnatal neglect or other maltreatment), it elicits a host of responses to organize the brain to develop along a specific pathway that can be either adaptive or maladaptive (3).

Both of these chapters, in their own right, cover fascinating aspects of stress-trauma research. As clinicians, we can only really fully appreciate the diverse spectrum of clinical symptomatology in men and women with stress-related disorders if we understand it in the broader context of developmental and neurobiologic influences that intervene across the lifespan.

REFERENCES

1. Troisi A. Gender differences in vulnerability to social stress: a Darwinian perspective. Physiol Behav 2001;73:443–449.
2. Kirschbaum C, Bartussek D, Strasburger CJ. Cortisol responses to psychological stress and correlations to personality traits. Pers Individ Diff 1992;13:1353–1357.
3. Teicher MH, Andersen SL, Polcari A, et al. The neurobiological consequences of early stress and childhood maltreatment. Neurosci Biobehav Rev 2003;27(1–2):33–44.

Childhood

Section II Summary
Commentary from the United States
Mani N. Pavuluri

The four chapters in this section share common themes and raise pertinent questions: What does epidemiology teach? How can it be urgently translated ino service? And where should future research be headed?

Manassis highlights the critical point that anxiety symptoms may not be pathological at subclinical level while depression, even at a subsyndromal level, raises the risk for depression by threefold. It is important to translate these findings to real-life practice. The Virginia twin study, for instance, highlights the need to intervene early with depressed girls. Cross-cultural studies show a consistency of gender difference in depression/anxiety in Asia but not in Africa. Understanding of these differences needs to be linked with gender role orientation and cultural context. The results of biologic research in depression/anxiety should be taken as spring boards for future effortsóthe final word on effectiveness and safety of SSRIs in children and adolescents, for instance, is not yet in (1). With respect to interpersonal psychotherapy, it is particularly effective in girls, who tend more than boys to internalize conflicts (2).

Bradley and Zucker have reviewed gender identity disorder (GID) from a clinical and research standpoint, highlighting Canadian and Dutch studies. Both these cultures being western, where unisex style of dressing and "tomboyish" behavior is accepted, it is plausible that girls get referred later than boys while this may not be so in other cultures. Most of the conclusions are based on maternal information and show a need for stronger support for mothers and daughters alike. Studies on rhesus monkeys give new insights into the timing of hormonal manipulation in utero that results in masculinization (3). Similarly, preliminary results indicate 5 alpha reductase deficiency leading to GID in girls (4). No systematic data exist in developing countries where GID may be hidden. Levy introduces the multiple obstacles in identifying behavior disorder such as referral bias, rater bias and fundamental differences in subtypes of attention deficit hyperactivity disorder (ADHD). It would be safe to say that a cross culturally uniform over-representation of the inattentive subtype of ADHD is noted in girls. Data from available studies do not resolve the question of whether neurocognitive profiles are gender specific or linked to the inattention subtype of ADHD. An important point to highlight is that boys outnumber girls even among those with the inattention subtype Higher heritability and a possible polygenic multiple threshold model has been proposed in females but replication is needed. New data point to gender based differences in neuroanatomy of the brain with smaller amygdalae in female brains compared to male (5). Future studies will determine the relevance of this finding.

Lipman and Offord's chapter on conduct disorder (CD) reports an intriguing epidemiological profile where girls equal boys in the clinic population. This is good news and bad news. Are there more boys in the community with CD not being referred to clinics? Are boys accepted as being somewhat aggressive and boisterous? Is society's threshold for tolerance of externalizing behavior in girls too low? But the good news for girls is that they appear to obtain services readily. Social aggression in girls is critical to address in future treatment studies as it comes in the way of opportunities to succeed and pursue leadership roles. Gender-specific treatment strategies will greatly improve the quality of life for young women. Several epidemiological studies tend to focus on maternal risk factors for child disorders probably because mothers are readily accessible for interviewing. Paternal factors need to be pursued as well.

In conclusion, a few critical issues can be highlighted in interpreting the data presented here. First, epidemiological findings are derived from only a few selected countries and cultures. Second, findings suggest the usefulness of gender-specific treatment. Third, more biological studies need to be carried out to validate external phenocopies and to better understand etiopathology.

REFERENCES

1. Riddle, MA. Paroxetine and the FDA. J Am Acad Child Adolesc Psychiatry 2004;43:128–130.
2. Mufson L, Moreau D, Weissman MM, et al. Modification of interpersonal psychotherapy with depressed adolescents: phase I and II studies. J Am Acad Child Adolesc Psychiatry 1994;33:695ñ705.
3. Goy RW, Bercovitch FB, McBrair MC. Behavioral masculinization is independent of genital masculinization in prenatally androgenized female rhesus macaques. Horm Behav 1988; 22:552–571.
4. Imperato-McGinley J, Guerrero L, Gautier T, et al. Steroid 5-alpha reductase deficiency in man: an inherited form of male pseudohermaphroditism. Science 1974;186:1213–1215.
5. Koshibu K, Levitt P, Ahrens ET. Sex-specific, postpuberty changes in mouse brain structures revealed by three-dimensional magnetic resonance microscopy. Neuroimage 2004;22: 1636–1645.

CHAPTER 4

Depression and Anxiety in Girls

Katharina Manassis

This chapter focuses on epidemiology, proposed etiologic factors, and developmental changes evident in anxiety and depression in children and adolescents. Emerging concepts that may enhance understanding and treatment of these disorders will also be described. In all sections, differences between the sexes will be highlighted when present.

EPIDEMIOLOGY

PREVALENCE

Anxiety and depression are among the most prevalent psychiatric disorders in childhood [10.5% of school-aged children are affected in Ontario (1)]. Many studies emphasize that the long-term morbidity and disability associated with these disorders is severe [reviewed in (2)]. In adolescents, depression is also associated with increased mortality due to suicide (1).

Until recently, childhood anxiety and depression were underreported. There is some debate as to whether the apparent increase in these conditions in recent years is due to stresses in children's lives or is an artifact of better reporting. Whichever is the case, many affected children still experience lengthy delays in seeking and obtaining treatment. The large Ontario epidemiologic study concluded that up to 80% of children with these disorders are never treated (1). Moreover, a substantial number of anxious children experience comorbid depression, and the risk of this comorbidity increases with age and lack of intervention (3). In contrast to children with either disorder alone, children with comorbid anxiety and depression often suffer sequelae well into adulthood and are relatively less responsive to treatment (4). These findings underscore the need to identify anxious and depressed children at an early age, to improve their functioning, and to reduce the risk of comorbidity and long-term impairment.

Sex differences in rates of anxiety and depression are not consistently found in childhood, but there is a clear female preponderance (about 2:1 for depression) in both conditions by adolescence [see (5)]. Possible reasons for this shift in sex distribution are discussed below (see also Chapter 12, on depression and anxiety in adulthood).

MEASUREMENT

Measurement difficulties may contribute to underidentification and treatment delay in these conditions. Several well-validated self-report inventories exist for anxiety and depression [for example, the Multidimensional Anxiety Scale for Children (6); Children's Depression Inventory (7)]. However, correspondence among informants is consistently fair to poor [reviewed in (8)], with parents tending to report more overt, behavioral symptoms and children reporting more distressed feeling states. In some cases, a child may fail to report symptoms despite evidence of disorder. Alternatively, the child may recognize symptoms although adults in his or her environment do not and hence referral for assessment and treatment is unlikely to occur. Therefore, in clinical practice, symptoms that either the parent or the child endorse merit investigation.

Symptom inventories are also limited by low specificity because many children with noninternalizing types of psychopathology have elevated scores. Such inventories are best used as part of a more thorough diagnostic assessment that provides an estimate of severity and (when repeated) a means of evaluating progress objectively.

Anxiety and depression require somewhat different thresholds for concern. Certain fears are developmentally normative [reviewed in (9)], and mild anxiety enhances academic performance on some tasks. Avoidance of risk can also be adaptive in certain circumstances (for example, reducing risk of accident-related injuries). Therefore, anxiety is considered pathologic only if it is very distressing or results in substantial impairment. By contrast, the presence of depressive symptoms, even at subclinical levels, always merits concern. Large-scale longitudinal studies of children with elevated depression scores on self-report found a threefold increased risk for subsequent depression compared to other children (10,11).

ETIOLOGY: BIOLOGIC FACTORS

In many cases, biologic factors contribute to the emergence of anxiety and depression. It is recognized, however, that the outcome is usually determined by the interaction between biologic vulnerability and psychosocial factors that increase or ameliorate that vulnerability. The next two sections describe key vulnerabilities and factors studied as well as proposed interactions.

HERITABILITY OF CHILDHOOD ANXIETY AND DEPRESSION

Twin and adoption studies have shown that genetic factors account for at least 50% of the variance in the transmission of mood disorders, although specific genes are only now being identified (12). Children of depressed parents have a threefold lifetime risk of major depression and are also more vulnerable to anxiety disorders. Therefore, some authors have suggested that what is inherited is a general tendency to internalize problems and that environmental factors influence which symptoms are manifested.

The Virginia Twin Study has yielded some interesting findings with respect to the relationship between anxiety and depression in girls (13). Using over 600 female twin pairs (about two thirds monozygotic and one third dizygotic), the authors found three distinct patterns. Early overanxious disorder (OAD) and simple phobias were linked to specific genetic vulnerability to depression after age 14; shared environmental factors influenced symptoms of depression before age 14 and later separation anxiety and simple phobias; and shared environmental influences on depression after age 14 also increased vulnerability to concurrent OAD and separation anxiety. The association between early OAD and later depression is consistent with models suggesting a temporal progression from anxiety to depression. Interestingly, these findings suggest that the progression may be based, at least in part, on a common genetic risk rather than a depressive response to untreated anxiety symptoms. Other studies have since confirmed shared environmental influences as more salient in prepubertal depression, with greater heritability in adolescent depression (14). Genetic susceptibility to adolescent depression in response to environmental adverse events was also demonstrated in this sample.

Family and twin studies have both found a definite familial contribution to childhood anxiety disorders [reviewed in (2)]. Anxiety disorder rates were elevated in children of parents with anxiety disorders or mixed anxiety-depression. Conversely, parents of children with school refusal were found to have elevated rates of anxiety and depressive disorders. While several twin studies have established a genetic contribution to childhood anxiety, further studies will clarify the degree of genetic versus environmental contribution to specific anxiety disorders. In a recent twin study, for example, Topolski and others (15) found that shared environmental effects played a moderate role in separation anxiety disorder but not in OAD. In contrast, genetic influences appeared to predominate in OAD. Specific genetic loci are now being researched.

TEMPERAMENTAL SUBSTRATES

The constitutional factor examined most extensively in relation to childhood anxiety is a trait termed "behavioral inhibition" [reviewed in (16)]. Behavioral inhibition is an aspect of temperament measurable in the laboratory, characterized by a tendency to restrict exploration and avoid novelty. Human and primate studies have confirmed the heritability of this trait, and its physiologic basis. Inhibited children show evidence of chronically high sympathetic arousal, leading to the hypothesis that inhibition occurs when there is a reduced threshold to arousal in the amygdala, a part of the limbic system.

Many children "outgrow" behavioral inhibition, probably because of their parents' encouraging them to enter new situations, which results in desensitization. There may be sex differences, however, in the degree of encouragement of exploratory behavior parents offer. In many cultures, girls are expected to be more reticent than boys, resulting in inhibited behavior being socially sanctioned and thus likely to persist. Persistent inhibition, in turn, has been linked prospectively to an increased risk of subsequent anxiety disorders in middle childhood and specifically to social phobia in adolescence.

Perhaps because they typically have a later onset, less study has been devoted to temperamental antecedents of mood disorders.

COGNITIVE BIASES

Cognitive biases have been implicated in childhood depression [reviewed in (17)]. For example, longitudinal studies have shown that children with a negative cognitive style experience prolonged dysphoric mood when exposed to stresses such as poor grades or peer rejection. Such dysphoric mood may predispose to depression. Negative cognitive style and self-perceptions are also found during depressive episodes, but it is unclear whether these are part of the depressed state or represent long-term traits. Modeling, critical or rejecting familial relationships, and stressful life events all have been proposed as contributing to negative cognitions in depressed children.

Cognitive biases, in particular attentional and interpretational biases, are also thought to play a role in many anxiety disorders, with relative specificity depending on the type of bias [reviewed in (18)]. For example, when doing a timed color-naming task of both neutral and threatening words, spider-phobic children had slowed color-naming times when shown spider-related words (e.g., web) but not neutral words (e.g., fly). Anxious children were also faster to react to a probe preceded by a threatening rather than a neutral word on dot-probe tasks, showing selective attention to threat cues.

Interpretation bias has been evidenced in studies comparing anxious versus nonanxious children's interpretation of homophones (e.g., dye or die) and ambiguous stories. Results indicated that anxious children were more likely to interpret ambiguous situations in a threatening way. Parent–child interactions can, however, influence children's tendency to interpret ambiguous material as threatening.

Dichotic listening tasks that examined cerebral laterality have also found differences between anxious and depressed children relative to normal controls. My colleagues and I (19) found enhanced perception of emotional tone of voice in anxious children compared to normal children, regardless of ear or hemisphere of presentation. Pine and colleagues (20) found that depressed adolescents showed an increased right ear/left hemisphere advantage for fused words.

In summary, there is emerging evidence that cognitive biases in attention and perception likely have some physiologic basis, but interpretation biases may also be subject to the influence of parental modeling and other parent–child interactions. None of the cognitive bias studies found gender differences, but parental expectations of girls might still play a role in interpretation bias.

SPECIFIC BIOLOGIC VULNERABILITIES

Following upon work in adults, several hormones have been studied in relation to childhood depression. [reviewed in (12)]. Because most studies are cross-sectional, it is often unclear whether these constitute vulnerability factors or markers of the depressed state. Blunted response of growth hormones to insulin-induced hypoglycemia has been found to persist upon remission, suggesting that this may be more of a trait marker. Findings regarding growth hormone without stimulation are equivocal, though. Findings in children are also inconsistent for the dexamethasone-suppression test, a common marker for depression in adults. Lower cortisol levels after infusion of L-5-hydroxytryptophan have been found in children with early-onset major depression. Depressed girls have been found to have elevated prolactin levels compared to girls who are not depressed. None of these findings is specific enough to constitute a "test" for depression (often requested by families), but they continue to be of research interest to better understand the disorder and obtain potential markers for treatment response.

Panic disorder has been linked to an exaggerated fear of suffocation due to a biologic and possibly heritable hypersensitivity in the brain's receptors for carbon dioxide [reviewed in (21)]. Differential sensitivity in the receptors of anxious versus control children is shown by carbon dioxide panic provocation challenge studies; evidence of higher than average incidences of anxiety disorders in asthmatic children; and lower incidences of anxiety symptoms in children with faulty carbon dioxide receptors. It is possible that these overly sensitive receptors trigger isolated panic attacks, which are thought to cue conditioning experiences and in turn phobic avoidance.

"Anxiety sensitivity" has been found to be a specific predictor of onset of adolescent panic [reviewed in (22)]. This construct, measurable by self-report inventories, consists of the tendency to respond with anxiety to sensations of autonomic arousal. To address this response in the cognitive-behavioral treatment of panic, patients are helped to reinterpret sensations of autonomic arousal as benign rather than threatening.

MEDICAL AND CHROMOSOMAL CONDITIONS ASSOCIATED WITH ANXIETY OR DEPRESSION

Several medical conditions have been linked to childhood anxiety or depression [see (23)]. The sudden onset of anxiety or depression in a previously outgoing child should alert the clinician to explore a medical or traumatic etiology. Hyperthyroidism commonly produces anxiety states, and hypothyroidism can contribute to depression. Medications that are sympathomimetic (for example, Ventolin inhalers for controlling asthma) can contribute to anxiety. Endocrine conditions affecting adrenal steroids have been linked to mood disorders. In girls, consumption of caffeinated beverages, particularly diet colas, often contributes to anxiety. Many over-the-counter diet aids also contain stimulants that can exacerbate anxiety. Pediatric chronic illnesses have also been linked to depression, with both child and illness characteristics contributing to the vulnerability [reviewed in (24)].

Turner syndrome is a condition found in phenotypic girls who have monosomy of the X chromosome. It is characterized by gonadal failure, short stature, and some associated medical abnormalities. Many girls with Turner's syndrome suffer symptoms of anxiety and depression [reviewed in (25)]. In the past, these symptoms were thought to reflect low self-esteem secondary to the condition. Recent studies, however, suggest that these symptoms persist even when affected girls are treated with growth hormone to address short stature. Differences in executive cognitive functions and brain anatomy distinguished monozygotic twins discordant for Turner syndrome (26), and may account for difficulty modulating negative affect in this population.

ETIOLOGY: PSYCHOSOCIAL FACTORS

EARLY ATTACHMENT

Attachment theory proposes that infants are predisposed to behave in ways that enhance proximity to their caregivers, and caregivers are prone to behave reciprocally (27). When parent–infant attachment is secure (as demonstrated in the laboratory), the primary caregiver eventually serves as a "secure base" from which the infant can explore the world, returning at times of distress. Insecure attachment, however, has been linked with childhood anxiety symptoms concurrently and with anxiety disorders prospectively (28). Security or insecurity of attachment has been found to be relatively independent of child temperament. Interventions that promote secure attachment relationships therefore have the potential to prevent some anxiety problems in temperamentally vulnerable children.

The influence of early attachment on brain development has been the subject of increased study recently [reviewed in (29)]. Studies of animals and human beings have both confirmed that adverse early relational experiences can result in activation and eventually alteration of the functioning of the hypothalamic-pituitary-adrenal (HPA) axis. Physiologic responses to stress are thus changed. Furthermore, the altered HPA functioning influences the development of brain pathways linked to anxiety and depression, increasing vulnerability to these disorders. Maternal depression is known to be associated with high rates of insecure attachment and risk of adolescent depression. While modeling of depressive cognitions and impaired parenting likely contribute to this association, the findings suggest that alterations of the HPA axis may also play a role.

PARENTING AND FAMILY INTERACTIONS ASSOCIATED WITH ANXIETY OR DEPRESSION

Depressed adults regularly report more conflict than do normal adults as well as more rejection, more communication problems, and less support in their childhood families of origin [reviewed in (12)]. Given that these reports are retrospective, however, it is unclear to what extent they are biased by the cognitive distortions associated with depression. In depressed children, the possibility of bidirectional effects must also be considered. For example, a sullen, irritable child with depression may elicit rejecting or conflicted interactions with parents, but these interactions may, in turn, worsen the child depression. Children of depressed mothers may be at particular risk, however, both because of modeling of depressive behaviors and cognitions and because of high rates of insecure attachment (see above).

In children with anxiety disorders, observational studies of parent–child interactions have supported a link between anxiety and overprotective parenting. For example, Hudson and Rapee (30) found that mothers of anxiety-disordered children were more controlling and intrusive during a puzzle task than mothers of nonanxious children. They proposed a bidirectional relationship such that the parent of an anxious child may be more likely to become overinvolved with the child in an effort to reduce and prevent the child's distress. In turn, this behavior would reinforce the child's anxiety by promoting beliefs that the world is a dangerous place from which the child needs protection and over which he or she has no control. The parent's own anxiety is also likely to compound this maladaptive pattern of behavior.

Parental modeling has also been implicated in the development of anxiety disorders in children. For example, adult social phobics have retrospectively reported their families as encouraging isolation and constraining contacts with neighbors, relatives, and acquaintances [see (31)]. In addition to minimizing or discouraging social networking, parents may also provide children with information that heightens anxiety about certain situations.

Sex differences in parental overprotection and anxious modeling have not been studied, but the tendency to perceive girls as more frail and vulnerable than boys may exaggerate these behaviors by anxious parents in relation to their daughters.

PEER INFLUENCES

Peer relationships have been studied most in relation to social anxiety. Ginsburg and colleagues (32) found that peer acceptance is predictive of lower levels of social anxiety in youth. Similarly, the highest levels of social anxiety were found among peer-neglected and peer-rejected middle-school students. Withdrawal from peers may interfere with the attainment of social skills and relationships, which may lead to further increases in social anxiety. Peer relationship problems are also increased in depressed children compared to controls (33), and victims of bullying have been shown by teacher and parent report to be vulnerable to both anxiety and depressive symptoms (34).

CULTURAL INFLUENCES

Cultural factors have been examined more in relation to childhood anxiety than depression. These factors likely influence definitions of the degree and type of fearfulness that are considered "abnormal," parenting practices that may increase or decrease fearfulness, and differences in expected levels of fearfulness.

Research using the Fear Survey Schedule for Children–Revised (9) has provided useful information about differences in fearfulness (severity, prevalence, and content) across cultures. This research has shown that children and adolescents from Nigeria, Kenya, and China report a greater number of fears than children from Western cultures such as Australia, the United States, and the United Kingdom. Ollendick proposed that the higher rates of fearfulness may be associated with increased fostering of inhibition and compliance in African and Asian cultures in comparison to Western cultures.

The greater prevalence of anxiety disorders and fearfulness in female samples is explained in part by cultural factors. [reviewed in (35)]. Although Western and Asian cultures have shown clear sex differences between girls and boys, with girls reporting higher levels of fear than boys, there is a lack of sex differences in reported fearfulness among African children. In many cultures, anxiety or fear is generally considered less socially acceptable in men than in women. Generally, men experience more pressure from the environment to behave bravely in situations of both ambiguous and certain threat. In contrast, avoidance behavior in women is considered far more acceptable and is perhaps even encouraged. In adult and child studies, gender role orientation has been associated with fearfulness: individuals who score high on measures of femininity also score high on measures of fearfulness, while individuals scoring high in masculinity report low levels of fearfulness.

STRESSFUL LIFE EVENTS

Stressful life events have been linked to the onset of depression in both child and adult studies [see (12)]. Both severe events such as exposure to the suicide of someone close and nonsevere events such as poor grades or relationship problems have been cited. Adolescents may also perceive some events as more severe than an adult would. In the year prior to onset of depression, significantly larger numbers of stressful events are reported by depressed youth than by normal controls.

Several studies have found higher rates of aversive life events in clinically anxious children [reviewed in (33)]. Specific events include the occurrence of parental separations and divorce, death of a family member, family conflict, and repeated changes of school. Many anxious children, however, do not experience elevated rates of stressors, and many youth survive trauma without clinically significant psychological problems. The negative impact of these stressful events is thought to depend on factors that amplify or buffer their effects. Factors that appear to reduce the negative impact of aversive events upon children include availability of social support and problem-focused coping strategies (36).

CHANGES WITH DEVELOPMENT

CHANGES IN MANIFESTATION OF DEPRESSION AND ANXIETY

Differences in manifestation of disorder in prepubertal versus adolescent individuals have been a major focus of study in depression. There is an ongoing debate as to how similar or dissimilar depression in young children is relative to adolescent and adult forms of the disease. Birmaher and colleagues (37) found that depressive symptomatology, duration, severity, rates of recovery and recurrence, and family psychiatric history were similar for prepubertal and postpubertal probands. High family loading and protracted clinical course were evident in both groups. Other authors have emphasized neuroendocrine differences between these groups, with prepubertal depressed children often lacking the HPA axis abnormalities common in depressed adults [reviewed in (37)]. Perinatal insults and motor delays have also been linked to juvenile-onset depression (38). Still others have tried to identify particularly vulnerable subgroups of depressed children. For example, Wickramaratne and colleagues (39) found that prepubertal depressives with familial loading had a higher risk of recurrence and continuity of depression into adulthood, but this was not true of those with onset after puberty. While there appear to be developmental differences in some aspects of depression, there is some clinical consensus that children with early onset and a positive family history for depression merit ongoing follow-up for the emergence of further psychopathology.

Both fears and anxiety disorders show changes with development [see (40)]. In young children, fears tend to be more concrete, such as fear of loud noises, strangers, separation, and physical injury, while in adolescence, social evaluative concerns and more abstract worries are prominent. Separation anxiety disorder is clearly more prevalent in early childhood when there is high dependency on parents, while generalized anxiety disorder, panic disorder, and social phobia show an increase from childhood to adolescence. These findings suggest that age influences the presentation of specific anxiety disorders.

One factor potentially underlying these age differences is the child's cognitive development. For example, concerns of negative evaluation by an audience are considered central to the disorder of social phobia (41). Such concerns are only possible when a child can, to a degree, consciously evaluate his or her own performance. That ability has been found to be present in most 8-year-olds but not in most 5-year-olds. Similarly, certain cognitive developments may also be required before the onset of panic disorder is possible. One of the core features of panic disorder is a fear of losing control, going crazy, or dying during the panic attack. Nelles and Barlow (42) suggested that these symptoms do not occur in children because their ability to predict catastrophic consequences from physical symptoms is limited. That is, children are less able to make the cognitive leap from a certain physical symptom to loss of control or death and thus are less likely to develop panic disorder.

Children with anxious and depressive comorbidity also appear to be a highly vulnerable group [reviewed in (4)], and this comorbidity increases with increasing age. Comorbid children are more impaired than children with either disorder alone, and when followed longitudinally, are more poorly adjusted in early adulthood. Brady and Kendall (3) have proposed a temporal relationship between anxiety and depression, with older, more impaired anxious children having a high risk of developing comorbid depression. This idea is appealing because it suggests that early intervention with anxious children may prevent subsequent depression. Other authors, however, have examined familial factors in explaining anxious/depressive comorbidity. Certain parenting styles (for example, so-called "affectionless control") have been linked to both disorders in children (43). A genetic basis for the comorbidity has also been proposed [reviewed in (44)]. Parents of comorbid children have higher rates of mood disorders than parents of anxious children, and twin studies suggest that separate genes may account for anxiety/depression rather than depression alone.

PUBERTY AND SEX DIFFERENCES

The emergence of differences between the sexes in the rates of anxiety and depression at puberty has been a remarkably consistent finding [reviewed in (5)]. Girls begin to show much higher rates of these disorders than boys, and this difference persists into adulthood. Psychosocial and biologic (predominantly hormonal) mechanisms for this change have been proposed. Correlations between pubertal development and low mood have been cited repeatedly and can be accounted for by either mechanism (hormones or negative social consequences of pubertal development). Findings from epidemiologic surveys and from twin studies suggest that differences between the sexes in anxiety may precede puberty (45). It is unclear, though, whether this prepubertal difference represents non-pathologic fearfulness in girls, or true anxiety disorders (35).

Psychosocial factors proposed to contribute to internalizing disorders in post-pubertal girls include: self-consciousness about body image, history of sexual trauma, stressful life events, peer problems, a poor sense of self-competence (compared to boys), women being more likely to acknowledge negative feeling states (i.e., artifactual), and depressing aspects of the female gender role in society [reviewed in (5)]. Findings for many of these factors are inconsistent, and some appear contributory but cannot entirely account for gender differences. For example, controlling for differential rates of sexual trauma reduced but did not eliminate the associations between gender and anxiety and depression (46). The association between self-competence and internalizing disorders initially appears more robust. Gender differences in trait anxiety are markedly attenuated, and gender differences for depression become insignificant when this factor is controlled (47). It is unclear, however, whether low self-competence is an antecedent or a result of anxiety and depression in girls.

Cyclic withdrawal of gonadal steroid hormones with the menstrual cycle, particularly estrogen, has been linked to postpubertal girls' and women's vulnerability to anxiety and depression (48). Gonadal steroids modulate GABA-A receptors, linked to anxiety and may protect the brain from the neurotoxic effects of stress hormones. Changes in gonadal steroids with pregnancy, however, have been linked to increased risk for certain types of anxiety (particularly obsessive compulsive disorder, OCD) (49). Other authors have linked changes in adrenal hormones occurring earlier in development to a risk for anxiety disorders. Dorn and colleagues (50) found that, among children aged 6 to 9, those with premature adrenarche had a 44% rate of anxiety disorders and higher self-reported depression. Parker and Brotchie (5) have recently proposed an elegant stress-diathesis model to account for postpubertal differences in both anxiety and depression. They argue that children of both sexes with a temperamental tendency toward "neuroticism" (defined as high limbic activation in response to stress, similar to Kagan's "behavioral inhibition" construct) are vulnerable to anxiety or depression. At puberty, however, hormonal influences on the brain may render females with this trait more vulnerable to social stress, increasing their risk for anxiety and depression.

CHANGES IN COPING STYLES

Much as children's expression of anxiety and depression may change with development, their ability to manage negative emotion evolves over time as well. There are a limited number of ways of managing unpleasant emotions, and those one uses habitually have been termed "coping styles." Use of avoidant coping strategies (for example, trying to avoid thinking about a problem or actually avoiding the problematic situation) rather than active ones (for example, seeking guidance or trying to solve the problem) has been linked to anxiety in numerous studies [see (51)]. Depressive coping, on the other hand, is characterized by "learned helplessness," a tendency to give up on solving a problem without even trying.

When coping strategies are used repeatedly, they can become entrenched over time. This entrenchment may explain the phenomenologic shift from apparently fluid, highly comorbid anxiety disorders in early childhood to clearer, more persistent disorders in adolescence and early adulthood. Gender differences in the rate of anxiety disorders that emerge in adolescence have been recently linked to coping style. Byrne (52) found similar coping strategies in boys and girls at age 7, but dramatic differences at age 12, with boys using strategies that more effectively reduced anxiety and girls using less effective strategies. Both early attachment relationships and social sanctioning or discouragement of different coping behaviors have been implicated in the type of coping style an individual develops (53). Many cognitive-behavioral interventions with anxious or depressed youth focus on providing a repertoire of alternative, more effective coping responses.

EMERGING CHALLENGES IN CLINICAL PRACTICE

Treatments for childhood anxiety and depression have generally been adaptations of adult treatment models. They are, unfortunately, not always based on knowledge of developmental processes in children. Recent controversy surrounding the use of certain antidepressants in children has focused attention on this problem, but it is relevant to other clinical treatments as well.

SELECTIVE SEROTONIN REUPTAKE INHIBITORS IN CHILDREN

There has been extensive media coverage of the finding of increased suicidal ideation in some depressed adolescents taking selective serotonin reuptake inhibitors (SSRIs) compared to those taking placebos. Major regulatory bodies (for example, the Food and Drug Administration in the United States; Health Canada) have issued warnings pertaining to these medications. A further concern is the discrepancy between published data on these medications (suggesting a favorable risk/benefit profile) and unpublished data that contradict these findings (54). Families have been understandably concerned by this controversy, and many have either discontinued administration of a child's SSRI or expressed reluctance about pursuing SSRI treatment. While more study is clearly needed, clinicians must continue to practice and advise their patients using the best available information. In this regard, the points in the following paragraphs are worth noting:

Rates of suicidal ideation in the adolescents treated with SSRIs, while higher than placebo, were still relatively low [3% to 5%; (54)]. Thus, the vast majority of adolescents taking these medications do *not* experience suicidal ideation.

It is unclear whether or not the relationship between SSRIs and suicidal thoughts is causal; other factors may account for the association.

There is a paucity of rigorous, controlled studies demonstrating efficacy for SSRIs in children and adolescents, but some clearly show benefit.

All studies reporting increased suicidality with SSRIs have examined adolescents suffering from primarily mood disorders. They have not examined children or adolescents with obsessive compulsive disorder or other debilitating anxiety disorders. It is unclear whether or not suicidal ideation occurs in these conditions, which are also regularly treated with SSRIs.

There are risks associated with failing to treat severe mood and anxiety disorders that may be as great or greater than the potential risk of suicidal ideation with SSRIs.

There are risks associated with sudden discontinuation of treatment with SSRIs (relapse of symptoms; a flulike "discontinuation syndrome" with many SSRIs).

Medical alternatives to SSRIs in childhood anxiety and depression (for example, tricyclics or benzodiazepines) have not been shown consistently efficacious relative to placebos [reviewed in (12)], and also have potentially serious side effects (cardiac arrhythmias in the former; addictive potential in the latter).

Evidence-based psychological treatments (for example, cognitive-behavioral therapy) may not be sufficient to alleviate symptoms in severely affected children and are not always readily available.

In the absence of definitive information, Health Canada (55) has provided what appears to be prudent advice: clinicians must weigh the risks and benefits of SSRIs in each case, discuss them with the child and family, and monitor all children and teens taking these medications on a regular basis. Sudden discontinuation of SSRIs is not advised.

PSYCHOLOGICAL TREATMENTS

Cognitive-behavioral treatment (CBT) that combines anxiety management training with enactive exposure has been extensively studied in relation to anxious children. Its brevity and reproducibility (through the use of standardized manuals) facilitate outcome studies. Several groups of investigators have done randomized controlled trials in mixed anxious samples, based on adaptations of Philip Kendall's "Coping Cat" treatment model (56), for both group and individual interventions. Efficacy has been demonstrated repeatedly, with added benefits demonstrated in some studies when parents were involved in treatment.

The long-term effects of CBT on developmental outcomes in anxious children remain to be elucidated, most studies having followed children for only a year or less. Furthermore, the treatment's high reliance on verbal ability limits its utility in less verbal children, and the transportability of CBT from academic centers to the community has not yet been demonstrated. Lack of availability of CBT in the community is a further clinical challenge.

Cognitive-behavioral therapy has also been found efficacious in child and adolescent depression in randomized comparisons with control treatments [reviewed in (57)]. Unfortunately, results at longer-term follow-up have been variable. Relapse rates are reported to be high (up to 40%), and a substantial proportion of children (about 30%) do not respond to treatment. Studies have also been criticized for selecting only mildly depressed children for participation, and for other methodologic flaws. Predictors of poor treatment response have included parent–child conflict, older age, social impairment, lower self-esteem, severe depression, and the presence of one or more comorbid conditions. There are few existing trials of family intervention with depressed children and adolescents. To date, these suggest that family intervention is likely superior to wait-list control, but not clearly superior to CBT. Studies of treatments that combine CBT with the most successful family interventions appear worthwhile. Given the high rates of relapse in adolescent depression, the role of family intervention in relapse prevention merits further study as well.

Interpersonal therapy (IPT) is another brief, manual-based therapy for adolescent depression. Its focus is on accepting and managing interpersonal roles and conflicts and changes in this domain. Although a recent randomized controlled trial showed promising results (58), the sample size was small and not ethnically diverse, limiting the generalizability of the findings. Given the interpersonal challenges of adolescence, further study of IPT is definitely warranted. Moreover, several interpersonal factors have been found to predict symptoms of depression in female adolescents (59). Also, CBT's greater emphasis on examining one's personal thoughts, with less emphasis on solving interpersonal problems, may not be appealing to all adolescents. If efficacy is replicated in more diverse populations, IPT may be a valuable treatment option for adolescents who are experiencing interpersonal stresses or who are more amenable to discussing relationships than cognitions.

COMORBIDITY AND TREATMENT

Comorbidity among childhood internalizing disorders and between internalizing disorders and other psychopathology is highly prevalent. In children with multiple comorbidities, the most disabling symptoms must be prioritized, and families require encouragement to persevere with treatment until the child is returned to age-appropriate functioning in most areas [reviewed in (60)]. Studies of comorbid samples are rare, as most treatment protocols target "pure" disorders.

Combined medical and psychological treatments are often used for children with comorbid disorders, but it is unclear whether these provide additive benefits or may, potentially, be less effective as one treatment interferes with the other. In childhood anxiety disorders, one review (61) suggested a somewhat higher response rate in studies where pharmacotherapy and behavior therapy were combined than in studies where either was examined alone. Randomized comparisons of single and combined treatments, however, have not been published. Optimum treatment combinations may also vary by disorder and degree of severity.

PREVENTING DISORDERS

Dadds and colleagues (62), in large randomized controlled trials in Australia, were able to demonstrate reduced anxiety symptoms and reduced onset of new anxiety disorders in symptomatic children using school-based cognitive-behavioral interventions with some parental involvement. Barrett and Turner (63) have demonstrated the feasibility of teaching this type of intervention to school personnel. Caution is warranted in interpreting these results, however, because the children were not clinically identified. While subclinical levels of anxiety may be amenable to school-based interventions, it is unrealistic to expect school personnel to address the needs of children with severe anxiety disorders. Primary prevention of depression has not been consistently found effective but promising studies are reported below. Targeted interventions have focused on two groups: children at risk due to familial depression and children with elevated scores on self-report inventories for depression.

Beardslee and colleagues (64) did a randomized trial of a manualized psychoeducational intervention with children of depressed parents. They intervened with families as children were entering adolescence, providing education about depression to all family members and attempting to increase positive interactions between parents and children. While benefits were demonstrated for both lecture-based and clinician-facilitated programs, parents reported more changes in child behaviors and attitudes in the clinician-facilitated version.

In children reporting depressive symptoms, Jaycox and colleagues (65) did a controlled study of a school-based group intervention using cognitive and social problem-solving techniques. They found reduced depressive symptoms in the treatment condition up to two years after treatment. Clarke and colleagues (66) did a large controlled trial of a school-based cognitive-behavioral group intervention for children self-reporting elevated depressive symptoms. They demonstrated a reduced incidence of affective disorders in the treatment condition during the 12 months following the study (notably, 26% of the children in the control condition developed affective disorders).

Preventing recurrence of depression is a particular challenge. From 40% to 70% of depressed adolescents experience recurrent episodes, and long-term impairment in functioning is worse in those with recurrent disorder [see (12)]. Conflict in the family environment has been identified as a significant predictor of recurrence (57), suggesting that family-based interventions could potentially have a long-term benefit even if they add little to acute treatment efficacy.

SUMMARY OF GENDER-SPECIFIC ISSUES AND DIRECTIONS FOR FURTHER RESEARCH

Anxiety and depression in girls and boys can be understood as resulting from the interaction of biologic and environmental vulnerabilities. Nevertheless, girls face some unique challenges in both of these areas of vulnerability. Certain disorders associated with anxiety and depression (for example, Turner syndrome) are unique to girls. The dramatic change in gender distribution for internalizing disorders at puberty likely bears some relationship to hormonal changes. Social pressures faced by girls at this time, particularly those related to body image and personal competence, may also play a role. Some families' greater tolerance for fearful behavior and greater protectiveness toward girls than boys may perpetuate the girls' anxiety and reduce the families' seeking help for their anxious daughters. Avoidant coping styles that support anxiety can also develop on this basis. Given the evidence for a temporal relationship between anxiety and depression, anxious girls may also be predisposed to later depression. Other developmental issues meriting further study include identifying specific genes or interactions between genes and the environment that might predispose individuals to anxiety or depression; identifying protective/resiliency factors for anxiety and depression; and identifying developmental trajectories of risk, which may differ by gender.

When treatment is sought for girls with internalizing disorders, their less disruptive presentation compared to that of boys may result in less aggressive management. Given the limited study of pharmacotherapy in anxious and depressed children, it is not clear whether there are gender differences in response. Psychological intervention for these disorders has focused on cognitive-behavioral therapy, with good results for treatment completers of both genders. However, girls may have a greater focus on interpersonal relationships than boys, suggesting they may also benefit (or be more motivated to complete) therapy with this focus. To date, such interpersonal therapy has received limited study. Finally, it will be important to determine how to best prevent relapse of childhood internalizing disorders in order to reduce their persistence into adulthood and associated long-term morbidity.

REFERENCES

1. Offord DR, Boyle MH, Fleming JE, et al. Ontario Child Health Study: Summary of selected results. Can J Psychiatry 1989;34:483–491.
2. Bernstein GA, Borchardt CM, Perwien AR. Anxiety disorders in children and adolescents: a review of the past 10 years. J Am Acad Child Adolesc Psychiatry 1996;35:1110–1119.
3. Brady EU, Kendall PC. Comorbidity of anxiety and depression in children and adolescents. Psychol Bull 1992;111:244–255.
4. Manassis K, Menna R. Depression in anxious children: possible factors in comorbidity. Depress Anxiety 1999;10:18–24.
5. Parker GB, Brotchie HL. From diathesis to dimorphism: the biology of gender differences in depression. J Nerv Ment Dis 2004;192:210–216.
6. March J. Multidimensional Anxiety Scale for Children (MASC). Toronto: Multi Health Systems, Inc., 1998.
7. Kovacs M. Children's Depression Inventory Manual. North Tonawanda, NY: Multi Health Systems, 1992.
8. Klein RG. Parent–child agreement in clinical assessment of anxiety and other psychopathology: a review. J Anx Dis 1991;5:187–198.
9. Ollendick TH. Reliability and validity of the Revised Fear Survey Schedule for Children. Behav Res Ther 1983;21:685–692.
10. Gotlib IH, Lewinsohn PM, Seeley JR, et al. Negative cognition and attributional style in depressed adolescents: an examination of stability and specificity. J Abnorm Psychol 1993;102:607–615.
11. Weissman MM, Fendrich M, Warner V, et al. Incidence of psychiatric disorder in offspring at high and low risk for depression. J Am Acad Child Adolesc Psychiatry 1992;31:640–648.
12. Birmaher B, Ryan ND, Williamson DE, et al. Childhood and adolescent depression: a review of the past 10 years (pt 1). J Am Acad Child Adolesc Psychiatry 1996;35:1427–1439.
13. Silberg J, Rutter M, Neale M, et al. Genetic moderation of environmental risk for depression and anxiety in adolescent girls. Br J Psychiatry 2001;179:116–121.
14. Scourfield J, Rice F, Thapar A, et al. Depressive symptoms in children and adolescents: changing etiological influences with development. J Child Psychol Psychiatry 2003;44:968–976.
15. Topolski TD, Hewitt JK, Eaves LJ, et al. Genetic and environmental influences on child reports of manifest anxiety in symptoms of separation anxiety and overanxious disorders. Behav Genetics 1997;27:15–28.
16. Kagan J, Reznick JS, Gibbons J, et al. Inhibited and uninhibited types of children. Child Dev 1989;60:838–845.
17. Hilsman R, Garber J. A test of the cognitive diathesis-stress model of depression in children: academic stressors, attributional style, perceived competence, and control. J Pers Soc Psychol 1995;69:370–380.
18. Manassis K, Hudson J, Webb A, et al. (AABT special section on childhood anxiety). Development of childhood anxiety disorders: beyond behavioral inhibition. Cog Behav Practice 2004;11:3–12.
19. Manassis K, Tannock R, Masellis M. Cognitive differences between anxious, normal, and ADHD children on a dichotic listening task. Depress Anxiety 1996;2:279–285.
20. Pine DS, Kentgen LM, Bruder GE, et al. Cerebral laterality in adolescent major depression. Psychiatry Res 2000;93:135–144.
21. Klein DF. False suffocation alarms, spontaneous panics, and related conditions: an integrative hypothesis. Arch Gen Psychiatry 1993;50:306–317.
22. Silverman WK, Ginsburg GS, Goedhart AW. Factor structure of the childhood anxiety sensitivity index. Behav Res Ther 1999;37:903–917.
23. Manassis K. An approach to intervention with childhood anxiety disorders. Can Fam Physician 2004;50:379–384.
24. Burke P, Elliott M. Depression in pediatric chronic illness: a diathesis-stress model. Psychosomatics 1999;40:5–17.
25. Lagrou K, Xhrouet-Heinrichs D, Heinrichs C. Age-related perception of stature, acceptance of therapy, and psychosocial functioning in human growth hormone-treated girls with Turner's syndrome. J Clin Endocrinol Metab 1998;83:1494–1501.
26. Reiss AL, Freund L, Plotnick L. The effects of X monosomy on brain development: monozygotic twins discordant for Turner's syndrome. Ann Neurol 1993;34:95–107.
27. Bowlby J. Attachment and Loss: Attachment. New York: Basic Books, 1973.
28. Warren SL, Huston L, Egeland B, et al. Child and adolescent anxiety disorders and early attachment. J Am Acad Child Adolesc Psychiatry 1997;36:637–644.
29. Beatson J, Taryan S. Predisposition to depression: the role of attachment. Aust NZ J Psychiatry 2003;37:219–225.
30. Hudson JL, Rapee RM. Parent–child interactions and the anxiety disorders: an observational analysis. Behav Res Therapy 2001;39:1411–1427.

31. Rapee RM, Melville LF. Recall of family factors in social phobia and panic disorder: comparison of mother and offspring reports. Depress Anxiety 1997;5:7–11.

32. Ginsburg GS, LaGreca AM, Silverman WK. Social anxiety in children with anxiety disorders: relation with social and emotional functioning. J Abnorm Child Psychol 1998;26:175–185.

33. Goodyer I, Wright C, Altham P. The friendships and recent life events of anxious and depressed school-aged children. Br J Psychiatry 1990;156:689–698.

34. Snyder J, Brooker M, Patrick MR, et al. Observed peer victimization during early elementary school: continuity, growth, and relation to risk for child antisocial and depressive behavior. Child Dev 2003;74:1881–1898.

35. Ginsburg GS, Silverman WK. Gender role orientation and fearfulness in children with anxiety disorders. J Anx Dis 2000;14:57–67.

36. Compas B. Coping with stress during childhood and adolescence. Psychol Bull 1987;101: 393–403.

37. Birmaher B, Williamson DE, Dahl RE, et al. Clinical presentation and course of depression in youth: does onset in childhood differ from onset in adolescence? J Am Acad Child Adolesc Psychiatry 2003;43:63–70.

38. Jaffee SR, Moffitt TE, Caspi A, et al. Differences in early childhood risk factors for juvenile-onset and adult-onset depression. Arch Gen Psychiatry 2002;59:215–222.

39. Wickramaratne PJ, Greenwald S, Weissman MM. Psychiatric disorders in the relatives of probands with prepubertal-onset or adolescent-onset major depression. J Am Acad Child Adolesc Psychiatry 2000;39:1396–1405.

40. Schniering CA, Hudson JL, Rapee RM. Issues in the diagnosis and assessment of anxiety disorders in children and adolescents. Clin Psychol Rev 2000;20:453–478.

41. Rapee RM, Heimberg RG. A cognitive-behavioral model of anxiety in social phobia. Behav Res Ther 1997;35:741–756.

42. Nelles WB, Barlow DH. Do children panic? Clin Psychol Rev 1988;8:359–372.

43. Rapee RM. Potential role of childrearing practices in the development of anxiety and depression. Clin Psychol Rev 1997;17:47–67.

44. Hewitt JK, Silberg JL, Rutter M, et al. Genetics and developmental psychopathology: 1. Phenotypic assessment in the Virginia Twin Study of Adolescent Behavioral Development. J Child Psychol Psychiatry 1998;38:943–963.

45. Lewinsohn PM, Gotlib IH, Lewinsohn M, et al. Gender differences in anxiety disorders and anxiety symptoms in adolescents. J Abnorm Psychol 1998;107:109–117.

46. Kessler RC. Gender differences in major depression: epidemiological findings. In: E. Frank, ed., Gender and Its Effects on Psychopathology. Washington, DC: American Psychiatric Press, 2000:61–84.

47. McCauley Ohannessian C, Lerner RM, et al. Does self-competence predict gender differences in adolescent depression and anxiety? J Adolesc 1999;22:397–411.

48. Seeman MV. Psychopathology in women and men: focus on female hormones. Am J Psychiatry 1997;154:1641–1647.

49. Zohar AH. The epidemiology of obsessive-compulsive disorder in children and adolescents. Child Adolesc Psychiatr Clin N Am 1999;8:445–460.

50. Dorn LD, Hitt SF, Rotenstein D. Biopsychological and cognitive differences in children with premature vs. on-time adrenarche. Arch Pediatr Adolesc Med 1999;153:137–146.

51. Ledoux JE, Gorman JM. A call to action: overcoming anxiety through active coping. Am J Psychiatry 2001;158:1953–1955.

52. Byrne B. Relationship between anxiety, fear, self-esteem, and coping strategies in early adolescence. Adolescence 2000;35:201–215.

53. Main M, Kaplan N, Cassidy J. Security in infancy, childhood and adulthood: a move to the level of representation. Monographs of the Society for Research in Child Development 1985;50(1–2, Serial no 209):66–104.

54. Whittington CJ, Kendall T, Tonagy P, et al. Selective serotonin reuptake inhibitors in childhood depression: systematic review of published versus unpublished data. Lancet 2004;363:1341–1345.

55. Health Canada 2004: www.hc-sc.gc.ca/hpfb-dgpsa/tpd-dpt/sap_ssri

56. Kendall PC, Flannery-Schroeder E, Panichelli-Mindel SM, et al. Therapy for youths with anxiety disorders: a second randomized clinical trial. J Cons Clin Psychol 1997;65:366–380.

57. Birmaher B, Brent DA, Kolko D, et al. Clinical outcome after short-term psychotherapy for adolescents with major depressive disorder. Arch Gen Psychiatry 2000;57:29–36.

58. Mufson L, Moreau D, Weissman MM, et al. Modification of interpersonal psychotherapy with depressed adolescents: phase I and II studies. J Am Acad Child Adolesc Psychiatry 1994;33: 695–705.

59. Milne LC, Lancaster S. Predictors of depression in female adolescents. Adolescence 2001;36: 207–223.

60. Manassis K, Monga S. A therapeutic approach to children and adolescents with anxiety disorders and associated comorbid conditions. J Am Acad Child Adolesc Psychiatry 2001;40:115–117.

61. Kearney CA, Silverman WK. A critical review of pharmacotherapy for youth with anxiety disorders: things are not as they seem. J Anx Dis 1998;12:83–102.
62. Dadds MR, Holland DE, Laurens KR, et al. Early intervention and prevention of anxiety disorders in children: results at follow-up. J Consult Clin Psychol 1999;67:145–150.
63. Barrett P, Turner C. Prevention of anxiety symptoms in primary school children: preliminary results from a universal school-based trial. Br J Clin Psychol 2001;40(pt 4):399–410.
64. Beardslee WR, Gladstone TR, Wright EJ, et al. A family-based approach to the prevention of depressive symptoms in children at risk: evidence of parental and child change. Pediatrics 2003;112:119–131.
65. Jaycox LH, Reivich KJ, Gillham J, et al. Prevention of depressive symptoms in school children. Behav Res Ther 1994;32:801–816.
66. Clarke GN, Hawkins W, Murphy M, et al. Targeted prevention of unipolar depressive disorder in an at-risk sample of high school adolescents: a randomized trial of a group cognitive behavioral intervention. J Am Acad Child Adolesc Psychiatry 1995;34:312–321.

SUGGESTED READINGS

REVIEWS OF DEVELOPMENTAL ISSUES IN CHILDHOOD DEPRESSION AND ANXIETY

Birmaher B, Ryan ND, Williamson DE, et al. Childhood and adolescent depression: a review of the past 10 years (pt 1). J Am Acad Child Adolesc Psychiatry 1996;35:1427–1439.
Manassis K, Hudson J, Webb A, et al. (AABT special section on childhood anxiety). Development of childhood anxiety disorders: beyond behavioral inhibition. Cog Behav Practice 2004;11:3–12.
Parker GB, Brotchie HL. From diathesis to dimorphism: the biology of gender differences in depression. J Nerv Ment Dis 2004;192:210–216.

BOOKS ABOUT PROMOTING HEALTHY DEVELOPMENT IN ANXIOUS/DEPRESSED CHILDREN

(Note: although written in layman's language, these books are also useful for professionals.)
Manassis K. Keys to Parenting Your Anxious Child. Hauppauge, NY: Barron's Educational Series, 1996.
Manassis K, Levac AM. Helping Your Teenager Beat Depression. Bethesda, MD: Woodbine House, 2004.

CHAPTER 5

Gender Identity Disorder in Girls

Susan J. Bradley, Kenneth J. Zucker

This book is about women's mental health, but the distinction between one sex and the other is not always clear, an observation that is best illustrated by a discussion of gender identity disorder (GID) (1,2). This chapter begins with the current diagnostic criteria in use for GID and explains what is known about the prevalence of the disorder in boys and girls. The chapter provides an overview of the clinical picture in girls specifically and then discusses the course of the disorder and its possible outcomes. We touch briefly on intervention, but there is little empirical evidence bearing on its effectiveness. We then address the overlap between gender identity disorder and sexual orientation and discuss the literature that attempts to understand GID and homosexuality. Finally, we relate the development of GID to other disorders involving difficulties with affect regulation and we suggest possibilities for further research. The focus in this chapter is on GID in girls. However, in examining the literature on girls, we also explore the literature generally and then point out differences between boys and girls.

DEFINITIONS

The term "gender identity disorder" refers to that class of disorders in which an individual exhibits "a strong and persistent identification" with the opposite sex and "persistent discomfort" (dysphoria) with his or her own sex or "sense of

inappropriateness in the gender role of that sex". In children, such an identification is revealed in statements about either being or wishing to be the other
sex, in dressing as and taking on the roles of the other sex, and in a preference for
the playthings and play activities typically enjoyed by the other sex. Young children's discomfort with their own sex is seen in avoidance or dislike of the activities and dress of their own sex. By contrast, in adolescents and adults, gender
identification and dysphoria are manifested by a desire to be the other sex and the
concomitant involvement in "passing" as the other sex. This includes attempts at
disguising same-sex features and showing sexual interest in same-sex individuals. The same-sex attraction is experienced as "heterosexuality" because of these
individuals' cross-gender identification. To separate the gender identity disorders
from more minor or fleeting cross-gender interests or role-taking, cross-gender
behaviors must be persistent, affect several aspects of behavior, and result in distress or functional impairment (1,2).

PREVALENCE

The gender identity disorders are considered relatively rare, but there are no epidemiologic studies to provide accurate estimates of prevalence. Recent studies,
based on referrals to GID clinics in Holland, estimate the prevalence in adults to
be 1:10,000 to 1:30,000 (3,4). Sex ratios among adults are roughly equal, while
among children the prevalence, determined by referrals to GID clinics, is substantially higher in boys than in girls, between 3 to 1 and 6 to 1 (5). Given the
lack of epidemiologic data and subsequent reliance on rates of referral to GID
clinics, it is quite possible that these figures are distorted by factors such as
greater social sanction with respect to cross-gender behavior in boys than in girls.
For a discussion of this issue, see Zucker and Bradley (6). In studies from our
clinic, the Gender Identity Clinic for Children and Adolescents in Toronto, and
from the Gender Clinic of the University Medical Centre of Utrecht in Holland,
mothers of girls with GID report more cross-gender symptoms than do mothers
of boys. Girls are older at age of referral, suggesting that the sex ratio is skewed
by a greater tolerance for cross-gender behavior in girls (4,6).

Examining data from the standardization sample of the Child Behavior Checklist (CBCL) (7), a widely used parent-report instrument, 6% of nonreferred boys
are reported by their mothers as "behaving like the opposite sex" at age 4 to 5, but
such reports diminish to only 0.7% for boys 12 to 13 years old. In contrast, almost
12% of nonreferred girls "behave like the opposite sex," and this percentage remains reasonably stable into early adolescence. Examining the other gender-related
item, "wishes to be the opposite sex," mothers of nonreferred boys report low levels of this behavior (0 to 2%) throughout childhood, while mothers of girls report
it for 5% aged 4 to 5, a prevalence that declines to about 2% to 3% when girls
reach early adolescence. Children referred to mental health clinics for other problems are generally reported as displaying relatively higher levels of both "cross-
gender behavior" and "the wish to be the opposite sex." For referred girls "behaving like the opposite sex," there is only a modest decline, from 18.6% at ages 4–5
to 16.5% at ages 12–13. The item "wishes to be the opposite sex" is reported for
6.5% of girls referred at ages 4–5, 8.3% at ages 8–9, and 4.2% at ages 12–13.

What these data tell us is that cross-gender behaviors and wishes are not
uncommon and, among children referred for clinical problems, appear to be
more prevalent in girls than in boys. It is, however, impossible to estimate how

common the full syndrome of GID may be. What is interesting is that, in middle childhood, a significant number of girls wish to be boys, and that this wish is more common among girls already manifesting other clinical problems. Because these data were collected in the 1970s and we do not have current data, we cannot determine whether this is a cohort effect.

Although GID has been studied most systematically in Western countries, there is evidence that cross-gender behavior occurs in many, if not most, cultures. In some cultures, individuals who assume a cross-gender role are given special status. In other cultures, however, especially where there are religious proscriptions against such behavior, cross-gender behavior is highly stigmatized (8).

CLINICAL PRESENTATION

CHILDHOOD

Characteristically, girls with GID begin to exhibit interest in cross-gender activities when they are preschoolers, at a time when most children display awareness of sex and gender differences and begin to label themselves accordingly (10). Children are not usually referred for consultation, however, until those behaviors impress a parent or teacher with their pervasiveness and when they are accompanied by statements about wishing to be the opposite sex or statements that suggest the child believes she is a boy. Despite parents' attempts to dissuade their daughter from either wishing she were a boy or believing she is a boy, in many cases the girl adheres tenaciously to her wish or belief. Not infrequently, one of the greatest points of conflict occurs when parents attempt to persuade their daughter to wear a dress for a special occasion. The intensity of the child's refusal may begin to convince the parents that her belief about being a boy is not "just a passing phase." Requests by girls to have their hair cut short are characteristic. Occasionally, younger girls' play behavior may include simulation of being male by using brooms and other objects as a pretend penis. For more complete case information, see Zucker and Bradley (5).

Associated behaviors include traditional "tomboyish" interests, such as playing with guns or balls, and a variety of outdoor activities. Playmates are typically boys or occasionally other "tomboyish" girls. The activity level of these girls, according to parental report, is higher than that for sisters without GID, girls who are controls in clinical studies, and normal girls. Furthermore, activity is higher than that of GID boys and approaches the level of the general population of boys (5).

The majority of GID girls develop resistant or avoidant behavior that makes parenting a challenge. Clinically, some of these behaviors appear to arise from a mother's being depressed, having difficulty being emotionally available to her daughter, and being unable to set limits. In other situations, GID girls meet criteria for attention deficit hyperactivity disorder (ADHD) and present behavioral challenges because of their hyperactivity and impulsivity. Quite regularly, there is conflict between parents and child and evidence of oppositional defiant behaviors. The parents of such a girl are often in conflict over the management of their daughter with respect to both the cross-gender behavior and other unwanted behavior. The extent of both internalizing and externalizing behavior increases in the period between preschool age and school age (5). Although this increase in symptoms partially correlates with increases in peer difficulties (10), it is also possible that it reflects the increased conflict that ensues once a child's oppositional behavior is left uncontrolled by parents. For a more complete analysis of associated behavior problems, see Zucker (10).

Most girls with GID express the fantasy of "protecting other females." This appears to be related to their wish to be male and often occurs in the context of a perceived marital conflict in which the child perceives the male parent as the powerful one and the female parent as the vulnerable one. Many of these girls are anxious but may mask their overt anxiety by "macho" type behavior.

ADOLESCENCE

Girls with GID who present for help in adolescence have sometimes displayed the same pattern of behavior from early childhood. Generally in those situations parents have been overwhelmed or distracted by other issues and have not seen their daughter's cross-gender behaviors as a high priority. In some instances, however, the extent of earlier cross-gender behavior has been modest and the full-blown GID syndrome appears to have either intensified with puberty or in the context of a trauma. Many of these girls appear depressed at the time of assessment, and it may be difficult to understand the factors that have been most salient in the onset of their cross-gender wishes. Several referrals have occurred following a sexual assault in which the trauma of the assault has reinforced the sense of female vulnerability.

Many girls with GID come to clinical attention when they make efforts to pass as males; some even convince girlfriends that they are male. Concern about the risks they face with such behavior may lead school authorities or parents to seek help. Adolescent GID girls continue to relate more comfortably to male peers with whom they share interests in sports and video games. Their clothing is typically very casual, often emulating "rap" characters. Short hair and baseball caps are characteristic.

Associated behavior problems in adolescent girls are more prevalent than in childhood, as are poor peer relations (10).

FAMILY PSYCHOPATHOLOGY

Generally, there is a high prevalence of anxiety, mood, and substance abuse disorders in the families of children with GID (5). Such families appear very similar to families of other children referred to mental health clinics.

CHILD CASE EXAMPLE

Sara was 5 when first seen in the Child and Adolescent Gender Identity Clinic in Toronto. She was the younger of two girls living with their mother. The father had committed suicide when Sara was 3 years 9 months old. It was thought that he suffered from an undiagnosed bipolar disorder, as had his father.

Sara's mother indicated that the child had always been "boyish" and interested in boy's activities. However, she dates the intensification of Sara's preoccupation with boy's roles and dress to around age 3½. This appears to have followed a dramatic fight between the parents in which the father "lost it" and physically attacked the mother. The children witnessed the attack and were very frightened by it. When the father committed suicide, Sara, for a time, believed that her mother had killed him in retaliation for his attack on her. She had been close to her father, who was her main caregiver, the mother working outside of the home. Sara expressed much anger at her mother following the father's death. The mother experienced a serious bout of depression following the father's suicide and was hospitalized for three weeks.

The mother reported that Sara was unplanned and difficult as an infant. She cried a lot and slept poorly. When she became mobile, she was hyperactive and constantly into things. She frequently wandered off and she got lost several times, apparently with little overt fear. Both parents found her difficult and were regularly in battles with her over control and limits.

At the time of assessment, the mother was concerned that Sara might have bipolar disorder or ADHD in addition to GID.

Sara was adamant about being a boy and insisted that others address her with her chosen boy's name. She refused to wear girls' clothes but eventually agreed to wearing a girls' bathing suit since her mother would not allow her to swim in boys' bathing trunks. She often pretended she had a penis and tried urinating standing up, like a boy. She insisted on having her hair cut very short. In a laboratory free play situation, she gravitated to boys' toys, particularly a dart gun, and dressed up as a soldier. Although she was apparently doing well at school, she appeared to show some difficulty understanding and processing academic material, often responding in unusual ways that seemed to reflect her preoccupation with being a boy. However, it was also not clear if she had fully understood what was being asked.

Sara was referred back to the referring agency with recommendations for stimulant medication to treat her hyperactivity and consideration of an atypical antipsychotic for her aggression and overly intense reactions to stimuli. Individual therapy was recommended to help Sara deal with her anger and her belief that she needs to be male to feel secure. Support for her mother concerning management of the daughter's difficult behavior was also recommended.

ADOLESCENT CASE EXAMPLE

Ali presented to our clinic at age 15 having emigrated with her family (parents and three older siblings) from a Middle Eastern country three years previously. She was requesting sex reassignment surgery.

She indicated being first aware of cross-gender feelings between ages 8 and 9. In her country of origin, gender sex-typed rules and dress codes were quite strict. She reported no cross-dressing until she arrived in Canada, where she perceived the dress codes and expectations for sex-typed behavior as more free. At that time, she began to cross dress and preferred playing with boys. She described role playing male roles when younger and having tomboyish interests. She was also described as "always getting her own way."

On entering high school, she presented herself as a boy. She was not discovered until one day her name was called out on the public address system and "she" was asked to report to the office. This "deception" caused enough fuss that she transferred to an alternate school in which her cross-gender behavior was understood from the start and accepted by the administration.

At the time of assessment, she had been dating two girls, both of whom (it was assumed) regarded her as a male. She was sexually attracted to females but regarded lesbianism as "gross." Her cultural community regarded homosexuality negatively.

Ali displayed a depressed mood at the time of assessment but was not suicidal and had no evidence of anxiety or conduct problems, no psychotic features, and denied having experienced sexual abuse. On the gender interview, there was evidence of significant confusion between a masculine and feminine identification. Projective testing showed preoccupations with powerful male figures, themes of being trapped and pleading for help. She scored in the below average to mildly retarded range on standard intellectual testing. Her sister, who filled out the CBCL on Ali, reported elevations in the clinical range on scores in anxious-obsessive, somatic complaints, depressed-withdrawn, immature-hyperactive, delinquent, and cruel domains.

Ali's family was split and angry about her cross-gender behavior. Her father accepted it, while her mother and the eldest sister, who had raised Ali, were very upset by her behavior. The inquiry about Ali's growing up revealed a family with high levels of conflict. The father was very negative about his wife, referring to her as uneducated, harsh, unable to discipline the children, and constantly yelling. The patient described her father as scary when violent. She reported many efforts to protect her mother and older sister from his violence.

Ali had little insight into her condition and was not very amenable to supportive therapy. She was considered at high risk for continuing to want sex reassignment surgery. This was problematic because several of her associated difficulties were likely to prevent her from stabilizing her life adequately to meet the criteria for sex reassignment.

COURSE AND OUTCOMES

There have been limited follow-up studies of girls with GID. Based on our experience in our Toronto clinic and on experience in the clinic in Utrecht, the course is variable (10). Some of these girls appear to relinquish their desire to be the opposite sex and assume a more typically female identification. Others continue with some cross-gender identification into adolescence. Based on follow-up studies of boys with GID and our own limited follow-up, we speculate that many of these girls will adopt a lesbian orientation, but, again, there are few data to confirm or refute this assumption.

Adolescents with GID appear more fixed in their cross-gender identity than younger girls (5,12). Although we do not have systematic follow-up data, more of the adolescents appear to move toward sex reassignment surgery despite psychotherapeutic efforts to help them explore their need for a cross-gender identity. In contrast to males with GID, females seem better able to adapt to masculine roles and jobs following sex reassignment surgery (13).

As with offspring of families with anxiety, mood, and substance abuse disorders, there are high levels of these disorders in the GID population in adolescence and adulthood and these disorders, as much as the presence of GID, may interfere with adaptive functioning (5).

INTERVENTION

Given the few researchers working in this area and the relatively small number of children in any one clinic, there has been little empirical study of intervention strategies. Generally, efforts are directed at helping families support girls with GID to feel better about being female and less in need psychologically of a cross-gender identity. In addition, because of the associated behavioral difficulties, work is usually directed at diminishing the conflict between parents and child as well as between the child's parents. For some children, individual therapy is believed to be helpful in order to examine the fantasy about protecting females from male aggression. Clearly, in situations where there has been trauma, dealing with the effects of trauma is clinically indicated.

In adolescence, supportive therapy is important. This is intended to assist the girl in deciding whether sex reassignment surgery is her best option and whether treatment of her depression or reaction to trauma may, in time, diminish her desire for SRS. For those adolescents in whom the cross-gender identification seems quite fixed, use of puberty-delaying hormones may be indicated (12). This may allow some reduction in pressure to move toward SRS and permit the adolescent to shift gradually and more safely to passing as the other sex. In Holland, in contrast to North America, there is more support for cross-gender living and an earlier move to hormone replacement and surgery in adolescence is advocated (12,14).

ETIOLOGY

There are few systematic studies of etiology of female GID. As indicated above under "Course and Outcomes," many children with GID ultimately develop a homosexual sexual orientation. Retrospective studies of homosexual adults suggest that many displayed cross-gender interests and behavior as children (15). However, not all did, and there are no studies that clearly document what proportion of individuals with a homosexual orientation would have met criteria for GID in childhood. Thus, homosexuality and GID are not synonymous, as has sometimes been suggested. However, because of the clear connection between GID and homosexuality, there has been interest among GID researchers in examining those factors that are thought to play a role in the development of homosexuality. In this section, we will briefly review some of the literature related to homosexuality, specifically where it may provide etiologic links relevant to GID.

BIOLOGIC FACTORS

There is evidence from animal studies that levels of cross-gender behavior in young offspring can be manipulated through altering exposure to androgens in utero. This work led to the prenatal hormone theory, which posits that sex-dimorphic patterns of behavior result from brain patterning that occurs with exposure to androgens at various critical periods of brain development (16). A confounding factor in transferring this theory to human development has been the presence of genital masculinization in intersex conditions. Ambiguous genitalia were seen as eliciting ambivalence from caregivers and contributing to the child's reactions. However, work in rhesus macaques has shown that hormonal manipulation can affect aspects of behavior, such as mounting and rough play, without inducing genital masculinization and that these effects are dependent on the timing of hormonal manipulation (17). However, despite years of research, largely on male homosexuality, evidence that "brain patterning" plays a significant role in human sexuality or GID is modest. There is some evidence from studies of intersex conditions suggesting that exposure to androgens in utero may play a contributory role in gender role behavior in girls.

Congenital adrenal hyperplasia (CAH) is an intersex disorder in which affected females are exposed to abnormally high levels of androgens in utero because their adrenals lack the hormone that converts cortisone precursors to cortisone. This cortisone deficiency results in lack of the normal feedback at the level of the hypothalamus and an increase in levels of adrenocorticotrophic hormone (ACTH), which in turn increases the adrenal production of androgen. There are two variants, simple virilizing and salt-wasting CAH, the latter being generally more severe and tending to produce more masculinization in utero. Girls with CAH, particularly of the salt-wasting type, show higher levels of activity and more tomboyish interests and behavior than do their nonaffected sisters. As adults, they are somewhat slower in their overall psychosexual development and have higher levels of homoerotic fantasy but not homosexual behavior. Their gender identity is typically female although there may be a somewhat higher level of referral for GID than would be expected from the number of these disorders in the population. (For reviews see 16,18,19.)

There is also some evidence supporting a correlation between maternal testosterone in utero and masculine role behavior in girls. In a normative sample, following 679 children (50.3% males) from early in the pregnancy through childhood, Hines and coauthors (20) found a linear relationship between prenatal maternal testosterone (T) levels and masculine gender role behavior in girls but not boys. Although the girls classified behaviorally as "masculine" had higher maternal testosterone levels, the amount of the variance explained by the hormonal difference was small.

As noted above, conjecturing about the role that exposure to elevated levels of testosterone in utero may play is confounded in intersex cases by the presence of genital ambiguity at birth. What is interesting, however, is that girls with intersex conditions who had virilized genitals at birth and who, it is presumed, were exposed to elevated levels of testosterone in utero, displayed sex role behavior that was less masculine overall than that of our sample of girls with GID, who were physically normal (21). This suggests that, whatever role the exposure to testosterone in utero plays, it is less powerful than other factors in the development of GID in girls.

As reported above, girls with GID do display a higher activity level than their sisters without GID, similar to that of boys who are controls in the studies (5). Whether this reflects a hormonal effect or is simply a temperamental variable is difficult to ascertain. It does seem to permit these girls to relate comfortably to boys and to share their interests.

The only other area that tends to support a testosterone effect in utero involves the length of the second and fourth digits in the hand, known as the 2D:4D ratio. Typically males have a low (less than 1) 2D:4D ratio and females have a high (greater than 1) ratio (22). In at least three studies (23,24,25), lesbians as well as males and females with CAH (26) have been found to have a low ratio (27). Although a recent large study failed to confirm this finding in lesbian women (27), the Hall and Love (23) study examining twins concordant and discordant for sexual orientation did find a lower 2D:4D ratio in the lesbian as opposed to the heterosexual twin, suggesting higher in utero androgen exposure in the lesbian cotwins. This has not been studied systematically in GID, although masculine lesbian women have a lower ratio than feminine lesbian women (28). Although some might argue that the exposure to testosterone in utero at higher than normal levels makes a female more likely to be masculine or sexually attracted to females, this is most likely a relatively small effect. It may, however, contribute to the higher activity level seen in CAH girls and possibly in girls with GID.

Other putative biologic factors include the effects of maternal stress in utero. In animals, stress in utero tends to lead to reversals of sex typical characteristics in males. This is less marked in females (29). In the Avon Longitudinal Study of Parents and Children, subjects in a large sample of children were followed from 18 or 32 weeks of gestation to 42 months after birth. The authors could find no influence of stress on gender role behavior in boys and only a very modest effect in girls (30). However, from this same study, there is evidence that maternal stress during pregnancy does appear to increase stress reactivity in offspring. This may play a role in the development of psychopathology more generally, and contribute to the development of GID. See below and Bradley (31) for a more thorough discussion.

Following findings of a later birth order for males with GID (32), there has been interest in examining this effect in females with GID. There has been only one small study (n = 22) conducted in females with GID in comparison with clinical controls. Girls with GID were earlier in their birth order than the controls (33). This is the mirror opposite of the findings in boys with GID and homosexual men, who are born later in their birth order with an excess of brothers (32). If an early birth order effect exists in girls with GID, it is hard to find an adequate biologic explanation for such an effect. In males the late birth order effect has been posited to represent an autoimmune reaction that increases with prior male births. Equally possible is that both the male and female findings may represent psychosocial effects related to the child's position in the family.

Studies of handedness in homosexual men do suggest a higher rate of non–right handedness. A similar finding has been reported in GID boys. Although not as strong as the findings in males, there is some evidence for a higher rate of non–right-handedness in lesbian women (34,35). When taken together, it is hard to frame a gender-related theory that accounts for non–right-handedness in homosexual males *and* females except that such atypicality may simply reflect developmental anomalies resulting from in utero effects. The finding of a higher rate of non–right-handedness also occurs in individuals with other forms of psychopathology and suggests a more general developmental interference effect (36).

Lastly, girls with GID are perceived to be more "rugged" or "handsome" than are control girls. This is in contrast to boys with GID, who are rated as cute or beautiful (37). These data are difficult to interpret, likely representing the child's efforts to create an identity, as much as they measure something more intrinsic to the child's physiognomy.

PSYCHOSOCIAL FACTORS

Because there have been no systematic comparative studies examining psychosocial variables, this section must draw on systematic clinical observation and psychometric test results from our clinic and the Utrecht group.

Although dated, the work of Money and the Hampsons from the 1950s continues to provide the best extant information concerning the capacity of the parenting system to override biologic variables (38). These early investigators examined the gender identity outcomes for intersex infants and generally concluded that sex of assignment and rearing, particularly if decided before the child is 18 months old, predicts eventual gender identity in later childhood and adulthood. Despite controversy and some discrepant findings, particularly with respect to individuals with 5-alpha-reductase deficiency who, raised as girls, convert to a male gender identity with appearance of male secondary sex characteristics at puberty (39), these findings continue to be accepted as generally valid. With respect to children with GID, all of the physically normal children were assigned appropriately at birth. What has been much more difficult to assess is whether the parents might have been ambivalent about the child's sex. In a study by Green examining variables related to outcome in GID boys, the finding was that parents failed to discourage the cross-gender behavior (40). This has been typical of our experience in our clinic in families of boys and girls with GID. Another factor that appeared salient in Green's work on GID in boys was that parents of boys with GID spent less time with them than did parents of controls with their sons. This is consistent with our observations in both boys and girls. We believe that these relationship difficulties reflect parental psychopathology or difficulties parents experience in rearing a particular child. Regardless of their origins, parent–child relationship difficulties likely play a role in the ambivalent rearing received by the child with GID.

As with other groups of children referred to mental health clinics, we have found relatively high levels of attachment insecurity in boys with GID (41). Our sample of girls has not been examined systematically using empirically based measurements of attachment. However, we have reported high levels of depression in mothers of girls with GID, particularly at the time when these girls were infants or toddlers, the putative time when the child's attachment and identification with the mother would be expected to be most affected by the mother's mental state (5). Mothers of girls with GID appear to have experienced higher than expected levels of sexual and physical abuse and it is our perception that this experience has affected the way these women feel about being safe as females, a fear that we believe is somehow transmitted to their daughters. This perception of being vulnerable as a female is reinforced when these girls witness their fathers or older male siblings acting out their anger in explosive and threatening behaviors. We believe that these girls are traumatized by these experiences and "identify with the aggressor" as a way of recapturing a sense of safety.

We have presented a formulation that attempts to capture this array of biologic and psychosocial factors (5). GID is a rare phenomenon and requires the presence of a number of factors, some of which are common to other forms of psychopathology and others that are unique to GID. Children with GID can be presumed to carry a vulnerability for affective instability or stress reactivity. This is reflected in the family histories of anxiety, mood, and substance abuse disorders. Furthermore, these children are recognized as sensitive, a trait that is part of the picture of stress reactivity seen in animal studies and studies of inhibited children. For a more complete discussion, see Bradley (31). This trait predisposes individuals to later anxiety and depression. The early rearing experience of these children is often one of insecure attachments related to maternal depression, parental conflict, and parent–child conflict. These factors are relatively common in the development of childhood psychopathology. What may be unique in the experience of girls who develop GID is their perception of their mother as relatively vulnerable, especially in the face of male aggression. This dynamic combined with the high level of activity of girls with GID may enable the fantasy solution of being strong, powerful, invulnerable, and able to protect other females as a male. The parents' lack of overt discouragement of the fantasy, acted out in her cross-gender behavior and role taking, permits this fantasy to become a part of her identity. When the girl with GID is permitted to continue using this fantasy into adolescence, she may gradually consolidate an identity that is relatively stable, the more so as it serves to control anxiety. This makes it difficult to give up, because doing so would leave the girl feeling very insecure. This viewpoint helps to explain the relative immutability of GID in adolescent and adult individuals.

FUTURE DIRECTIONS

Research on GID in girls is relatively complex, given the small sample sizes in any one clinic. However, as psychophysiologic measures of stress reactivity become more available, it is possible to think of ways of testing some of our presumptions. Recent work on individuals who have been traumatized or maltreated suggests hypoactivity and hyperactivity of the hypothalamic pituitary adrenal axis (HPA) (42,43). Moreover, there is now evidence that some individuals who are inhibited show increases in excitability of the amygdala related to genetic polymorphisms of the serotonin transporter (SERT), and that this same polymorphism also predisposes to vulnerability to depression (44,46). These findings suggest that examination of children with GID with respect to functioning of the HPA axis and arousability of the amygdala or genetic testing for SERT polymorphisms could prove relevant.

The other important research direction involves comparison of girls with GID and girls with other anxiety disorders but without GID on family dynamic variables, such as maternal experience of male aggression both historically and currently. Lastly, in light of the fact that adolescents with GID present with high levels of depression and trauma, it would also be useful to compare them with populations of depressed adolescents without GID as well as with traumatized adolescents without GID.

Use of a concrete fantasy solution, such as we propose occurs in GID, is relatively uncommon in the development of psychopathology generally. There are some parallels in women with eating disorders (see Chapter 8, "Eating Disorders and Body Image in Adolescence," by Bulik and Reba in this book). What causes an individual to resort to such dramatic and concrete solutions to inner distress is not well understood. Are there cognitive predispositions that facilitate the use of such strategies? In the past, questions have been raised about GID being a delusional disorder. Generally individuals with GID do not manifest the other phenomena typically associated with psychotic disorders. Is it possible that their solution binds their anxiety in a way that protects them from displaying more psychotic symptoms? Although these questions remain difficult to answer, in order to adequately understand the disorder, it may be necessary to explore more fully the cognitive strategies employed by individuals who develop GID.

Clearly, further testing of variables such as the 2D:4D finger ratio, birth order, and handedness in GID females deserves attention and may contribute to understanding how vulnerability in utero may interact with rearing effects.

Intervention in adolescents, as noted above, has been largely supportive, directed at helping the adolescent clarify whether the wish for sex reassignment surgery (SRS) is fixed or malleable. It is possible to consider using medications to reduce stress reactivity, such as the selective serotonergic reuptake inhibitors (SSRIs), or even atypical antipsychotics early on in the course of treatment, to examine whether reducing anxiety might make it more possible for adolescents with GID to relinquish their need for such a dramatic solution to distress.

Lastly, prediction of which individuals who present with a request for SRS are most likely to persist in their wish has been hampered by the lack of follow-up studies of this population, whether first presenting in childhood or in adolescence. Systematic recruitment of girls presenting with GID into longitudinal studies would provide answers that could assist in treatment (47).

CONCLUSIONS

Gender identity disorder in girls is a relatively rare, and somewhat understudied area. Although efforts have been made to find a simple biologic explanation to the puzzle of this firmly held conviction (that is not quite a delusion), this work has not proven fruitful. It appears that this syndrome arises from a complex interplay of biologic and psychosocial variables. The conviction is relatively more mutable in early childhood but assumes increasing rigidity with time. Factors that offer hope for intervention include locating the vulnerability to anxiety in this population (as in the study of the SERT polymorphism) and further study of the biologic reactions to trauma assuming early intervention in trauma can reduce the likelihood of later symptomatology.

REFERENCES

1. American Psychiatric Association. Diagnostic and Statistical Manual of Mental Disorders. 4th Ed, text rev. Washington, DC: Author, 2000.
2. World Health Organization. International Statistical Classification of Diseases and Related Health Problems. 10th rev. Geneva: Author, 1992.
3. Bakker A, van Kesteren PJM, Gooren LJG, et al. The prevalence of transsexualism in the Netherlands. Acta Psychiatr Scand 1993;87:237-238.
4. Zucker KJ, Bradley SJ, Sanikhani M. Sex differences in referral rates of children with gender identity disorder: some hypotheses. J Abnorm Child Psychol 1997;25:217–227.
5. Zucker KJ, Bradley SJ. Gender Identity Disorder and Psychosexual Problems in Children and Adolescents. New York: Guilford, 1995.
6. Cohen-Kettenis PT, Owen A, Kaijser VG, et al. Demographic characteristics, social competence, and behavior problems in children with gender identity disorder: a cross-national, cross-clinic comparative analysis. J Abnorm Child Psychol 2003;31:41–53.
7. Achenbach TM, Edelbrock C. Manual for the Child Behavior Checklist and Revised Child Behavior Profile. Burlington, VT: University of Vermont, Department of Psychiatry, 1983.
8. Herdt G, ed. Third Sex, Third Gender: Beyond Sexual Dimorphism in Culture and History. New York: Zone Books, 1994.
9. Martin CL, Ruble DN, Szkrybalo J. Cognitive theories of early gender development. Psychol Bull 2002;128:903–933.
10. Zucker, KJ. Gender identity disorder. In: Bell-Dolan D, ed. Behavioral and Emotional Problems in Girls. New York: Kluwer Academic/Plenum Press, 2005:285–319.
11. Zucker KJ, Owen A, Bradley SJ, et al. Gender-dysphoric children and adolescents: a comparative analysis of demographic characteristics and behavioral problems. Clin Child Psychol Psychiatry 2002;7:398–411.
12. Cohen-Kettenis PT, van Goozen SHM. Sex reassignment of adolescent transsexuals: a follow-up study. J Am Acad Child Adolesc Psychiatry 1997;36:263–271.
13. Pfäfflin F, Junge A. Geschlechts-umwandlung: Abhandlungen zur transsexualität. New York: Schattauer, 1992.
14. Gooren L, Delemarre-van de Waal H. The feasibility of endocrine interventions in juvenile transsexuals. J Psychol Human Sexual 1996;8:69–84.
15. Bailey JM, Zucker KJ. Childhood sex-typed behavior and sexual orientation: a conceptual analysis and quantitative review. Dev Psychol 1995;31:43–55.
16. Collaer ML, Hines M. Human behavioral sex differences: a role for gonadal hormones during early development? Psychol Bull 1995;118:55–107.
17. Goy RW, Bercovitch FB, McBrair MC. Behavioral masculinization is independent of genital masculinization in prenatally androgenized female rhesus macaques. Horm Behav 1988;22:552–571.
18. Meyer-Bahlburg HFL. Gender and sexuality in classic congenital adrenal hyperplasia. Endocrin Metab Clin North Am 2001;30:155–172.

19. Zucker KJ. Intersexuality and gender identity differentiation. Annu Rev Sex Res 1999;10:1–69.

20. Hines M, Golombok S, Rust J, et al. Testosterone during pregnancy and gender role behavior of preschool children: a longitudinal, population study. Child Dev 2002;73:1678–1687.

21. Zucker KJ, Allin S, Babul-Hirji R, et al. Assessment of gender identity and gender role behavior: a comparison of girls with gender identity disorder, girls exposed prenatally to gender-atypical levels of androgens, and control girls. Poster session presented at the First World Congress: Hormonal and Genetic Basis of Sexual Differentiation Disorders, Tempe, AZ, May 2002.

22. Garn SM, Burdi AR, Babler WJ, et al. Early prenatal attainment of adult metacarpal-phalangeal rankings and proportions. Am J Phys Anthropol 1975;43:327–332.

23. Hall LS, Love CT. Finger-length ratios in female monozygotic twins discordant for sexual orientation. Arch Sex Behav 2003;32:23–28.

24. Rahman Q, Wilson GD. Sexual orientation and the 2nd to 4th finger length ratio: evidence for organising effects of sex hormones or developmental instability? Psychoneuroendocrinology 2002;28:288–303.

25. Williams TJ, Pepitone ME, Christensen SE, et al. Finger-length ratios and sexual orientation. Nature 2000;404:455–456.

26. Brown WM, Hines M, Fane BA, et al. Masculinized finger length ratios in human males and females with congenital adrenal hyperplasia. Horm Behav 2002;42:380–386.

27. Lippa RA. Are 2D:4D finger-length ratios related to sexual orientation? Yes for men, no for women. J Pers Soc Psychol 2003;85:179–188.

28. Brown WM, Finn CJ, Cook BM, et al. Differences in finger length ratios between self-identified "butch" and "femme" lesbians. Arch Sex Behav 2002;31:123–127.

29. Ward IL, Weisz J. Differential effects of maternal stress on circulating levels of corticosterone, progesterone, and testosterone in male and female rat fetuses and their mothers. Endocrinology 1984;114:1635–1644.

30. Hines M, Johnston KJ, Golombok S, et al. Prenatal stress and gender role behavior in girls and boys: a longitudinal, population study. Horm Behav 2002;42:126–134.

31. Bradley SJ. Affect Regulation and the Development of Psychopathology. New York: Guilford, 2000.

32. Blanchard R. Birth order and sibling sex ratio in homosexual versus heterosexual males and females. Ann Rev Sex Res 1997;8:27–67.

33. Zucker KJ, Lightbody S, Pecore K, et al. Birth order in girls with gender identity disorder. Euro Child Adolesc Psychiatry 1998;7:30–35.

34. Green R, Young R. Hand preference, sexual preference, and transsexualism. Arch Sex Behav 2001;30:565–574.

35. Lalumiére ML, Blanchard R, Zucker KJ. Sexual orientation and handedness in men and women: a meta-analysis. Psychol Bull 2000;126:575–592.

36. Previc FH. Nonright-handedness, central nervous system and related pathology, and its lateralization: a reformulation and synthesis. Dev Neuropsych 1996;12:443–515.

37. McDermid SA, Zucker KJ, Bradley SJ, et al. Effects of physical appearance on masculine trait ratings of boys and girls with gender identity disorder. Arch Sex Behav 1998;27:253–267.

38. Money J, Hampson JG, Hampson JL. Imprinting and the establishment of gender role. Arch Neurol Psychiatry 1957;77:333–336.

39. Imperato-McGinley J, Guerrero L, Gautier T, et al. Steroid 5-alpha reductase deficiency in man: an inherited form of male pseudohermaphroditism. Science 1974;186:1213–1215.

40. Green R. Sexual Identity Conflict in Children and Adults. New York: Basic, 1974.

41. Birkenfeld-Adams AS. Quality of attachment in young boys with gender identity disorder: a comparison to clinic and nonreferred control boys. Unpublished doctoral dissertation, York University, Downsview, Ontario 1999.

42. Cicchetti D, Rogosch FA. Diverse patterns of neuroendocrine activity in maltreated children. Dev Psychopath 2001;13:677–693.

43. Gunnar MR, Vazquez DM. Low cortisol and a flattening of expected daytime rhythm: potential indices of risk in human development. Dev Psychopath 2001;13:515–538.

44. Hariri A, Mattay VS, Tessitore A, et al. Serotonin transporter genetic variation and the response of the human amygdala. Science 2002;297:400–403.

45. Caspi A, Sugden K, Moffitt TE, et al. Influence of life stress on depression: moderation by a polymorphism in the 5-HTT gene. Science 2003;301:386–389.

46. Schwartz CE, Wright CI, Shin LM, et al. Inhibited and uninhibited infants "grown up": adult amygdalar response to novelty. Science 2003;300:1952–1953.

47. Smith YLS, van Goozen SHM, Cohen-Kettenis PT. Adolescents with gender identity disorder who were accepted or rejected for sex reassignment surgery: a prospective follow-up study. J Am Acad Child Adolesc Psychiatry 2001;40:472–481.

CHAPTER 6

Developmental Pathways of ADHD

Florence Levy

PREVALENCE OF ATTENTION DEFICIT HYPERACTIVITY DISORDER

Of interest to women's mental health, most prevalence studies of attention deficit hyperactivity disorder (ADHD) have reported a significant excess of boys over girls, with ratios varying from 18:1 to 4:1 (1). The actual prevalence depends on whether the classification system used is categorical or dimensional. It also depends on the choice of informant, the age and gender composition of the population studied, and the instrument used to measure impairment. Widely divergent estimates of prevalence, from 4% to 17% of the population, have been reported (estimates are lower, 0.8% to 1.7%, for hyperkinetic disorder, the term used by the *International Classification of Diseases*, 10th edition, ICD-10) (1). All questionnaire estimates show an excess of ADHD in boys. There is less consistency with respect to the influence of age and comorbidity. In general, interview studies suggest a decline in prevalence with age. The Buitelaar review found high rates of comorbidity of ADHD and oppositional defiant disorder (25%), conduct disorder (15%), anxiety (25%), and depression (25%) (1). Studies of externalizing and internalizing comorbidity patterns in children aged 6 to 12 years old (with ADHD combined and ADHD inattentive subtypes) indicate significant comorbidity between ADHD combined subtype and oppositional defiant disorder or conduct disorder (2).

Possible explanations for the male excess are rater bias, referral bias, threshold differences, and behavioral or learning differences between the sexes. Faraone and colleagues (3) have found that boys have an increased risk over girls for ADHD diagnosed according to criteria of the *Diagnostic and Statistical Manual of Mental Disorders*, 3rd edition (DSM-III) only in families that exhibit antisocial disorders. These investigators postulate that gender differences might be important in that they provide clues to the genetic heterogeneity of ADHD.

In terms of etiology, Rhee and colleagues (4,5) have compared the constitutional variability model with the polygenic multiple threshold model. The latter assumes a continuum of liability with a higher threshold for girls, while the constitutional variability model implies unique male susceptibility. Evidence for male susceptibility is buttressed by the fact that the birth of boys is associated with relatively more labor and delivery problems and boys show greater immaturity at birth. Boys exhibit greater degrees of overactivity and inattention. In this way of thinking, girls with ADHD represent a brain-damaged group. The polygenic model postulates that those of the sex that is less frequently affected (females in the case of ADHD) should have more affected relatives than those of the more frequently affected sex. Indeed, Rhee and colleagues have shown that cotwins and cosiblings of girls with ADHD have a higher number of ADHD symptoms on average (mean = 5.54, sd = 4.35) than the cotwins and cosiblings of boys with ADHD (mean = 4.24, SD = 4.0), a finding supportive of the polygenic multiple threshold model (4).

In their review of gender differences in prevalence and in the association of ADHD and hyperkinetic disorder (HKD), Heptinstall and Taylor (6) point to a number of inconsistencies and contradictions in the literature, namely that population samples and clinic-referred samples differ in their characteristics. A study on the discriminant validity (e.g., relationship to criteria external to the defining symptoms) of DSM-IV ADHD in a nationally representative Australian sample of 3,597 children, aged 6 to 17 years, found a prevalence of 7.5% (6.9% if only those with impairment are included) for ADHD (7). The inattentive subtype was found to be more common than the combined and hyperactive-impulsive subtypes. This study, which included parent-rated impairment measures, concluded that ADHD was more prevalent among males in all three subtypes, with the male to female ratio for combined type being approximately twice that of hyperactive-impulsive and inattentive type (7).

In their meta-analysis of gender differences in ADHD (8), Gaub and Carlson found that among population samples not referred to clinics girls with ADHD displayed lower levels of inattention, internalizing behavior, and peer aggression than boys with ADHD, but clinic-referred samples showed similar gender levels of both impairment and comorbidity. According to observations of classroom behavior of 403 boys and 99 girls with ADHD, boys engaged in more rule-breaking and externalizing impulsive behaviors (disruptive behavior disorders, or DBD) than did girls (9). It was also found that children with ADHD and DBD manifested more interference with classroom routine behaviors than did children with ADHD and anxiety, although comorbid anxiety did not always inhibit the rate of disruptive behavior.

A recent meta-analysis by Gershon has pointed out that identification of ADHD in females is difficult, as fewer females than males are evaluated in specialized clinics (10). While epidemiologic samples estimate gender differences at 3:1, clinical samples range closer to 9:1. This supports the Australian epidemiologic findings: male:female ratio of 1.7:1 for hyperactive-impulsive types and 4.6:1 for combined types, respectively, somewhat lower and somewhat higher than in previous community-based studies. Combined subtypes had higher scores on the anxious/depressed scale of the Achenbach Child Behavior Checklist (CBCL), and on all three externalizing scales of the CBCL. Combined type symptoms were rated as causing greater disruption to family activities than inattentive and hyperactive-impulsive symptoms. All children with combined type symptoms met criteria for impairment, compared with 93% of the inattentive and 86% of the hyperactive-impulsive types (7).

Comparing results with those of Gaub and Carlson, Gershon (10) examined potential moderators of effect size estimates of the male:female ratio. These include publication status, referral source, rater effects, assessment of IQ, age of subjects, and diagnostic system used. He found that ADHD females manifested significantly fewer externalizing problems, but significantly more internalizing problems than ADHD males. Girls performed worse on full scale and verbal IQ. Teachers rated girls as less inattentive and having fewer externalizing problems than boys. Clinically referred samples, as was expected, tended to manifest more severe symptoms than community samples. This study also found a possible gender bias in rating scales, all tending to score boys higher than girls. Large gender differences persist, however, even when this is taken into account.

HERITABILITY DIFFERENCES

Sex differences in prevalence are not explained by heritability differences between girls and boys. Rietveld and colleagues (11) studied a large community sample of twins 3 to 12 years old for overactive behavior and attention problems. They used a cross-sectional twin design controlling for developmental, gender, and rater contrast contributions. They found that heritability ranged from 68% to 76% across age groups. In general, patterns of additive genetic, dominance, and unique environmental effects were similar in boys and girls, with a rater contrast effect found at 3 years of age.

DEVELOPMENTAL RISKS

Boys may be more vulnerable than girls to many developmental and social problems (12). For instance, girls in general have superior literary skills and are more aware of and more explicit about their feelings, while boys are said to lack an emotional vocabulary.

An interesting animal study reported by Andersen and Teicher found sex differences in dopamine receptor density. They found greater lateralized D_2 dopamine receptor density in young male rats, which was thought to parallel the appearance of motor symptoms (13). The presence of ADHD has significant developmental implications, which may differ in girls compared to boys, with boys manifesting more comorbid externalizing problems. This can give rise to difficulties with socialization throughout preschool and the primary school years. On the other hand, the tendency for girls with inattention to experience anxiety is also likely to interfere with school adjustment. The transition through adolescence into adulthood is a particularly vulnerable phase for children with ADHD. This may have particularly significant implications for girls; vulnerability to adolescent pregnancy is an example.

Rucklidge and Tannock found that females with ADHD (aged 13 to 16) were more significantly impaired than female controls on most measures of psychosocial functioning, including self-reported depression (14). When compared to males, there were no significant differences in major Axis I clinical disorders, but females reported more overall distress, anxiety, and depression and a more external locus of control than males. On the WISC-III, males had lower scores on processing speed, while females had lower vocabulary scores. The authors concluded that having ADHD may be more psychologically impairing for females.

Dalsgaard and colleagues (15) report on a 20-year (1969–1989) follow-up of 218 children, initially aged 4–15 years, who received pharmacologic treatment with methylphenidate or dexamphetamine because of inattention and hyperactivity. Interestingly, gender was the most important predictor of psychiatric admission in adulthood, with women most at risk; 32% of the female sample had an adult admission. Girls with ADHD plus conduct problems had a much higher risk of adult psychiatric admission than those without conduct disorder (60% of those with an initial diagnosis of ADHD with conduct disorder, compared with 22.6% of those with an ADHD diagnosis). However, antisocial personality development was not predicted by gender, IQ, duration of stimulant treatment, or degree of childhood ADHD symptomatology. The study suggests a relatively poorer outcome for girls with ADHD, particularly those with comorbid conduct disorder.

ETIOLOGIC RISKS

Etiologic risks were investigated by Biederman and colleagues (16) in two clinical samples of children who met full DSM-III criteria for ADHD at the time of referral. The study used a three-stage ascertainment procedure and contrasted subjects to healthy controls. The investigators found Rutter's indicators of adversity to be significantly associated with the risk for ADHD, but the cumulative adversity risk did not differ by gender. For substance use disorders, there was a significant gender-by-diagnosis interaction, indicating that ADHD was a significantly weaker risk factor for substance use in boys than it was in girls. However, girls did seem relatively protected with respect to global functioning and learning disability, whereas boys seemed more vulnerable to adverse outcomes. The authors suggested that twin and adoption studies of adversity effects would be a useful way to separate genetic and environmental effects.

Biederman et al. (17) also investigated the discrepancy in the male:female ratio between clinic-referred (10 to 1) and community-referred (3 to 1) samples of children with ADHD. They studied 140 boys and 140 girls with ADHD and 120 boys and 120 girls without ADHD for indicators of social adversity, IQ, reading, and arithmetic achievement. They found that ADHD in girls was more likely to be predominantly of the inattentive subtype and less likely to be associated with a learning disability in either reading or mathematics. The risks for ADHD-associated impairment were similarly elevated in boys and girls, but gender-specific baseline risks may have resulted in different rates of psychiatric morbidity. Despite this, they again found that there was a significantly increased risk for substance use disorders in girls compared with boys among children referred to ADHD clinics.

ADOPTEE AND TWIN STUDIES

Attention deficit hyperactivity disorder (ADHD) has been shown to be a highly heritable disorder, with increasing numbers of studies investigating genetic factors (18). A study was conducted of adoptees between 18 and 47 years of age who were separated from their biologic families within a few days of birth. At least one biologic parent was diagnosed with antisocial personality or substance abuse or both. With the use of structural equation modeling, it was found that, in the males, oppositional defiant disorder (ODD) was predicted by an antisocial biological background but not by an adverse adoptive environment. Conduct disorder (CD), on the other hand, was predicted by adoptive environment alone. For females, the results were somewhat different. A biologic background or biologic-environmental interactions predicted both ODD and CD (19).

A study of 2,082 twin pairs found that the overlap of conduct problems and ADHD was explained by common genetic and nonshared environmental factors (20). Together with our finding of very low, shared environmental influences on ADHD (18), this study suggests different etiologic factors for different behavior syndromes. Waldman and colleagues (21) sampled the first wave of the Australian Twin Study on 2,600 3-year-old to 15-year-old male and female same-sex and opposite-sex twins, and similar age nontwin siblings. A multivariate genetic analysis, using Cholesky decomposition, indicated that, while there was considerable overlap in the genetic and environmental influences on ADHD, CD, and ODD, the influences of shared environment on CD was much greater than on ODD. Thus, twin studies suggest separate etiologic subgroupings of ADD/ADHD and ODD/CD symptom profiles.

MOLECULAR GENETICS

The candidate gene approach to searching for putative genes responsible for these disorders is based on postulated neurotransmitter mechanisms. Molecular genetic approaches have been tried in relation to dopaminergic [dopamine transporter (DAT), dopamine D4 receptor (DRD4), and dopamine D5 receptor (DRD5)] genes as well as adrenergic, serotonergic, and nicotinic receptor genes (22). Comorbidity with learning disability has given rise to renewed interest in "reading" genes. For example, Grigorenko et al. described an association of phonetic awareness with a site on chromosome 6 and an association of whole word reading with a site on chromosome 15 (23). Reviewing twin and genetic studies of dyslexia, these researchers point out the complexities resulting from varied definitions and cognitive models of dyslexia (24). However, despite the developmental variability of the phenotype, there is emerging evidence suggesting that phonologic abilities constitute a core set of reading-related processes predictive of accuracy and speed of reading. Twin studies found reading performance to be highly heritable in both proband (0.82) and control (0.66) twins (25). Molecular genetic investigations have pursued an association between autoimmune disturbances and dyslexia (26). Findings from an affected sib-pair study have provided evidence for linkage between reading disability and DNA markers localized to 6p21.3 (the HLA region or "neighborhood"). Reproducible genetic findings should enable treatments in the future to be more individually tailored in terms of gene–phenotype relationships.

GENDER DIFFERENCES IN COMORBIDITY

Sharp and colleagues, studying a clinical sample of 42 girls and 56 boys with ADHD combined type, found few gender differences in ADHD ratings, comorbidity, and treatment response (27). An earlier study by Berry et al. had found that, within an ADD *with* hyperactivity group, girls demonstrated more severe cognitive impairments than boys, particularly in language function (28). Girls were also comparatively younger at the time of referral. Boys manifested more disruptive behaviors. In contrast, within the ADD *without* hyperactivity group, the girls were significantly older than the boys and demonstrated lower self-esteem. The sample came from children being evaluated at a learning disorders unit and a pediatric neurology clinic. An inventory paralleling DSM-III criteria was used. While the sample may have been biased by its referral source, the study results suggest subtype differences between genders in behavior, cognition, and comorbidity.

My colleagues and I obtained data from a large sample of twins and siblings consisting of 2,173 males (mean age 10.69 years) and 2,197 females (mean age 10.75) years, from the Australian Twin Study of ADHD (29). Through mailed DSM-I–based questionnaires, we investigated patterns of comorbidity in the three DSM-IV subtypes of ADHD: 1) predominantly inattentive, 2) predominantly hyperactive-impulsive, and 3) combined, with oppositional defiant disorder, conduct disorder, separation disorder, speech, and reading problems. The findings indicated there were no significant gender differences in comorbidity for externalizing disorders but separation anxiety was greater in females than males in the inattentive subtype. The greater separation anxiety in inattentive girls could be a manifestation of developmental immaturity, possibly suggesting a different etiology or developmental path for this subtype in girls. These results may reflect the community source of the sample given that boys manifest more externalizing disorder in clinical samples.

LEARNING SUBTYPES

Willcutt and colleagues utilized a community sample of 373 twin pairs ranging from 8 to 18 years old in which at least one twin exhibited a history of learning disability, to examine the etiology of inattention and hyperactivity-impulsity (Hyp/Imp). Their results showed that extreme inattention scores were highly heritable whether or not the proband exhibited extreme Hyp/Imp. In contrast, the heritability of extreme Hyp/Imp increased as a linear function of the number of inattention symptoms exhibited. The conclusion was that extreme Hyp/Imp might be attributable to different etiologic influences depending on the presence or absence of extreme inattention (30).

The same research team also showed that approximately 95% of the phenotypic covariance between reading disability (RD) and symptoms of inattention was attributable to common genetic influences, whereas the same was only true of 21% of the phenotypic overlap between RD and Hyp/Imp (31).

TREATMENT

Treatment for boys and girls is essentially similar. Sharp and colleagues found that girls exhibited beneficial effects of stimulant medications similar to those exhibited by boys (27). They suggested that both methylphenidate and dextroamphetamine should be tried if response to one or the other was not optimal. Recent developments of slow-release stimulant medications allow single daily dose regimens, but their comparative value remains to be evaluated.

IMPLICATIONS FOR CARERS

Caring for a child who has ADHD is both demanding and unrelenting, particularly for mothers, many of whom may be single or lacking in support. This has implications for individuals and for policy. At the individual level, parents are called upon to support and treat a child who demands more care and structure for a longer period of time than other children. Single mothers may have several children for whom they carry responsibility and are likely to be stressed, with little financial or social support. In addition, ADHD medications tend to be expensive, particularly the recent slow-release preparations. Thus, at the policy level, provision should be made to support families whose children need care and whose treatment involves great expense relative to other children. In these respects, ADHD should be regarded as a developmental disability. There are also educational implications for increased support at primary and high school levels, including remediation for language and learning problems. Children from low socioeconomic status and deprived backgrounds are particularly at risk, as they often lack access to treatment or remedial programs.

FUTURE APPROACHES

Gender differences in subtypes, including comorbidity, can be identified by twin and genetic approaches, while pharmacogenomic studies may, in the future, identify differences or similarities in medication response. Also, further prospective outcome studies such as that of Dalsgard and colleagues (15) should help to identify similarities and differences between developmental pathways for girls and those for boys.

REFERENCES

1. Buitelaar JK. Epidemiological aspects and what we have learned over the last decade. In: Hyperactivity and Attention Disorders of Childhood, Sandberg S, ed. Cambridge: Cambridge University Press, 2002:30–63.
2. Eiraldi RB, Power TJ, Maguth Nezu C. Patterns of comorbidity associated with subtypes of attention-deficit/hyperactivity disorder among 6- to 12-year-old children. J Am Acad Child Adolesc Psychiatry 1997;36:503–514.
3. Faraone SV, Biederman J, Keenan K, et al. Separation of DSM-III attention deficit disorder and conduct disorder: evidence from a family genetic study of American child psychiatric patients. Psychol Med 1991;21:109–121.
4. Rhee SH, Waldman ID, Hay DA, et al. Sex differences in genetic and environmental influences on DSM-III-R Attention Deficit Hyperactivity Disorder (ADHD) J Abnorm Psychol 1999;108:24–41.
5. Rhee SH, Waldman ID, Hay DA, et al. Aetiology of sex differences in the prevalence of DSM-III-R ADHD: a comparison of two models. In: Levy F, Hay DA, eds. Attention Genes and ADHD. Philadelphia: Brunner-Routledge, 2001.
6. Heptinstall E, Taylor E. Sex differences and their significance. In: Hyperactivity and Attention Disorders of Childhood, Sandberg S, ed. Cambridge: Cambridge University Press, 2002:99–125.
7. Graetz BW, Sawyer M, Hazell PL, et al. Validity of DSM-IV ADHD subtypes in a nationally representative sample of Australian children and adolescents. J Am Acad Child Adolesc Psychiatry 2001;40:1410–1417.
8. Gaub M, Carlson CL. Gender differences in ADHD: a meta-analysis and critical review. J Am Acad Child Adolesc Psychiatry 1997;36:1036–1045.
9. Abikoff HB, Jensen PS, Arnold LL, et al. Observed classroom behavior of children with ADHD: relationship to gender and comorbidity. J Abnorm Child Psychol 2002;30:349–359.

10. Gershon J. A meta-analytic review of gender differences in ADHD. J Attention Dis 2002;5:143–154.
11. Rietveld MJH, Hudziak JJ, Bartels M, et al. Heritability of attention problems in children: I. Cross-sectional results from a study of twins, age 3–12 years. Am J Med Genet 2003;117B:102–113.
12. Kraemer S. The fragile male. Br Med J 2000;321:1609–1612.
13. Andersen SL, Teicher MH. Sex differences in dopamine receptors and their relevance to ADHD. Neurosci Biobehav Rev 2000;24:137–141.
14. Rucklidge JJ, Tannock R. Psychiatric, psychosocial, and cognitive functioning of female adolescents with ADHD. J Am Acad Child Adolesc Psychiatry 2001;40:530–540.
15. Dalsgaard S, Mortensen PB, Frydenberg M, et al. Conduct problems, gender, and adult psychiatric outcome of children with attention-deficit hyperactivity disorder. Br J Psychiatry 2002;181:416–421.
16. Biederman J, Faraone SV, Monuteaux MC. Differential effect of environmental adversity by gender: Rutter's index of adversity in a group of boys and girls with and without ADHD. Am J Psychiatry 2002;159:1556–1562.
17. Biederman J, Mick E, Faraone SV, et al. Influence of gender on attention deficit hyperactivity disorder in children referred to a psychiatric clinic. J Am Acad Child Adolesc Psychiatry 2002;159:36–42.
18. Levy F, Hay DA, McStephen M, et al. Attention-deficit hyperactivity disorder: a category or a continuum? Genetic analysis of a large-scale twin study. J. Am Acad Child Adolesc Psychiatry 1997;36:737–744.
19. Langbehn DR, Cadoret RJ, Yates WR, et al. Distinct contributions of conduct and oppositional defiant symptoms to adult antisocial behavior: evidence from an adoption study. Arch Gen Psychiatry 1998;55:821–829.
20. Thapar A, Harrington R, McGuffin P. Examining the comorbidity of ADHD-related behaviours and conduct problems using a twin study design. Br J Psychiatry 2001;179:224–229.
21. Levy F. Molecular genetics of ADHD: prospects for novel therapies. Expert Rev Neurother 2002;2:491–497.
22. Waldman ID, Rhee SH, Levy F, et al. Causes of the overlap among symptoms of ADHD, oppositional defiant disorder, and conduct disorder. In: Levy F, Hay D, eds. Attention, Genes and ADHD. Philadelphia: Brunner-Routledge, 2001.
23. Grigorenko EL, Wood FB, Meyer MS, et al. Susceptibility loci for distinct components of developmental dyslexia on chromosomes 6 and 15. Am J Human Genet 1997;60:27–39.
24. Grigorenko EL. Developmental dyslexia: an update on genes, brains, and environments. J Child Psychol Psychiatry 2001;1:91–125.
25. Alarcon M, DeFries JC. Reading performance and general cognitive ability in twins with reading difficulties and control pairs. Pers Individ Diff 1997;22:793–803.
26. Cardon LR, Smith SD, Fulker DW, et al. Quantitive trait locus for reading disability on chromosome 6. Science 1994;266:276–279.
27. Sharp WS, Walter JM, Marsh WL. et al. ADHD in girls: clinical comparability of a research sample. J Am Acad Child Adolesc Psychiatry 1999;38:40–47.
28. Berry CA, Shaywitz SE, Shaywitz BA. Girls with attention deficit disorder: a silent minority? A report on behavioral and cognitive characteristics. Pediatrics 1985;76:801–809.
29. Levy F, Hay D, Bennett K, et al. (Submitted). Gender differences in ADHD subtype comorbidity.
30. Wilcutt EG, Pennington BF, DeFries JC. Etiology of inattention and hyperactivity/impulsivity in a community sample of twins with learning difficulties. J Abnorm Child Psychol 2000;28:149–158.
31. Willcutt EG, Pennington BF, DeFries JC. A twin study of comorbidity between reading disability and attention-deficit/hyperactivity disorder. Am J Med Genetics (Neuropsychiatr Genetics) 2000;96:293–301.

SUGGESTED READINGS

Faraone SV, Biederman J, Chen WJ, et al. Genetic heterogeneity in attention-deficit hyperactivity disorder (ADHD): gender, psychiatric comorbidity, and maternal ADHD. J Abnorm Psychol 1995;104:334–345.
Neuman RJ, Heath AC, Reich W, et al. Latent class analysis of ADHD and comorbid symptoms in a population sample of adolescent female twins. J Child Psychol Psychiatry 2001;42:933–942.
Rhee SH, Waldman ID, Hay DA, Levy F. Aetiology of sex differences in the prevalence of DSM-III-R ADHD: a comparison of two models. In: Levy F, Hay DA, eds. Attention Genes and ADHD. Philadelphia: Brunner-Routledge, 2001.
Sharp WS, Walter JM, Marsh WL, et al. ADHD in girls: clinical comparability of a research sample. J Am Acad Child Adolesc Psychiatry 1999;38:40–47.

CHAPTER 7

Conduct Disorders in Girls

Ellen L. Lipman, David R. Offord*

WHAT IS IT?

Conduct disorder, as defined by the *Diagnostic and Statistical Manual of Mental Disorders*, 4th edition (DSM-IV), identifies individuals with "a repetitive and persistent pattern of behavior in which the basic rights of others or major age-appropriate societal norms or rules are violated" (see Table 7.1) (1). These behaviors manifest as aggression to people and animals (e.g., physical fights, cruelty to animals), destruction of property (e.g., fire setting), deceitfulness, or theft (e.g., breaking into someone's house), and/or other serious violations of rules (e.g., often truancy from school). To meet DSM-IV criteria for the disorder, at least three of 15 possible behaviors must have been present in the past 12 months, with at least one in the past six months. Specifiers include type, based on age of onset (childhood onset or adolescent onset), and severity, based on number or harmfulness of symptoms (mild, moderate, severe). Conduct disorder differs from delinquency, which refers to involvement with the police and/or court system for breaking the law. Delinquents make up a portion of the individuals with conduct disorder.

In this chapter, we focus on girls with conduct disorder, a group that has been understudied. The aim of this chapter is to present updated prevalence estimates, review biologic and psychosocial risk and protective factors, and outline course and long-term outcomes.

*Deceased

93

TABLE 7.1

DSM-IV Diagnostic Criteria for Conduct Disorder

A. A repetitive and persistent pattern of behavior in which the basic rights of others or major age-appropriate societal norms or rules are violated as manifested by the presence of three (or more) of the following criteria in the past 12 months, with at least one criterion present in the past 6 months:

Aggression to People and Animals
　　(1) often bullies, threatens, or intimidates others
　　(2) often initiates physical fights
　　(3) has used a weapon that can cause serious physical harm to others (e.g., a bat, brick, broken bottle, knife, gun)
　　(4) has been physically cruel to people
　　(5) has been physically cruel to animals
　　(6) has stolen while confronting a victim (e.g., mugging, purse snatching, extortion, armed robbery)
　　(7) has forced someone into sexual activity

Destruction of Property
　　(8) has deliberately engaged in fire setting with the intention of causing serious damage
　　(9) has deliberately destroyed others' property (other than by fire setting)

Deceitfulness or Theft
　　(10) has broken into someone else's house, building, or car
　　(11) often lies to obtain goods or favors or to avoid obligations (i.e., "cons" others)
　　(12) has stolen items of nontrivial value without confronting a victim (e.g., shoplifting, but without breaking and entering; forgery)

Serious Violations of Rules
　　(13) often stays out at night despite parental prohibitions, beginning before age 13 years
　　(14) has run away from home overnight at least twice while living in parental or parental surrogate home (or once without returning for a lengthy period)
　　(15) is often truant from school, beginning before age 13 years

B. The disturbance in behavior causes clinically significant impairment in social, academic, or occupational functioning.

C. If the individual is age 18 years or older, criteria are not met for antisocial personality disorder.

Specifiers
1. Type based on age at onset:
　　a. Childhood-onset type: onset of at least one criterion characteristic of conduct disorder prior to age 10 years
　　b. Adolescent-onset type: absence of any criteria characteristic of conduct disorder prior to age 10 years
2. Severity:
　　a. Mild: few if any conduct problems in excess of those required to make the diagnosis and conduct problems cause only minor harm to others
　　b. Moderate: number of conduct problems and effect on others intermediate between "mild" and "severe"
　　c. Severe: many conduct problems in excess of those required to make the diagnosis or conduct problems cause considerable harm to others

Adapted from American Psychiatric Association, Diagnostic and Statistical Modified Manual of Mental Disorders 4th Ed. Washington, DC: 1994:90–91.

PREVALENCE AND IMPAIRMENT

PREVALENCE

The prevalence of conduct disorder varies according to populations sampled (clinical or community), age of child, gender, and the informant. Within clinical populations, conduct disorder is among the most common reasons for referral. Data collected using the Brief Child and Family Phone Interview (2) on over 10,000 children and adolescents 6 to 18 years old who were referred to a children's mental health center in Ontario between March 2000 and June 2003 demonstrate that 37.7% of parents endorse behaviors consistent with conduct disorder at the time of intake (see Table 7.2). Rates vary slightly by gender, with girls demonstrating slightly higher rates (girls 39.7%, 40.0%, and 39.3% for 6–18, 6–11, and 12–18 years, respectively; boys 36.4%, 36.3%, and 36.5% for the same age ranges).

General population estimates based on epidemiologic studies of behavior problems for children and adolescents 4–18 years old throughout the world range from 0.0 to 11.9% (median 2.0%) (3). Canadian data from the Ontario Child Health Study, a community-based study of 4- to 16-year-olds in Ontario completed in 1983 with follow-up in 1987, estimated prevalence at 5.5% for 4- to 16-year-olds in Ontario. Prevalence rates vary by age and gender, with higher rates reported for boys than girls and in older than younger children (girls 2.7%, 1.8%, and 4.1% for 4–16, 4–11, and 12–16 years, respectively; boys 8.1%, 6.5%, and 10.4% for the same ages) (4).

Although the prevalence of conduct disorder in the general or in specific populations is important, several issues must be recognized. First, the prevalence of a disorder depends on the threshold and therefore is somewhat arbitrary. For example, DSM-IV requires three of 15 symptoms for diagnosis (1). Changing the threshold to two or four of 15 symptoms will increase or lower the prevalence of disorder respectively. Second, within the system of psychiatric classification, diagnostic criteria for conduct disorder have changed over time, as some criteria have been modified and others added or withdrawn. Changing the behaviors required to meet criteria for conduct disorder can also influence prevalence.

Understanding differences in the rates of conduct disorder between girls and boys has been of interest to researchers in the field. It has been suggested that these differing rates reflect true differences in conduct disorder between girls and boys that arise because of differing social and cultural expectations for each sex (5). Others have argued that the establishment of DSM criteria for conduct disorder came primarily from studies of boys, and that a different definition should be used for girls with conduct disorder (6). For example, in a sample of girls representative of the general population in Quebec who demonstrated persistent antisocial behaviors from ages 6 to 10 years, only 3% met DSM-III-R criteria for conduct disorder (7), prompting the investigators to question the adequacy of the definition or criteria for conduct disorder for girls. Ideas for modification of the definition include setting gender-specific thresholds for conduct disorder or including different behaviors in the criteria for disorder (6). One investigation testing the prevalence of conduct disorder using gender-specific thresholds among children with comorbid attention deficit hyperactivity did not support a difference in diagnostic threshold by gender (8).

TABLE 7.2

Rates of Conduct Disorder and Other Disorders[a] Among Children Referred to Children's Mental Health Clinics in Ontario (May 2000 to June 2003)

Age (years)	Disorder (%) by Age and Gender[b]											
	Conduct		Attention		Oppositional Defiant Disorder		Separation Anxiety		Generalized Anxiety Disorder		Mood	
	F	M	F	M	F	M	F	M	F	M	F	M
6–18	37.7		42.6		51.8		20.5		20.5		40.8	
(n)	(10,065)		(10,119)		(10,098)		(10,060)		(10,052)		(10,028)	
6–18	39.7	36.4	44.7	41.3	56.4	48.9	22.4	19.3	22.3	19.4	43.9	38.8
(n)	(1,548)	(2,245)	(1,752)	(2,562)	(2,208)	(3,025)	(876)	(1,189)	(870)	(1,194)	(1,708)	(2,383)
6–11	40.0	36.3	46.9	38.9	54.3	47.8	26.8	18.7	23.3	19.3	36.9	36.6
(n)	(771)	(1,414)	(909)	(1,523)	(1,052)	(1,864)	(517)	(727)	(450)	(749)	(706)	(1,419)
12–18	39.3	36.5	42.5	45.6	58.3	51.0	18.2	20.4	21.7	19.7	50.8	42.7
(n)	(777)	(831)	(843)	(1,039)	(1,156)	(1,161)	(359)	(462)	(420)	(445)	(1,002)	(964)

[a]Classification of disorder based on scores on Brief Child and Family Phone Interview set at >2 standard deviations above mean score of general population sample of children aged 6–18 years.
[b] F= female, M= male.

Many of the behaviors included in conduct disorder reflect physical or direct aggression, which is more common among boys and in minor forms considered normal. Up to about 4 years of age, girls and boys generally show equal rates of aggressive behaviors. After that, rates of physically aggressive behaviors increase in boys. Data from the 1994 National Longitudinal Survey of Children and Youth (NLSCY), a long-term survey of child development and well-being in Canada, that examined physical aggression among girls and boys, suggest that differences among girls and boys may emerge earlier, since mean physical aggression scores were found to be elevated among boys as early as ages 2 to 3 years (9).

The concept of indirect or social aggression (harm caused in the context of social relationships) is thought to better represent female aggression. Peer interactions for girls in early and middle childhood are generally with other girls, and formation of close relationships is important during this developmental stage, so attempts to hurt others through disruption or control of peer relationships are potent aggressive behaviors. Girls rate social aggression as being more harmful than boys do, and rate it as harmful as physical aggression (10). In interpersonal problem situations, aggressive girls prefer relationally or indirectly aggressive solutions, whereas aggressive boys prefer overtly physical or directly aggressive solutions.

The National Longitudinal Survey of Children and Youth collected information on both physically and socially aggressive behaviors. These are demonstrated in Table 7.3 (4). Higher rates of physically aggressive behaviors are reported for boys than for girls in both age groups (4–7 and 8–11 years old). Female:male ratios of direct aggression behaviors range from 26.3% to 76.4%, with the biggest female:male discrepancy emerging for the most aggressive behavior, "physically attacks people" (lowest ratio of 0.5:1.9 or 26.3%). Female:male ratios for 8-year olds to 11-year-olds are slightly greater, with "physically attacks people" remaining at the lowest ratio (41.2%). The behavior "threatens people," the least aggressive behavior in the direct aggression list, is greater among girls in the older age group (female:male ratio, 171.4%). Rates of indirect or social aggression are higher among girls than boys in both age groups (4–7 and 8–11 years), with rates of socially aggressive behaviors reported increasing with age for girls compared with boys.

IMPAIRMENT

A heavy burden of suffering is associated with conduct disorder. This is due to the high prevalence; the associated impairments in behavioral, social, and academic functioning; the persistence of difficulties for many into the adult years; and the substantial costs of resources utilized by individuals with conduct disorder, their families, and their victims in the health and judicial systems to name a few.

Comorbidity is common among children and adolescents with conduct disorder. Other disruptive behavior or externalizing disorders, attention deficit hyperactivity disorder, and oppositional defiant disorder are among the most frequent comorbid conditions. The internalizing disorders, mood and anxiety disorders, also can co-occur. In a Canadian general population sample of children 4 to 11 years old from the National Longitudinal Survey of Children and Youth, under half of children with conduct disorder had it as a single disorder (11). Parents reported that over one third of children with conduct disorder had comorbid hyperactivity

TABLE 7.3

Prevalence of Indirect and Direct Aggression Symptoms[a] by Age[b] and Gender[c]

	Prevalence (%)					
	Age					
	4–7			8–11		
Symptoms	F	M	F:M Ratio	F	M	F:M Ratio
Indirect Aggression						
When mad at someone,						
Tries to get others to dislike that person	1.8	1.5	1.20	2.8	1.8	1.56
Becomes friends with another as revenge	1.9	1.3	1.46	2.4	0.8	3.00
Says bad things behind the person's back	1.6	1.6	1.00	2.3	2.2	1.05
Says to others: "Let's not be with her/him"	2.3	1.5	1.53	2.8	1.5	1.87
Tells the person's secrets to a third person	1.9	1.0	1.90	2.0	1.1	1.82
Direct Aggression						
Gets into fights	3.2	5.1	0.63	3.8	4.7	0.81
When another child accidentally hurts her/him (such as by bumping into her/him), assumes the child meant to do it and then reacts with anger and fighting	5.5	7.2	0.76	4.4	6.9	0.64
Physically attacks people	0.5	1.9	0.26	0.7	1.7	0.41
Threatens people	0.8	1.1	0.73	1.2	0.7	1.71
Is cruel, bullies, or is mean to others	0.5	1.1	0.46	0.4	0.6	0.67
Kicks, bites, hits other children	0.4	1.6	0.25	0.5	1.1	0.45

[a]Prevalence estimates from National Longitudinal Survey of Children and Youth (Cycle 1, 1994). Note prevalence estimates ≤ 2.0 are unstable, and should be interpreted with caution.
[b]Age in years.
[c]F= female, M= male.

Adapted from Offord DR, Lipman EL. Emotional and behavioural problems: frequency by age, gender and income level and co-occurrence with other problems. In: Growing Up in Canada. National Longitudinal Survey of Children and Youth. Human Resources Development Canada, Statistics Canada, Ottawa. Catalogue no 89-550-MPE, 1996:121.

(38.0%), one third had difficulties with comorbid feelings of anxiety and depression (35.5%), and one fifth had difficulties with both hyperactivity and anxious/depressive feelings (19.0%) (see Figure 7.1) (11). Comorbid anxious and depressive feelings are more common in girls than boys, particularly as girls become adolescents.

Rates of comorbid conditions are often higher in clinical populations (see Table 7.4). Conduct disorder occurs concommitantly with a range of disorders, with the highest rates of comorbidity occurring with difficulties with attention and oppositional behavior. Rates of comorbidity between conduct disorder and difficulties with attention, oppositional behavior, and mood were generally elevated among girls compared with boys. For example, attention difficulties and conduct disorder co-occurred in 61.0%, 64.0%, and 58.1% of girls 6–18, 6–11, and 12–18

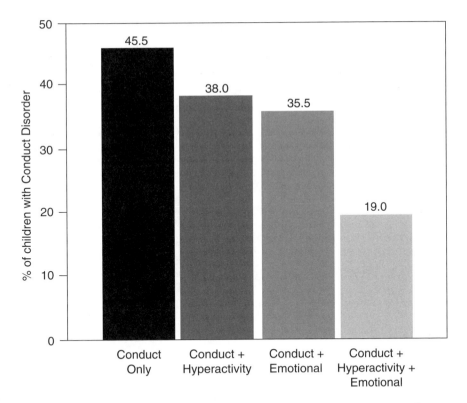

FIGURE 7.1 ● Comorbidity of hyperactivity and emotional disorder in a general population sample aged 4 to 11 years. Emotional disorder is indicated by the responses "seems unhappy, sad, depressed," "not as happy as other children," "too fearful or anxious," "worried," "cries a lot," "nervous, high-strung, tense," "trouble enjoying her/himself," "appears miserable, unhappy, tearful, or distressed." (Figure adapted from Offord DR, Lipman EL. Emotional and behavioural problems: frequency by age, gender and income level and co-occurrence with other problems. In: Growing up in Canada. National Longitudinal Survey of Children and Youth. Human Resources Development Canada, Statistics Canada, Ottawa. Catalogue no 89-550-MPE, 1996:124.)

years old, respectively, while rates for boys were 58.6%, 56.4%, and 62.5% for the same ages (see Table 7.4).

Other difficulties that commonly co-occur with conduct disorder are academic difficulties and impairment in social relationships. Data from the NLSCY demonstrate that among children with one or more behavioral or emotional problems, one tenth (12.1%) had academic difficulties (repeating a grade), one tenth (10.8%) had difficulties in social relationships, and 1.5% had both academic and social difficulties (11).

Among girls, the risk of anxiety and depression increases in adolescence, so increased rates of comorbidity for these disorders with conduct disorder are expected. This is described as a gender paradox, since the gender with the lower prevalence of conduct disorder (girls) is at higher risk to develop a more rare comorbid condition. Substance use (e.g., alcohol and marijuana) is elevated among adolescent girls with conduct disorder compared with boys (12) and may be influenced by depressive symptoms.

In addition to the gender paradox described above, other patterns of comorbidity may influence girls and boys differently. For example, boys with conduct

TABLE 7.4

Rates of Comorbidity[a] with Conduct Disorder[a] Among Children Referred to Children's Mental Health Clinics in Ontario (May 2000 to June 2003)

Age (years)	Comorbid Disorder[a] (%) by Age and Gender[b]									
	Attention		Oppositional Defiant Disorder		Separation Anxiety		Generalized Anxiety Disorder		Mood	
6–18	59.6		74.0		21.6		19.4		49.3	
(n)	(2,258)		(2,801)		(815)		(729)		(1,852)	
	F	M	F	M	F	M	F	M	F	M
6–18	61.0	58.6	78.2	71.1	20.6	22.3	20.5	18.5	51.0	48.5
(n)	(942)	(1,316)	(1,209)	(1,592)	(317)	(498)	(316)	(413)	(783)	(1,069)
6–11	64.0	56.4	76.4	70.4	23.5	21.7	21.4	19.7	44.1	47.0
(n)	(492)	(797)	(588)	(993)	(180)	(306)	(164)	(277)	(337)	(658)
12–18	58.1	62.5	80.0	72.2	17.7	23.2	19.7	16.5	57.8	49.9
(n)	(450)	(519)	(621)	(599)	(137)	(192)	(152)	(136)	(446)	(411)

[a]Classification of disorder based on scores on Brief Child and Family Phone Interview set at >2 standard deviations above mean score of general population sample aged 6 to 18 years.
[b] F= female, M= male.

disorder and attention deficit hyperactivity disorder (ADHD) have a worse outcome than boys with conduct disorder alone. Less is known about ADHD and conduct disorder in girls, although it has been suggested that girls with ADHD have a higher than expected chance of conduct disorder, despite a lower prevalence rate of both disorders in girls. Anxiety disorders may also influence girls and boys differently. Boys with early anxiety only have a decreased rate of conduct problems later, while those with both anxiety and aggression do worse. Further work is needed to try to understand these complex relationships among disorders and related influences of gender.

RISK AND PROTECTIVE FACTORS

RISK FACTORS

A substantial number of risk and protective factors have been identified for conduct disorder. The information that follows is not an exhaustive list, and is divided broadly into biologic and psychosocial factors. Emphasis is on newer and novel work in this area.

Biologic risk factors that have been identified to be associated with conduct disorder include physiologic arousal, prenatal and perinatal factors, and genetic factors. Physiologic underarousal has been measured in children with conduct disorder as manifested by decreased sensitivity to pain, lower resting heart rate, and decreased cortisol levels. Only heart rate studies have included girls (13). Among girls with aggression measured at age 11, there was a significant association with low resting heart rate at age 3, even after controlling for biologic, psychological, and psychiatric confounding factors (13). Girls with conduct disorder admitted to a psychiatric inpatient unit had significantly lower heart rates than other inpatients without conduct disorder (14). Physiologic underarousal in youth has been shown to be associated with later criminality (15).

Prenatal and perinatal risk factors have been associated generally with behavior problems in children. Maternal substance use, specifically smoking during pregnancy and persistent smoking during and after pregnancy, has been associated with conduct disorder in girls and boys. A strong dose–response relationship has been demonstrated, with the strength of association between smoking and conduct problems as great or greater among girls as boys (16). In comparison with children whose mothers were nonsmokers during pregnancy, the odds of childhood-onset conduct problems were greater among girls of mothers who smoked during pregnancy than among boys (relative odds with increasing levels of maternal smoking were 2.17–3.04 for girls and 1.47–2.07 for boys) (16). The association between conduct problems and omega-3 fatty acid intake is also of interest. It has been demonstrated that increased levels of dietary intake of fish and polyunsaturated fatty acids are associated with decreases in hostile and aggressive behaviors in young adults (17). Lower consumption of omega-3 fatty acids from seafood during pregnancy has also been associated with increased maternal depressive symptoms, even after accounting for other risk factors associated with depression during pregnancy and more broadly. Following these lines of investigation, current work is examining whether varying levels of omega-3 fatty acid consumption during pregnancy are associated with varying levels of conduct problems in children, and whether this varies by gender.

Antisocial behaviors tend to aggregate in families, and genetic factors have been implicated in some disruptive behavior disorders (e.g., ADHD). Familial aggregation of conduct problems has been demonstrated in the general population and in clinical populations, although this may represent genetic or environmental factors or an interaction between the two. One study of girls demonstrated patterns of familial association for comorbid conduct disorder and ADHD, although no pure conduct disorder group was studied and the number of girls with this comorbid condition was small (18). Several twin studies have examined the influence of genetic factors and conduct disorder, but issues of variation related to developmental stage, informant, and measurement and their impact of the genetic factors and conduct disorder remain to be resolved.

Other biologic risk factors for conduct disorder that are the topic of active investigation include abnormalities in neurotransmitters (e.g., low levels of serotonin in the central nervous system and aggression), neuroanatomical variations (e.g., frontal lobe damage or dysfunction), and other neurochemicals (e.g., decreased salivary cortisol levels, testosterone). Child temperament is also thought to have a biologic basis, to be related to later externalizing problems, and to differ in girls and boys. Children who had a "difficult to manage" temperament measured at age 3 have higher rates of delinquency at age 11 (19).

Psychosocial risk factors will be divided into family, peer, and community risk factors. Family risk factors include parental psychopathology, parenting practices, attachment, and stressful events. Parental psychopathology may work through multiple mechanisms (as above). In addition to parental antisocial behaviors as a risk factor for conduct disorder, maternal depression is associated with child disruptive behavior. A recent meta-analysis of observational studies of depression and parenting revealed a strong association between maternal depression (either current or lifetime) and negative and coercive behaviors (20), and coercive parenting has been linked with child difficulties (see below). Lower engagement and fewer positive interactions were also demonstrated (20). Work in this field is influenced by debate over the extent to which maternal depressive symptomatology influences mothers' ratings of their children's behavior, and relationships between maternal depression and child behavior problems may be bidirectional.

Parenting practices characterized by lack of warmth or involvement, poor supervision, parent–child conflict, and discipline styles that are inconsistent or harsh have been found to be associated with disruptive behaviors in children. Coercive parent–child interactions take place in many families of children with conduct problems and have been linked to child difficulties across a range of developmental stages. The relationship between parenting practices and child behavior is bidirectional, and interventions that focus on parenting practices have shown some success among children with conduct disorder and their families. Many of the studies in this area have been done with males, and since parents tend to interact differently with their daughters and sons, the relationship between coercive parenting practices and outcomes may be different for girls' than for boys' outcomes. One study examining girls and boys from preschool to school age found that coercive parent–child interactions in the preschool years predicted continued aggressive behavior at school age for boys but not for girls (21). Further work is needed to identify whether coercive parenting and other parenting practices may influence the development of conduct disorder in girls.

Attachment between a child and parent depends on the child's perception of parental availability and responsiveness to his or her needs. Attachment quality is thought to influence a child's internal representational models of relationships, which develop during the first year of life, and a child's future relationships. Insecure attachment types (insecure-avoidant, insecure-ambivalent/resistant, insecure-disorganized/disoriented) are thought to develop from inconsistent and unresponsive parenting practices, and insecure attachment has been linked to difficulties with anger and in social relationships in young children. However, findings from the work in this area are inconsistent, and more study is needed.

Stressful events classified as family risk factors include marital conflict, high levels of family stress, large family size, parental separation or divorce, and child abuse and neglect. The first four factors listed have been associated with later violence, aggressive behavior, or criminal conviction in some studies, although not consistently. Child abuse and neglect have been associated with conduct disorder in children, and this is thought to be partially mediated through the development of difficulties in social information processing, which may occur as a consequence of abuse (see below). Difficulties with violence and criminality later in life have also been documented. Differences between girls' and boys' responses to child abuse or neglect and the association with conduct disorder require further investigation, with attention to specific factors related to the abuse (e.g., whether the abuse was physical or sexual, severity and duration of the abuse, and relationship of the perpetrator to the child).

Peer risk factors include social information processing, peer group characteristics, and peer group status. Social information processing refers to how children process information about social interactions and relates to child social adjustment. Evidence has been found that some aggressive children process social information differently than nonaggressive children. They overattend to aggressive cues, underattend to nonaggressive or prosocial cues, and attribute hostile intent in ambiguous situations. This hostile attributional bias results in a reactive aggressive response by the child which she or he feels is justified. Difficulties in social information processing have been demonstrated in children as young as 4 years old, and more impairment in social information processing is thought to be related to increased aggression. Aggressive behaviors demonstrated by children vary by gender, with aggressive girls utilizing relational aggression while aggressive boys utilize physical aggression (22).

Peer group characteristics influence conduct problems. Within same-sex peer groups, girls are more likely to demonstrate relational or indirect aggression, whereas boys are more likely to demonstrate physically aggressive behaviors. Aggressive preschoolers are more likely to associate with other aggressive children, and this may continue through adolescence. Deviancy training may occur within groups of aggressive youth by their encouraging and reinforcing one another's deviant behavior, and it may lead to delinquency and other difficulties (e.g., substance use). Girls with early pubertal maturation more commonly associate with deviant peers (23), although whether early puberty in and of itself represents a risk factor among girls for conduct disorder and other psychopathology is a matter of debate (24). Notably, peer group influence likely varies as a result of developmental stage, with increasing influence as children move into adolescence.

Peer group status, specifically rejection by the peer group, is often an issue for aggressive children. For girls, relational aggression is a powerful predictor of rejection, whereas for boys, physical aggression is a strong predictor of rejection. Since social relationships are of such great importance for girls, peer rejection may act as a more important risk factor for conduct disorder for girls than for boys. Children who are reactively aggressive are rated as being disliked more than children with proactive aggression. Although children with proactive aggression may be liked initially, the friendships they establish do not remain stable over time.

Community risk factors are broadly defined to include factors related to the context within which the child lives and which are outside of the family. These include socioeconomic characteristics, neighborhood characteristics, and school characteristics. Low socioeconomic status has been associated repeatedly with conduct problems. In the Ontario Child Health Study, conduct disorder was significantly associated with low income as well as other markers of low socioeconomic status (e.g., welfare status, subsidized housing, unemployment, and overcrowding). In the National Longitudinal Survey of Children and Youth, the prevalence of one or more behavioral or emotional problems, including conduct problems, increased as income decreased (11). The mechanisms through which low socioeconomic status influences child behavior are incompletely understood but likely include indirect pathways such as parenting, since poverty increases stress on parents and may decrease social support and mood as well as their ability to use optimal parenting strategies.

Certain neighborhood characteristics are more common among children with conduct-disordered behaviors. Growing up in a neighborhood that is disadvantaged often means living in a public housing project; exposure to violence and drug use; and lack of or poor quality child care, schools, health care, and adult-run recreational activities. In Canada, because of the nation's social welfare system, there is generally less variability in the quality of schools and health care than there is in the United States.

School characteristics may influence child aggressive behaviors. It is known that certain school features (such as good management practices in the school overall and in the classroom, and a balance of children achieving at various levels) have an impact on behavior and academic achievement. This effect is independent of the characteristics of the children at school entry. Schools may find it helpful to the children to be aware of the potential negative impact of labeling children as conduct disordered. Rather than only reacting to difficult behaviors, schools may be able to help children by providing nonstigmatizing programs universally or various targeted levels to foster prosocial behavior.

PROTECTIVE FACTORS

Protective factors for conduct disorder are sometimes the absence or opposite of the risk factors above, although some specific factors have been identified. These include resilient temperament, academic skills, child competence at a skill, child involvement with prosocial peers and organizations, noncoercive supportive and authoritative parenting practices, and a relationship with at least one supportive adult.

COURSE AND LONG-TERM OUTCOMES

COURSE

The age of onset of conduct disorder has been found to influence its developmental course. DSM-IV describes childhood-onset conduct disorder as starting earlier than 10 years of age, and adolescent-onset conduct disorder as starting at 11 years of age and up (1). These subtypes have been upheld in studies, although the data are based largely on males and it is not clear that 10 years of age is the optimal cutoff. Childhood-onset conduct disorder is thought to have a more chronic course than adolescent-onset disorder. Childhood-onset disorder is associated with numerous difficulties in adulthood, including substance use, violent criminal behavior, and partner abuse. It is also associated with an elevated number of biologic, familial, and other psychosocial risk factors. Adolescent-onset disorder is described as generally being less serious and more transitory and lacking the associated early risk factors of childhood-onset disorder.

Conduct disorder in boys may follow either the childhood-onset or the adolescent-onset pathway. Risk of serious adult difficulties for adolescent-onset conduct disorder exceeds that of controls but is less severe than that of childhood-onset disorder; it includes difficulties with employment and mental health. The majority of girls with conduct disorder are described as having a "delayed-onset," with behaviors manifesting during adolescence. However, retrospective studies of age of onset suggest that a number of girls do have childhood onset of the disorder (25). Prospective studies of the onset of conduct disorder among girls are lacking.

A number of theories have been proposed to understand the development of conduct disorder in girls. One model proposes that fewer girls exhibit childhood-onset disorder because of the biologic, cognitive, and social strengths exhibited by most girls during this developmental period (e.g., strong language skills and more prosocial responses) (26). Another theory notes that some girls subsequently diagnosed with adolescent-onset conduct disorder have risk factors similar to those of boys with childhood-onset disorder (e.g., biologic or family risk factors) but do not develop problematic behaviors until adolescence, when the behaviors appear as resistance to authority and attempts at increased autonomy (27). A further theory suggests that girls do have difficulties with childhood-onset conduct disorder but, because the definition of conduct disorder focuses on directly aggressive behaviors, the diagnosis does not capture these girls, who more commonly show relational aggression (28).

LONG-TERM OUTCOMES

Long-term outcome outcomes for conduct disorder are best evaluated using prospective general population studies. The Cambridge Study in Delinquent Development prospectively followed boys in a London working-class area from ages 8 to 32, and found aggression, unemployment, and drug and alcohol use in adulthood (29). Prospective data on girls with conduct disorder are lacking, although other studies have found that longer-term outcomes for girls with conduct disorder include antisocial personality disorder and other psychiatric disorders, early pregnancy and relationships with antisocial partners, criminal behavior, and mortality (30). Adult psychiatric morbidity has been documented in girls with conduct disorder, with rates ranging from 14% to 60% in various studies. Antisocial personality is common; it occurs in up to about one third of girls with conduct disorder. Other adult psychiatric disorders may be more common, including substance use and suicidal behavior, although not necessarily depression.

Sexual promiscuity and teen pregnancy are often correlated with conduct disorder in girls. Several studies have demonstrated that ratings of aggression completed among girls in grade school predicted early pregnancy. Girls' aggression also predicted their poor verbal and emotional responsiveness as mothers and developmental delays in their children. Delayed childbearing may not be superior, as female offenders choose a male offender more often than a male offender chooses a female offender.

High rates of criminality (33%–50% depending on the study design and sample) have been documented for girls with conduct disorder based on self-report and official (arrest) data. Delinquent girls have even more elevated rates of adult crime (up to 96%). Rates of adult crime among girls with conduct disorder exceeded those of girls with other psychiatric disorders and control girls.

Among studies of the adult outcomes of girls with conduct disorder, mortality rates varied from 0% to 11%. Although the intervals of follow-up varied considerably (from as few as 2 years to as many as 30 years), deaths occurred in early adulthood for most of the women who died.

Other adult difficulties that may occur among girls with conduct disorder include general difficulties with adult functioning, poor academic achievement, unemployment, and high rates of service utilization (e.g., physicians, welfare, child protection).

CONCLUSION

Conduct disorder is a common psychiatric disorder in the general population and in clinical populations and is associated with a variety of impairments, including comorbid psychiatric disorders and difficulties with academic and social functioning. Rates of conduct disorder are greater among boys than among girls. This may reflect the choice of behaviors included in the definition, as girls and boys tend to display differing forms of aggressive behaviors. While numerous biologic and psychosocial risk and protective factors for conduct disorder have been identified, work in understanding these factors for girls is handicapped by the paucity of studies that have included girls and by mixed findings that may relate to study methodology or the developmental stage of study participants. Similarly, study of long-term outcomes in girls has been inadequate. Improving our understanding of conduct disorder in girls is important, and more research is required in this significant area of study.[a]

REFERENCES

1. American Psychiatric Association. Diagnostic and Statistical Manual of Mental Disorders. 4th Ed. Washington, DC: 1994:85–91.
2. Cunningham CE, Pettingill P, Boyle M. Brief Child and Family Phone Interview Interviewer's Manual. Hamilton, Ontario: Canadian Centre for Studies of Children at Risk, 2001.
3. Lahey BB, Miller TL, Gordon RA, et al. Developmental epidemiology of disruptive behavior disorders. In: Quay HC, Hogan AE, eds. Handbook of Disruptive Behavior Disorders. New York: Kluwer Academic/Plenum Press, 1999:23–48.
4. Offord DR, Boyle MH, Szatmari P, et al. Ontario Child Health Study. II. Six-month prevalence of disorder and rates of service utilization. Arch Gen Psychiatry 1987;44:832–836.
5. Zahn-Waxler C. Warriors and worriers: gender and psychopathology. Dev Psychopathol 1993; 5:79–89.
6. Zoccolillo M. Gender and the development of conduct disorder. Dev Psychopathol 1993; 5:65–78.
7. Zoccolillo M, Tremblay R, Vitaro F. DSM-III–R and DSM-III criteria for conduct disorder in girls. Specific but insensitive. J Am Acad Child Adolesc Psychiatry 1996;35:461–470.
8. Doyle AE, Biederman J, Monteaux M, et al. Diagnostic threshold for conduct disorder in girls and boys. J Nerv Ment Dis 2003;191:379–386.
9. Tremblay RE, Boulerice B, Harden PW, et al. Do children in Canada become more aggressive as they approach adolescence? In: Growing Up in Canada. National Longitudinal Survey of Children and Youth. Human Resources Development Canada, Statistics Canada, Ottawa. Catalogue no 89-550-MPE, 1996:127–137.
10. Galen BR, Underwood MK. A developmental investigation of social aggression among children. Dev Psychol 1997;33:589–600.
11. Offord DR, Lipman EL. Emotional and behavioural problems frequency by age, gender, and income level and coocurrence with other problems. In: Growing Up in Canada. National Longitudinal Survey of Children and Youth. Human Resources Development Canada, Statistics Canada, Ottawa. Catalogue no 89-550-MPE, 1996:119–126.
12. Fergusson DM, Horwood LJ, Lynskey MT. The comorbidities of adolescent problem behaviors: a latent class model. J Abnorm Child Psychol 1994;22:339–354.
13. Raine A, Venables PH, Mednick SA. Low resting heart rate at 3 years old predisposes to aggression at age 11 years: evidence from the Mauritius Child Health Project. J Am Acad Child Adolesc Psychiatry 1997;36:1457–1464.
14. Rogeness GA, Cepeda C, Macedo CA, et al. Differences in heart rate and blood pressure in children with conduct disorder, major depression, and separation anxiety. Psychiatry Res 1990;33:199–206.
15. Raine A, Venables PH, Williams M. Relationships between central and autonomic measures of arousal at age 15 years and criminality at 24 years. Arch Gen Psychiatry 1990;47:1003–1007.
16. Maughan B, Taylor C, Taylor A, et al. Pregnancy, smoking, and childhood conduct problems: a causal association? J Child Psychol Psychiatry 2001;42:1021–1028.
17. Iribarren C, Markovitz JH, Jacobs DR, et al. Dietary intake of n-3, n-6 fatty acids and fish: relationship with hostility in young adults—the CARDIA study. Eur J Clin Nutr 2004;58:24–31.
18. Faraone SV, Biederman J, Monteaux MC. Attention deficit disorder and conduct disorder in girls: evidence for a familial subtype. Biol Psychiatry 2000;48:21–29.
19. White JL, Moffitt TE, Earls F, et al. How early can we tell? Predictors of childhood conduct disorder and adolescent delinquency. Criminology 1990;28:507–533.

[a] *Dr. Lipman is supported by an Intermediate Research Fellowship from the Ontario Mental Health Foundation. The authors also wish to acknowledge Ms. Marjorie Waymouth and Ms. Donna Bohaychuk for help with the BCFPI, and Dr. Harriet MacMillan and Dr. Darren Holub for helpful comments.*

20. Lovejoy MC, Graczyk PA, O'Hare E, et al. Maternal depression and parenting behavior: a meta-analytic review. Clin Psychol Rev 2000;20:561–592.
21. McFayden-Ketchum SA, Dodge KA. Problems in social relationships. In: Mash EJ, Barkley RA, eds. Treatment of Childhood Disorders, 2nd Ed. New York: Guilford, 1998:338–365.
22. Crick NR, Werner NE. Response decision processes in relational and overt aggression. Child Dev 1998;69:1630–1639.
23. Stattin H, Magnusson D. Pubertal Maturation in Female Development. Hillsdale, NJ: Erlbaum, 1990.
24. Kennan K, Loeber R, Green S. Conduct disorder in girls: a review of the literature. Clin Child Fam Psychol Rev 1999;2:3–19.
25. Tolan PH, Thomas P. The implications of age of onset for delinquency risk II. Longitudinal data. J Abnorm Child Psychol 1995;23:157–181.
26. Keenan K, Shaw DS. Developmental and social influences on young girls' early problem behavior. Psychol Bull 1997;121:95–113.
27. Silverthorn P, Frick PJ. Developmental pathways to antisocial behavior: the delayed-onset pathway in girls. Dev Psychopathol 1999;11:101–126.
28. Crick NR, Grotpeter JK. Relational aggression, gender, and social-psychological adjustment. Child Dev 1995;66:710–722.
29. Farrington DP. Childhood aggression and adult violence: early precursors and later life outcomes. In: Pepler DJ, Rubin KH, eds. The Development and Treatment of Childhood Aggression. Hillsdale NJ: Erlbaum, 1991:189–197.
30. Pajer KA. What happens to "bad" girls? Review of the adult outcomes of antisocial adolescent girls. Am J Psychiatry 1998;155:862–870.

Adolescence

Section III Summary
Commentary from New Zealand
Leah K. Andrews, M. Louise Webster

Western culture seems determined to portray adolescence as a time of great turmoil. Sex, substance use, crime, and anti-social behavior are supposedly the norm, young people never talk to their parents except to make unreasonable demands, and adolescent women in particular are seen as being at the mercy of their hormones and societal pressure, with mood swings so typical as to be unremarkable. Adolescents seem to symbolize both the best and the worst of our worlds. But what is the evidence for any of this?

Adolescence as a developmental phase for study has a relatively short history. One of the first notable books on the topic was G. Stanley Hall's 1904 Adolescence: Its Psychology and Its Relations to Anthropology, Sociology, Sex, Crime and Education (1). It is clear that Hall acknowledged the multiple influences on adolescent behavior and emotional outcomes. Some traditional cultures have not seen adolescence as a distinct developmental phase, yet current processes of globalization have had a significant impact on how societies manage transitions for youth. Such issues are highlighted by researchers in New Zealand studying Samoan girls' views of themselves (2) in a culture where adolescence is not generally recognized, or in New Zealand Maori rangatahi (teenagers') discussion of their body image (3).

A steep rise in many "adult-type" mental health problems occurs at adolescence, and gender differences in prevalence of disorder also become far more marked than in childhood. Suicide attempts, anxiety and depressive disorders, and eating disorders are all more common in adolescent girls than boys (4). Adolescent girls have traditionally shown lower rates of substance abuse, antisocial behavior, and completed suicide, but even these rates are rising to match those of boys (5). Although no gender difference is found in attachment security in early childhood, in adolescent girls we find a higher rate of emerging borderline personality disorder and a greater vulnerability to developing post-traumatic stress disorder (6).

Powerful media portrayals of young women's lives also play a significant role in their socialization. In many societies, a huge shift has occurred from the expectation that women's lives would be devoted to family to the idea that combined career and childrearing are possible for all. The social construction of adolescence in girls is beyond the focus of this book, but it has a strong role in parental and institutional uncertainty in interpreting, labeling, and managing the behavior and emotions of young women.

Evidence-based approaches are teaching us to be far more cautious about data. We are learning that studies that don't separate findings by gender may not provide answers for women's health. Likewise, we need to consider how the age and culture of subjects in studies may influence results. The chapters in this section are exciting because they begin to address these important matters.

Bulik and Reba's Chapter 8 on eating disorders and body image in adolescence shows a wide appreciation of the complexities of adolescent girls' lives, particularly the issue of culture and exposure to Western media and its interaction with genetic factors in the production of eating problems.

Differences between the sexes in the onset and course of psychosis are also explored by Addington and Schultze-Lutter, who speculate on the role of stress and the hypothalamic-pituitary axis in Chapter 9.

Adolescent girls who abuse substances are influenced by a complex web of biologic, family, peer, and sociocultural influences, and these influences are explored in a reasoned and probing manner in Chapter 10.

In Chapter 11 on the neurobiologic correlates of disorders of emotional regulation, Lanius, Bluhm, and Pain draw interesting parallels between chronic post-traumatic stress disorder and borderline personality disorder, suggesting that girls are especially vulnerable because they are more likely to experience sexual abuse.

Finally, we must remember the success of young women; large-scale surveys of adolescent girls show that the majority are fine. In a self-report survey of almost 10,000 secondary school students in New Zealand, 80% of students felt healthy, did not engage in risky behaviors, and reported positive connections to school, family, and peers (7). Much can be learned by studying the factors that promote such positive outcomes.

REFERENCES

1. Hall G. Adolescence: Its Psychology and Its Relations to Anthropology, Sociology, Sex, Crime and Education. New York: Appleton; 1904.
2. Tupuola A-M. "Adolescence": myth or reality for Samoan women? Beyond the stage-like toward shifting boundaries and identities. Unpublished Ph.D. dissertation. Wellington, NZ: Education, Victoria University of Wellington, 1998.
3. Moewaka-Barnes H, Borell B. Not too fat and not too skinny: a study of body perceptions and influences with female rangatahi. Auckland, New Zealand: Whariki Research Group, Alcohol and Public Health Research Unit, University of Auckland.; 2002.
4. Fergusson D, Horwood L. The Christchurch Health and Development Study: review of findings on child and adolescent mental health. Aust NZ J Psychiatry 2001;35(3):287–296.
5. McCabe K, Rodgers C, Yeh M, et al. Gender differences in childhood onset conduct disorder. Dev Psychopathology. 2004;16(1):179–192.
6. Allen J, Land D. Attachment in adolescence. In: Cassidy J, Shaver PR, eds. Handbook Of Attachment, Theory, Research and Clinical Implications. New York: Guilford, 1999.
7. Adolescent Health Research Group. New Zealand youth: a profile of their health and well-being. University of Auckland. Available at: www.youth2000.ac.nz. Accessed November 24, 2004.

Eating Disorders and Body Image in Adolescence

Cynthia M. Bulik, Lauren Reba

*E*lla developed anorexia nervosa when she was 12, about six months after she had her first period. Before this, she was a popular girl, never one to be in cliques but someone who got along with just about everybody. Her teachers praised her for her intellect and creativity. Her coaches held her up as a model of self-discipline. Her pastor valued her volunteer work at church. When she started losing weight, her friends were at first envious and wanted to know her secret. Then she became more and more withdrawn. She dropped all her activities, except running, until her running coach refused to let her train with the team anymore. Over the next five years, she was hospitalized six times for anorexia nervosa, each time gaining weight and then losing it all again soon after discharge. She lost all her friends, and her parents' marriage nearly broke up over disagreements about her care. At 17, during one of her hospitalizations, something finally clicked. Hospitalized with her on the service was a 55-year-old woman whose bones were as brittle as lace from years of anorexia. Ella realized that she, too, would end up that way unless she made changes immediately. Gradually she put on weight, although she was still plagued by a loathing of her body and fear of gaining too much weight.

She started menstruating again at 18 and became interested in relationships for the first time. As she watched her college mates interact with guys at parties and other social events, she realized that she had missed her entire adolescence. She had never faced any of the developmental tasks or used the critical interpersonal tools that are typically honed during the teenage years. She felt like a child in an adult's body and began to appreciate how much of life had been lost to anorexia nervosa.

FACTS AND FEATURES

Anorexia and bulimia nervosa are serious mental illnesses that strike primarily during adolescence and young adulthood. They are serious and potentially lethal disorders that are influenced by both genetic and environmental factors (1). Anorexia nervosa has the highest mortality of all psychiatric disorders (2). Important questions about these disorders are as yet unanswered: What is their nature and to what extent are body image and body dissatisfaction core psychopathologic features? Why are anorexia and bulimia nervosa markedly more common in women, and why is Westernization associated with increases in disordered eating behavior? The answers to these questions will require sophisticated studies that are able to address the complex interplay among genetic, environmental, and cultural factors.

ANOREXIA NERVOSA

Anorexia nervosa is the eating disorder that is visible, although individuals with the disorder often go to extremes to hide their increasingly emaciated bodies. Girls with anorexia nervosa are unable to maintain a normal healthy body weight, commonly dropping to below 85% of their ideal weight. Young girls who are still growing fail to attain expected standards in weight (and often height as well). These individuals fear gaining weight or becoming fat, and they experience their bodies as overweight even when they are emaciated. They place critical importance on their shape and weight; self-esteem is completely enmeshed with body esteem. Amenorrhea is unreliable as a diagnostic criterion given the frequency with which physicians prescribe birth control pills to regulate the menses of women with anorexia nervosa. Moreover, data from several studies suggest that there are no meaningful differences between women with anorexia nervosa who do and those who do not menstruate (3).

Estimates from around the world place the lifetime prevalence of anorexia nervosa between 0.1% and 1.0% (4–9). Although the media make it seem as if there is an epidemic of anorexia nervosa, the data are conflicting, with some studies suggesting that the incidence is increasing (10–15) and others reporting stable rates (16–20). Epidemiologic studies reveal that the peak age of onset is between 15 and 19 years old (21); however, there are anecdotal reports of increasingly frequent presentations in prepubertal children (22), as well as new onset cases in midlife and late life (23,24).

BULIMIA NERVOSA

Bulimia nervosa is the invisible eating disorder, as it afflicts girls and women of all weights and shapes. Symptomatically, bulimia is marked by recurrent binge eating, which is conventionally defined as eating an unusually large amount of food in a discrete period of time and feeling that eating during these episodes is out of control. Binge eating is accompanied by compensatory behaviors ranging from excessive exercise and fasting (nonpurging bulimia nervosa) to more active measures such as self-induced vomiting and laxative, diuretic, or emetic abuse. Like anorexia nervosa, self-evaluation for an individual with bulimia nervosa hinges on shape and weight.

Bulimia nervosa is more common than anorexia nervosa and is reported to occur in 1% to 2.8% of women (25–32). Like anorexia, bulimia nervosa is overwhelmingly more common in women and unequally distributed throughout the age spectrum (4). Age of onset is most commonly late teens to early twenties (33). Females are disproportionately afflicted; the gender ratio is 9:1 (34). However, adjustment of the diagnostic criteria to include methods of compensatory behaviors more typical of males leads to a narrowing of the gender ratio (35).

SUBTHRESHOLD CONDITIONS

Concerns about shape and weight are emerging at increasingly younger ages in girls. By high school, isolated symptoms of eating behaviors are already commonplace (http://www.cmwf.org/programs/women/adoleshl.asp), with one third of high school girls reporting they are overweight, 58% reporting they have dieted, and 18% reporting bingeing and purging (8% daily or weekly). As public health education increasingly targets childhood obesity, we need to be careful that this does not encourage disordered eating behaviors and unhealthy eating practices.

GENDER AND EATING DISORDERS

Prepubertal anorexia nervosa is uncommon (but possibly increasing in frequency), and there are very few documented cases of prepubertal bulimia nervosa (36). Isolated symptoms such as dieting, weight dissatisfaction, and binge eating are clearly present in preadolescence (37–40). One theory that has received some support in the literature is that early menarche may increase the risk of developing bulimia nervosa. This theory holds that the greater body fat associated with maturation is at odds with the cultural ideal of thinness and leads to weight loss behaviors (41), which in turn increase the risk of developing eating disorders. Some prospective studies found that body fat percentage as well as Tanner staging predicted the development of eating problems and bulimia nervosa (37,38,41), although such findings are not universal (39). Retrospective studies have also shown that early menarche is more common in women with bulimia nervosa than in healthy women or psychiatric controls (42).

IMPACT OF EATING DISORDERS ON DEVELOPMENT

As illustrated by the clinical vignette of Ella, anorexia and bulimia nervosa have the capacity to arrest psychological, social, and even physical development when they occur in adolescence. Associated features of eating disorders such as depression, anxiety, social withdrawal, difficulty eating in social situations, self-consciousness, fatigue, and medical complications lead to social withdrawal and isolation. The psychological profile of young and older adults with anorexia nervosa is uneven. In some areas, they achieve age-appropriate functioning, but developmental lacunae are evident, reflecting the experiences that were missed and the developmental tasks that were never addressed.

BODY IMAGE, CULTURE, AND EATING DISORDERS

Historically, anorexia and bulimia nervosa were considered to be disorders of white upper-middle-class girls and women. Although data suggest that anorexia nervosa remains less frequently diagnosed in African American than in Caucasian women (43), this may reflect underdetection. Dissatisfaction with the size or shape of one's body is often thought to be the psychological motivator for dieting behavior (44), the first step on the slope of disordered eating behavior. This dissatisfaction is hypothesized to be secondary to increases in body fat associated with female pubertal development (45) and is the driving force for the onset of dieting behavior (46–50). Prospective studies have found that the greater the dissatisfaction with the body and the stronger the drive for thinness, the more problem eating is seen in nonclinical samples (37,39,41). In a 10-year follow-up study, drive for thinness and perfectionism were found to be the strongest predictors of bulimic symptomatology in university women (51). Several studies have attempted to place the core eating disorders features of body image and body dissatisfaction into a cultural context, since body image and body dissatisfaction are influenced not only by individual and family values but also by wider cultural perspectives.

Many theories have arisen to explain the development and presence of these phenomena in ethnically diverse populations. These explanatory constructs implicate exposure to and acceptance of Western value systems. Kuba and Harris (52) cite the term "acculturation" to define the process of change from the values of the culture of origin to the integration of the values and beliefs of the host culture. Through immigration or the global infusion of Western influence, a shift in cultural context occurs that may affect the perception of one's body and may lead to the development of eating disorders (52). Opposing theories suggest that the established body ideals of one's ethnic group of origin exert the main influence on the development of body dissatisfaction and eating disorders (53–55). Other theories implicate other universal environmental triggers (56).

IMMIGRATION AND ACCULTURATION

One valuable approach to understanding the role of culture on the development of body dissatisfaction and disordered eating is to study individuals undergoing immigration or acculturation experiences. Exploring the contextual factors that lead to eating disorders in first-generation Mexican American college-aged women, Kuba and Harris (52) suggest that, although intrapsychic issues contribute to eating disorders, the individual's response is related to macro, ethnocultural factors. Their observations suggest that a complex combination of variables, including level of acculturation, immigration, socioeconomic status, peer group identification, and family factors contribute to concern about weight and to disordered eating. In this population, family rigidity, maternal dominance, perceived maternal rejection, familial overconcern with food, or strained familial interaction were the most significant predictors of both bulimic symptoms and body dissatisfaction.

Possible overarching explanations include conflicting cultural demands, especially between Mexican American women's academic and career accomplishments and possible traditional familial ideals, or a strained mother–daughter relationship influenced by conflicting ethnic identities (57).

The concept of acculturation is particularly controversial when used with Native American and African American populations, for whom the more accurate concept is identification with majority cultural values (52). For example, Native American adolescent girls seem to present with compulsive eating behaviors and a greater acceptance of higher body weight than other ethnic groups. One explanation is that, for Native American girls forging their self-identity, body image standards and food consumption practices of their traditional ethnic culture play a more dominant role than presiding American ideals of thinness and dieting (58). Although research has shown that African American women with strong ethnic identity are somewhat protected from the thin ideal standards of the dominant American culture (59), they are nevertheless exposed to the pressure to attain their ethnic group's ideal body image. In a college study of African American and Caucasian women, Perez and Joiner (55) found that, regardless of race, body image symptoms correlate with bulimic symptoms; for example, women who see themselves as divergent from their ethnic group's ideal body size endorse more bulimic symptoms. African American women tend to perceive themselves as underweight, whereas Caucasian women tend to see themselves as overweight. In turn, in African American female populations, a decreased acceptance of majority ideals with respect to thinness and an increased identification with ethnic standards that value a heavier figure correlate with a distorted body image and disordered eating behavior precisely because a discrepancy exists between what one "should be" and what one is.

However, findings supporting the effects of acculturation on disordered eating and body dissatisfaction have not been universally upheld (53,54). Observing eating disorder symptoms and body image in Iranian and Iranian American female college students, Abdollahi and Mann (53) found that participants in Tehran reported as much disordered eating as participants in Los Angeles, and they concluded that neither exposure to Western media nor acculturation to Western norms appeared to be related to disordered eating and body image concerns. Further, in comparing body image and eating behavior between Taiwanese American and Taiwanese women, Tsai and colleagues (54) found that Taiwanese women in Taiwan had greater body dissatisfaction and disordered eating attitudes than their expatriate counterparts. A possible explanation for this may lie in the relationship of the generally small physical build of the Taiwanese woman in contrast with the larger size of the average American woman. In terms of body image, the modal Taiwanese American woman fits the Western model of thinness more closely than her American contemporaries, and thus feels less societal pressure to control her weight. Further, it is possible that other stressors present in Iranian and Taiwanese culture, such as political disquiet or modernization respectively, may equal or supersede the effects of acculturation in the development of disordered eating.

Compounded, these findings reinforce the notion that a complex collection of variables, including specific environmental pressures to adapt or react to a new system of cultural values (52,57), as well as the simultaneous need to meet non-Western aesthetic ideals (53,54), contribute to distorted body image or to the development of an eating disorder. Moreover, in complex Western societies, majority ideals frequently coexist alongside strong ethnic identities. Further studies of individuals with "a foot in two cultures" will no doubt reveal more about both risk and protective factors for eating disorders and body image concerns.

IMPOSED CULTURE

Recent studies in non-Western societies have shown an increasing influence of Western culture, through media, technology, and use of English (60), on female adolescents (61,62). Focusing on a population of urban and rural Egyptian girls aged 11 to 19, Jackson and colleagues (63) observed a strong correlation between the silhouette shapes the girls chose to represent their body type and their calculated body mass index (BMI) values. These data differ from studies of Western teenage females, who often perceive themselves as overweight when BMI values suggest otherwise. However, more than their rural counterparts, girls residing in Cairo desired a slimmer body shape for themselves than they believed their mothers wanted for them, which suggests the more prevalent global influences on adolescents in an urban context and the eroded importance of traditional Egyptian ideals of larger body size in the younger generation of females. Evaluating the impact of Western television on disordered eating among indigenous girls in Fiji, Becker and colleagues (64) found that indicators of disordered eating were far more prevalent following exposure to Western media. This study concluded that Western media may have a negative impact on body image and eating behaviors of media-naïve populations with long-held cultural ideals.

In observing body image issues in relationship to eating attitudes in South African schoolgirls, Caradas and colleagues (65) found that Black and White girls identified with different ideal body types. Although Black girls had higher BMI than White or mixed girls, White girls desired a significantly smaller ideal body type and showed greater dissatisfaction with present body size. However, a comparative percentage of all girls had scores indicative of eating disorder pathology. Given massive socioeconomic changes and relatively recent abolishment of apartheid legislation, young South Africans are currently becoming exposed to new belief systems and thereby may be more susceptible to developing new perspectives on body ideals. Still, with a much larger population of Black South Africans never attending secondary school, this study, which focused on secondary school girls, may not be representative of abnormal eating attitudes and associated body image of the population at large.

In terms of the etiology of eating disorders, globalization may have a particularly detrimental effect on "developing" societies in transition between traditional cultural norms and newly imposed Western influences. However, research has yet to explain why certain cultures seem to be more immune to the influx, through media and technology, of Western standards of beauty and diet. A possible explanation may involve an intricate balance of factors including established ethnic identity, the state of societal transition, and the willingness of members of a given population to embrace Western ideals. Future research needs to focus on developing instruments specific to the practices of a given culture with which to measure body image and eating issues.

UNIVERSAL ENVIRONMENTAL TRIGGERS

Some features of body discrepancy, the difference between the self and the cultural ideal, may have a universally negative impact. Examining the effects of weight-related teasing on body image and eating disturbance in Swedish and Australian adolescent girls, Lunner and colleagues (56) found that BMI predicted teasing and body dissatisfaction, and body dissatisfaction predicted level of eating restraint. The same results were found across all samples and partially replicated previous research in U.S. populations. Such cross-cultural findings have significant implications for developing prevention and treatment programs to reduce negative social stigma and associated teasing behavior, and to develop strategies for deflecting teasing in order to protect against the development of unhealthy eating practices in youth (56).

If teasing universally mediates the relation between BMI and body dissatisfaction in the development of disturbed eating, future research may have the potential to develop prevention and treatment interventions focused on teasing prevention and deflection as yet another tool in the battle against eating disorders.

THE GENE–ENVIRONMENT NEXUS IN EATING DISORDERS

The question remains how body image and body dissatisfaction influence risk for developing eating disorders. In light of powerful recent findings on the contribution of genetic factors to anorexia and bulimia nervosa, body image and body dissatisfaction may represent the node at which environment and culture exert their influence by increasing the risk for genetically vulnerable individuals to express an underlying predisposition to eating disorders.

SUMMARY OF GENETIC FINDINGS IN EATING DISORDERS

Over the past decade, family studies have consistently shown that eating disorders run in families with a relative risk of 10 to 12 (66,67). Population-based twin studies have shown that the observed familial patterns are largely a product of the additive effects of genes (1,9,29,68). In addition, linkage studies have begun to identify chromosomal regions that may harbor susceptibility loci for anorexia and bulimia, and association studies are beginning to isolate specific candidate genes that may influence risk (69–78). Together, these findings have forced the reappraisal of genetic factors as etiologic agents in eating disorders and led to the exploration of new mechanisms through which environment and culture exert their influence.

ENVIRONMENTAL MAIN EFFECTS

Although historically the dominant view, evidence for environmental causal main effects on eating disorders is lacking (1,79). Exposure to thin body ideals and dieting behaviors are nearly universal in industrialized countries (48,80); however, the prevalence of eating disorders remains lower than 5%, far lower than the percentage of individuals exposed to the putative environmental risk factors. The most likely avenue through which environment influences the risk for eating disorders is via complex patterns of gene–environment interplay.

GENE–ENVIRONMENT INTERPLAY

The genetic findings in eating disorders are convincing, but they do not paint the entire picture. Twin studies indicate that a substantial portion of variance in liability to eating disorders rests with nonshared environmental influences (81). However, as mentioned previously, factors such as acculturation, identification with majority culture, and universals such as scorn and derision influence body image and satisfaction, which subsequently increase the likelihood of disordered eating behaviors in order to match shape and weight to a perceived cultural ideal. Nonetheless, when cultures undergo rapid Westernization or when new putative risk exposures are introduced, eating disorders and disordered eating behaviors are not inevitably expressed. For example, in a study in Fiji Becker et al. (64) found that not all young girls developed body dissatisfaction and disordered eating after the introduction of television. One possibility is that there is something about the exposure (e.g., increase in behaviors such as unhealthy dieting) that influences the expression of an underlying genetic predisposition. The risk for expression of the trait is proportional to the degree of genetic risk.

IMPLICATIONS FOR PREVENTION AND TREATMENT

The fact that both genetic and environmental factors contribute to risk for eating disorders aids us in developing appropriate prevention and treatment interventions. Genetic research may ultimately unveil novel biologic pathways that can further elucidate the underlying pathophysiology of eating disorders and ultimately lead to new drug targets. Environmental and cultural studies will further identify environmental exposures that influence eating disorder risk. In addition, novel melded approaches will unravel gene–environment interplay. An example of a melded approach (to depression) is provided by Caspi and colleagues (82). They showed that a functional polymorphism in the promoter region of the serotonin transporter gene (5-HT T) moderated the influence of stressful life events. In this example, an individual's genotype influenced susceptibility to the negative effects of major life stressors such as loss. Such paradigms can easily be applied to future research in anorexia and bulimia nervosa.

The family, twin, and genetic data all point toward offspring of women with eating disorders being a group who could benefit from targeted prevention trials. Such interventions are best directed toward both mothers [who struggle with feeding and body-related issues with their children (83)] and their offspring.

PROTECTIVE ALLELES AND PROTECTIVE ENVIRONMENTS

In addition to focusing on genes and environments that increase risk, it is also worthwhile to explore the role of protective alleles and protective environments. For example, Slof and colleagues (84) reported that persistent thinness throughout the life span is associated with low rates of eating disorders in women. Individuals who report low healthy weight throughout childhood, adolescence, and adulthood have a relatively late age at menarche, low rates of dieting and binge eating, more health satisfaction, higher self-esteem, and lower perfectionism and body dissatisfaction than peers. When genes for persistent thinness are identified, they will likely be associated with a decreased risk for the development of eating disorders.

Likewise, prevention studies in offspring of individuals with eating disorders will assist with identifying environments that inhibit the development of disordered eating attitudes and behaviors. In many ways, a sole focus on risk factors can be limiting. Exploring protective genes and protective environments can open up new avenues of inquiry and fresh approaches to an unsolved problem.

CONCLUSION

Sociocultural processes clearly influence body image and body esteem among young girls (85). Simultaneously, genetic factors clearly influence risk both for eating disorders and for related traits such as body dissatisfaction (86,87). Body dissatisfaction can trigger disordered eating behavior and negative affect and be the first step along the path toward eating disorders. Prevention and treatment interventions aimed at bolstering body satisfaction and esteem—possibly by defocusing self-esteem evaluation away from body-based issues—and providing youth with successful defensive strategies to buffer the impact of teasing and cultural pressures toward ultrathinness could serve to derail the downward spiral from body dissatisfaction to eating disorders, especially in genetically vulnerable individuals.

REFERENCES

1. Bulik C, Sullivan P, Wade T, et al. Twin studies of eating disorders: a review. Int J Eat Disord 2000;27:1–20.
2. Sullivan PF. Mortality in anorexia nervosa. Am J Psychiatry 1995;152:1073–1074.
3. Watson T, Andersen A. A critical examination of the amenorrhea and weight criteria for diagnosing anorexia nervosa. Acta Psychiatr Scand 2003;108:175–182.
4. Hoek HW. The incidence and prevalence of anorexia nervosa and bulimia nervosa in primary care. Psychol Med 1991;21:455–460.
5. King MB. Eating disorders in a general practice population: prevalence, characteristics and follow-up at 12 to 18 months. Psychol Med Monogr Suppl 1989;14:1–34.
6. Meadows GN, Palmer RL, Newball EU, et al. Eating attitudes and disorder in young women: a general practice based survey. Psychol Med 1986;16:351–357.
7. Wells JE, Bushnell JA, Hornblow AR, et al. Christchurch Psychiatric Epidemiology Study Part I: Methodology and lifetime prevalence for specific psychiatric disorders. Aust NZ J Psychiatry 1989;23:315–326.
8. Whitehouse A, Cooper P, Vize C, et al. Prevalence of eating disorders in three Cambridge general practices: hidden and conspicuous morbidity. Br J Gen Pract 1992;42:57–60.
9. Walters EE, Kendler KS. Anorexia nervosa and anorexic-like syndromes in a population-based female twin sample. Am J Psychiatry 1995;152:64–71.
10. Eagles J, Johnston M, Hunter D, et al. Increasing incidence of anorexia nervosa in the female population of northeast Scotland. Am J Psychiatry 1995;152:1266–1271.
11. Jones D, Fox M, Babigan H, et al. Epidemiology of anorexia nervosa in Monroe County, New York: 1960–76. Psychosom Med 1980;42:551–558.
12. Lucas AR, Beard CM, O'Fallon WM, et al. Anorexia nervosa in Rochester, Minnesota: a 45-year study. Mayo Clin Proc 1988;63:433–442.
13. Moller-Madsen S, Nystrup J. Incidence of anorexia nervosa in Denmark. Acta Psychiatr Scand 1992;86:187–200.
14. Szmukler G, McCance C, McCrone L, et al. Anorexia nervosa: a psychiatric case register study from Aberdeen. Psychol Med 1986;16:49–58.
15. Willi J, Grossman S. Epidemiology of anorexia nervosa in a defined region of Switzerland. Am J Psychiatry 1983;140:564–567.
16. Hall A, Hay P, Eating disorder patient referrals from a population region 1977–1986. Psychol Med 1991;21:697–701.

17. Hoek H, Bartelds A, Bosveld J, et al. Impact of urbanization on detection rates of eating disorders. Am J Psychiatry 1995;152:1272–1278.
18. Jorgensen J. The epidemiology of eating disorders in Fyn County, Denmark, 1977–1986. Acta Psychiatr Scand 1992;85:30–34.
19. Nielsen S. The epidemiology of anorexia nervosa in Denmark from 1973 to 1987: a nationwide register study of psychiatric admission. Acta Psychiatr Scand 1990;81:507–514.
20. Willi J, Giacometti G, Limacher B. Update on the epidemiology of anorexia nervosa in a defined region of Switzerland. Am J Psychiatry 1990;147:1514–1517.
21. Lucas AR, Beard CM, O'Fallon WM, et al. 50-year trends in the incidence of anorexia nervosa in Rochester, Minn.: a population-based study. Am J Psychiatry 1991;148:917–922.
22. Gowers S, Crisp A, Joughin N, et al. Premenarcheal anorexia nervosa. J Child Psychol Psychiatry 1991;32:515–524.
23. Inagaki T, Horiguchi J, Tsubouchi K, et al. Late onset anorexia nervosa: two case reports. Int J Psychiatry Med 2002;32:91–95.
24. Beck D, Casper R, Andersen A. Truly late onset of eating disorders: a study of 11 cases averaging 60 years of age at presentation. Int J Eat Disord 1996;20:389–395.
25. Bushnell J, Wells J, Hornblow A, et al. Prevalence of three bulimia syndromes in the general population. Psychol Med 1990;20:671–680.
26. Drewnowski A, Hopkins SA, Kessler RC. The prevalence of bulimia nervosa in the US college student population. Am J Public Health 1988;78:1322–1325.
27. Garfinkel PE, Lin E, Goering P, et al. Bulimia nervosa in a Canadian community sample: prevalence and comparison of subgroups. Am J Psychiatry 1995;152:1052–1058.
28. Johnson-Sabine E, Wood K, Patton G, et al. Abnormal eating attitudes in London schoolgirls—a prospective epidemiological study: factors associated with abnormal response on screening questionnaires. Psychol Med 1988;18:615–622.
29. Kendler KS, MacLean C, Neale MC, et al. The genetic epidemiology of bulimia nervosa. Am J Psychiatry 1991;148:1627–1637.
30. King M. Eating disorders in general practice. Br Med J 1986;293:1412–1414.
31. Rand CSW, Kuldau JM. Epidemiology of bulimia and symptoms in a general population: sex, age, race, and socioeconomic status. Int J Eat Disord 1992;11:37–44.
32. Schotte DE. Stunkard AJ. Bulimia vs. bulimic behaviors on a college campus. JAMA 1987;258:1213–1215.
33. Soundy T, Lucas A, Suman V, et al. Bulimia nervosa in Rochester, Minnesota from 1980 to 1990. Psychol Med 1995;25:1065–1071.
34. American Psychiatric Association, Diagnostic and Statistical Manual of Mental Disorders. 4th Ed. Washington, DC, 1994.
35. Anderson CB, Bulik CM. Gender differences in compensatory behaviors, weight and shape salience, and drive for thinness. Eat Behav 2004;5:1–11.
36. Stein S, Chalhoub N, Hodes M. Very early-onset bulimia nervosa: report of two cases. Int J Eat Disord 1998;24:323–327.
37. Graber J, Brooks-Gunn J, Paikoff R, et al. Prediction of eating problems: an 8-year study of adolescent girls. Dev Psychol 1994;30:823–834.
38. Killen J, Taylor C, Hayward C, et al. Pursuit of thinness and onset of eating disorder symptoms in a community sample of adolescent girls: a three-year prospective analysis. Int J Eat Disord 1994;16:227–238.
39. Leon G, Fulkerson J, Perry C, et al. Personality and behavioral vulnerabilities associated with risk status for eating disorders in adolescent girls. J Abnorm Psychol 1993;102:438–444.
40. Sands R, Tricker J, Sherman C, et al. Disordered eating patterns, body image, self-esteem, and physical activity in preadolescent school children. Int J Eat Disord 1997;21:159–166.
41. Attie I, Brooks-Gunn J. Development of eating problems in adolescent girls: a longitudinal study. Dev Psychol 1989;25:70–79.
42. Fairburn CG, Welch SL, Doll HA, et al. Risk factors for bulimia nervosa. a community-based case-control study. Arch Gen Psychiatry 1997;54:509–517.
43. Striegel-Moore R, Dohm F, Kraemer H, et al. Eating disorders in white and black women. Am J Psychiatry 2003;160:1326–1331.
44. Stice E. Review of the evidence for a sociocultural model of bulimia nervosa and exploration of mechanisms of action. Clin Psychol Rev 1994;14:633–661.
45. Marino DD, King JC. Nutritional concerns during adolescence. Pediatr Clin North Am 1980;27:125–139.
46. Cash T, Henry P. Women's body images: the results of a national survey in the U.S.A. Sex Roles 1995;33:19–28.
47. Hawkins R, Clement P. Binge-eating: measurement problems and a conceptual model. In: Hawkins R, Fremouw W, Clement P, eds. The Binge-Purge Syndrome: Diagnosis, Treatment and Research. New York: Springer, 1984:229–251.

48. Rodin J, Silberstein L, Streigel-Moore R. Women and weight: a normative discontent. In: Sonderegger T, ed. Psychology and Gender: Nebraska Symposium on Motivation. Lincoln: University of Nebraska Press, 1985.

49. Tiggemann M. Gender differences in the interrelationships between weight dissatisfaction, restraint, and self-esteem. Sex Roles 1994;30:319–330.

50. van Strien T. Dieting, dissatisfaction with figure, and sex role orientation in women. Int J Eat Disord 1989;8:455–463.

51. Joiner TE Jr, Heatherton TF, Rudd MD, et al. Perfectionism, perceived weight status, and bulimic symptoms: two studies testing a diathesis-stress model. J Abnorm Psychol 1997; 106:145–53.

52. Kuba S, Harris D. Eating disturbances in women of color: an exploratory study of contextual factors in the development of disordered eating in Mexican American women. Health Care Women Int 2001;22:281–298.

53. Abdollahi P, Mann T. Eating disorder symptoms and body image concerns in Iran: comparisons between Iranian women in Iran and in America. Int J Eat Disord 2001;30:259–268.

54. Tsai G, Curbow B, Heinberg L. Sociocultural and developmental influences on body dissatisfaction and disordered eating attitudes and behaviors of Asian women. J Nerv Ment Dis 2003;191:309–318.

55. Perez M, Joiner TJ. Body image dissatisfaction and disordered eating in black and white women. Int J Eat Disord 2003;33:342–350.

56. Lunner K, Werthem E, Thompson J, et al. A cross-cultural examination of weight-related teasing, body image, and eating disturbance in Swedish and Australian samples. Int J Eat Disord 2000;28:430–435.

57. Comez-Diaz L, Greene B. Women of color: integrating ethnic and gender identities in psychotherapy. New York: Guilford, 1994.

58. Smith J, Krejci J. Minorities join the majority: eating disorders among Hispanic and Native American youth. Int J Eat Disord 1991;10:179–186.

59. Parker S, Nichter M, Nicter M, et al. Body image and weight concerns among African American and Caucasian adolescent females: differences that make a difference. Hum Org Sum 1995; 54:103–114.

60. Katzmarzyk P, Malina R, Song T, et al. Television viewing, physical activity, and health-related fitness of youth in the Quebec Family Study. Adolesc Health 1998;23:318–325.

61. Wang M, Ho T, Anderson J, et al. Preference for thinness in Singapore—a newly industrialized society. Singapore Med J 1999;40:502–507.

62. Field A, Camargo C, Taylor C, et al. Overweight, weight concerns, and bulimic behaviors among girls and boys. J Am Acad Child Adolesc Psychiatry 1999;38:754–760.

63. Jackson R, Rashed M, Saad-Eldin R. Rural–urban differences in weight, body image, and dieting behavior among adolescent Egyptian schoolgirls. Int J Food Sci Nutr 2003;54:1–11.

64. Becker A, Burwell R, Gilman S, et al. Eating behaviours and attitudes following prolonged exposure to television among ethnic Fijian adolescent girls. Br J Psychiatry 2002;180: 509–514.

65. Caradas A, Lambert E, Charlton K. An ethnic comparison of eating attitudes and associated body image concerns in adolescent South African schoolgirls. J Hum Nutr Diet 2001;14:111–120.

66. Lilenfeld L, Kaye W, Greeno C, et al. A controlled family study of restricting anorexia and bulimia nervosa: comorbidity in probands and disorders in first-degree relatives. Arch Gen Psychiatry 1998;55:603–610.

67. Strober M, Freeman R, Lampert C, et al. Controlled family study of anorexia nervosa and bulimia nervosa: evidence of shared liability and transmission of partial syndromes. Am J Psychiatry 2000;157:393–401.

68. Wade T, Neale MC, Lake RI, et al. A genetic analysis of the eating and attitudes associated with bulimia nervosa: dealing with the problem of ascertainment. Behav Genet 1999;29:1–10.

69. Collier DA, Arranz MJ, Li T, et al. Association between 5-HT2A gene promoter polymorphism and anorexia nervosa. Lancet 1997;350:412.

70. Enoch MA, Kaye WH, Rotondo A, et al. 5-HT2A promoter polymorphism—1438G/A, anorexia nervosa, and obsessive-compulsive disorder. Lancet 1998;351:1785–1786.

71. Nacmias B, Ricca V, Tedde A, et al. 5-HT2A receptor gene polymorphisms in anorexia nervosa and bulimia nervosa. Neurosci Lett 1999;277:134–136.

72. Devlin B, Bacanu SA, Klump KL, et al. Linkage analysis of anorexia nervosa incorporating behavioral covariates. Hum Mol Genet 2002;11:689–696.

73. Koronyo-Hamaoui M, Danziger Y, Frisch A, et al. Association between anorexia nervosa and the hsKCa3 gene: a family-based and case control study. Mol Psychiatry 2002;7:82–85.

74. Urwin R, Bennetts B, Wilcken B, et al. Anorexia nervosa (restrictive subtype) is associated with a polymorphism in the novel norepinephrine transporter gene promoter polymorphic region. Mol Psychiatry 2002;7:652–657.

75. Grice DE, Halmi KA, Fichter MM, et al. Evidence for a susceptibility gene for anorexia nervosa on chromosome 1. Am J Hum Genet 2002;70:787–792.
76. Westberg L, Bah J, Rastam M, et al. Association between a polymorphism of the 5-HT2C receptor and weight loss in teenage girls. Neuropsychopharmacol 2002;26:789–793.
77. Bulik CM, Devlin B, Bacanu SA, et al. Significant linkage on chromosome 10p in families with bulimia nervosa. Am J Hum Genet 2003;72:200–207.
78. Hu X, Murphy F, Karwautz A, et al. Analysis of microsatellite markers at the UCP2/UCP3 locus on chromosome 11q13 in anorexia nervosa. Mol Psychiatry 2002;7:276–277.
79. Brownell KD. Dieting and the search for the perfect body: where physiology and culture collide. Behav Therapy 1991;22:1–12.
80. Striegel-Moore R, Silberstein LR, Rodin J. Toward an understanding of risk factors for bulimia. Am Psychol 1986;41:246–263.
81. Klump KL, Wonderlich S, Lehoux P, et al. Does environment matter? A review of nonshared environment and eating disorders. Int J Eat Disord 2002;31:118–135.
82. Caspi A, Sugden K, Moffitt T, et al. Influence of life stress on depression: moderation by a polymorphism in the 5-HTT gene. Science 2003;301:386–389.
83. Mitchell-Gieleghem A, Mittelstaedt ME, Bulik CM. Eating disorders and childbearing: concealment and consequences. Birth 2002;29:182–191.
84. Slof R, Mazzeo S, Bulik CM. Characteristics of women with persistent thinness. Obes Res 2003;11:971–977.
85. Stice E, Shaw HE. Role of body dissatisfaction in the onset and maintenance of eating pathology: a synthesis of research findings. J Psychosom Res 2002;53:985–993.
86. Wade T, Martin N, Tiggemann M. Genetic and environmental risk factors for the weight and shape concerns characteristic of bulimia nervosa. Psychol Med 1998;28:761–771.
87. Klump KL, McGue M, Iacono WG. Age differences in genetic and environmental influences on eating attitudes and behaviors in preadolescent and adolescent female twins. J Abnorm Psychol 2000;109:239–251.

CHAPTER 9

Prodromal Phase of Psychosis in Adolescent Women

Jean Addington, Frauke T. K. Schultze-Lutter

Schizophrenia is one of society's costliest medical conditions. The disorder usually evolves during the developmentally crucial time of late adolescence and early adulthood. Although the diagnosis is not made until psychotic symptoms appear, it has long been known that in the majority of cases psychosis is preceded by identifiable signs and symptoms, making schizophrenia the only disorder in which the prodrome adds to diagnosis (1). One of the most important and exciting new concepts in psychiatry is that detection and intervention very early in the course of schizophrenia (and other psychotic illnesses) offers hope for realizing substantive improvements in the outcome of schizophrenia spectrum disorders. Current work in schizophrenia focuses on either the late preonset or early postonset phases of schizophrenia.

Postonset studies and early psychosis programs aim to detect and treat schizophrenia close to onset in order to minimize the duration of untreated psychosis (DUP). Reducing DUP may prevent future severity of symptoms, chronicity, or collateral damage from the disorder. Treatment in the initial prodromal phase includes all of these aims as well as the potential to delay or prevent the expression of the manifest disorder; that is, the onset of psychotic symptoms. Aiming at shortening the duration of untreated illness (DUI), the preonset studies are somewhat more controversial because they actually address the future risk of schizophrenia, the probable but uncertain development of a disorder. However, in the putatively prodromal phase of a psychotic illness, symptoms are already severe and disability has already begun. Current research studies suggest that a putatively prodromal state is beginning to be defined such that there may be enough predictive power for the disorder to be tested as a new diagnostic threshold (2–4).

The purpose of this chapter is to consider what is known about the prepsychotic period, which typically occurs in adolescence, and its special relevance for young women. It needs to be stated, however, that, because early detection and intervention is a rather new area, little consideration has hitherto been given to gender-specific issues.

AGE OF ONSET AND EARLY PHASES OF PSYCHOSIS

Early intervention for individuals experiencing their first episode of psychosis has a high likelihood of resulting in remission of psychotic symptoms. However, it is common for patients in remission following a first episode of schizophrenia to experience persistent difficulties in everyday functioning. A large percentage of such individuals have difficulty working and find themselves disabled and unable to support themselves (5,6). It is believed that this disability develops in the years preceding the onset of psychotic symptoms, the prodromal period, in which social withdrawal and the evolution of negative symptoms form the base upon which psychotic symptoms subsequently develop (7).

One of the major retrospective studies of the onset of schizophrenia, the Mannheim Age, Beginning, Course (ABC) study (8), showed that 73% of 232 patients hospitalized for first-episode schizophrenia had experienced a prodromal phase with negative and nonspecific symptoms. Twenty-seven percent reported an acute illness onset with positive symptoms (7%) or positive and negative symptoms occurring within one month (20%). No gender differences were observed in this aspect of the prodrome. On average, the prodromal phase lasted five years and was followed by a psychotic prephase of 1.1 years, which was characterized by the first occurrence and escalation of positive symptoms. Thus, independent of gender, before the first inpatient treatment for schizophrenia, the majority of individuals were ill for more than six years.

In line with the finding of the Determinants of Outcome study by the World Health Organization (WHO) (9), the ABC study found an average three to four years difference between males and females in the milestones of the early course (i.e., first sign, first negative symptom, first positive symptom, first episode, and first admission), with men reaching each of these milestones earlier than women (8). The distribution of age of onset of the illness (i.e., occurrence of the first sign) showed an early and steep increase for men, with a pronounced peak between 15 and 25 years of age and a decrease in the later years. In women, the increase was less steep, with the peak lower and later, between 15 and 30 years of age. A brief decline in incidence thereafter was followed by a second, lower peak around menopause, age 45 to 49. In adolescence and early adulthood, men are at a twofold risk of morbidity for schizophrenia in comparison to women. Consequently, studies of adolescent schizophrenia tend to report a male:female ratio of 2:1. This ratio has also been observed in first-episode studies (5,6). In a Canadian sample of 361 first-episode subjects, there was a significant gender difference in age of onset (5,6). Males were significantly younger for the onset of a schizophrenia spectrum disorder and of schizophrenia. However, no other gender differences such as DUP, symptoms, insight, social, or cognitive functioning have been observed in this first-episode group (5,6).

The gender difference in age of onset does not exist in subjects who have a family history of schizophrenia (10). Similarly, women with schizophrenia with a history of prenatal and perinatal complications show an onset age similar to that of men (11). One explanation for the gender disparity in age of onset of schizophrenia is a putative protective effect of estrogen that can be overridden by genetic and other factors (12,13). Support for the estrogen hypothesis is offered by commonly occurring premenstrual, postpartum, and postmenopausal exacerbations of schizophrenia, by the relative freedom from relapse during pregnancy, and by the approximately threefold increased risk of schizophrenia during the 90 days after childbirth (14), as well as by the significant relationship between age of menarche and age at onset of schizophrenia in women. A late age of menarche has been reported to be related to an earlier onset (15). For women lacking additional risk factors, schizophrenia is not necessarily a disorder that first shows itself in adolescence, as it almost always is in men. (Jayashri Kulkarni addresses gender issues in adult schizophrenia more fully in Chapter 14 of this book.)

THE PREPSYCHOTIC PHASE: RESULTS FROM FIRST-EPISODE AND HIGH-RISK RESEARCH

Häfner found gender similarity in patterns of course, symptomatology, and neuropsychological functioning in schizophrenia (8) and concluded that it was "important to analyze gender differences in variables more distant to the disease process" (p. 204). Such an opportunity exists in early detection and intervention research in the initial prodrome of first-episode psychosis.

The term "prodrome" is retrospective because, until psychotic illness develops, no prodrome can be said to have existed (16). The prodrome refers to the time between the appearance of mental state features that represent a change from a person's premorbid functioning until the onset of frank psychosis (16). Approximately 80% to 90% of patients with schizophrenia report a variety of symptoms (including changes in perception, beliefs, cognition, mood, affect, and behavior) that preceded psychosis; and only 10% to 20% develop psychotic symptoms without any apparent significant prodromal period (8,17). Nonspecific symptoms and negative symptoms usually emerge first, followed by attenuated positive symptoms (13). These earliest signs do not differ significantly between men and women (8). The most pronounced gender difference has been found for social behaviors. Men more often than women present a history of drug or alcohol abuse and social disability. They are also more likely to show inadequate personal hygiene, reduced interest in acquiring a job, social inattentiveness, lack of free-time activities, and deficits in communication (8). These results fit with findings from genetic high-risk and birth-cohort studies that indicate clear gender-specific differences in social behavior: girls developing schizophrenia were introverted throughout childhood into adolescence; boys were disagreeable and less socially integrated, but only in the later school grades (18). These very early aberrations do not seem to interfere with social role performance prior to the onset of the first sign of the illness but, by the time of first admission, a functional advantage for young women is already evident (8). Further examination of study data reveals a significant interaction of gender and preillness social behaviors as a determinant of the medium-term social outcome of schizophrenia (19).

GENERAL CRITERIA OF THE INITIAL PRODROME OR ULTRAHIGH-RISK STATE

High-risk groups selected by positive family history of a first-degree relative with schizophrenia have long been identified in schizophrenia research, and several prospective longitudinal studies are currently ongoing (20). In these genetic high-risk studies, the risk of converting to psychosis is still relatively low, approximately 10% to 20% (20). However, if prepsychotic intervention is the goal, then we need to reach those whose risk of converting to psychosis is much higher than 10% to 20%.

Based on clinical observations and retrospective research on the prodromal phase of first-episode psychosis, the so called ultrahigh-risk (UHR) criteria of the initial prodrome of psychosis were developed and prospectively refined at the Personal Assessment and Crisis Evaluation (PACE) Clinic in Melbourne (4). The criteria include the recent onset of a functional decline plus genetic risk, or recent onset of subthreshold or brief threshold psychotic symptoms. Using these new criteria, the risk of converting to psychosis increases from 10% to 20% in the genetic high-risk group to approximately 40% to 60%. This has been reported in several studies (21).

Criteria focusing mainly on symptoms, which resemble psychotic symptoms phenomenologically and thus possess a certain face-validity, are currently the most widely applied in early detection and intervention research. Reliability of these criteria has been excellent, and studies using these criteria support the view that prodromal persons are symptomatic (22) and at high and imminent risk for psychosis (23). Twelve-month transition rates of 34% to 50% in studies utilizing the UHR criteria have hitherto been reported from two naturalistic follow-up studies (4,24).

Another approach to the early detection of schizophrenia is offered by the German "basic symptom" concept (25). Basic symptoms are subtle, subclinical, self-experienced disturbances in drive, stress tolerance, affect, thinking, speech, perception, and motor action, first operationalized for their presence or absence in the Bonn Scale for the Assessment of Basic Symptoms (BSABS) (26). They have been assessed for their predictive accuracy for schizophrenia in the prospective Cologne Early Recognition (CER) project (2). Ten cognitive-perceptive basic symptoms were found to be early predictors of schizophrenia (2). Overall, approximately 80% of the subjects with at least two basic symptoms developed schizophrenia; 23.9% by 12 months, 46.3% by the second year, and 60.8% by the third.

Because we are dealing with degrees of risk for onset rather than certainty of onset, the mental state characterized as a prodrome is best termed an "at risk mental state" (27). Those who meet criteria for this state will, in this chapter, be considered at ultrahigh risk for developing psychosis.

MALE AND FEMALE DIFFERENCES IN THE ULTRAHIGH-RISK PERIOD

Few studies have examined prospectively individuals who may putatively be prodromal for psychosis. In a follow-up monitoring study, Yung et al. (23), observed no gender differences in those who developed psychosis from the prodromal state compared to those who did not. Furthermore, the CER study (2) found no significant gender differences in regard to transition rates, age at onset of illness or psychosis, duration of the prodrome, prominent clinical picture at first examination, subscale totals of the seven basic symptom clusters, or distribution of hallucinations and delusions.

However, preliminary baseline results of a prospective evaluation study of a new instrument for the quantitative assessment of basic symptoms, the Schizophrenia Prediction Instrument, Adult version (SPI-A), showed at least some statistical trends for psychopathologic gender differences in putatively prodromal subjects, although not for the distribution of UHR and basic symptom criteria, average 12-month transition rates, or age. Female prodromal subjects (n = 47) tended to report more severe attenuated positive symptoms on the Structured Interview for Prodromal Syndromes (SIPS) (24), whereas male prodromal subjects (n = 100) reported more severe scores on the PANSS Negative Syndrome Scale. In general, similar to a first-episode group, these putatively prodromal individuals showed a pattern of slight, essentially insignificant gender differences. The higher scores for women were in self-experienced distress, as well as cognitive difficulty, body perception problems, perception, and motor disturbances.

INTERVENTION STUDIES

Several clinical trials have attempted to intervene either with medication (28) or cognitive-behavior therapy (29) or both in order to prevent the development of psychosis in those at risk (30). Results of these very early studies are either preliminary or have not yet been published. As with many groundbreaking studies, sample sizes are small and, therefore, it is difficult to draw firm conclusions. In the PACE clinic in Melbourne, Australia, 59 UHR subjects were randomized to either six months of active treatment or six months of needs-based intervention (30). The active treatment included low-dose risperidone plus cognitive-behavior therapy, and the needs-based intervention was case management or support, as needed. Fifty-eight percent of the subjects were male and 42% female. After treatment, 10 of the control group and three of the treatment group had converted to psychosis; the number in the treatment group increased to six within six months of the treatment ending. Fourteen percent of the males in this trial converted, in comparison to 32% of the females (Lisa Phillips; personal communication). It is not clear why there should be a gender difference of this magnitude and whether it may be related to sampling issues, often a problem in small sample studies. For instance, more females than males may have sought help closer to onset.

A second trial, the PRIME (Prevention through Risk Identification Management and Education) study, was a randomized double-blind parallel study of 60 prodromal subjects comparing the efficacy of a low-dose antipsychotic (olanzapine) versus placebo in preventing or delaying the onset of psychosis (28). At initial presentation, these subjects were symptomatic and seeking help; they had a broad range of attenuated positive and negative symptoms in line with the UHR criteria. The sample consisted of 21 females and 39 males. For the most part, differences across gender were minimal. No significant differences were observed, for example, on demography, prodromal type, premorbid functioning, or scores on the General Assessment of Functioning (GAF). In terms of initial presenting symptoms rated on a range of scales (22), males scored significantly higher than females on conceptual disorganization, motor symptoms, mannerisms, poor abstraction, blunted affect, and negative symptoms. Females scored significantly higher on dysphoria, depression, sadness, tension, and sleep disturbance.

The Early Detection and Intervention Evaluation (EDIE) trial was recently completed in Manchester, UK. It is a single-blind randomized trial of CBT with individuals meeting UHR criteria assessed with the PANSS (29). In this trial, 70% of the subjects were male and 30% were female. At one year, 10 subjects had converted to psychosis [eight males (80%) and two females (20%)].

In an ongoing study of ultrahigh-risk individuals at the Recognition and Prevention (RAP) Clinic in New York (31), three groups have been identified based on symptom presentation in a clinical high-risk group. Although there are more males than females in all three groups, this difference is dramatically increased in the group that includes only those with nonspecific attenuated negative symptoms such as social isolation and deterioration of school functioning. This may be a result of an ascertainment bias attributing more dysfunction to such symptoms in adolescent boys than girls. It may be a function of the small sample size (31).

These studies are among the first to examine young adults and adolescents in the prepsychotic phase. Much of the work in this area to date has been in identifying factors that might predict conversion to a full-blown psychotic illness for those who appear to be at ultrahigh risk—that is, those who have an increased vulnerability to developing a psychotic illness beyond genetic heritage. Thus, in this early phase of research, gender issues have not been fully addressed. Most sample sizes are too small for a scientific gender analysis. Differences noted may be due to ascertainment bias, recruitment strategies, or small sample size. However, the first very preliminary results are in line with what was described for gender differences in manifest psychosis, which, in turn, broadly reflect general differences between genders regardless of schizophrenia or psychosis (8,32).

PATHWAYS TO CARE

Few studies have examined the specific path that individuals experiencing a first episode of psychosis or meeting UHR criteria use to gain access to treatment (33,34). Thus, knowledge about attempts made by these individuals to seek help is sparse. One study to date has examined pathways to care in the prodromal period (33). The majority (85%) of 86 individuals with a schizophrenia spectrum disorder reported concerning behaviors both in the period prior to the onset of the psychosis and during the period of untreated psychosis. Despite having concerns, half of the sample did not make any attempt to seek help prior to the onset of psychotic symptoms. The biggest concerns of this group (all of whom developed a psychotic illness) were drug use, depression, a decline in functioning, and decreased social contact. Those who sought help during the prodrome presented with concerns such as depression, a decline in functioning, and the beginnings of hallucinations and delusional or paranoid thinking (17%). Family physicians were contacted more often than psychologists, psychiatrists, or teachers in the prepsychotic phase. Although individuals made one to four contacts in an attempt to obtain help, only two of 86 individuals were successful in receiving care (33). In the prodromal period, females made more attempts to seek help than males although, once psychotic, there were no gender differences in the number of attempts made prior to receiving help. Unfortunately, the sample sizes were too small to determine if females sought help from different sources than males or whether they had different reasons for seeking help. Since substance abuse and aggressive behavior are relatively increased in males, understanding different help-seeking reasons and approaches would aid in developing improved detection and access to care for these early cases.

In a retrospective study on 82 inpatients with first-episode schizophrenia (73% males and 27% females), only one third had sought help for their mental problems in the prodromal phase even if the problems were already severe (35). The longer the duration of the prodromal phase, the greater was the number of symptoms. For individuals seeking help, those first contacting a private psychiatric or psychotherapeutic center (36.7%) had less attenuated positive symptoms than those first contacting a psychiatric hospital (13.3%) or the police (8.3%). No relationship was found for duration of untreated illness and gender, education, or marital status (35).

Independent of gender, help-seeking approaches of potentially prodromal subjects will depend on multiple interacting factors, such as problem severity, problem denial, level of substance use, homelessness, cultural factors, the person's propensity to seek help, available coping strategies, subjective burden of symptoms, accessibility of services, individual attitudes toward seeking help for mental problems and toward psychological/psychiatric services, availability of alternative support, key reference persons' interpretation of observable changes, and fear of stigmatization (34). Gender differences among these factors are not yet fully understood because studied parameters, such as contact rates, have led to often inconsistent results (see, e.g., 36).

THE IMPACT OF THE "AT RISK MENTAL STATE" ON THE DEVELOPMENTAL TRAJECTORY

The onset of psychosis may complicate or interfere with many of the developmental tasks that the young adult is attempting to accomplish at this time (37,38). Typical developmental tasks of early adulthood include individuating from the family; developing interests, hobbies, and skills; discovering and experimenting with sexuality; forming and maintaining relationships; and engaging in further or higher education and vocational activities. As was shown in the ABC study (8), persons with first-episode schizophrenia fell behind age- and gender-matched controls in the performance of these crucial social roles only after the onset of first mental problems. This was, on average, one year before the onset of the first psychotic symptom—that is, during the initial prodromal phase.

Identity formation is yet another major task of young adults. According to Erikson (40) developing a meaningful self-concept is central to identity formation. A vital component of this process is social interactions with significant others (38). It is through such interactions that the young person is able to glean some sense of how he or she is perceived by others. Young persons approaching adulthood become more dependent on peers for these interactions than on family members. Clearly, these important social interactions are often missed if, because of the emergence of psychosis, the individual begins to withdraw from friends and peers or is hindered in making friends. This pattern has been described by Jones (18). Girls who later developed schizophrenia were observed to be introverted, while boys were noted to diminish their social networks by exhibiting disagreeable and antisocial behavior.

Another important component in the development of a positive identity is good self-esteem and a sense of self-worth (37). Poor self-esteem is typically characterized by low confidence, a sense of being the target of the poor opinion of others, and sensitivity to criticism. Poor self-esteem results in an inconsistent frame of reference within which to accommodate and assimilate experiences of self and others. Such negative affects and cognitions may result in avoidance of the very situations that could potentially enhance self-esteem.

A third step toward developing a positive identity is role formation, which often involves determining one's vocational or career path. Role diffusion is not unusual for the adolescent struggling with these developmental tasks, a problem that again is compounded by the emergence of psychosis.

We can easily imagine the often devastating effects that psychosis and the early prepsychotic phase can have on what is a normal struggle with these developmental tasks. As these young individuals develop a psychosis, they often fall out of step with their peers, become socially isolated, develop an altered self-perception, and become unable to complete their education. The potential for achievements is reduced and, as the gap between these individuals and their peers widens, catching up becomes more difficult. The potential for achievement is further reduced if, because of difficulties they are experiencing, these individuals delay completion of education or vocational training. Thus, failure or difficulty in accomplishing these developmental tasks, along with experiences of stigma related to mental illness, has a major impact on the young person over and above the "at risk mental state" or psychosis itself.

FUTURE DIRECTIONS AND OPPORTUNITIES

Research groups (39) are now poised to make major efforts to continue advances in the full spectrum of biologic, epidemiologic, psychological, and sociological research into this time of ultra high risk for psychosis. Adoption of this broad perspective will aid the translation of new evidence into clinical advances that will enhance prevention, care, and recovery. Increased recognition that the prevalence, the course, and the early manifestation of discrete mental illnesses differ in women and men serves to advance knowledge and to aid accurate diagnosis, effective treatment, and, ultimately, prevention. While this is important, gender differences in psychiatric disorders are less likely to reflect illness-specific processes than general differences in male and female physiology, living circumstances, life experiences, and social roles (14).

There are two directions in which to focus our attention. The first is in terms of research that will help us better understand schizophrenia and other psychotic illnesses. An examination of gender differences within the prospective studies with those at ultrahigh risk of developing psychosis can, in the long term, lead to improved theoretical specifications of the mechanisms underlying the onset of psychosis. We have the opportunity to examine the course of the prodrome and the timing, in terms of both biologic and psychosocial development, of the onset in both males and females. Areas under study where gender differences may help advance the understanding of psychosis and its development are, for example, the biologic effects of stress as mediated by the hypothalamic-pituitary-adrenal (HPA) axis (40). (See Chapter 3 by Elaine Walker and Zainab Sabuwalla.) A further question, assuming a stress-diathesis model, is whether there are specific stressors or protectors for young women that may impact the onset of the illness. Gender differences may exist in factors that predict conversion from a high-risk state to psychosis; such information would aid preventive approaches.

The second direction for prodrome studies is to increase our understanding of the mechanisms of action of both biologic and psychological treatments and how they may affect young men and women differently in terms of safety and effectiveness. Such interventions should be based on the different developmental needs and concerns of males and females. In developing interventions to prevent or delay onset, there may be specific issues that need to be addressed in young women if we are to impact maximally on the environmental influences on their vulnerability to psychosis. Longitudinal studies will provide opportunities to study potential neuroprotective effects of estrogen, as in possible variations of symptoms across the menstrual cycle and the interaction of estrogen levels and early use of antipsychotic medications.

CONCLUSION

The focus of this chapter has been to consider what is known about the prepsychotic period in schizophrenia and its relevance for young women. As studies in the rather new field of early detection and intervention develop, it is vital to consider gender differences both to help increase our understanding of schizophrenia and to design prevention and intervention strategies that may have relevance for the needs of both sexes. Focusing attention on the exciting scientific developments in the field of early psychosis will facilitate the development of evidence-based practice and ultimately lead to necessary changes in mental health care delivery internationally.

REFERENCES

1. American Psychiatric Association. Diagnostic and Statistical Manual of Mental Disorders, 4th Ed. Washington, DC: 1994.
2. Klosterkötter J, Hellmich M, Steinmeyer EM, et al. Diagnosing schizophrenia in the initial prodromal phase. Arch Gen Psychiatry 2001;58:158–164.
3. McGlashan TH. Psychosis treatment prior to psychosis onset: ethical issues. Schizophr Res 2001;51:47–54.
4. Phillips LJ, Yung AR, McGorry PD. Identification of young people at risk of psychosis: validation of personal assessment and crisis evaluation clinic intake criteria. Aust NZ J Psychiatry 2000;34 (Suppl.):164–169.
5. Addington J, Leriger E, Addington D. Symptom outcome one year after admission to an early psychosis program. Can J Psychiatry 2003;48:204–207.
6. Addington J, Young J, Addington D. Social outcome in early psychosis. Psychol Med 2003;33:1119–1124.
7. Häfner H, Löffler W, Maurer K, et al. Depression, negative symptoms, social stagnation and social decline in the early course of schizophrenia. Acta Psychiatr Scand 1999;100:105–118.
8. Häfner H. Gender differences in first-episode schizophrenia. In: Frank E, ed. Gender and Its Effects on Psychopathology. Washington, DC: American Psychiatric Press, 2000:187–228.
9. Jablenski A, Sartorius N, Ernberg G, et al. Schizophrenia: manifestations, incidence and course in different cultures. A World Health Organization ten-country study. Psychol Med (Monograph Suppl 20). Cambridge: Cambridge University Press, 1992.
10. DeLisi L, Bass N, Boccio A, et al. Age of onset in familial schizophrenia. Arch Gen Psychiatry 1994;51:334–335.
11. Könnecke R, Häfner H, Maurer K, et al. Main risk factors for schizophrenia: increased familial loading and pre- and peri-natal complications antagonize the protective effect of oestrogen in women. Schizophr Res 2000;44:81–93.
12. Seeman MV, Lang M. The role of estrogens in schizophrenia gender differences. Schizophr Bull 1990;16:185–193.
13. Häfner H, Hambrecht M, Löffler W, et al. Is schizophrenia a disorder of all ages? A comparison of first episodes and early course across the life-cycle. Psychol Med 1998;28:351–365.
14. Gold J. Gender differences in psychiatric illness and treatments. A critical review. J Nerv Ment Dis 1998;186:769–775.

15. Cohen RZ, Seeman MV, Gotowiec A, et al. Earlier puberty as a predictor of later onset of schizophrenia in women. Am J Psychiatry 1999;156:1059–1064.
16. Yung AR, McGorry PD, McFarlane CA, et al. Monitoring and care of young people at incipient risk of psychosis. Schizophr Bull 1996;22:283–303.
17. Yung AR, McGorry PD. The prodromal phase of first-episode psychosis: past and current conceptualizations. Schizophr Bull 1996;22:353–370.
18. Jones PB. Risk factors for schizophrenia in childhood and youth. In: Häfner H, ed. Risk and Protective Factors in Schizophrenia: Towards a Conceptual Model of the Disease Process. Darmstadt: Steinkopff, 2002:141–162.
19. Schultze-Lutter F, Löffler W, Häfner H. Testing models of the early course of schizophrenia. In: Häfner H, ed. Risk and Protective Factors in Schizophrenia: Towards a Conceptual Model of the Disease Process. Darmstadt: Steinkopff, 2002:229–242.
20. Cornblatt B, Obuchowski M. Update of high-risk research: 1987–1997. Int Rev Psychiatry 1997;9:447.
21. Yung AR, Phillips LJ, Yuen H, et al. Psychosis prediction: a 12-month follow-up of a high-risk ("prodromal") group. Schizophr Res 2003;60:21–32.
22. Miller TJ, Zipursky R, Perkins DO, et al. A randomized double blind clinical trial of olanzapine vs placebo in patients at risk for being prodromally symptomatic for psychosis II: recruitment and baseline characteristics of the "prodromal" sample. Schizophr Res 2003;61:19–30.
23. Schaffner KF, McGorry PD. Preventing severe mental illnesses: new prospects and ethical challenges. Schizophr Res 2001;51:3–15.
24. Miller TJ, McGlashan TH, Rosen JL, et al. Prospective diagnosis of the initial prodrome for schizophrenia based on the structured interview for prodromal syndromes: preliminary evidence of interrater reliability and predictive validity. Am J Psychiatry 2002;159:863–865.
25. Huber G, Gross G. The concept of basic symptoms in schizophrenic and schizoaffective psychoses. Recenti Prog Med 1989;80:646–652.
26. Gross G, Huber G, Klosterkötter J, et al. Bonner Skala für die Beurteilung von Basissymptomen (BSABS; Bonn Scale for the Assessment of Basic Symptoms). Berlin: Springer, 1987.
27. McGorry PD, Yung A, Phillips L. Ethics in early intervention in psychosis: keeping up the pace and staying in step. Schizophr Res 2001;51:17–29.
28. McGlashan TH, Zipursky R, Perkins DO, et al. A randomized double blind clinical trial of olanzapine vs placebo in patients at risk for being prodromally symptomatic for psychosis I: study rationale and design. Schizophr Res 2003;61:7–18.
29. Morrison T, Bentall R, French P, et al. Early detection and intervention for psychosis in primary care. Acta Psychiatr Scand 2002;413 (Suppl.):44.
30. McGorry PD, Yung AR, Phillips LJ, et al. A randomized controlled trial of interventions designed to reduce the risk of progression to first-episode psychosis in a clinical sample with subthreshold symptoms. Arch Gen Psychiatry 2002;59:921–928.
31. Cornblatt BA, Lencz T, Smith CW, et al. The schizophrenia prodrome revisited: a neurodevelopmental perspective. Schizophr Bull 2003;29:633–652.
32. Spauwen J, Krabbendam L, Lieb R, et al. Sex differences: normal or pathological? Schizophr Res 2003;62:45–49.
33. Addington J, van Mastrigt S, Hutchinson J, et al. Pathways to care: help seeking behavior in first episode psychosis. Acta Psychiatr Scand 2002;106:358–364.
34. Lincoln C, Harrigan S, McGorry PD. Understanding the topography of the early psychosis pathways: an opportunity to reduce delays in treatment. Br J Psychiatry 1998;172:21–25.
35. Köhn D, Niedersteberg A, Wieneke A, et al. Frühverlauf schizophrener ersterkrankungen mit langer dauer der unbehandelten erkrankung - eine ergleichende studie. Fortschr Neurol Psychiatr 2004;72:88–92.
36. Saarento O, Räsänen S, Nieminen P, et al. Sex differences in the contact rates and utilization of psychiatric services. A three-year follow–up study in northern Finland. Eur Psychiatry 2000;15:205–212.
37. Erikson EH. Identity, Youth and Crisis. New York: Norton, 1968.
38. Muuss RE. Theories of Adolescence. New York: McGraw-Hill, 1988.
39. Auther AM, Lencz T, Smith CW, et al. Overview of the first annual workshop on the schizophrenia prodrome. Schizophr Bull 2003;29:625–631.
40. Corcoran C, Walker E, Huot R, et al. The stress cascade and schizophrenia: etiology and onset. Schizophr Bull 2003;29:671–692.

CHAPTER 10

Substance Use, Abuse, and Dependence in Adolescent Girls

Sheila B. Blume, Monica L. Zilberman, Hermano Tavares

About 40 years ago, one of the authors (S.B.B.) admitted a 15-year-old boy into the state hospital alcoholism rehabilitation unit she directed. He came from a family with multigenerational alcohol problems and had started to drink regularly at 12. This patient was so unusual that she considered publishing a case report. How hard it would have been to imagine that within the next few decades, the treatment of alcohol and other drug problems would become a routine part of pediatrics and adolescent medicine, and not only for boys (at that time substance abuse was assumed to be almost entirely confined to the male), but for nearly equal numbers of girls.

The trend for younger and younger onset of substance use disorders was noted in the United States in the 1970s and 80s. Nevertheless, repeated annual studies of tobacco, alcohol, and other drug use by teens in the United States that began in the 1970s found a general decrease in rates of use until about 1990. The rates remained stable until about 1995, after which adolescent substance use increased steadily and significantly as the twentieth century came to a close. The University of Michigan's annual Monitoring the Future Study (MTF), a survey of tens of thousands of secondary school students in grades 8 to 12 (ages 14 to 18 years), documents these trends (1). MTF data also yield evidence of convergence of the rates of use between boys and girls.

Despite differences in different parts of the world, these trends are not limited to Western or European cultures. We must assume that twenty-first-century health-care practitioners throughout the world will continue to need an understanding of the diagnosis and treatment of substance use disorders in girls and women as well as of the interaction of these disorders with the other complex physical, psychological, and developmental issues of women's lives.

EPIDEMIOLOGY

The 2002 MTF survey, involving 43,700 students in 394 schools throughout the United States, found that over half the students had taken at least one illicit drug by the time they completed high school. The survey brought some good news evidenced by a modest decline in the use of some drugs compared to the previous year, particularly of MDMA ("ecstasy") and, to a lesser degree, of cannabis. Other drugs, including cocaine and heroin, held steady, while tranquilizers and barbiturates showed some increase. By twelfth grade 57% of students had already tried cigarettes, 27% were current smokers, and 62% reported having been drunk at least once in their lifetime. Although prevalence estimates of substance use in this survey tend to be higher for male students than for female students, the magnitude of gender differences has become smaller over time. Rates of cigarette smoking are now the same for boys and girls (1,2). In view of adolescent girls' increased difficulty in quitting smoking compared to boys (3), this is a cause for concern. It is also estimated that 26% of high school girls binge drink (defined as consuming five or more drinks at one sitting), 20% currently use marijuana, 4% use cocaine, and another 4% use inhalants (4).

The National Household Survey on Drug Abuse (NHSDA), conducted annually in the United States, also provides evidence for gender convergence regarding alcohol use initiation among adolescents, showing that from the 1950s to the 1990s the male:female ratio (MFR) of starting to drink among adolescents aged 10–14 slowly decreased from 4:1 to 1:1. It is not surprising, then, that a MFR of 1:1 was found for alcohol dependence in the 12-year-old to 17-year-old group in 1999. Even more disturbing is the predominance of early cocaine use among girls. MFRs for lifetime cocaine and crack use in the 12–17 age bracket were 0.7:1 and 0.5:1, respectively, in 1996 (5).

These trends, also observed in other parts of the world (6), imply that the previously identified pattern of women starting substance use later in life than men (a protective factor in terms of progression to substance dependence) is no longer the case. Added to this concern is the fact that, partly due to gender differences in drug metabolism, women develop substance-related medical complications more rapidly than men do, including, in some cases, substance dependence.

PATTERNS OF SUBSTANCE USE

Substance use is starting at progressively younger ages in recent generations, and this drop in age of onset is more marked for girls, particularly for alcohol (the most consumed substance in adolescence) and tobacco. Physically, girls tend to have smaller body sizes and lower tolerances compared to boys, putting them at greater risk for alcohol-related problems even at lower levels of consumption. Similarly, smoking is now as frequent in girls as in boys, but girls are more likely to carry over nicotine addiction into adulthood. Also, girls who begin to smoke are likelier than boys to develop nicotine dependence and do this more rapidly. Substance use differs between girls and boys in many ways, including reasons for use. Girls most often initiate substance use as a coping mechanism, whereas boys usually are motivated by curiosity. Boys who are risk takers and crave excitement are therefore the most likely to become early substance users. While girls who fit this description also use substances, many are quite the opposite—shy, anxious, depressed, troubled girls who find that alcohol, in particular, helps them cope with the stresses of teenage life.

A matter of current debate is the "gateway theory," postulating that particular substances (usually tobacco and alcohol) act as introductory drugs that pave the way to further substance use. This theory was first applied to cannabis use in adolescents. Opponents argue that the association is an artifact of the higher prevalence of alcohol and tobacco use at earlier ages. Although not all persons who smoke, drink, or use cannabis will progress to harder drug use, evidence suggests that the risk for progression is increased for those who start before age 15 (4).

CHARACTERISTICS OF SUBSTANCE ABUSE AND DEPENDENCE IN ADOLESCENT GIRLS

Girls commonly prefer wine or spirits, whereas boys more often drink beer. Adolescents in general are more likely to be intermittent or binge drinkers and users than to drink or use drugs in a pattern of consuming small amounts throughout the day.

Rebellious adolescents, some of whom have a history of attention deficit or hyperactivity disorder and/or conduct disorder, often drink and use drugs in groups that openly defy adult norms. They have a high prevalence of associated behaviors such as early and risky sexual activity, shoplifting, truancy, and un- planned pregnancy. However, girls who use substances to cope with internal mood states or social discomfort may carefully conceal their drinking or use of il- legally obtained prescription medications or other illicit drugs.

Girls with substance-related problems seldom reach the attention of medical or mental health professionals for the substance use alone, except in cases of al- cohol poisoning or other toxic states such as hyperthermia related to the use of MDMA. They are more often seen because of menstrual irregularities, injuries or vague physical complaints, failing school performance, or family problems, so that it is up to the clinician to maintain a high index of suspicion and inquire care- fully about substance use. Adolescent girls often minimize their use of alcohol and drugs, as well as rationalizing that "everybody does it." Those who are focused on body image and the desire to be thin rationalize the use of cigarettes or stimulant drugs as helping them lose weight. Those who use alcohol or pre- scription drugs to cope with depression are at increased risk for suicide, so that it is particularly important to evaluate substance use in depressed teens.

Sexual assault, including date rape, is a hazard to which adolescent girls are exposed. Alcohol and other drug use (particularly sedative drugs) by both rapist and victim increase the risk of this traumatic event.

Alcohol-impaired driving is also a concern for adolescent girls in the United States given that motor vehicle crashes are currently the most frequent cause of death in the U.S. for persons aged 15 to 20. Because of their inexperience behind the wheel and sensitivity to alcohol, alcohol-involved teen drivers have a rate of crashes that is more than twice as high as that for alcohol-involved drivers aged 21 or older (7).

RISK FACTORS

PSYCHOLOGICAL FACTORS

Psychological factors have a major influence on adolescent girls' substance use and progression to abuse/dependence. The National Center on Addiction and Substance Abuse at Columbia University (CASA) (4) released a comprehensive study of American girls and young women (8–22 years of age), documenting that high school girls are more likely than boys to report feeling depressed, hopeless, and sad, and to consider and attempt suicide. Such feelings, as mentioned above, are related to substance use among girls. These girls are also more likely to report negative feelings and suicidal behavior than girls who have never used substances.

College women who drink to relieve shyness, to feel high, or to get along better on dates are likelier to develop drinking problems later in life than women who did not report this pattern in college. In a 27-year follow-up of a large college drinking study, they were found the most likely group to develop alcohol abuse/dependence in adulthood, even when compared to women who had reported overt alcohol-related problems while in college (8).

Girls with problems of substance use present to treatment with increased rates of psychiatric symptomatology and diagnoses (including mania and attention deficit and conduct disorders). In addition to these disorders, girls with substance use disorders also have higher rates of depressive, eating, and psychotic symptomatology, whereas affective and eating symptomatology are not increased among boys with substance use problems and disorders (9). Diagnoses of mental disorders may be classified as primary or secondary, depending on age of onset, with the earlier disorder classified as primary (although not necessary causative of the secondary disorder). Overall, the available evidence suggests that depressive and anxiety symptomatology more often precedes alcohol abuse or dependence (so-called secondary alcoholism) in girls and women, while in men the alcoholism is more often primary. Thus psychological factors are likely to have a greater etiologic significance for women than for men (10).

As pointed out under characteristics of substance use and dependence, personality factors, particularly impulsivity, also represent risk factors for substance use problems. Antisocial and deviant behaviors are associated with substance use initiation and maintenance as well as poorer treatment outcome (11). Among girls, borderline personality features may represent additional risk by combining two risk factors (impulsivity and anxiety/depressive traits) (12). Further, self-esteem issues impact substance use patterns, particularly for girls.

A large population-based study of adolescent twins investigated the relationship between conduct disorders and attention deficit hyperactivity disorder (ADHD) and substance use problems in adolescents. Conduct disorder was found to increase the risk of substance use and abuse in adolescents. Although ADHD per se was not associated with increased risk of substance use disorders, girls with ADHD were at slightly higher risk than boys (13). Also, the severity of inattention in childhood may predict substance use outcomes (14).

In adolescents, as in adults, substance use disorders are related to trauma, and recent studies have found an increasing prevalence of substance use disorders comorbid with post-traumatic stress disorder (PTSD) among adolescents. The risk of PTSD is three times higher in adolescents with substance use disorders compared to those without these diagnoses (15). Trauma, particularly sexual abuse, is a factor in substance use and abuse among girls. Conversely, substance-abusing girls are at higher risk for several forms of physical, sexual, and psychological abuse, a fact that leads to a vicious circle of trauma initiating substance use and abuse, which in turn lead to further trauma.

Childhood abuse of all kinds is more common in the histories of both girls and women with substance use problems (compared to their counterparts who do not abuse substances), which suggests that the effect of childhood trauma is longlasting among women (16,17).

Girls are more likely than boys to worry about body image and to try to control their weight by various, often unhealthy means, such as smoking, fasting, vomiting, or taking laxatives or diet pills. Data from the CASA study show that adolescents who are dieting to control weight are more likely to smoke and drink than are girls who are not dieting.

SOCIOCULTURAL FACTORS

Several sociocultural factors affect substance use initiation and progression. In terms of ethnicity, for instance, the MTF survey shows drug use is highest among Native American girls and lowest among Black and Asian American girls (1).

Parental and sibling substance use are potent predictors of substance use among children and adolescents. Parental smoking, for example, is associated with increased risk of adolescent smoking, while parental smoking cessation significantly reduces children's risk of smoking (18). Cross-cultural research shows that family composition itself has an impact on smoking behavior among adolescents, those living with both biologic parents smoking less than others (19).

Popular media have significantly contributed to the increase of girls' substance use. Special "women's" brands of cigarettes have been developed and marketed, their advertisements stressing thinness and independence. Alcohol marketing campaigns have also been directed to girls and young women, and the beverage industry has released products that appeal to girls. Examples include sweet fruit-flavored wines and "alcopops," a sugary combination of fruit ice and alcohol at about 5% concentration, stronger than most beers. The movie industry since the 1920s has impacted smoking initiation among girls and young women by representing women's smoking behavior as related to ideals of elegance and independence. This connection may be felt even more strongly by adolescents searching for role models than by more mature women.

GENETIC FACTORS

Genetic factors are related to substance initiation, use, abuse, and dependence, in adolescents as well as adults (see Chapter 13 of this book). There is evidence that the relative contribution of genetic and environmental factors is different across genders. For instance, for women, genetic factors play a more significant role in smoking initiation than in smoking maintenance (20).

In evaluating a girl for any health or behavior problem, it is very useful to obtain a family history of substance use, including information about not just the parental generation but grandparents and siblings. A positive history puts a girl at increased risk for substance problems, even if she does not live with the relative (e.g., an absent alcoholic father).

SCREENING AND DIAGNOSIS

Early detection of substance use problems among adolescents is important for the prevention of further disability. Thus screening should be an integral part of primary as well as specialist care (21). A number of screening tools have been developed for the adolescent population. Although none of them is specific for girls, preliminary research suggests that they apply equally to girls and boys. The CRAFFT (22) comprises six yes/no questions and is convenient to incorporate into the history-taking interview. A significant problem with substance use is indicated by two or more positive answers. (The name of the tool is taken from the key words in the six questions: car, relax, alone, forget, family, trouble; see Table 10.1).

The Substance Use/Abuse Scale from the Problem Oriented Screening Instrument for Teenagers (POSIT) is a self-administered 17-item measure that was developed for the detection of substance use problems in primary adolescent care. It distinguishes severe substance users from nonusers by means of yes/no questions such as, "Do you miss out on activities because you spend too much money on drugs or alcohol?" and "During the past month, have you driven a car while you were drunk or high?" A score of 1 or more (range: 0–17) is considered indicative that further evaluation should be undertaken (23).

Many female adolescents who have substance-related problems satisfy a diagnosis of substance abuse or dependence according to the American Psychiatric Association's *Diagnostic and Statistical Manual of Mental Disorders*, 4th edition (DSM-IV), or fit into the category of harmful use or dependence syndrome in the International Statistical Classification of Diseases and Related Health Problems, 10th revision (ICD-10). A DSM-IV diagnosis of abuse describes a maladaptive pattern of substance use over time that puts the patient at risk or has already created problems although those problems have not met criteria for substance dependence. Dependence involves satisfying at least three of seven criteria within the past 12 months. These include indications of impaired control over use, such as persistent desires or the inability to cut down or stop using the substance, or

TABLE 10.1

The CRAFFT Questions* — A Brief Screening Test for Adolescent Substance Abuse

C— Have you ever ridden in a *car* driven by someone (including yourself) who was "high" or had been using alcohol or drugs?

R— Do you ever use alcohol or drugs to *relax*, feel better about yourself, or fit in?

A— Do you ever use alcohol or drugs while you are by yourself, *alone*?

F— Do you ever *forget* things you did while using alcohol or drugs?

F— Do your family or *friends* ever tell you that you should cut down on your drinking or drug use?

T— Have you ever you gotten into *trouble* while you were using alcohol or drugs?

© Children's Hospital Boston, 2001

*Reproduced with permission from the Center for Adolescent Substance Abuse Research, CeASAR, Children's Hospital Boston. For more information, contact info@CRAFFT.org, or visit www.crafft.org.

Source: Knight JR, Sherritt L, Shrier LA, et al. Validity of the CRAFFT substance abuse screening test among adolescent clinic patients. Arch Pediatr Adolesc Med 2002;156:607–614.

use for longer periods or in greater quantities than intended, spending a great deal of time in activities related to the substance, life problems due to this use, continued use in spite of recognizing these problems, and criteria for tolerance and withdrawal that indicate physiologic dependence. Physiologic dependence is not necessary for a dependence diagnosis if three or more of the other criteria are satisfied. The ICD-10 diagnostic categories are roughly equivalent to the DSM categories of abuse and dependence.

PHASES OF TREATMENT

Approaches to the adolescent girl may be divided into three phases, although in any one case they may overlap or change in sequence.

IMMEDIATE TREATMENT

The first challenge is to accomplish as complete an assessment as possible of the multiple problems facing the patient while developing a rapport that will mature into a therapeutic alliance. The patient's goals may be simple. She may just wish to relieve the current pressures from family, school, or the justice system (depending on the referral source). In developing mutually agreed preliminary goals, this initial motivation should be taken into account. For the treatment professional, the initial goals are to deal with any immediate threats to life and health and to devise a treatment plan with the appropriate level of care. The American Society of Addiction Medicine (ASAM) Patient Placement Criteria are helpful in choosing the proper level of care by considering multiple factors. Guidelines written specifically for adolescents are included (24).

The treatment professional's goals also include interrupting the use of substances as quickly as possible. This involves working with the patient's current motivation to establish the connection between her use of substances and immediate problems, and agreeing on the need to stop using alcohol or drugs. She need not agree to a goal of lifetime abstinence at this point, but she must be willing and able to try to abstain in the short term with the help of a therapist or program. The program can be one of the mutual help groups such as Alcoholics Anonymous (AA) or Narcotics Anonymous (NA), both of which have young people's groups, all-female groups, and beginner's groups in many places.

Patients who are physiologically dependent on one or more substances may require medication to treat a withdrawal syndrome, especially in the case of dependence on alcohol, a sedative, or an opiate. Sedatives such as phenobarbital, benzodiazepines such as chlordiazepoxide, or opiates, including methadone and buprenorphine, may be prescribed as detoxification treatment. (See caveats in the next section, however.) Because adolescents are more likely to use multiple substances than adults, a wider range of withdrawal symptoms can be expected for them. Detoxification may be performed on an outpatient basis, preferably in an intensive or partial hospital setting, or as an inpatient, according to the needs of the case.

Most clinicians recommend that smoking cessation be a part of the overall treatment of adolescents for alcohol or other drug abuse or dependence. Although it can be more difficult for a patient to quit smoking in an outpatient setting than in a residential treatment setting, being nicotine-free should be an accepted part of the long-range goals established with the patient.

Family involvement should be encouraged at every stage of treatment. Al-Anon and Nar Anon are useful mutual help programs from which family members will profit.

SHORT-TERM TREATMENT

Once treatment has begun, the goals include educating the patient about the effects of substances and the disorders of abuse and dependence (including relapse triggers and techniques to prevent relapse), and about the risks of switching addictions, for example from one drug to another or to a behavioral addiction such as pathologic gambling or compulsive shopping. This involves exploring and improving coping skills and often requires finding a new, nonusing peer group. Mutual help groups are often instrumental in providing such a group and in teaching and reinforcing these new ideas. The patient must be helped to develop an altered self-concept, that of a person in successful recovery from a life-threatening illness, rather than a rebel, a loser, or an incompetent. Self-esteem is built in learning about herself and her disease, in staying clean and sober day by day, and in improving her functioning in school, work, and family. All-female addiction therapy groups, if available, are preferred by many clinicians, especially for young women who have a history of sexual abuse. Sometimes mixed-sex adolescent therapy groups can be supplemented by special-issue women's or girls' groups to work on these problems.

Some colleges and universities sponsor "clean and sober" support meetings and substance-free dormitories. Some high schools also run support groups for recovering substance users or for children of alcoholics and addicts. The treating professional should be aware of all of the resources available in the patient's community.

During this phase, a stable internal motivation to remain substance-free should be fostered based on an understanding of the role of alcohol and drugs in the young woman's earlier life problems and the rewards of remaining sober. The treatment professional should not assume that the patient's motivation is constant, as it may fluctuate, so that frequent "motivation checks" are as important as asking, "How are you doing?"

Comorbid physical and psychiatric conditions should be treated at the same time as the substance use disorder whenever possible. When prescription medications are used in treating these conditions, it is important to avoid the use of drugs that have an abuse potential, such as benzodiazepines, sedatives, and opiates. Girls who suffer from substance-related disorders are at high risk for secondary iatrogenic addictions. Teaching methods to reduce tension and anxiety without medication, such as deep relaxation, yoga, or other exercise, can be very helpful in this group. Encourage continuing involvement of the patient's family in the treatment because family members also need education about the nature of substance use disorders and about recovery.

Medications used as adjuncts to therapy in the treatment of alcohol dependence in adults, such as naltrexone and acamprosate, have not been well studied in adolescent populations although some clinicians do prescribe them for this age group. Disulfiram, a drug that causes a toxic interaction with alcohol if the patient drinks, is not usually used in adolescents because of their impulsivity and the risk of adverse reactions. Maintenance of an opiate agonists (methadone or buprenorphine) as a treatment for opiate dependence is not appropriate for younger adolescents but may be considered in older adolescents or young adults who have failed at other treatments. In the United States, current regulations place the minimum age for methadone treatment at 18.

Relapses are to be expected early in treatment, especially if the care is in an outpatient setting and the patient is still exposed to her usual environment. The challenge is to interrupt the substance use as quickly as possible and to learn from analyzing the relapse. What were the triggers? How did the planned response fail? What could have been done differently? It is important not to consider relapse a failure of treatment or failure of the patient. However, relapse is a signal to reevaluate the treatment plan. Serious or repeated relapses may indicate the need for a more intensive level of care.

LONG-TERM TREATMENT

If the patient's initial treatment has taken place in a residential or partial hospital setting, the long-term aspect of her care is usually called aftercare, although to the patient it is often the most crucial period of recovery. In this phase, she must put into daily practice the lessons learned earlier in treatment, including coping with life problems without using substances and resisting the pressure from peers to resume use. Again, motivation should be assessed regularly. The patient should be helped to develop an emergency plan to avoid use in the case of a sudden, unexpected challenge. She should be encouraged to monitor her mood and feel comfortable in seeking help from a variety of sources if she feels she needs it. If a girl or young woman in treatment for substance use disorder says to her therapist, "You're the only one who understands me" or "You're the only one who can help me," this is a signal that her treatment is lacking in resources. It is important for her to recognize that many others in her life (such as members of support groups or other staff members within a treatment program or in the community) can understand and help her in a crisis.

Continued psychotherapy, either individually or in young persons' groups, may be indicated for some patients, while others may be managed with less intensive treatment but with close monitoring in case more intensive treatment becomes necessary. Ongoing participation in mutual help or other support groups is also important. In addition to friendship, support, and reminders of the need to stay sober, the patient is likely to find herself able to use her experiences to help others in earlier stages of recovery and thereby enhance her self-esteem. Groups based on the 12-step program of Alcoholics Anonymous stress the spiritual aspects of recovery along with physical, mental, and social factors, which is also a great help to many adolescents.

The treatment professional should be aware that others in the patient's family may also have substance problems and should try to link these family members with treatment for themselves wherever possible.

RESEARCH ON TREATMENT

Only recently have researchers investigated the factors that influence treatment outcome among adolescents. The Drug Abuse Treatment Outcomes Studies for Adolescents (DATOS-A) showed that comorbidity (particularly conduct disorders) is associated with increased problem severity before treatment and with worse outcomes but also with increased motivation for treatment (25). Length of stay in treatment and participation in aftercare are both related to better outcomes. Thus increasing treatment retention and completion and developing programs that are relevant and attractive to adolescents represent critical challenges in treating this population (11,26). Research suggests that adolescent girls and boys have similar long-term substance use outcomes (27), but girls may have greater improvement in terms of psychological adjustment following treatment (28). Similar to adult women, adolescent girls entering addiction treatment are reported to have more substance use issues, mental and physical health problems, and HIV sexual risk behaviors. Hence the girls need a more comprehensive assessment and more targeted information and behavior change strategies. Trauma-related issues should also be screened and addressed as they enter treatment, making use of a safe setting and sensitive questioning. Addressing these issues is critical for their adherence to treatment (29). Eating disorders and body image issues may be dealt with along with substance use, since many female adolescents (even those without a diagnosable comorbid eating disorder) may stick to nicotine, cocaine, and other stimulants to control weight. Further, it is not uncommon that the stress involved in recovering from an addiction problem will trigger the recurrence of an eating problem that had been subclinical or in remission. Alternative ways of dealing with weight (nutrition facts and regular exercise) should be explored (30).

Adolescents with substance-related disorders may be pregnant or have a history of one or more pregnancies. Education about sex, birth control, and about the effects of alcohol and other drug use on the developing fetus are another important feature of treating these patients.

Treatment options for adolescents include both inpatient and outpatient models, often based on the 12-step philosophy. All-youth therapeutic communities are also available. In making decisions about treatment options, the treatment philosophy of providers and an assessment of severity level should be considered in addition to setting (31). Since psychiatric comorbidity is more often the rule than the exception in treating young women with substance use problems, treatments designed to address both conditions simultaneously may particularly fit this population's needs (32).

Given the impact that family factors play in substance use behavior among adolescents, and the disruptive effects of the adolescent's problems on other family members, involvement of the family is usually very helpful in treating adolescents. Family therapy may be indicated, usually as an adjunct to treatment for addiction. Available research supports the effectiveness of including a family treatment component in addiction treatment for adolescents (31).

PREVENTION

One of the most important goals of prevention is to obviate entirely, or at least delay, the onset of use of all substances of abuse. The earlier the use, the greater the risk of problems. For alcohol this may be related to the detrimental effects of alcohol on the still-developing brain (33). Persons who begin drinking before age 15 are four times more likely to develop alcohol dependence at some time in their lives than those who have their first drink at age 20 or older (34). These findings hold up in various ethnic and cultural settings. For example, studies in Colombia have shown that early tobacco use is associated with later marijuana and other illicit drug use and drug-related problems. Early marijuana use, in turn, is associated with behavior, work, and school problems and violence (35).

Primary care physicians are in a unique position for the early detection of substance-related problems. Therefore, medical training should place more emphasis on the importance of substance use, particularly for female adolescents (since, as mentioned, substance use poses greater risk for young women's health and well-being).

Prevention programs directed to youth should include issues that are unique to adolescent girls and young women, including date rape and other abuse, substance use during pregnancy, and the increased sensitivity of girls to alcohol and other drugs. Some factors found by research to be associated with greater effectiveness of prevention programs are strengthening family support, encouraging school connectedness and positive role models, and acquisition of life skills and social skills. Ideally, prevention programs should start early in school. Particularly for girls, programs starting in grades 4 to 8 (before substance use begins) are more effective than programs starting later in school (4).

Although the inclusion of topics related to emotions and feelings management is helpful, this should not be the primary focus of prevention, even for girls. For both girls and boys, such programs are not as effective as more comprehensive programs. Gains from prevention programs may differ between girls and boys depending on time elapsed, with girls showing improvements later (after the conclusion of the program), and boys showing improvements earlier (during the course of the program).

Elementary and high school settings are important for prevention in many other ways. Rules about smoking, alcohol, and drugs, and their enforcement, set a tone for student attitudes. After-school activities that are substance-free are preventive. Research has shown that girls who involve themselves in team sports are less likely to use substances, although this is not true for boys.

Colleges and universities have established a variety of preventive measures that involve rules about underage drinking (both on campus and off campus), education about substance use and abuse for students and campus leaders, and relationships with the outside community. The most difficult element in prevention on campuses is changing the college culture that supports underage and binge drinking as a norm. Polls find that students tend to overestimate the amount of alcohol that their friends and fellow students consume, so one factor in educating students is correcting that false impression and providing accurate information about drinking and drug use on campus and its consequences. Another is offering confidential help to students who think they may have a problem or who are children of alcoholic or addicted parents.

Additional important resources for prevention and early intervention are the criminal justice system and the family courts. Careful screening of adolescents and families involved in these systems can lead to early intervention and diversion from the criminal to the treatment system.

Community attitudes toward the enforcement of laws relating to substance use, such as sales of tobacco and alcohol to minors, smoking and drinking at sports events and other public places, and laws prohibiting drunk driving or drinking while driving, are likewise important elements in prevention.

Whereas the advertising of alcohol and tobacco can increase the rates of early use, media campaigns can also play an important role in counteracting substance use. Media messages to young people, some of them using female celebrities such as athletes and singers as positive role models for adolescent girls, can help deliver prevention messages, although more research establishing the effectiveness of media campaigns is clearly needed (4). Changes in the depiction of smoking and use of alcohol and other drugs in movies, songs, and magazines and other literature aimed at young readers are necessary to help alter the attitudes of adolescents about the use of these substances. Health professionals can and should take an activist stance about the need for prevention, both in their own communities and on a national and international level. For the sake of future generations, a wide perspective on youth substance use and abuse is essential.

REFERENCES

1. Wallace JM Jr, Bachman JG, O'Malley PM, et al. Gender and ethnic differences in smoking, drinking and illicit drug use among American 8th, 10th and 12th grade students, 1976–2000. Addiction 2003;98:225–234.
2. Johnson LD, O'Malley PM, Bachman JG. Monitoring the future national results in adolescent drug use: overview of key findings, 2002. NIH Publication no 03-5374. Bethesda, MD: National Institute on Drug Abuse, 2003.
3. Patton GC, Carlin JB, Coffey C, et al. The course of early smoking: a population-based cohort study over three years. Addiction 1998;93:1251–1260.
4. National Center on Addiction and Substance Abuse at Columbia University (CASA). The formative years: pathways to substance abuse among girls and young women ages 8–22, 2003. Available at: www.casacolumbia.org.
5. Greenfield SF, O'Leary G. Gender differences in substance use disorders. In: Lewis-Hall F, Williams TS, Panetta JA, et al., eds. Psychiatric Illness in Women: Emerging Treatments and Research. Washington, DC: American Psychiatric Publishing, 2002:467–533.
6. Zilberman ML, Tavares H, el-Guebaly N. Gender differences and similarities: prevalence and course of alcohol and other substance related disorders. J Addict Dis 2003;22(4):61–74.
7. Yi H, Williams GD, Dufour MC. Trends in alcohol-related fatal traffic crashes, United States: 1977–99. Surveillance Report 56. National Institute on Alcohol Abuse and Alcoholism, Division of Biometry and Epidemiology, 2001.
8. Fillmore KM, Bacon SD, Hyman M. The 27-year longitudinal panel study of drinking by students in college. 1979 Report to National Institute of Alcoholism and Alcohol Abuse. Contract no ADM 281–76–0015, Washington, DC, 1979.
9. Shrier LA, Harris SK, Kurland M, et al. Substance use problems and associated psychiatric symptoms among adolescents in primary care. Pediatrics 2003;111(6 Pt 1):699–705.
10. Zilberman ML, Tavares H, Blume SB, et al. Substance use disorders: sex differences in psychiatric comorbidities. Can J Psychiatry 2003;48:5–15.
11. Latimer WW, Newcomb M, Winters KC, et al. Adolescent substance abuse treatment outcome: the role of substance abuse problem severity, psychosocial, and treatment factors. J Consult Clin Psychol 2000;68:684–696.
12. Ralph N, McMenamy C. Treatment outcomes in an adolescent chemical dependency program. Adolescence 1996;31:91–107.
13. Disney ER, Elkins IJ, McGue M, et al. Effects of ADHD, conduct disorder, and gender on substance use and abuse in adolescence. Am J Psychiatry 1999;156:1515–1521.
14. Molina BS, Pelham WE Jr. Childhood predictors of adolescent substance use in a longitudinal study of children with ADHD. J Abnorm Psychol 2003;112:497–507.
15. Giaconia RM, Reinherz HZ, Hauf AC, et al. Comorbidity of substance use and post-traumatic stress disorders in a community sample of adolescents. Am J Orthopsychiatry 2000;70:253–262.
16. Pedersen W, Skrondal A. Alcohol and sexual victimization: a longitudinal study of Norwegian girls. Addiction 1996;91:565–581.
17. Simpson TL, Miller WR. Concomitance between childhood sexual and physical abuse and substance use problems: a review. Clin Psychol Rev 2002;22:27–77.
18. Bricker JB, Leroux BG, Peterson AV Jr, et al. Nine-year prospective relationship between parental smoking cessation and children's daily smoking. Addiction 2003;98:585–593.
19. Bjarnason T, Davidaviciene AG, Miller P, et al. Family structure and adolescent cigarette smoking in eleven European countries. Addiction 2003;98:815–824.
20. Li MD, Cheng R, Ma JZ, Swan GE. A meta-analysis of estimated genetic and environmental effects on smoking behavior in male and female adult twins. Addiction 2003;98:23–31.
21. Center for Substance Abuse Treatment (CSAT). Screening and assessing adolescents for substance use disorders: treatment improvement protocol (TIP) series 31. Rockville, MD: U.S. Department of Health and Human Services Publication no (SMA) 99-3282, 1999. Available at: http://hstat.nlm.nih.gov.
22. Knight JR, Sherritt L, Shrier LA, et al. Validity of the CRAFFT substance abuse screening test among adolescent clinic patients. Arch Pediatr Adolesc Med 2002;156:607–614.

23. Rahdert ER. The Adolescent Assessment/Referral System Manual. DHHS Publication no (ADM) 91-1735. Rockville, MD: U.S. Department of Health and Human Services, ADAMHA, National Institute on Drug Abuse, 1991.
24. American Society of Addiction Medicine (ASAM). ASAM Patient Placement Criteria for the Treatment of Substance-Related Disorders, 2nd Ed.-Rev. Chevy Chase, MD, 2001.
25. Hser YI, Grella CE, Collins C, et al. Drug-use initiation and conduct disorder among adolescents in drug treatment. J Adolesc 2003;26:331–345.
26. Hser YI, Grella CE, Hubbard RL, et al. An evaluation of drug treatments for adolescents in four US cities. Arch Gen Psychiatry 2001;58:689–695.
27. Winters KC, Stinchfield RD, Opland E, et al. The effectiveness of the Minnesota Model approach in the treatment of adolescent drug abusers. Addiction 2000;95:601–612.
28. De Leon G, Jainchill N. Residential therapeutic communities for female substance abusers. Bull NY Acad Med 1991;67:277–290.
29. Stevens SJ, Murphy BS, McKnight K. Traumatic stress and gender differences in relationship to substance abuse, mental health, physical health, and HIV risk behavior in a sample of adolescents enrolled in drug treatment. Child Maltreat 2003;8:46–57.
30. Zilberman ML, Tavares H, Blume S, et al. Towards best practices in the treatment of women with addictive disorders. Addict Disord Their Treatment 2002;1:39–46.
31. Center for Substance Abuse Treatment (CSAT). Treatment of adolescents with substance use disorders: treatment improvement protocol (TIP) series 32. Rockville, MD: U.S. Department of Health and Human Services Publication no 99-3283, 1999. Available at: http://hstat.nlm.nih.gov.
32. Jorgensen ED, Salwen R. Treatment of dually diagnosed adolescents: the individual alliance within a day treatment model. In: Approaches to Drug Abuse Counselling. Rockville, MD: National Institute on Drug Abuse, National Institute of Health Publication no 00-4151, 2000. Available at: http://www.drugabuse.gov/ADAC/ADAC6.html.
33. Spear LP. The adolescent brain and the college drinker: biological basis of propensity to use and misuse alcohol. J Stud Alcohol Suppl 2002;(14):71–81.
34. Grant BF, Dawson DA. Age at onset of alcohol use and its association with DSM-IV alcohol abuse and dependence: results from the National Longitudinal Alcohol Epidemiologic Survey. J Subst Abuse 1997;9:103–110.
35. Siqueira LM, Brook, JS. Tobacco use as a predictor of illicit drug use and drug-related problems in Colombian youth. J Adolesc Health 2003;32:50–57.

CHAPTER 11

The Origins of Emotion Regulation: Clinical Presentation and Neurobiology

Ruth A. Lanius, Robyn L. Bluhm, Clare Pain

Post-traumatic stress disorder (PTSD), chronic complex PTSD, and borderline personality disorder (BPD) are disorders that show significant clinical overlap; the terminology used to describe their most prominent features is also similar. Asmundson et al. (1) note that PTSD involves four identifiable symptom factors—intrusions, avoidance, dissociation or numbing, and hyperarousal—precipitated by terrifying experiences that threaten death, serious injury, or loss of physical integrity. The three major symptom factors consistently identified in BPD are impaired relatedness (unstable relationships, identity disturbance, and emptiness), behavioral dysregulation (impulsiveness and deliberate self-harm), and affect dysregulation (labile mood and excessive anger, associated with threatened abandonment) (2,3). However, in contrast to PTSD, a history of trauma is not required for a diagnosis of BPD and trauma is not inevitably present (4,5). Several symptoms of BPD and PTSD have similar features, for example, excessive irritability and anger, estrangement and chronic emptiness, emotional reactivity to specific trauma cues and in general, and dissociative symptoms. The BPD criteria generally require more marked persistence, pervasiveness, or relational instability than occur in PTSD, but current symptom levels can be similar (4). In addition, recurrent suicidal threats or behavior, recurrent self-injury, severe impulsivity, markedly unstable relationships, interpersonal manipulation, and avoidance of abandonment are features of complex PTSD and BPD rather than of PTSD alone (4).

The extent to which PTSD and BPD are related to each other and etiologically to trauma is a source of controversy, and we suggest that a better understanding of the genesis, psychology, and neurobiology of the effects of exposure to trauma, especially during early development, will help to elucidate the relationship between them. Deficits in regulation of emotion observed in each of these disorders are central to their clinical presentation. Explication of the mechanisms of emotion regulation and dysregulation will provide new research directions and, ultimately, a better understanding of the relationship between PTSD and BPD. We note that the diagnostic criteria of both PTSD and BPD fail to capture the full clinical picture of most chronically traumatized individuals, and that the attempt to include such a disorder (disorder of extreme stress not otherwise specified, or DESNOS) in the *Diagnostic and Statistical Manual of Mental Disorders*, 4th edition (DSM-IV) failed. This too contributes to the difficulty in clarifying the important clinical similarities and differences between PTSD and BPD.

The chapter provides an overview of the epidemiology of trauma, PTSD, and BPD and then discusses the proposed role of early life experience in the development of trauma-related psychopathology. Following a brief review of the literature on attachment in infancy and its effects on adult attachment style, we review the work of Allan Schore on the neurobiology of attachment (6). Whereas Schore concentrates on the importance of stressful experiences during infancy on the development of the ability to regulate one's emotions, we suggest that the potential for traumatic experiences to affect the developing brain may extend into adolescence and adulthood. In discussing the clinical and biologic aspects of trauma in adults, we draw on the neuroimaging literature and suggest that pathologic neural functioning in PTSD and BPD occurs in relation to pathologic emotional experiences and the subject's response to them over time.

WHAT IS TRAUMATIC STRESS?

POST-TRAUMATIC STRESS DISORDER

The quintessential trauma-related disorder is post-traumatic stress disorder (PTSD). PTSD cannot be diagnosed in the absence of exposure to an event (or events) that cause the individual to fear for his or her life or safety, or that of another person, and to respond with feelings of intense fear, helplessness, or horror. However, differences in clinical presentation are common in PTSD patients, and comorbidity is common. Substance use disorders (7–9), persistent anxiety and affective disorders (10,11), eating disorders (12), borderline personality disorder (13,14), physical health impairments (15), and a significantly increased use of medical and mental health services (16) have all been associated with a diagnosis of PTSD.

The National Comorbidity Survey showed that as many as one in two individuals in the general population experiences trauma at some point in life (17). Between 10% and 25% of people exposed to psychological trauma subsequently develop PTSD, a disorder that can have debilitating effects on every facet of daily living, including sleep, work or school, and interpersonal relationships (see Chapter 16 by Kaminer and Seedat in this book) (17,18). Yet these statistics mask important gender differences in the epidemiology of PTSD. Gavranidou and Rosner (19) reviewed the literature on the epidemiology of PTSD and found that three themes were consistently reported: men are more likely than women to experience a traumatic event; the types of traumatic events experienced tend to be different for women than for men; and women are more likely than men to develop PTSD subsequent to exposure to trauma (see Chapter 16). In fact, the national comorbidity survey suggests that the lifetime prevalence of PTSD is 10.4% for women and 5% for men.

Yehuda (20) notes that the most salient characteristics of events that lead to PTSD are their severity, duration, type, and predictability. Thus, it seems that the difference in prevalence between genders may be due, in part, to differences in the types of traumatic events experienced by women and men. In particular, women are more likely than men to be abused and to experience sexual abuse as children. Men, by contrast, tend to experience traumatic events such as physical attacks and serious accidents more commonly as adults. Thus, there are differences in the types of "interpersonal" or "social" traumatic events, although there are no gender differences in the reporting of events such as natural disasters or sudden death of a partner or friend (21). Because of this, Gavranidou and Rosner (19) suggest that one explanation for the difference in prevalence of PTSD between men and women is that women are more likely to suffer events that "are subject to heavily negative social sanction." Interestingly, Brewin, Andrews, and Valentine (22) reported in a meta-analysis of risk factors for PTSD that the gender effect, although substantial among civilians, was not significant in combat settings.

All of this discussion about the nature of trauma and the impact of traumatic events on an individual's understanding of herself and her place in the world requires a discussion of what *counts* as a traumatic event. DSM-IV defines a traumatic event in terms of its emotional impact on the individual who experiences it. As described above, a traumatic event is one that causes fear for the life or safety of oneself or another individual and causes a reaction of fear, helplessness, or horror. Two individuals might experience the same event differently. Thus, an event such as a relatively minor accident or a perceived danger of assault might not be traumatic for one individual but might well be experienced as a life-threatening and traumatic event by another individual. In fact, in some cases, individuals with PTSD report precipitating events that seem minor to observers but that clearly are a source of great distress to them (23,24). This has led clinicians to believe that, in many cases, the ability to cope with relatively "minor" traumas depends on the individual's history. In particular, women with a history of childhood abuse or neglect may lack the ability to cope with sudden stressful experience (23,24).

BORDERLINE PERSONALITY DISORDER

The term "borderline personality" was first used in 1938 by Adolph Stern to describe patients who could be diagnosed neither as neurotic nor as psychotic and who were therefore not appropriate candidates for psychoanalysis. During the 1950s and 1960s, the concept of borderline personality disorder was strongly influenced by object-relations theory. Analysts described the disorder as stemming not from the "classic" Freudian Oedipus complex but from difficulties during an earlier, narcissistic phase. The importance of Winnicott's "good enough" mothering and later Bowlby and Ainsworth's "secure" mother–infant attachment is emphasized in Wirth-Cauchon's (25) recent work: "The fragile process of relating to and differentiating from the mother in the pre-oedipal period is the primary site for the construction of a sense of self or identity. Thus, any aberrations in 'good enough' mothering will prove disastrous for the fragile emerging self." While the current criteria for the diagnosis of BPD concentrate solely on symptomatology and do not discuss this purported etiology, the historical association of the disorder with early difficulties in the relationship with caregiver(s) is influential.

The prevalence of BPD in the general population has been estimated to be 1.3% (26). However, one survey (27) found that in a primary care population, the lifetime prevalence of BPD was 6.4%. Moreover, prevalence of BPD is dramatically higher in psychiatric populations: estimates for psychiatric inpatients range from 15% to 20% (28) to up to 63% (29). DSM-IV-TR also reports gender differences in the diagnosis of BPD, with approximately 75% of diagnoses occurring in women. Like PTSD, BPD is associated with extensive use of the mental heath system, as compared with other personality disorders and major depressive disorder (30). Individuals with BPD are also at high risk of self-injury or suicide (4,29).

There is a high degree of comorbidity between BPD and PTSD. In a sample of BPD patients Zanarini, et al. (31), found that 56% had comorbid PTSD. Shea et al. (32) reported that 68% of PTSD patients in their sample also had BPD. Partly because of this comorbidity, it has been hypothesized that both disorders should be considered trauma-spectrum disorders (13,14), although this suggestion is controversial. Other authors, however, deny that BPD and PTSD are variants of the same disorder (5,31), but suggest instead that BPD predisposes individuals to vulnerability to the effects of trauma, thus placing them at risk of developing PTSD as well (33). This separation of the two disorders is congruent with the current diagnostic position of PTSD as an axis I disorder and BPD as an axis II disorder.

We suggest that this controversy can only be resolved by approaching the problem of psychological trauma from a number of different perspectives. Traditionally, the concept of psychological trauma was associated etiologically with hysteria by Freud but was developed quite differently by Janet, whose work has been "rediscovered" by van der Hart and van der Kolk (34–36) in the last few years, proffering possible theoretical underpinnings to dissociative phenomena. The development of attachment theory through the midtwentieth and twenty-first centuries continues to refine our understanding. However, more recently, clinicians who work from a more biologic perspective have begun to develop techniques for elucidating biologic markers associated with PTSD and BPD. These biologic approaches, which include neuroimaging and endocrinology, promise to give a new insight into the etiology of trauma-related disorders. One of the central themes of this chapter is that in order to develop an understanding of trauma and of trauma-related psychiatric disorders, it will be necessary to integrate the insights of those disciplines that have investigated trauma; no one approach on its own can be sufficient to allow us to understand or to treat the effects of trauma. In the following sections, we will discuss trauma-related disorders in terms of a deficiency in emotion regulation, from both a clinical and a neurobiologic perspective. We will describe work that links early life experiences to the process of brain maturation after birth and then turn to a consideration of neuroimaging studies that elucidate brain function associated with emotional experience in both PTSD and BPD.

ATTACHMENT AND EARLY DEVELOPMENT

Psychodynamic approaches to trauma have emphasized the importance of early experiences and their permanent effects on the developing infant. The role of mother–infant attachment has been accentuated, with deviations from "good enough" mothering etiologically linked to a number of later diagnoses, most notably borderline personality disorder.

Traditionally, developmental theorists have focused on the importance of early relationships, primarily with the mother, in helping an infant to learn how to moderate her own affective states. Taylor, Bagby, and Parker (37) noted, "studies on attachment styles in infancy and childhood have confirmed that the sensitivity and responsiveness of the primary caregiver to the child's emotional states is a major determinant of the way the child learns to regulate distressing affects and to relate to other people." Securely attached children are better able than their insecurely attached counterparts to respond both behaviorally and emotionally to changing conditions in their environment (38). Such psychological theories of attachment have recently begun to be integrated with research in developmental neurobiology, primarily by Schore (6), who has offered an account of infant development that considers the effects of an infant's environment, particularly her social environment, on brain development. Schore emphasizes that the genetically encoded developmental sequence, which provides the basis for our biologic and psychological characteristics, is not completed at the time of our birth. Rather, the most advantageous unfolding of this sequence is dependent upon the infant's interaction with the environment. In the case of biologic development, this point seems obvious; without proper nutrition and the opportunity to move about and explore the environment, the infant's growth and development will be suboptimal. However, the same is true for the infant's psychological development, in particular for the emergence of a sense of self. In Schore's view, "The relationship between the dynamics of early interactional development and the ontogeny of the emergent function for self-regulation is perhaps the most fundamental problem of development."

This interaction begins as early as 2 months of age. By this time, and peaking at 9 or 10 months, the infant and her mother respond to each other's facial expressions. On the basis of the mother's ability to modulate the infant's response to her facial expression, the infant learns to tolerate increasingly intense positive emotions. By the age of about 10 months, when the infant is beginning to interact more with the environment, the mother's responses to her child's emotional state teach the infant to modulate her own emotions. Schore draws on the work of developmental psychologists who observe these mother–child interactions to argue that "the mother induces a mood modification in the infant (39) and is directly influencing the infant's learning of 'how to feel,' 'how much to feel,' and 'whether to feel' about particular objects in the environment." Schore further cites studies that indicate that this relationship promotes the maturation of specific neural circuits in the brain that are necessary for appropriate emotion regulation in the adult. The infant brain, particularly the prefrontal cortex, is a locus of great change. The development and maturation of neural circuits occur throughout infancy and are dependent upon environmental conditions; Schore believes that if these environmental conditions are outside of a certain normal range, the effects on the infant's development are permanent.

It should be noted that these effects of disruptions in neurobiologic and emotional development, in addition to persisting into adulthood and complicating the adaptation to ongoing stress and trauma, could be transmitted to the next generation. There is evidence that infant attachment types correlate with adult attachment patterns, which, in turn, can predict parenting style and the attachment behavior of the next generation of infants (40). Both categories of insecure attachment (insecure-avoidant and insecure-ambivalent) may be seen as adaptive responses to suboptimal caregiving. However, Holmes (41) suggests that disorganized attachment is a third variant of insecure attachment, which coexists with all three attachment categories (secure, insecure-avoidant, insecure-ambivalent) and is by definition nonadaptive; he notes the links between disorganized attachment and psychopathology are much more evident. Disorganized attachment represents an approach-avoidance dilemma of the child who both needs and fears the parent as a source of safety and simultaneously of threat.

Disorganized attachment in a child is highly correlated with unresolved attachment status in a parent (the adult equivalent of disorganized attachment) and with specific parental behaviors that move beyond the inattentiveness and insensitivity that give rise to insecure-ambivalent or insecure-avoidant attachments (42). The behaviors of the parent are both frightening and frightened; there is a disrupted "dissociative" aspect to the parent's capacity to maintain her own affective continuity, which disables her ability to read her child's cues and respond appropriately (41). Fonagy et al. (43) noted that this repetitive failure of a mother to read her child's cues leads to attachment insecurity with an impoverished capacity for the child to mentalize; that is, to have a theory of mind. The same authors noted that resilience to psychological stress is linked to the development of a secure attachment with the concomitant capacity to mentalize. It is this self-reflective ability to take into account the motivational causes underlying the behaviors of self and others that seems to be the achievement of a secure attachment and the locus of psychological resilience (43). Any developmental impairment of this could be salient to the later emergence of either BPD or PTSD.

REGULATION OF EMOTION

The previous section highlighted the importance of a secure attachment relationship to the development of the infant's nervous system and the infant's ability to learn to modulate his or her own emotional reactions to the world. It was further suggested that the absence of such a foundation in early life contributes substantially to the development of or at least the susceptibility to trauma-related disorders, including BPD, in adulthood. While Schore's work emphasizes the importance of experiences in infancy, recent work suggests that the development of the critical areas of the prefrontal cortex continues throughout childhood and adolescence (44,45). It is important to note that the process of learning to regulate one's emotions also continues throughout childhood, adolescence, and importantly from the clinical standpoint, adulthood.

While most adults do reach a socially acceptable level of skill at emotion regulation, certain psychological disorders, including BPD and PTSD, can be described as being, in large part, disorders of emotion regulation. In the case of BPD, the experience of affect dysregulation, along with an associated instability of interpersonal relationships, are core diagnostic features in the DSM-IV. In the case of PTSD, the link to emotion dysregulation is not overtly stated in the DSM-IV. Some clinicians have argued that the current diagnostic category of PTSD must be reorganized and expanded to allow differentiation between individuals who are suffering the aftereffects of a single traumatic experience and those who have experienced chronic traumatization. To this end, Herman (46) has argued for the creation of a new diagnosis, complex PTSD, while van der Kolk et al. (36) and Pelcovitz et al. (47) have suggested the term DESNOS (Disorders of Extreme Stress Not Otherwise Specified) be used to designate the disorder following chronic traumatization in which emotion dysregulation is a central characteristic. The current diagnostic criteria for PTSD do not differentiate between individuals who have experienced a single traumatic event and those who have had multiple traumatic experiences; a significant subset of those currently diagnosed with PTSD have been chronically traumatized and would likely meet criteria for complex PTSD or DESNOS (47). We suggest that the current diagnostic criteria obscure both the clinically and biologically important differences between "simple" and "complex" cases of PTSD and also the fundamental importance of emotion regulation in this disorder.

Unlike the case in BPD, the deficits in emotion regulation associated with PTSD appear, at least at first glance, to be concerned solely with the traumatic experience. Reminders of a traumatic event evoke sustained psychological and physiologic arousal that the patient is unable to modulate or control. However, this hyperreactivity can, in many cases, become generalized so that the patient reports feeling constantly on edge and easily startled. Moreover, in addition to these hyperreactivity symptoms, a second symptom cluster in PTSD emphasizes withdrawal and emotional numbing following the experience of a traumatic event. Patients avoid not only reminders of their trauma, but also work, social relationships, and leisure activities. In this respect patients with PTSD and BPD are very similar because individuals in both diagnostic groups have difficulty attaining, containing, and sustaining their own affective responses, a problem that limits and usually severely impacts on their function.

In situations in which patients are currently experiencing or vividly remembering a traumatic event, two different types of response are possible and these appear to parallel the symptom clusters in PTSD of intrusive re-experiencing, and avoiding and numbing. The first involves an overwhelming experience of emotions, while the second represents a pathologic state of "no emotions." Bremner et al. (48) hypothesized that the first of these two subtypes of immediate response to traumatic events is characterized by intrusive memories and hyperarousal and the other response is predominantly dissociative.

In the next sections, we will review the neuroimaging literature on emotional states in healthy subjects, patients with PTSD, and patients with BPD in order to examine and compare neural pathways involved.

NEUROIMAGING OF EMOTIONAL STATES

Several PET neuroimaging studies have examined patterns of brain activity associated with the experience of emotional states, including sadness, anxiety, happiness, and disgust in normal subjects. George et al. (49,50) induced emotion in subjects by having them recall autobiographical events associated with sad emotion while viewing emotionally congruent faces; they found that the emotion activated a much larger predominantly left-sided anterior paralimbic region in women than in men. PET studies by Liotti et al. (51), Mayberg et al. (52), and Lane et al. (53) have also implicated anterior paralimbic regions with transient sadness in healthy women, including activation in the subgenual cingulate area (BA 25) and areas of the insula (51,52). Liotti et al. (51) found that sadness induced by autobiographical memory scripts was associated with activation of the subgenual cingulate area (BA 25) and dorsal insula as well as the inferior parietal areas (BA 40). Lane et al. (53) also found script-driven sadness to be associated with activation of the anterior insula. In addition, deactivation of frontal areas including the right prefrontal cortex (BA 9) (51) and right dorsal prefrontal cortex (BA 46/9) and dorsal anterior cingulate gyrus (BA 24) (52) has also been reported.

Studies have also investigated the neural correlates of anxiety using script-driven imagery or viewing affect-appropriate faces or both. In response to faces plus scripts, anxiety was associated with increased regional cerebral blood flow (rCBF) in the left superior temporal gyrus, the left inferior frontal cortex, the left anterior cingulate, and bilateral cuneus. In contrast, decreased rCBF was found in the right medial frontal gyrus, the right prefrontal cortex, and the right parietal cortex (54). Liotti et al. (51), using script-driven imagery, reported that anxiety was associated with activation of the ventral insula and the orbitofrontal and anterior temporal cortices. Deactivation was seen in the parahippocampal gyri and the inferior temporal cortex (BA 20/37).

Damasio et al. (55) suggest that areas involved in the mapping and regulation of internal organism states such as the somatosensory cortices and upper brainstem nuclei are activated when subjects recall personal life episodes marked by sadness, happiness, anger, or fear. They hypothesize that a strong link exists between homeostasis and emotional experience that is underpinned by both unconscious and conscious processes. Altered activity in any part of the network of brain regions involved in these processes may underlie the emotional symptoms of BPD and PTSD. In the next section, we will outline neuroimaging studies in patients with these disorders and show that there is a significant overlap in the areas involved in emotion and those implicated in PTSD and in BPD.

NEUROIMAGING IN PTSD AND BPD

POST-TRAUMATIC STRESS DISORDER

Hyperarousal Response to Trauma Reminders

In recent years a number of studies have investigated the patterns of neural activity associated with patients' experience of PTSD symptoms. Because the diagnosis of PTSD is associated largely with transient states, such as physiological or emotional reactivity upon exposure to reminders of a traumatic event, many of these studies have used symptom-provocation paradigms to evoke such states. The majority of these studies have focused on subjects who have become what we have described as "hyperaroused" in response to reminders of their trauma. This response is characterized by physiologic and emotional reactivity, often accompanied by memories with vivid sensory characteristics or even full-blown flashbacks of the traumatic event. However, a minority of subjects has responded to reminders of their traumatic experiences with a dissociative response (56), reporting that they feel disconnected from their bodies or their emotions. Studies in our laboratory have also shown that these two types of responses are extremes and that some subjects have a response that includes aspects of both (57).

A number of reviews of the neuroimaging literature in PTSD have been published recently (57–60); thus in this chapter we summarize the key brain areas implicated in PTSD and discuss their potential roles in emotion regulation and dysregulation.

Anterior cingulate cortex. The majority of the neuroimaging studies in PTSD have implicated the anterior cingulate cortex as playing a major role in PTSD (57–60). This region has also been shown to be involved in the representation of subjective experience and emotion. Lane et al. (61) have reported positive correlations between scores on the Levels of Emotional Awareness Scale and cerebral blood flow in BA 24 of the anterior cingulate gyrus during film-induced and recall-induced emotion. Thus, it is possible that the abnormalities in anterior cingulate functioning observed in PTSD underlie the emotion dysregulation seen in this disorder, including both the re-experiencing of emotionally distressing memories and the avoidance of emotional stimulation also observed in these patients.

Medial prefrontal cortex. The medial prefrontal cortex has also been implicated in the pathophysiology of PTSD (reviewed in 57–60). Moscovitch and Winocur (62) have suggested that the role of the medial prefrontal cortex in the retrieval of episodic memories is to ensure that "currently relevant memories can be differentiated from memories that may have been relevant once but are no longer" (62). Although these authors do not link this suggestion to the re-experiencing of memories seen in patients with PTSD, their suggestion has clear relevance to the alterations in activity seen in the medial prefrontal cortex of PTSD patients during traumatic recollections.

Thalamus. The thalamus acts as the principal synaptic relay station for information reaching the cortex (63); with the exception of olfactory information, all sensory input is routed through the thalamus to the cerebral cortex. Thalamic dysfunction in PTSD has been shown in a number of studies but not consistently in all studies (57). The thalamus has also been suggested to be involved in mediating the interaction between attention and arousal (64), both of which are clearly relevant to the phenomenology of traumatic stress syndromes. High levels of arousal during traumatic experiences have been hypothesized to lead to altered thalamic sensory processing (65), which in turn results in a disruption of transmission of sensory information to the frontal cortex, cingulate gyrus, amygdala, and hippocampus. Krystal et al. (66) hypothesized that this mechanism underlies dissociative symptoms and may be one of the mechanisms underlying flashbacks in PTSD.

Amygdala. Although amygdala dysfunction has been reported in some PTSD neuroimaging studies, these findings have not always been consistent across studies (57–60). The amygdala is reciprocally connected with many areas of the brain, including the hypothalamus, hippocampus, neocortex, and the thalamus. Le Doux (67) has shown that the amygdala plays a crucial role in fear conditioning and also is implicated in contextual learning. Moreover, the basolateral amygdala has been shown to play a role in stress-mediated alterations of memory, including memory consolidation after an event (68).

Neuroimaging of Dissociative Responses in PTSD and Other Disorders

The neuroimaging literature of dissociation in PTSD to date has been sparse. However, several studies have examined brain activation patterns in pharmacologically induced depersonalization, depersonalization disorder, and dissociative identity disorder (DID). These studies give an indication of the key brain areas that appear to be involved in dissociation.

Temporal cortex. Much of the study of the role of the temporal cortex in dissociative phenomena come from work on epilepsy patients. Penfield and Rasmussen (69) found that the patients tend to report dissociative experiences in response to stimulation of the middle and superior temporal gyrus during neurosurgery. More recently, Teicher et al. (70) have investigated the relationship between current temporal lobe symptoms and early abuse. Neuroimaging studies of PTSD (56) and depersonalization disorder (71) also indicate that the temporal cortex plays an important role in dissociative experiences.

Parieto-occipital cortex. Several neuroimaging studies of psychiatric conditions [depersonalization disorder (71), PTSD (56) and DID (72)] report alterations in activity in the posterior parietal and occipital cortices. These areas play a role in multimodal integration and may reflect the reported dysregulation of visual and sensory experience during dissociation (73,74).

The corticolimbic model of dissociation. Sierra and Berrios (75) have proposed a corticolimbic model of depersonalization. They postulate that depersonalization involves corticolimbic disconnection, whereby left medial prefrontal activation with reciprocal amygdala inhibition results in hypoemotionality and decreased arousal, and right dorsolateral prefrontal cortex activation with reciprocal anterior cingulate inhibition leads to attentional difficulties and emptiness of mental contents. In support of their model, these authors cited evidence for medial prefrontal involvement in both the monitoring and modulation of emotions. In this model, once a threshold of anxiety is reached, the medial prefrontal cortex inhibits emotional processing on limbic structures (the amygdala), which in turn leads to a dampening of sympathetic output and reduced emotional experiencing. Finally, several studies suggest that the prefrontal cortex has inhibitory influences on the emotional limbic system; among these are PET studies showing a negative correlation between blood flow in the left prefrontal cortex and the amygdala (76,77). Our findings partially lend support to the above model. We found that patients with dissociative PTSD had increased activation in the dorsolateral prefrontal cortex (BA 9) and the medial frontal cortex (BA 10) and did not exhibit increased amygdala activation. Increased activation of the medial prefrontal cortex may underlie the lack of autonomic response observed in some of these patients (78).

Borderline Personality Disorder

In comparison with PTSD, relatively few imaging studies have been conducted in patients with BPD. However, there is a small but growing literature on functional abnormalities associated with BPD. As with the PTSD studies, these experiments often involve inducing particular emotions in subjects and observing alterations in brain functioning.

Two studies (79,80) have compared emotional responses to pictures of negative stimuli and to pictures of emotional faces, respectively, in persons with BPD to the responses in healthy control subjects. Using slides of neutral and unpleasant stimuli, Herpertz et al. (80) found that, in response to the unpleasant pictures, BPD subjects showed activation in the left and right fusiform gyrus (BA 37), left and right amygdala, right inferior frontal gyrus (BA 47), and left medial frontal gyrus (BA 10). Control subjects, by contrast, showed activation in the medial temporal gyrus (BA 39) and left medial occipital gyrus (BA 39).

Donegan et al. (79) examined neural responses to neutral, happy, sad, and fearful faces. BPD patients responded with an increase in left amygdala activation to the neutral, fearful, and sad faces. The response to neutral faces may be explained by the reported tendency of BPD patients to project negative attributes onto the neutral faces.

Schmahl et al. (81,82) conducted script-driven imagery research in patients with BPD using sexual abuse and abandonment scripts. Because of the tendency of BPD patients to fear real or imagined abandonment, the first study used personalized scripts of abandonment situations to provoke a symptomatic state. All of the women in this study (n = 20) had a history of childhood sexual abuse. Of these, 10 met criteria for BPD. Exposure to abandonment scripts resulted in an increase in blood flow in the right dorsolateral prefrontal cortex (BA 10, 46, 47) and right cuneus (BA 19) in women with BPD but not in control subjects. The control group showed decreased blood flow in the left superior frontal gyrus (BA 8), right middle and superior frontal gyrus (BA 6, 8, 10). Decreased blood flow was observed in BPD subjects in the bilateral anterior cingulate gyrus; this decrease was significantly greater than the right hemispheric decrease seen in the control group (BA 24,32). Exposure to abuse scripts was associated with decreased blood flow in the right anterior cingulate gyrus (BA 24) and orbitofrontal cortex. Given the important role of the anterior cingulate gyrus and orbitofrontal cortex in emotion regulation, it may be that dysfunction in these areas underlies the emotion dysregulation often observed in patients with borderline personality disorder.

CONCLUSION

In this chapter we have emphasized the similarities in symptoms between PTSD and BPD and noted that for neither PTSD or BPD alone are the current diagnostic criteria adequate to describe the chronically traumatized individual. Because of these limitations, we included some consideration of the informal diagnosis of DESNOS in developing our hypothesis that emotional dysregulation is a central feature of these disorders. We believe that the development of new diagnostic criteria will improve clinicians' capacity to recognize the effects of early trauma as they are manifested in adulthood.

Current research into attachment patterns in both infants and adults, combined with insights from developmental neurobiology and functional neuroimaging, has the potential to reshape our understanding of PTSD and of BPD and to distinguish between various trauma-related disorders in a richer, and more clinically useful, way than has been previously available. We briefly reviewed the literature on the neural structures involved in emotional experience, in PTSD and in BPD and suggest that the link between traumatic experience and clinical symptomatology can best be drawn by research into the role of emotion regulation in trauma-related disorders. Further research examining this hypothesis must address the effects of trauma across the life span and draw on the strengths of clinical, psychological, and biologic research.

REFERENCES

1. Asmundson GJ, Frombach I, McQuaid J, et al. Dimensionality of posttraumatic stress symptoms: a confirmatory factor analysis of DSM-IV symptom clusters and other symptom models. Behav Res Ther 2000;38:203–214.
2. Skodol AE, Siever LJ, Livesley WJ, et al. The borderline diagnosis I: psychopathology, comorbidity, and personality structure. Biol Psychiatry 2002a;51(12):936–950.
3. Skodol AE, Gunderson JG, Pfohl B, et al. The borderline diagnosis II: biology, genetics, and clinical course. Biol Psychiatry 2002b;51(12):951–963.
4. Zlotnick C, Johnson DM, Yen S, et al. Clinical features and impairment in women with borderline personality disorder (BPD) with posttraumatic stress disorder (PTSD), BPD without PTSD, and other personality disorders with PTSD. J Nerv Ment Dis 2003;191:706–713.

5. Golier JA, Yehuda R, Bierer LM, et al. The relationship of borderline personality disorder to posttraumatic stress disorder and traumatic events. Am J Psychiatry 2003;160:2018–2024.

6. Schore AN. Affect Regulation and the Origin of the Self. Hillsdale, NJ: Erlbaum, 1994.

7. Chilcoat HD, Breslau N. Investigations of causal pathways between PTSD and drug use disorders. Addict Behav 1998a;23:827–840.

8. Chilcoat HD, Breslau N. Posttraumatic stress disorder and drug disorders: testing causal pathways. Arch Gen Psychiatry 1998b;55:913–917.

9. Chander G, McCaul ME. Co-occurring psychiatric disorders in women with addictions. Obstet Gyn Clin North Am 2003;30:469–481.

10. McCauley J, Kern DE, Kolodner K, et al. Clinical characteristics of women with a history of childhood abuse: unhealed wounds. JAMA 1997;277:1362–1368.

11. Hofmann SG, Litz BT, Weathers FW. Social anxiety, depression, and PTSD in Vietnam veterans. J Anx Dis 2003;17:573–582.

12. Lating JM, O'Reilly MA, Anderson KP. Eating disorders and posttraumatic stress: phenomenological and treatment considerations using the two-factor model. Int J Emerg Ment Health 2002;4:113–118.

13. Herman JL, Perry JC, van der Kolk BA. Childhood trauma in borderline personality disorder. Am J Psychiatry 1989;146:490–495.

14. McLean LM, Gallop R. Implications of childhood sexual abuse for adult borderline personality disorder and complex posttraumatic stress disorder. Am J Psychiatry 2003;160(2):369–371.

15. Felitti VJ, Anda RF, Nordenberg D, et al. Relationship of childhood abuse and household dysfunction to many of the leading causes of death in adults: the Adverse Childhood Experiences (ACE) Study. Am J Prev Med 1998;14:245–258.

16. Deykin EY, Keane TM, Kaloupek D, et al. Posttraumatic stress disorder and the use of health services. Psychosom Med 2001;63(5):835–841.

17. Kessler RC, Sonnega A, Bromet E, et al. Posttraumatic stress disorder in the National Comorbidity Survey. Arch Gen Psychiatry 1995;52:1048–1060.

18. Breslau N, Davis GC, Andreski P, Peterson E. Traumatic events and posttraumatic stress disorder in an urban population of young adults. Arch Gen Psychiatry 1991;48:216–222.

19. Gavranidou M, Rosner R. The weaker sex? Gender and post-traumatic stress disorder. Depress Anx 2003;17:130–139.

20. Yehuda R. Post-traumatic stress disorder. N Engl J Med 2002;346:108–114.

21. Breslau N. Epidemiologic studies of trauma, posttraumatic stress disorder, and other psychiatric disorders. Can J Psychiatry 2002;47:923–929.

22. Brewin CR, Andrews B, Valentine JD. Meta-analysis of risk factors for posttraumatic stress disorder in trauma-exposed adults. J Consult Clin Psych 2000;68:748–766.

23. Allen JG. Traumatic Relationships and Serious Mental Disorders. Chichester, UK: Wiley, 2001.

24. McFarlane AC, Golier J, Yehuda R. Treatment planning for trauma survivors with PTSD: what does a clinician need to know before implementing PTSD treatments? In: Yehuda R, ed. Treating Trauma: Survivors with PTSD. Washington, DC: American Psychiatric Publishing, 2002.

25. Wirth-Cauchon J. Women and Borderline Personality Disorder: Symptoms and Stories. New Brunswick, NJ: Rutgers University Press, 2001.

26. Torgerson S, Kringlen E, Cramer S. The prevalence of personality disorders in a community sample. Arch Gen Psychiatry 2001;58:590–596.

27. Gross R, Olfson M, Gameroff M, et al. Borderline personality disorder in primary care. Arch Intern Med 2002;162:53–60.

28. Widiger TA, Sanderson CJ. Personality Disorders. Philadelphia: Saunders, 1997.

29. Linehan MM. Cognitive-Behavioral Treatment of Borderline Personality Disorder. New York: Guilford, 1993.

30. Bender DS, Dolan RT, Skodol AE, et al. Treatment utilization by patients with personality disorders. Am J Psychiatry 2001;158:295–302.

31. Zanarini MC, Frankenburg FR, Dubo ED, et al. Axis I comorbidity of borderline personality disorder. Am J Psychiatry 1998;155:1733–1739.

32. Shea MT, Zlotnick C, Weisberg RB. Commonality and specificity of personality disorder profiles in subjects with trauma histories. J Personal Disord 1999;13:199–210.

33. Gunderson JG, Sabo AN. The phenomenological and conceptual interface between borderline personality disorder and PTSD. Am J Psychiatry 1993;150:19–27.

34. van der Hart O, Brown P, van der Kolk BA. Pierre Janet's treatment of posttraumatic stress. J Trauma Stress 1989a;2:379–396.

35. van der Hart O, Friedman B. A reader's guide to Pierre Janet on dissociation: a neglected intellectual heritage. Dissociation 1989b;2:3–16.

36. van der Kolk BA, Pelcovitz D, Roth S, et al. Dissociation, somatization, and affect dysregulation: the complexity of adaptation of trauma. Am J Psychiatry 1996;153:83–93.

37. Taylor GJ, Bagby RM, Parker JDA. Disorders of Affect Regulation. New York: Cambridge University Press, 1997.

38. Hesse E, Main M. Disorganized infant, child, and adult attachment: collapse in behavioral and attentional strategies. J Am Psychoanal Assoc 2000;48(4):1100–1127.

39. Feinman S. Social referencing in infancy. In: Shore AN, ed. Affect Regulation and the Origin of the Self. Hillsdale, NJ: Erlbaum, 1994.
40. Lyons-Ruth K, Yellin C, Melnick S, et al. Childhood experiences of trauma and loss have different relations to maternal unresolved and hostile-helpless states of mind on the AAI. Attach Hum Dev 2003;5:330–352.
41. Holmes J. Disorganized attachment and borderline personality disorder: a clinical perspective. Attach Hum Dev (in press).
42. Lyons-Ruth K, Jacobvitz D. Attachment disorganization: unresolved loss, relational violence, and lapses in behavioral and attentional strategies. In: Cassidy J, Shaver P, eds. Handbook of Attachment: Theory, Research, and Clinical Applications. New York: Guilford, 1999:520–554.
43. Fonagy P, Steele M, Steele H, et al. Attachment, the reflective self and borderline states: the predictive specificity of the adult attachment and pathologic emotional development. In: Goldberg S, Muir R, Kerr J, eds. Attachment Theory: Social, Developmental, and Clinical Perspectives. Hillsdale, NJ: Analytic, 2000:233–278.
44. Giedd JN, Blumenthal J, Jeffries NO, et al. Brain development during childhood and adolescence: a longitudinal MRI study. Nat Neurosci 1999;2:861–863.
45. Casey BJ, Giedd JN, Thomas KM. Structural and functional brain development and its relation to cognitive development. Biol Psychol 2000;54:241–257.
46. Herman J. Trauma and Recovery. New York: Basic, 1992.
47. Pelcovitz D, van der Kolk B, Roth S, et al. Development of a criteria set and a structured interview for disorders of extreme stress (SIDES). J Trauma Stress 1997;10:3–16.
48. Bremner JD, Narayan M, Staib LH, et al. Neural correlates of memories of childhood sexual abuse in women with and without posttraumatic stress disorder. Am J Psychiatry 1999;156: 1787–1795.
49. George MS, Ketter TA, Parekh PI, et al. Brain activity during transient sadness and happiness in healthy women. Am J Psychiatry 1995;152:341–351.
50. George MS, Ketter TA, Parekh PI, et al. Gender differences in regional cerebral blood flow during transient self-induced sadness or happiness. Biol Psychiatry 1996;40:859–871.
51. Liotti M, Mayberg HS, Brannan S, et al. Differential limbic-cortical correlates of sadness and anxiety in healthy subjects: implications for affective disorders. Biol Psychiatry 2000;48: 30–42.
52. Mayberg HS, Liotti M, Brannan SK, et al. Reciprocal limbic-cortical function and negative mood: converging PET findings in depression and normal sadness. Am J Psychiatry 1999;156: 675–682.
53. Lane RD, Reiman EM, Ahern GL, et al. Neuroanatomical correlates of happiness, sadness, and disgust. Am J Psychiatry 1997;154:926–933.
54. Kimbrell TA, George MS, Parekh PI, et al. Regional brain activity during transient self-induced anxiety and anger in healthy adults. Biol Psychiatry 1999;46:454–465.
55. Damasio AR, Grabowski TJ, Bechara A, et al. Subcortical and cortical brain activity during the feeling of self-generated emotions. Nat Neurosci 2000;3:1049–1056.
56. Lanius RA, Williamson PC, Boksman K, et al. Brain activation during script-driven imagery induced dissociative responses in PTSD: a functional magnetic resonance imaging investigation. Biol Psychiatry 2002;52:305–311.
57. Lanius RA, Bluhm R, Lanius U, Pain C. Neuroimaging of hyperarousal and dissociation in PTSD: heterogeneity of response to symptom provocation. Psychopharmacol Bull (in press).
58. Hull AM. Neuroimaging findings in post-traumatic stress disorder: systematic review. Br J Psychiatry 2002;181:102–110.
59. Pitman RK, Shin LM, Rauch SL. Investigating the pathogenesis of posttraumatic stress disorder with neuroimaging. J Clin Psychiatry 2001;62(Suppl 17):47–54.
60. Bremner JD. Neuroimaging studies in post-traumatic stress disorder. Curr Psychiat Rep 2002;4:254–263.
61. Lane RD, Reiman EM, Axelrod B, et al. Neural correlates of levels of emotional awareness: evidence of an interaction between emotion and attention in the anterior cingulate cortex. J Cog Neurosci 1998;10:525–535.
62. Moscovitch M, Winocur G. The frontal cortex and working with memory. In: Stuss DT, Knight RT, eds. Principles of Frontal Lobe Function. New York: Oxford University Press, 2002:188–209.
63. Kandel ER, Schwartz JH, Jessell TM. Principles of Neural Science. New York: Elsevier, 1991.
64. Portas CM, Rees G, Howseman AM, et al. A specific role for the thalamus in mediating the interaction of attention and arousal in humans. J Neurosci 1998;18:8979–8989.
65. Krystal JH, Bennett AL, Bremner JD, et al. Toward a cognitive neuroscience of dissociation and altered memory functions in posttraumatic stress disorder. In: Friedmen MJ, Charney DS, Deutsch AY, eds. Neurobiological and Clinical Consequences of Stress. Normal Adaptations to PTSD. New York: Raven, 1995:239–268.
66. Krystal JH, Bremner JD, Southwick SM, et al. The emerging neurobiology of dissociation: implications for the treatment of posttraumatic stress disorder. In: Bremner JD, Marmer CR, eds. Trauma, Memory, and Dissociation. Washington, DC: American Psychiatric Press, 1998:321–363.

67. Le Doux J. Synaptic Self: How Our Brains Become Who We Are. New York: Viking, 2002.

68. Cahill L. Modulation of long-term memory in humans by emotional arousal: adrenergic activation and the amygdala. In: Aggleton IP, ed. The Amygdala. New York: Oxford University Press, 2000:425–446.

69. Penfield W, Rasmussen T, eds. The Cerebral Cortex of Man: A Clinical Study of Localization of Function. 4th Ed. New York: Macmillan, 1957:157–181.

70. Teicher MH, Glod CA, Surrey J, et al. Early childhood abuse and limbic system rating in adult psychiatric outpatients. J Neuropsychiatry Clin Neurosci 1993;5:301–306.

71. Simeon D, Guralnik O, Hazlett EA, et al. Feeling unreal: a PET study of depersonalization disorder. Am J Psychiatry 2000;157:1782–1788.

72. Reinders AA, Nijenhuis ER, Paans AM, et al. One brain, two selves. Neuroimage 2003; 20(4):2119–2125.

73. Bremner JD, Krystal JH, Putnam F, et al. Measurement of dissociative states with the Clinician Administered Dissociative States Scale (CADSS). J Trauma Stress 1998;11:125–136.

74. Bernstein EM, Putnam FW. Development, reliability, and validity of a dissociation scale. J Nerv Ment Dis 1986;174:727–735.

75. Sierra M, Berrios GE. Depersonalization: neurobiological perspectives. Biol Psychiatry 1998; 44:898–908.

76. Davidson RJ, Sutton SK. Affective neuroscience: the emergence of a discipline. Curr Opin Neurobiol 1995;5:217–224.

77. Drevets WC, Videen TO, Price JL, et al. A functional anatomical study of unipolar depression. J Neurosci 1992;12:3628–3641.

78. Semple WE, Goyer PF, McCormick R, et al. Attention and regional cerebral blood flow in posttraumatic stress disorder patients with substance abuse histories. Psychiatry Res 1996;67:17–28.

79. Donegan NH, Sanislow CA, Blumberg HP, et al. Amygdala hyperreactivity in borderline personality disorder: implications for emotional dysregulation. Biol Psychiatry 2003; 54:1284–1293.

80. Herpertz SC, Dietrich TM, Wenning B, et al. Evidence of abnormal amygdala functioning in borderline personality disorder: a functional MRI study. Biol Psychiatry 2001;50:292–298.

81. Schmahl CG, Elzinga BM, Vermetten E, et al. Neural correlates of memories of abandonment in women with and without borderline personality disorder. Biol Psychiatry 2003;54:142–151.

82. Schmahl CG, Vermetten E., Elzinga BM, et al. Magnetic resonance imaging of hippocampal and amygdala volume in women with childhood abuse and borderline personality disorder. Psychiatry Res 2004;122:193–198.

Adulthood

Section IV Summary
Commentary from the Editor

Sarah E. Romans

The individual chapters in this section identify several common themes.

Current diagnostic classification systems are problematic and do not capture the subtleties of subtypes of disorder (phenotypes), or sensibly map comorbidity patterns. Perhaps further refinement could be achieved by returning to the basic criteria for separating disorders enunciated by the St. Louis group years ago: clinical description, laboratory studies, delimitation from other conditions, follow-up and family information (1).

All the authors emphasize the importance of sex and gender when considering how mental illnesses unfold. Complex social and biological mechanisms, acting simultaneously and interactively, affect women and men differently. The mental health of individuals needs to be understood in their interpersonal and sociocultural context. Internationally, 70% of those living in poverty and two thirds of the illiterate are women. One in four women is beaten by her husband or partner. Every day, 1,300 women die unnecessarily in childbirth or during pregnancy. The sociopolitical disadvantages that women experience are addressed by several other contributors in this volume (see particularly Astbury, Pandalangat, and C. C. Williams). Our thinking needs to be guided by a gender framework; the question should arise, "Does this apply equally for women and men?"

Abuse. Much recent research has focused on the adverse impact of abuse (physical, sexual, emotional, financial). A conceptual framework addressing the abuse of the submissive person in a dominant-submissive dyad provides many insights into factors that determine health outcomes (2).

This theme of abuse, which forms a strong thread through this section, also links to other parts of this book.

Service design and delivery. The contributors suggest that some psychiatric services have not helped women with mental disorders. Some are difficult to access and do not accommodate the unpaid and unacknowledged work that women do in the community; such as the care of children, the elderly and the ill, (3). A greater focus on the life circumstances of women with psychiatric problems gives a better fit for those in need of treatment.

The importance of a historical framework. This is implicit throughout the section. The authors all place the evolution of the concepts that currently frame the disorders that they discuss in a historical context. Kulkarni, in particular, traces how sexist attitudes toward women throughout the ages have shaped the way in which mental problems are defined and handled by successive generations.

Stigmatization. Mental health problems are often misunderstood in the general community. The tendency to view psychiatric disorders as strange, incomprehensible, dangerous, or untreatable has inflicted additional harm on people with psychiatric problems.

The importance of research. While firm commitment to quality research in developed nations is steadily advancing our knowledge, there are some factors that work against the comprehensive understanding of psychiatric disorders. Research is expensive and knowledge advances slowly. We need to acknowledge that each research design has weaknesses; even the most highly rated method, a prospective cohort study, which can give the best information about causal relationships, is limited by the ethical need to intervene when a medical problem is discovered. So, as the years go by, the cohort becomes less and less typical and the study's outcomes are therefore less generalizable. The most complete picture about any disorder will come from a careful amalgamation of results arising from diverse research strategies-cohort studies, cross-sectional surveys, and qualitative interviews strategies. By combining results from these projects, we can assemble a comprehensive picture.

Spirituality. Spirituality is one area of developing interest in mental health sciences which received little discussion in this section. This reflects the sparse research currently available. Spirituality is part of a person's deepest cultural beliefs and as such can be expected to show clear gender differences. A new diagnostic category entitled religious or spiritual problem has been included in the fourth edition of the Diagnostic and Statistical Manual of Mental Disorders (DSM-IV) and will spearhead research efforts in the coming years.

Taken together, these diverse chapters give a rich 2005 snapshot of our current knowledge on gender and mental health and show how we can integrate diverse but complementary spheres of knowledge.

REFERENCES

1. Feighner, JP, Robins, E, Guze, SB, et al. Diagnostic criteria for use in psychiatric research. Arch Gen Psychiatry 1972; 26(1):57-63.
2. Miller, JB. Toward a new psychology of women. Second ed. Boston: Beacon Press, 1986.
3. Waring, M. Counting for nothing: what men value and what women are worth. Wellington: Allen and Unwin, in association with Port Nicholson Press, 1988.

CHAPTER 12

Gender Differences in Depression and Anxiety Disorders

Gail Erlick Robinson

The objective of this chapter is to highlight sex and gender differences in the prevalence, etiology, presentation, and treatment of depression and anxiety disorders, with special emphasis on the effect of biologic sex and gender roles. The high female:male sex ratio in these conditions is one of the most replicated findings in epidemiology, yet one whose explanation remains uncertain.

Anxiety and depressive disorders are addressed together in this chapter because the distinction between them may be an artificial one. Medical historian Shorter and psychiatrist Tyrer suggest that the distinction originated with the development of the *Diagnostic and Statistical Manual of Mental Disorders,* 3rd edition (DSM-III) by the American Psychiatric Association (1). Before then, anxiety had been considered an integral part of depression but, with the arrival of the new diagnostic classification, the two became separate diagnoses. Despite the results of a nationwide household survey in the United Kingdom that showed mixed anxiety-depression to be the commonest form of affective disorder (2), the presence of a mixed syndrome is now viewed instead as comorbidity. Yet, over 90% of all depressed patients also have anxiety symptoms. In the Epidemiologic Catchment Area (ECA) study, 47% of the respondents meeting lifetime criteria for major depression also met criteria for a co-existing anxiety disorder (3). The National Comorbidity Study (NCS) also found that the presence of an anxiety disorder was associated with an increased risk for major depressive disorder (4).

Although the comingling of depression and anxiety is true for both sexes, comorbid anxiety disorder is more likely in depressed women than in depressed men (5).

EPIDEMIOLOGY

DEPRESSION

Prior to puberty, there are few differences in the prevalence of depression in males and females (6). (See Manassis, Chapter 4 of this book, on anxiety and depression in childhood.) By contrast, during their reproductive years, women show approximately twice the male frequency of depression. Importantly for the provision of optimum treatment, women are more likely than men to present with atypical depression, anxious depression, and seasonal affective disorder. There are no sex differences in the overall rates of bipolar disorders, but there are some important distinctions, The rapid cycling form of bipolar disorder is more prevalent in women, and women typically experience more episodes of depression relative to manic and hypomanic episodes. Also, the difficult clinical distinction between bipolar II (with hypomania and not mania) and personality disorders such as borderline personality disorder arises more frequently for women than men.

The preponderance of female depression has been found throughout the world, although the exact female:male ratios vary somewhat. As the number of symptoms increases, so does the female:male prevalence ratio. This ratio has, at times, been attributed to a variety of artifacts including women being more willing to talk about feelings; women coming more readily for help; and women's symptoms being more readily diagnosed as depression. Community surveys, however, have confirmed that the gender difference is found when the bias arising from help seeking is eliminated (3,7). This difference cannot be explained away, as some have speculated, by depressed men self-medicating with alcohol or drugs and, therefore, being diagnosed with substance abuse instead of a mood disorder.

ANXIETY

According to the ECA data, 13% of women compared to 6% of men met 6-month criteria for DSM-III Anxiety Disorders (3). The NCS study found that, not only was the 12-month prevalence of anxiety disorders significantly higher than the 12-month prevalence of substance abuse or affective disorders, but anxiety disorders were also more chronic (4). The majority of anxiety disorders, including specific phobias, agoraphobia with panic, panic disorders, and generalized anxiety disorders, are approximately twice as common in women (4). This difference in prevalence predates adolescence (by age 6, sex differences can already be seen) and increases over time.

DEPRESSIVE DISORDERS

ETIOLOGIC THEORIES OF DEPRESSION

Psychosocial Factors

Beginning at an early age, various psychosocial factors influence the occurrence of depression in women. Women are more likely to be sexually abused as children, and abused children are more likely to become depressed as adults (8). Prolonged separation from parents at an early age greatly increases the risk of depression in adult women, but this is also true for men. Women have a higher rate of victimization than men, and victimized women have high rates of depression. In the NCS data, however, Kessler (9) controlled for 24 types of life trauma and found that the sex ratio for depression was identical for those with and without previous trauma. Nevertheless, women are more likely to become depressed following stressful life events. (See Chapters 11 and 16 for response to trauma in women.)

As adults, women frequently struggle with role overload, the majority of women working full-time as well as doing 70% of the house and child care. Women are more likely to be depressed if they have young children at home, work outside the home (especially if they would rather stay at home), experience role conflict, or have trouble finding child care (10,11). These factors may contribute to the finding that marriage is not protective for women; married women are more likely to be depressed than married men or single women, the risk increasing further in unhappily married women. The explanation may lie in the fact that women are socialized to look after others, dismissing or minimizing their own needs. They are expected to handle things quietly without resorting to anger; as a consequence, they turn their feelings inward, which results in depression. As well, women are more often financially disadvantaged, and there is a particularly strong relationship between poverty in women and depression. (See Astbury, Chapter 27, in this book.)

Neurochemical and Anatomical Factors

Recent research has focused on the neurochemical and anatomical changes accompanying major depressive disorder (12). Although studies initially centered on the brain monoamine system, researchers more recently have looked at the role of cyclic adenosine monophosphate (cAMP) signal transduction cascade and cAMP-response element (CRE)–binding protein (CREB) (13). Brain-derived neurotrophic factor (BDNF), which protects against stress, appears to be an important gene product regulated by CREB (14). Clinical antidepressant efficacy mirrors the extent of expression of BDNF.

Activation of the hypothalamic-pituitary-adrenal (HPA) axis is commonly seen in depressed patients. There is evidence for elevated cortisol and corticotropin-releasing hormone (CRH) levels, nonsuppression on the dexamethasone suppression test, and a blunted adrenocorticotropic hormone (ACTH) response to CRH. Activation of the HPA axis appears to have prognostic value and is associated with increased risk of depression relapse and even suicide (15). CRH appears to modulate the general stress response as well as depression-related behaviors including appetite and sleep alterations and behavioral despair (16). Early life stress appears to produce longlasting changes in the regulation of CRH neurons and may, therefore, result in a biologic vulnerability to the subsequent development of depression, either directly or by means of increased reaction to stressors later in life. Patients with depression have been found to have volume reductions or other abnormalities in the prefrontal cortex and hippocampus, areas connected to the regulation of mood (17).

Research findings in animal models of depression have corroborated the profound effects of stress on intracellular signal transduction and on the expression of genes that drive fundamental neurotropic and neurotoxic processes, thereby demonstrating the link among environmental stressors, anatomical and neurochemical processes, and depression.

Hormonal Factors

Women's gonadal steroid hormones are thought to play an important role in the development of mood disorders (18). Mood often appears to fluctuate with the change of hormones. Times of low estrogen, such as the premenstrual and postpartum periods, are times of increased risk for mood disorder. (See Gold, Chapter 18 of this book.) It is possible that monthly cycling may trigger mood changes. We know that the brain is a major target organ for gonadal hormones. A complex interaction exists between gonadal hormones and neurotransmitters such as glutamate, gama-aminobutyric acid, acetylcholine, serotonin, dopamine, noradrenaline, adrenaline, and neuropeptides. Gonadal steroid hormones can affect the synthesis and release of these neurotransmitters, the expression of their receptors, and the membrane permeability of neurons.

Over the course of life, the risk of thyroid disease is four times higher in women than in men. Although thyroid abnormalities seen in depressed patients are probably transitory and stress-induced, subclinical hypothyroidism always needs to be ruled out in depressed women (19).

Genetic Factors

Although genetic factors play a large role in the vulnerability to mood disorders, they do not totally account for the occurrence of depression. Kendler and colleagues (20) found an estimated heritability for the liability to develop a major depressive disorder over a one-year period to be 41% to 46%; they found a lifetime estimated heritability of 70%. This research group postulates that what is inherited is a tendency to overreact to stressful life events. There is no evidence that men and women have a different genetic basis for unipolar depression; however, specific genetic risk factors may vary between men and women. For instance, specific genetic factors may be present in some women that predispose toward premenstrual mood disorder.

For children of bipolar patients, there is a 9% risk of developing the disorder compared to a 1% risk for the general population (21). Early reports of linkage of bipolar disorder to specific sites on the X chromosome have not been replicated. Similarly, reports of illness transmission from mother to child have not held up under scrutiny.

Personality Factors

Specific personality traits have been hypothesized as factors in the high prevalence of depression in women. Women as a group have been described as showing low self-esteem, low perceived control, pessimistic attributional styles, dependency, and overexpressiveness, factors that might result in depression or in being erroneously labeled as depressed. However, studies that carefully controlled for a previous history of depression found no significant association between these personality factors and depression (22). Duggan and colleagues (23), however, found that neuroticism was associated with both a one-year and a lifetime risk of depression and postulated that neuroticism predisposes to depression. More recently, Goodwin and Gotlib found that gender roles, and specifically neuroticism, may indeed play a key role (24). Because neuroticism is a very broad concept, it may be that these studies identified not so much personality factors as alterations in the response to stress, a probable determinant of vulnerability in women predisposed to depression.

Nolen-Hoeksema (25) has hypothesized an interesting relationship between women's coping styles and subsequent depression. She found that women are more likely than men to display a self-focused ruminative style of coping with feelings of sadness. Men's style of distracting themselves rather than ruminating appears, in Nolen-Hoeksema's studies, to be a more effective way of warding off depression.

SUBTYPES OF DEPRESSION

Dysthymic Disorder

Dysthymia affects from 3% to 6% of the population (4). There is no gender difference in children, but the prevalence rate for adult women (8.0%) is almost twice that of adult males (4.8%). The disorder usually begins gradually at an early age. Adolescent girls have been reported to have a greater number of symptoms and more problems with self-esteem than boys, who tend to show more aggressive behavior. Patients frequently suffer from comorbid illnesses such as anxiety or substance abuse. Forty percent have a coexisting major depression (double depression). Although the symptoms of dysthymia are not as severe as those of a major depression, they can nevertheless cause clinically significant distress and impairment in social, occupational, or other functioning.

Major Depressive Disorder (MDD)

MDD is 1.7 to 2.7 times more prevalent in women than in men (5). Girls begin to show an excess of depression over boys beginning around age 13. Ernst and Angst found that females had greater duration, recurrence, chronicity, and global manifestations of MDD than males during early to middle adulthood (26). However, when adjustments were made for recall bias in this retrospective study, these differences disappeared. Analysis of NCS and National Institute of Mental Health (NIMH) data has not found any differences in the course of MDD in men and women whether in recurrence rate, speed of recovery, or chronicity. But chronicity of depression appears to affect women more seriously than men, as manifested by more symptom reporting, poorer social adjustment, and poorer quality of life.

Women suffer more from atypical depression with psychomotor retardation, increased appetite and weight gain, and higher levels of somatic symptoms, ruminations, and feelings of worthlessness and guilt (27). They are also more likely than men to show comorbid generalized anxiety and panic disorders. Depressed women, more than men, also suffer from comorbid thyroid disorders, fibromyalgia, and migraines. No significant gender differences have been found in the risk of such sequelae of depression as early school leaving, having a child at a young age, marrying very early, or being unemployed. Early childbearing, however, when it does occur, leads to more severe consequences in women than in men.

Bipolar Disorder

Bipolar I disorder is equally prevalent in men and women (28). Bipolar II disorders, with episodes of depression and hypomania, occur more frequently in women. Although in 50% of cases in both men and women the onset occurs before age 25, among the other 50%, women generally have a later onset than men, onset in the fifth decade being more common in women.

Women with bipolar illness are more likely than men to have depressive or mixed episodes (29). They also tend toward more dysphoric than euphoric episodes of mania, but male bipolar patients are more likely to complete suicide.

As mentioned earlier, women, more often than men, are rapid cyclers (defined as having as four or more affective episodes per year). Although few have been well studied, a number of hypotheses have been presented to account for this excess of rapid cycling, among them the following: 1) because bipolar women tend to have more depressive episodes, they may more often take antidepressant medication, which increases the risk of developing a manic episode; 2) because women are generally more likely than men to be hypothyroid, subclinical hypothyroidism may initiate rapid cycling; 3) the mood-stabilizing effects of lithium may be offset by its thyrotoxic effect in women, thus making women less responsive; and 4) although there is no prospective evidence linking phases of the menstrual cycle to the onset of rapid cycling, a subset of women may be reactive to the effects of cycling reproductive hormones. No good evidence exists for any of these hypotheses.

Women with bipolar disorder have a 46% risk of developing a psychotic episode postpartum. (See Grigoriadis, Chapter 20 of this book.) This does not seem to be related to psychosocial stressors; these women may be particularly susceptible to the effects of sleep deprivation, which is common during the postpartum period.

Seasonal Affective Disorder (SAD)

The prevalence of SAD is related to latitude, with rates generally being higher in more northern locales (e.g., 4.3% at latitude 39 degrees versus 9.2% at 64 degrees (30). Subsyndromal SAD (S-SAD) shows similar variations from 13.5% to 28.3%. Multinational studies, however, show some variations that have been explained away on the basis of milder climates (e.g., Iceland with a combined SAD and S-SAD rate of only 11.3%) and the number of hours a person spends outdoors. Women have been found to be two to four times more likely than men to experience SAD. SAD has been attributed to both a dysfunction in the serotonin system and a phase delay in circadian rhythm (31).

Both bipolar disorder and MDD may present with a seasonal pattern. Typically, the individual becomes depressed in the fall, and the condition remits in the spring or summer. Patients usually complain of atypical symptoms, including increased appetite (sometimes especially for carbohydrates), weight gain, and hypersomnia. No gender differences have been shown in the course of the disorder.

TREATMENT OF DEPRESSIVE DISORDERS

Treatment of depressive disorders may require medication, psychotherapy, or a combination of these modalities. In considering medication in women, it is important to remember that drug distribution may differ in men and women because they have a different ratio of fat to muscle. As well, physiologic changes across the menstrual cycle influence gastric emptying and gastrointestinal transit time, which in turn affects the absorption and elimination of drugs. A premenstrual decrease in drug levels is common. As a result, some women need a premenstrual increase in medication in order to maintain the same drug levels across the cycle. It is also important to note whether the patient is taking oral contraceptives (OCs). Antidepressants such as fluoxetine, sertraline, paroxetine, and venlafaxine may increase the efficacy of OCs, whereas the mood stabilizers carbamazepine and topiramate decrease their efficacy. Plasma levels of tricyclic antidepressants may increase in women taking OCs, and doses of the antidepressant may need to be lowered.

Gender may affect choice of antidepressants. Several studies have found that, prior to menopause, women respond better to selective serotonin reuptake inhibitors (SSRIs) than to tricyclic antidepressants (TCAs) but, after menopause, this difference disappears (32). It has been suggested that this premenopausal and postmenopausal difference in drug response may be accounted for by the action of ovarian hormones in modulating the density of serotonin receptors in the hypothalamus, cortex, and nucleus accumbens as well as enhancing the antidepressant-induced down regulation of these receptors. A pooled analysis of 1,746 patients aged 18 to 65 found no differences in responses to TCAs or fluoxetine between men and women older and younger than 50 years (33). This analysis was marred, however, by its use of only one dose of open-label fluoxetine and by the small number of women in the over-50 group. Women may have more side effects from TCAs than men because of higher bioavailability and slower renal clearance. They are therefore more likely to discontinue treatment with TCAs than with SSRIs.

An analysis of studies comparing SSRIs and venlafaxine found no gender differences in response to either treatment (34). However, younger women appeared to respond better to SSRIs whereas venlafaxine was more beneficial in the older women.

The best approach to the treatment of dysthymic disorder seems to be a combination of medication and psychotherapy. Both men and women with MDD have been shown to respond to cognitive-behavioral therapy (CBT) and interpersonal therapy (IPT). Patients with more severe symptomatology may require antidepressant medication as well. Those with atypical depression respond best to monoamine oxidase inhibitor (MAOIs) (35). The addition of T_3 works better as an augmenting agent in women than in men (36). For the use of medication during pregnancy and breastfeeding, please see Chapters 19 and 20 of this book.

Reports have been mixed regarding the use of exogenous female sex hormones in the treatment of MDD in women (37). Some studies have shown an improvement in depressed postmenopausal women when estrogen replacement therapy (ERT) or hormone replacement therapy (HRT) was added to fluoxetine or sertraline but not venlafaxine. There is no agreement about the therapeutic benefit of estrogen alone in perimenopausal depression. Concerns about the increased risk of breast cancer, endometrial problems, heart attacks, and strokes in women taking ERT or HRT may limit use of these to cases of refractory depression.

Several studies have looked at the combination of psychotherapy and medication. Thase and colleagues (38) found a combination of IPT or CBT and a TCA was of greater benefit to men. This may be related to women's poorer response to TCAs. In contrast, Keller and colleagues (39) found that men and women responded equally when treated with a combination of nefazadone and CBT. In cases of chronic depression related to childhood trauma, Nemeroff's group (40) found that psychotherapy plus pharmacotherapy was marginally superior to psychotherapy alone.

ECT has been reported to be effective at lower doses, lead to less memory impairment (when treatment is unilateral on the right), and have a better acute response in women than in men. Thase and colleagues, however, report that women may have higher rates of relapse following ECT (41).

The main concern in the treatment of women with bipolar disorders is the need to prevent rapid cycling, as this has significant morbidity. Women should be monitored closely to detect the early signs of a rapid cycling period. If antidepressants cannot be avoided, SSRIs appear to have less chance of inducing a manic episode. Despite the lack of clear evidence for hypothyroidism being the cause of rapid cycling, some clinicians are using doses of levothyroxine up to 0.40 mg per day with some success even when thyroid laboratory findings are within normal ranges.

This should only be used in combination with mood-stabilizing medication to minimize the risk of inducing mania. Bone density should be monitored to ensure that there is no detrimental effect with high-dose levothyroxine.

Because women tend to have a greater number of depressive than manic episodes, mood stabilizers such as lithium and valproate, which are relatively ineffective at preventing depressive episodes, may not be the best choice. As well, valproate has been associated with the development of polycystic ovarian disease. Even though the evidence is not clear, it is probably wise to avoid its use in young women. Lamotrigine appears to be more effective at preventing depression (42). Lamotrigine also has the benefit of not interacting with oral contraceptives, whereas carbamazepine may reduce their efficacy. A combination of lithium and lamotrigine may be useful in managing rapid cycling bipolar disorder in women.

Atypical antipsychotics are being used more often as monotherapy or in combination with mood stabilizers. Certain side effects may be of particular concerns for women. Risperidone induces hypoprolactinemia, whereas olanzapine can cause significant weight gain.

Light therapy has proven to be effective in the prevention and treatment of SAD. The current recommendation is to expose the patient to 10,000-lux light intensity for 45 minutes twice a day. Side effects are rare and transient but may include irritability, headaches, eyestrain, and sleep disturbance. Improvement can be seen as early as within one week in some individuals. Antidepressants such as moclobemide, fluoxetine, sertraline, and citalopram have also been found to be effective alone or in combination with bright light therapy.

ANXIETY DISORDERS

Sex differences in anxiety begin at an early age (43). By age 6, the female:male ratio for anxiety is 2:1 (see Chapter 4). Although the duration of episodes does not differ between boys and girls, the severity of illness is greater in girls. Anxiety disorders have been associated with an increased risk of functional impairment, limited academic achievement, diminished occupational opportunities, impaired occupational performance, and elevated morbidity and mortality rates. As well, the presence of an anxiety disorder has been associated with elevated use rates for emergency medical and mental health-care services.

ETIOLOGIC THEORIES OF ANXIETY

Psychosocial Factors

Women who have a childhood history of separation from a parent or of parental marital separation have a greater risk of developing generalized anxiety disorder (GAD) as adults (44). Women with panic disorder report a greater frequency of childhood sexual abuse than women with other anxiety disorders. The onset of social phobia has been linked to the childhood experience of sexual assault by a relative and also to chronic exposure to verbal outbursts between parents. This association is true for women but not for men (45).

Neurochemical and Anatomical Factors

There is substantial evidence of overactivity in the central norepinephrine system in panic disorder and post-traumatic stress disorder (PTSD). In turn, the chronic stress resulting from the anxiety disorders leads to down regulation of postsynaptic alpha 2-receptor function. There appears to be postsynaptic 5-HT2A receptor and 5-HT1C sensitivity across anxiety disorders. Subsensitivity or dysregulation of gamma-aminobutyric acid (GABA) has also been found. Abnormalities in corticotropin-releasing factor (CRF) secretion have been identified in several anxiety disorders. Most anxiety disorders are associated with postsynaptic cholecystokinin receptor supersensitivity. In addition, there has been a consistent finding of lactate sensitivity in panic disorder patients. Neuroimaging studies have shown hippocampal atrophy in PTSD but not in panic disorder. (See Lanius, Bluhm, and Pain, Chapter 11 of this book.) The amygdala is activated during fear-conditioning procedures, suggesting that the amygdala is a key structure in the mediation of human anxiety (46). In persons with obsessive compulsive disorder (OCD) there appears to be a diffuse structural abnormality of the brain with an increase in total gray matter volume and a decrease in white matter (47). Gender differences have been seen in response to serotonergic probes in OCD, included here among the anxiety disorders. It may be that OCD is more related to serotonin dysregulation in women, but impairment of dopaminergic mechanisms is more common in men.

Hormonal Factors

The stress response is known to decrease during pregnancy. Placental CRF, prolactin, and oxytocin all inhibit the stress response at the level of the pituitary. No significant effect of menstrual cycle on symptom level in GAD has been reported, although women with GAD and comorbid premenstrual syndrome are reported to be symptomatic in both phases of the menstrual cycle (48).

Although some studies have found a worsening of anxiety symptoms in general, and in panic disorder in particular, in the midluteal phase of the menstrual cycle, to date, prospective studies have failed to find any significant association. Approximately equal percentages of women improve or deteriorate during this time. Postpartum, there is often a worsening in women with pre-existing panic disorder. Between 11% and 29% of women with panic disorder report that its first onset was during the postpartum period (49). Acute suppression of ovarian function, as in perimenopause, may also increase the risk of panic disorder. There is no evidence on the relationship between phobias and the female reproductive system.

Although retrospective studies have shown an increase of OCD symptoms in the late luteal phase, this research is of questionable validity. Between 13% and 39% of women report the first onset of OCD during pregnancy (50). For those with pre-existing OCD, 70% showed no change during pregnancy and equal numbers reported significant worsening or improvement during pregnancy. A postpartum increase in pre-existing OCD symptoms (as opposed to the onset of new symptoms) has been reported. In the six months following a miscarriage, OCD was found to occur eight times more frequently than in a control group who had not suffered miscarriages (51).

Genetic Factors

Genetic factors appear to play a strong role in the development of anxiety disorders. Kendler and colleagues, in their investigation of female twin pairs, found that genetics accounted for approximately 30% of the development of GAD (52). This work has provided strong evidence that GAD and depression may share a common genotype, the actual presentation being determined by environmental experiences. In panic disorder, women are reported to have a higher occurrence of a novel repeat genetic polymorphism on chromosome X than control subjects.

This is thought to mediate the expression of monoamine oxidase A (53). Twin studies suggest that, in general, environmental factors are much more important than genetic factors in the development of phobia, although, in generalized social phobia, there appears to be an important genetic contribution. In nongeneralized social phobia, twin studies have failed to find genetic transmission. OCD also appears to have a strong genetic component, and gender differences may exist in the nature of the genetic susceptibility (54).

Personality Factors

Sociotropy (an excess investment in interpersonal relationships) has been shown to be associated with trait anxiety in situations of social evaluation, physical danger, and ambiguous situations. An excessive concern with independence (autonomy) has been associated with trait anxiety in daily routines (55). Women with panic disorder more commonly meet criteria for a histrionic and cluster C personality diagnosis, particularly dependent personality; in contrast, men with panic disorder are more likely to be diagnosed as having schizoid or borderline personality disorders (56).

SUBTYPES OF ANXIETY DISORDERS

Just as the current classification systems require that we consider depressive conditions separately from anxiety, anxiety itself is currently subdivided into a number of separate conditions, which can co-occur in complex patterns.

Generalized Anxiety Disorder (GAD)

GAD occurs approximately twice as often in women as in men. The prevalence rate of GAD in women is 6.6% compared to 3.6% in men (4). It tends to be a chronic disorder with low remission rates and a prevalence rate that is constant throughout life. Mood disorders, panic disorder, and social anxiety are the most common comorbid disorders.

Women have a slightly later onset, a more chronic course, and greater symptom severity than men. This may be related to the fact that, in women, GAD is more likely to be complicated by a comorbid psychiatric disorder and is therefore associated with more functional impairment than in men. Even without comorbid disorders, people with GAD tend to have significant disability and are heavy users of medical services.

Panic Disorder and Agoraphobia

Panic disorder is one of the more prevalent psychiatric disorders, with a lifetime prevalence of 2.2% to 3.5%. In both the ECA and NCS studies, women were found to have two to four times the lifetime prevalence of men. Women have a 5.0% lifetime prevalence rate compared to 2% for men. Similar rates have been reported for the occurrence of panic disorder with agoraphobia. Women are twice as likely as men to meet criteria for agoraphobia without panic disorder (7% versus 3.5%).

Forty percent of women who have panic attacks during their childhood or adolescence develop a subsequent psychiatric disorder. Panic disorder appears to begin earlier in women and is most prevalent between the ages of 25 and 34 in women (compared to ages 30 and 44 in men). Postmenopausally, women improve, showing less anticipatory anxiety and fewer panic attacks and experiencing less severe attacks.

Women with panic disorder report greater levels of phobic avoidance, more reliance on family members as companions, and more functional impairment than do men. Yonkers and colleagues (57) found that men and women with pure panic disorder are equally likely to get well and have a similar age of onset and length of illness. However, women tend to have a greater number of relapses. This may be because women are more likely to have comorbid agoraphobia, which is associated with a poor outcome and an elevated lifetime risk for comorbid psychiatric disorders including depression, GAD, simple phobia, and somatization disorder (57).

Specific Phobia

Women are twice as likely as men to suffer from specific phobia (26% lifetime risk for women compared to 12% for men). Women have higher rates of situational and animal phobias and equal rates of health-related phobias.

Phobias generally have the earliest rate of onset of any anxiety disorders, with a mean age of 15 years. They tend to follow a chronic course, with frequent comorbidity including elevated rates of GAD and an increased vulnerability to subsequent major depression and addictive disorders. Phobias that continue into adulthood have approximately a 20% chance of remitting. There is little information about differences between men and women concerning clinical features or course of simple phobias (58).

Social Anxiety Disorder

The lifetime prevalence for social anxiety disorder is greater than 13%. The risk is 15.5% for women compared to 11.1% for men (4).

Social anxiety disorder usually begins before the age of 18; onset is rare after the age of 25. Although it tends to have a chronic and unremitting clinical course, those who experience remission tend not to relapse. Yonkers and colleagues found that nearly equal levels of women and men (38% versus 32%) experienced complete remission during an eight-year study (59).

There are two types of social anxiety disorder: generalized and nongeneralized. The most common type of nongeneralized social anxiety disorder is the fear of public speaking. The generalized subtype includes multiple fears related to performance and interactions in social situations. It is associated with greater chronicity, more functional impairment, and increased risk of comorbid disorders. Although there does not seem to be any gender difference in the prevalence of generalized versus nongeneralized type of social anxiety disorder or in their clinical courses, women appear to have greater symptom severity than men and a higher prevalence of concurrent agoraphobia (59).

Obsessive Compulsive Disorder (OCD)

The lifetime prevalence rate for OCD is 2% to 3% worldwide (4). Women appear to be 1.5 times more likely than men to develop OCD over their lifetime. The mean age of onset for men is 20 years as opposed to 25 years in women (60). Prior to the onset of puberty there is an excess of males with OCD. This is often associated with a tic disorder and a positive family history for OCD. After menarche, women begin to develop OCD at an increased rate, most frequently with a sudden onset. Generally, OCD patients follow a chronic clinical course with rare sustained remissions. There does not appear to be an association between gender and remission or outcome. As previously mentioned, the majority of women show no change in symptoms during pregnancy but may have a postpartum worsening.

The types of symptoms seen in OCD may vary with gender (60). Women are more likely to have symptoms related to contamination/cleaning or aggressive/checking dimensions whereas men more often have symptoms in the symmetry/ordering dimension. In women with OCD, there is a high rate of comorbid axis I disorder, including mood disorders, anxiety disorders, and eating disorders. The presence of a comorbid depression does not have a major impact on the prognosis of OCD; if the OCD symptoms improve, the depression often remits. OCD increases the severity of a comorbid eating disorder. Males with OCD are two to three times more likely than females to have comorbid Tourette syndrome or a tic disorder (60).

TREATMENT OF ANXIETY DISORDERS

The treatment of choice for GAD is one of the antidepressant medications that also have anxiolytic properties (SSRIs, venlafaxine, buspirone), although benzodiazepines have all been found to be effective in the short term. Despite greater evidence for the efficacy of antidepressants, benzodiazepines are more likely to be prescribed for women than antidepressant medication. There is no evidence of gender differences in response to medication, but few studies to date have specifically looked at this. A mixture of cognitive-behavioral therapy with interpersonal and experiential techniques has been used effectively (61).

Little information is available concerning the potential impact of gender on treatment response to panic disorder. The current treatment of choice is antidepressant medication such as SSRIs, tricyclic antidepressants, or MAOIs. High-potency benzodiazepines such as lorazepam and clonazepam are also effective. Contraceptive use in younger women or hormone replacement therapy in postmenopausal women has not been shown to have an effect on treatment response.

The first-line treatment for social anxiety disorder is an SSRI antidepressant. Treatment needs to be long term. Phobias tend to be undertreated, probably because they are rarely associated with significant impairment. Only 10% to 20% of people meeting the criteria for simple phobias receive appropriate treatment. The main feature of therapy for phobic disorder is exposure to the feared stimulus, accompanied, if required, by specific desensitization techniques. The combination of exposure-based therapy and cognitive-behavioral therapy, especially in a group setting, is particularly beneficial (62).

The treatments of choice for OCD continue to be SSRIs and clomipramine, but they lead to improvement in only 30% to 40% of patients. Patients who have a later age of onset tend to have a better response to treatment. Cognitive-behavior therapy has also been used.

SUMMARY AND FUTURE DIRECTIONS

During their reproductive years women are twice as likely as men to suffer from major depressive episodes. They also have more seasonal affective disorders and anxious and atypical depressions. There are also gender differences in the presentation and courses of these depressions. Although the prevalence of bipolar disorder is equal in men and women, women are more likely to have lows than highs and they are more likely to have the rapid cycling disorder. Genetic, psychosocial, hormonal, and neurochemical and anatomical factors have all been implicated in the etiology of depression. Further research is necessary to ascertain the combination of factors that increases women's risk of developing depression. Further information is needed about the impact of the menstrual cycle on the metabolism of psychotropic medications as well as gender differences in response. There are conflicting reports about the role of estrogen and HRT in the treatment of depressive disorders. Gender differences in response to newer treatments (e.g., transcranial magnetic stimulation, TMS) have yet to be determined.

Anxiety disorders also occur twice as frequently in women. Unlike depressive disorders, gender differences in anxiety disorders begin appearing by age 6. Systematic data concerning gender differences in underlying pathophysiology and treatment response are needed. Because anxiety and depressive disorders are frequently comorbid and show a similar response to treatment with antidepressants, questions are being raised as to the distinctiveness of these disorders. The classification system may need to be changed to reflect the overlap.

More research is needed as to the effect of pregnancy on the course of all depressive and anxiety disorders. As well, more information is needed about the safety of psychotropic medication and other treatments during pregnancy and breastfeeding.

REFERENCES

1. Shorter E, Tyrer P. Separation of anxiety and depressive disorders: blind alley in psychopharmacology and classification of disease. Br Med J 2003:327:158–160.
2. Jenkins R, Lewis G, Bebbington P, et al. The national psychiatric comorbidity surveys of Great Britain: initial findings from the household survey. Psychol Med 1997;27:775–799.
3. Regier D, Rae D, Narrow W, et al. Prevalence of anxiety disorders and their comorbidity with mood and addictive disorders. Br J Psychiatry 1998;34:24–28.
4. Kessler R, McGonagle K, Zhao S, et al. Lifetime and 12-month prevalence of DSM-3-R psychiatric disorders in the United States. Results from the National Comorbidity Survey. Arch Gen Psychiatry 1994;51:8–19.
5. Simonds VM, Whiffen VE. Are gender differences in depression explained by gender differences in co-morbid anxiety? J Affect Disord 2003;77:197–202.
6. Kuehner C. Gender differences in unipolar depression: an update of epidemiological findings and possible explanations. Acta Psychiatr Scand 2003;108:163–174.
7. Kessler RC, McGonagle KA, Swartz M, et al. Sex and depression in the National Comorbidity Survey I. Lifetime prevalence, chronicity and recurrence. J Affect Disord 1993;29:85–96.
8. Weiss EL, Longhurst JG, Mazure CM. Childhood sexual abuse as a risk factor for depression in women: psychosocial and neurobiological correlates. Am J Psychiatry 1999;156:816–828.
9. Kessler RC. Gender differences in major depression: epidemiological findings. In: Frank E, ed. Gender and Its Effects on Psychopathology. Washington, DC: American Psychiatric Association, 2000:61–84.
10. Bebbington PE, Dunn G, Jenkins R, et al. The influence of age and sex on the prevalence of depressive conditions: report from the National Survey of Psychiatric Comorbidity. Psychol Med 1998;28:9–19.
11. Wang JL. The difference between single and married mothers in the 12-month prevalence of major depressive syndrome, associated factors and mental health service utilization. Soc Psychiatry Psychiatr Epidemiol 2004;39:26–32.
12. Krystal JH, D'Souza DC, Sanacora G, et al. Current perspectives on the pathophysiology of schizophrenia, depression, and anxiety disorders. Med Clin North Am 2001;85:559–577.
13. Vaidya VA, Duman RS. Depression: emerging insights from neurobiology. Br Med Bull 2001;57:61–79.
14. Hashimoto K, Shimizu E, Iyo M. Critical role of brain-derived neurotrophic factor in mood disorders. Brain Res Brain Res Rev 2004;45:104–114.
15. Varghese FP, Brown ES. The hypothalamic-pituitary-adrenal axis in major depressive disorder: a brief primer for primary care physicians. Prim Care Companion J Clin Psychiatry 2001;3: 151–155.
16. Claes SJ. Corticotropin-releasing hormone (CRH) in psychiatry: from stress to psychopathology. Ann Med 2004;36:50–61.
17. Campbell S, Marriott M, Nahmias C, et al. Lower hippocampal volume in patients suffering from depression: a meta-analysis. Am J Psychiatry 2004;161:598–607.
18. Ostlund H, Keller E, Hurd YL. Estrogen receptor gene expression in relation to neuropsychiatric disorders. Ann NY Acad Sci 2003;1007:54–63.

19. Fountoulakis KN, Iacovides A, Grammaticos P, et al. Thyroid function in clinical subtypes of major depression: an exploratory study. BMC Psychiatry 2004;4:6.

20. Kendler KS, Neale MC, Kessler RC, et al. A longitudinal twin study of 1-year prevalence of major depression in women. Arch Gen Psychiatry 1993;50:843–852.

21. DePaulo JR, Jr. Genetics of bipolar disorder: where do we stand? Am J Psychiatry 2004; 161:595–597.

22. Hirschfeld RMA, Klerman GL, Clayton PJ, et al. Personality and gender-related differences in depression. J Affect Disord 1984;7:211–221.

23. Duggan C, Sham P, Lee AS, et al. Neuroticism: a vulnerability marker for depression: evidence from a family study. J Affect Disord 1995;35:139–143.

24. Goodwin RD, Gotlib IH. Gender differences in depression: the role of personality factors. Psychiatry Res 2004;126:135–142.

25. Nolen-Hoeksema S. The role of rumination in depressive disorders and mixed anxiety/depressive symptoms. J Abnorm Psychol 2000;109:504–511.

26. Ernst C, Angst J. The Zurich Study: XII. Sex difference in depression: evidence from longitudinal epidemiological data. Eur Arch Psychiatry Clin Neurosci 1992;241:222–230.

27. Quitkin FM. Depression with atypical features: diagnostic validity, prevalence, and treatment. Prim Care Companion J Clin Psychiatry 2002;4:94–99.

28. Arnold LM. Gender differences in bipolar disorder. Psychiatr Clin North Am 2003;26: 595–620.

29. Sit D. Women and bipolar disorder across the life span. J Am Med Women's Assoc 2004; 59:91–100.

30. Rosen LN, Targum SD, Terman M, et al. Prevalence of seasonal affective disorders at four latitudes. Psychiatry Res 1990;31:131–144.

31. Magnusson A, Boivin D. Seasonal affective disorder: an overview. Chronobiol Int 2003; 20:189–207.

32. Kornstein SG, Schatzberg AF, Thase ME, et al. Gender differences in treatment response to sertraline versus imipramine in chronic depression. Am J Psychiatry 2000;157:1445–1452.

33. Quitkin FM, Stewart JW, McGrath PJ, et al. Are there differences between women's and men's antidepressant responses? Am J Psychiatry 2002;159:1848–1854.

34. Entsuah AR, Huang H, Thase MF. Response and remission rates in different subpopulations with major depressive disorder administered venlafaxine, selective serotonin reuptake inhibitors, or placebo. J Clin Psychiatry 2001;62:869–877.

35. Benazzi F. Can only reversed vegetative symptoms define atypical depression? Eur Arch Psychiatry Clin Neurosci 2002;52:288–293.

36. Joffe RT, Levitt AJ, Bagby RM, et al. Predictors of response to lithium and triiodothyronine augmentation of antidepressants to tricyclic non-responders. Br J Psychiatry 1993;163:574–578.

37. Stoppe G, Doren M. Critical appraisal of effects of estrogen replacement therapy in symptoms of depressed mood. Arch Women Ment Health 2002;5:39–47.

38. Thase ME, Greenhouse JB, Frank E, et al. Treatment of major depression with psychotherapy or pharmacotherapy-psychotherapy combinations. Arch Gen Psychiatry 1997;54:1009–1015.

39. Keller MB, McCullough JP, Klein D. A comparison of nefazadone, cognitive behavioral analysis system of psychotherapy, and their combination for the treatment of chronic depression. N Engl J Med 2000;342:1462–1470.

40. Nemeroff CB, Heim CM, Thase ME, et al. Differential responses to psychotherapy versus pharmacotherapy in patients with chronic forms of major depression and childhood trauma. Proc Natl Acad Sci USA 2003;100:14293-14296.

41. Thase ME, Frank E, Kornstein SG, et al. Sex related differences in response to treatments of depression. In: Frank E, ed. Gender and Its Effects on Psychopathology. Washington, DC, American Psychiatric Publishing, 2000:103–129.

42. Calabrese JR, Faterni SH, Woyshville MJ. Antidepressant effects of lamotrigine in rapid cycling bipolar disorder. Am J Psychiatry 1996;153:1236.

43. Lewinsohn PM, Gotlib IH, Lewinsohn, et al. Gender differences in anxiety disorders and anxiety symptoms in adolescents. J Abnorm Psychol 1998;107:109–117.

44. Pigott TA. Anxiety disorders in women. Psychiatr Clin North Am 2003;25:621–672.

45. Magee W. Effects of negative life experiences on phobia onset. Soc Psychiatry Psychiatr Epidemiol 1999;34:343–351.

46. LaBar KS, Gatenby JC, Gore JC, et al. Human amygdala activation during conditioned fear acquisition and extinction: a mixed trial fMRI study. Neuron 1998;20:937–945.

47. Jenke MA, Breiter HC, Baer L, et al. Cerebral structural abnormalities in obsessive-compulsive disorder: a quantitative morphometric magnetic resonance imaging study. Arch Gen Psychiatry 1996;53:625–632.

48. McLeod D, Hoehn-Saric R, Foster G, et al. The influence of premenstrual syndrome on ratings of anxiety in women with generalized anxiety disorder. Acta Psychiatr Scand 1993;84:248–251.

49. Hertzberg T, Wahlbeck K. The impact of pregnancy and puerperium on panic disorders: a review. J Psychosom Obstet Gynaecol 1999;20:59–64.

50. Altshuler L, Hendrick V, Cohen L. Course of mood and anxiety disorders during pregnancy and the postpartum period. J Clin Psychiatry 1998;2:29–33.

51. Brier N. Anxiety after miscarriage: a review of the empirical literature and implications for clinical practice. Birth 2004;31:138–142.

52. Kendler K, Neale M, Kessler, et al. Generalized anxiety disorders in women: a population-based twin study. Arch Gen Psychiatry 1992;49:109–116.

53. Deckert J, Catalano M, Syagato Y, et al. Excess of high activity monoamine oxidase A gene promoter alleles in female patients with panic disorder. Hum Mol Genet 1999;8:621–624.

54. Pauls D, Alsobrook J. The inheritance of obsessive-compulsive disorder. Child Adolesc Psychiatr Clin North Am 1999;8:481–496.

55. Sato T, McCann D, Ferguson-Isaac C. Sociotropy-autonomy and situation-specific anxiety. Psychol Rep 2004;94:67–76.

56. Barzega G, Maina G, Venturello S, et al. Gender-related distribution of personality disorders in a sample of patients with panic disorder. Eur Psychiatry 2001;16:173–179.

57. Yonkers KA, Bruce SE, Dyck JR, et al. Chronicity, relapse and illness-course of panic disorder, social phobia, and generalized anxiety disorder: findings in men and women from eight years of follow-up. Depress Anxiety 2003;171:173–179.

58. Fredrikson M, Annas P, Fischer H, et al. Gender and age differences in the prevalence of specific fears and phobias. Behav Res Ther 1996;34:33–39.

59. Yonkers K, Dyck I, Keller M. An eight-year longitudinal comparison of clinical course and characteristics of social phobia among men and women. Psychiatr Serv 2001;52:637–643.

60. Lochner C, Hemmings SM, Kinnear CJ, et al. Gender in obsessive-compulsive disorder: clinical and genetic findings. Eur Neuropsychopharmacol 2004;14:105–113.

61. Borkovec TD, Newman MG, Castonguay LG. Cognitive-behavioral therapy for generalized anxiety disorder with integrations from interpersonal and experiential therapies. CNS Spectr 2003;8:382-389.

62. Heimberg RG, Liebowitz MR, Hope DA, et al. Cognitive behavioural group therapy vs. phenelzine therapy for social phobia: 12-week outcome. Arch Gen Psychiatry 1998;55:1133–1141.

SUGGESTED READINGS

Frank E. Gender and Its Effects on Psychopathology. Washington, DC: American Psychiatric Association, 2000.

Kornstein SG, Clayton AH. Women's Mental Health: A Comprehensive Textbook. New York: Guilford, 2002.

Stein DJ, Hollander E. Textbook of Anxiety Disorders. Washington DC: APPI, 2002.

Steinen M, Yonkers KA, Eriksson E. Mood Disorders in Women. London: Martin Dunitz, 2000.

CHAPTER 13

Substance Use and Abuse in Women

Monica L. Zilberman, Sheila B. Blume

Substance abuse is a major source of health problems worldwide. The National Comorbidity Survey (NCS), a large study of the United States population aged 15 to 54 years conducted at the beginning of the 1990s, suggests that approximately one fourth of Americans had already met criteria for a substance use disorder at the time they were surveyed (1). Although substance use disorders are currently more prevalent in men than in women, this was not always the case. During the nineteenth century, most Americans dependent on opiates were women (male:female ratio close to 1:2). Many of these women started opiate use on the advice of their physicians for a variety of complaints, much like the mother in Eugene O'Neill's play *Long Day's Journey into Night*. Substance use among women, often concealed, was silently accepted and tolerated by close relatives. This changed dramatically in the twentieth century with the advent of antidrug policies (2). The NCS estimates that now 8% of American women between the ages of 15 and 54 have a lifetime diagnosis of alcohol use disorders (male:female ratio of 2.5:1) and 6% have a diagnosis of other drug use disorders (male:female ratio of 1.6:1) (1). Although the current numbers are impressive, reports of abuse of or dependence on substances date back to ancient times. One such example comes from an ancient Egyptian quotation contained in the Anastasi Papyrus IV around 1500 BCE:

Beer makes him cease being a man. It causes your soul to wander, and you are like a crooked steering-oar in a boat that obeys on neither side, you are like a shrine void of its god, like a house void of bread. Now you are seated (still) in the house, and the harlots surround you, now you are standing and bouncing . . . now you stumble and fall over upon your belly, anointed with dirt. (3)

There is mention of substance abuse in the Hebrew bible, in Samuel, Book I, Chapter 1, where a priest mistakes a woman who is praying for a babbling drunkard and admonishes her to give up drinking.

Throughout history, excessive drinking and its consequences were traditionally attributed to individual choice and blamed on low moral standards. The notion that the desire to drink could be overwhelming and irresistible in some people for physiologic reasons is relatively recent. Dating from the nineteenth century, this notion is central to the modern disease concept of addiction, a term usually used as a synonym for dependence. Substance abuse is defined as the harmful use of a specific psychoactive substance. The next section presents general issues of substance use, abuse, and dependence, paving the path to sections dedicated to specific topics of substance use among women.

OVERVIEW OF SUBSTANCE USE, ABUSE, AND DEPENDENCE

For health professionals, establishing where recreational use of a substance ends and substance abuse starts is a challenge with important preventive and clinical implications. Any substance use pattern involves the complex interaction of pharmacologic, psychological, genetic, and sociocultural factors. Some substances are more liable than others to induce self-administration and thus lead to a pattern of abuse or dependence. (Nicotine, for instance, is associated with fast progression to dependence states, while alcohol dependence usually establishes itself only after several years of continued drinking.) Although initial substance use is often prompted by environmental and psychological factors (curiosity, peer pressure, "self-medication" of uncomfortable affective states), genetic factors have an important role in progression from recreational use to abuse or dependence. The problematic use of a substance represents a continuum from abuse to dependence. (Some prefer the term "substance misuse," because of the possible pejorative connotations of the term "abuse.") The continuum starting with substance use may lead to one or more substance-related problems, such as accidents, medical consequences, family and occupational problems, and eventually dependence. Dependence is a behavioral syndrome comprising (a) a strong desire to use the substance; (b) loss of control over substance use, which may be marked by the inability to abstain even in the face of various recurrent health, family, social, or occupational problems; and (c) signs of physiologic adaptation, such as tolerance and withdrawal. Physiologic adaptation (formerly known as physical dependence) is no longer considered a sine qua non criterion for dependence. In fact, substances like cannabis do not seem to be associated with a clear withdrawal syndrome (4), yet they clearly induce abuse and dependence. Further, as scientific knowledge has advanced, substances that were not formerly known to induce abuse have been shown to be strongly associated with dependence (nicotine is an example).

Substances of abuse vary widely in chemical structure but produce common behavioral syndromes. Both licit (often prescribed or even over-the-counter) substances and illicit substances are shown to have addictive properties. They can be classified for convenience into three groups: (a) central nervous system depressants: alcohol, barbiturates, benzodiazepines, inhalants, and opiates (opiates are sometimes classified in a separate category because their effects involve specific opiate receptors); (b) central nervous system stimulants: amphetamines, caffeine, cocaine, and tobacco (nicotine); (c) hallucinogens: cannabis, LSD, mescaline, psilocybin, and a wide variety of other substances, both natural and synthetic. Although each of these drugs has a different mechanism of action, they all stimulate the limbic system, including the nucleus accumbens and ventral tegmental area, a circuitry thought to be basic to the reinforcement of behavior and a final common pathway for addiction.

Knowledge about the neurobiology of addiction has improved dramatically with the use of neuroimaging techniques. Widespread brain structural changes have been associated with stimulant and opiate abuse, while frontal atrophy may appear in alcohol abuse. Functional techniques show altered regional cerebral activity associated with various substances. These techniques further reveal involvement of dopaminergic, serotonergic, opioid, and GABAergic systems in addiction (5).

Substance use and abuse are involved in a variety of problems, affecting directly or indirectly the health of users, family members, and society at large. Driving while intoxicated is one major cause of injuries and fatalities. Similarly, substance abuse is involved in most cases of domestic violence, including emotional, physical, and sexual abuse, affecting domestic partners, children, and the elderly. Legal and occupational problems related to substance use add to the global burden.

In addition to physical consequences, substance abuse is also associated with increased rates of conduct and personality disorders (mainly those characterized by intense impulsivity, such as antisocial and borderline personality disorders) and a number of psychiatric conditions, including affective, anxiety, and psychotic disorders. More than half of all persons with substance use disorders in the general population present at least one other psychiatric disorder (1). The risk of other addictive disorders is also greatly increased (polydrug abuse; eating disorders, particularly bulimia nervosa; and pathologic gambling, for instance). Women are at higher risk for psychiatric comorbidity in general and for developing iatrogenic substance abuse or dependence as well, because they are more likely to be prescribed hypnotics, analgesics, and sedatives by physicians. Worries about body image also put them at risk of abusing cocaine and amphetamines and other diet pills for the purpose of weight control.

SUBSTANCE USE IN WOMEN

Over the past several decades, health professionals and researchers alike have acknowledged that substance use manifests itself differently in women than in men. For many years the study of addiction was focused on men, and clinical approaches to the few women presenting for treatment were derived from what was known to work for men. Since the Second World War, the entry of women into the job market and into professions previously dominated by men, among other societal changes in women's roles, has very likely contributed to the narrowing of the distinction between women's and men's social roles and to broadened opportunities for women to drink and to use drugs. This contributes to the higher prevalence of substance use disorders among women observed in recent epidemiologic surveys (1). Gender differences are reported in a variety of areas, such as physiologic effects of substances, metabolic differences, physical and psychiatric comorbidities, and genetic and sociocultural factors. There are also important effects on women's reproductive health, pregnancy, and offspring. This section explores substance use issues that either express differently in women than in men or are unique to women.

PATTERNS OF SUBSTANCE USE

In spite of consistent lower levels of use (e.g., drinking or taking drugs less frequently and in lower quantities) compared to men, women develop substance abuse and dependence patterns more rapidly than substance-using men (6). Referred in the specialized literature as a "telescoping" effect, this phenomenon was first observed in the 1950s when it was noticed that women entered treatment with shorter histories of problem drinking than men, although the severity of symptoms was equal. At that point, some professionals found it intriguing that women, although starting to drink much later in life, were entering treatment at the same age as men. The age at which women start to drink has dropped dramatically since that time, being virtually the same for women as men since the 1990s, but the telescoping of alcohol problems among women remains a consistent feature. Women begin treatment for their alcohol disorder two to five years earlier than men, but this period also encompasses time spent dealing with personal feelings of shame and guilt (reinforced by social stigma), opposition of substance-abusing partners, and difficulties in finding treatment programs that can accommodate a woman's needs (such as child care and flexible hours of operation for women with children). Thus, it is possible that the magnitude of telescoping is underestimated. If it were not for the difficulties encountered by women in accessing addiction treatment, their admission would come earlier, resulting in even greater telescoping (6). A similar telescoping of substance-related problems in women is described for opiates, but data for cocaine are less consistent. Sex-related differences in the metabolism of alcohol and other drugs have been thought responsible, at least in part, for this telescoping effect (see below). However, a similar telescoping has been described for women who seek treatment for pathologic gambling, so that factors other than drug-related physiology must be involved (7).

Women and men also differ in the types of substances they are more likely to use. Although illegal drug use has been more commonly found in men, in recent years women are catching up with men; this is particularly noticeable among young people. The prevalence of prescription drug use (as well as abuse and dependence), however, continues to be higher for women than for men. Women are more likely to use and abuse pain relievers, tranquilizers, stimulants, and sedatives, for instance (8).

PHARMACOLOGIC FACTORS

Blood alcohol concentrations (BAC) are higher in women than in men consuming the same amount of absolute alcohol per unit of body weight. This is explained in part by women's lower body water content relative to men. Because the ingested alcohol is distributed in total body water and women have proportionately less water in their bodies, the alcohol is less diluted, thus increasing the BAC. As women age, there is a further increase in the body ratio of fat to water, enhancing the increased sensitivity to alcohol. Also, first-pass metabolism of alcohol at the gastric level occurs at lower rates in women. Even women who do not abuse alcohol have lower quantities of the enzyme alcohol dehydrogenase in their gastric mucosa, metabolizing less of the alcohol they ingest, compared to men. Thus, women's bodies absorb more of the alcohol they drink than do men's bodies, which further contributes to the increased BAC in women. In alcoholic women, there is a further decrease in gastric alcohol dehydrogenase, and virtually all of the alcohol ingested is absorbed (9). Whereas a man given a standard amount of absolute alcohol develops the same BAC on each occasion, a woman's BAC varies from day to day. Some but not all studies have found variation according to the menstrual cycle, with higher BAC in the premenstrual phase. Thus, a given dose of alcohol may produce more unpredictable BAC in a woman compared to a man. Women may also have more intense reactions when drinking the same amount as men, as acute alcohol tolerance is less marked in women (10). As mentioned above, this greater sensitivity to ethanol is thought responsible, at least in part, for the telescoping of the course of alcoholism in women.

Women also react differently to cocaine than do men, but the direction of the differences and their explanation are not clear. Greater subjective response in women than in men after intranasal cocaine administration has been reported, whereas higher and faster subjective responses, accompanied by higher plasma levels, in men than in women have also been observed. Others have found higher cocaine plasma levels in the follicular than in the luteal phase among women, although these levels were not accompanied by a higher subjective response to cocaine. It is hypothesized that the nasal mucosa of women in the luteal phase is more viscous, leading to decreased cocaine absorption and decreased plasma levels (11).

There has been less research on gender differences in the pharmacologic effects of other drugs, but there is evidence that the intensity of the acute response to cannabis and opiates may be influenced by sex hormones (11). Regarding tobacco, even with similar daily smoking patterns, women exhibit lower nicotine plasma levels, but they inhale more frequently and more intensely to achieve the same nicotine intake (12).

HEALTH CONSEQUENCES

Alcohol abuse is clearly associated with increased morbidity and mortality in women who drink excessively, compared both to women in the general population and to alcohol-abusing men. Women are at increased risk for hypertension, malnutrition, anemia, cardiovascular disease, fatty liver, cirrhosis, gastrointestinal hemorrhage, peptic ulcer, breast cancer, subarachnoid bleeding, decreased brain volume, and poor performance on attention and visuospatial tasks, to name a few conditions. Several of these problems develop faster and with lower total alcohol intake in women compared to men. It is possible that women's greater sensitivity to alcohol effects plays a role in the increased morbidity and mortality observed in women who abuse alcohol compared to men who abuse alcohol (13).

Although less studied, drugs other than alcohol (but commonly taken together) may directly or indirectly affect women's health. Intravenous injection of drugs is a potent risk factor for HIV infection, hepatitis B and C, syphilis, and other sexually transmitted diseases. Substance-injecting women combine two important risk factors: unprotected sex with an injecting partner and needle sharing. Drug injection and unprotected sex are more common when either or both partners are under the influence of alcohol or other drugs. Panic attacks are reported to be more frequent among women who smoke cannabis than among men (8).

The increase in tobacco smoking among women has led to renewed interest in the health-related consequences of its use. Women smokers are at increased risk for impaired immune response, cardiovascular disease, and cancer of the lung and bladder. This gender difference is due to a higher susceptibility to tobacco carcinogens in women. Recently, lung cancer mortality rates have risen to surpass breast cancer as the most frequent cause of death related to cancer among American women, whereas deaths associated with lung cancer in men have decreased (14). In women, tobacco smoking is also associated with increased rates of breast, ovarian, and cervical cancers.

EFFECTS ON SEXUAL FUNCTIONING AND THE REPRODUCTIVE SYSTEM

Heavy drinking is associated with several sexual and reproductive problems, including anovulation, decreased gonadal mass, and infertility. These problems seem to be due to increased testosterone plasma levels produced by increased rates of androstenedione conversion to testosterone in women's alcohol-damaged liver (10).

Sex responsiveness is impacted differently by alcohol in women and men. In women (but not in men), there is a negative association between the subjective experience of sexual arousal and the body's physiologic response, as measured in the laboratory, following alcohol ingestion. Although women reported feeling more aroused sexually, their actual physiologic response was significantly depressed in a dose–response relationship with the BAC. Similarly, it is more difficult for women to reach orgasm after drinking (latency is longer and intensity is decreased) (10).

Cocaine-induced hyperprolactinemia is involved in several changes in the menstrual cycle. Amenorrhea, galactorrhea, infertility, luteal phase dysfunction, and increased levels of luteinizing hormone have been reported. Conversely, cannabis use during the luteal phase produces transient but significant decreases in plasma levels of prolactin and luteinizing hormone (8). Nicotine inhibits the release of prolactin and luteinizing hormone. This may be the basis for the observed relationship between tobacco smoking and menstrual alterations, fertility problems, and early menopause among women smokers (15).

EFFECTS ON PREGNANCY AND OFFSPRING

Alcohol use during pregnancy poses significant risks for both the pregnancy and the offspring. Fetal alcohol syndrome (FAS) is currently the third most common cause of mental retardation in the United States after Down syndrome and spina bifida, and it is the only diagnosis among the three that is completely preventable. The estimated prevalence is 1 to 3 cases per 1,000 live births, and increased risk is associated with binge drinking, increased maternal age, and increased parity. The full syndrome is characterized by prenatal and postnatal growth retardation, central nervous system abnormalities (including microcephaly), facial dysmorphisms (with maxillary hypoplasia, shortened palpebral fissures, and epicanthal folds), and cardiac abnormalities. Other fetal alcohol effects may not be recognized if the full syndrome is not manifested; they include spontaneous abortion, reduced birth weight, and behavior changes (16). Safe levels for alcohol consumption during pregnancy have not been established and probably vary with the individual. Drinking during the breastfeeding period is associated with small but measurable negative effects in the newborn. Therefore, the most common recommendation for pregnant or nursing women (or those trying to get pregnant) is abstinence from alcohol (17). If a pregnant woman has been drinking heavily, interrupting the alcohol intake as early as possible improves the birth weight and health of the offspring.

Studies of the effects of cocaine use in the perinatal period document increased rates of obstetric and postpartum complications. These include abruptio placentae, meconium staining, premature rupture of membranes, and reduced birth weight and height. Although these effects have been studied extensively, it is difficult for researchers to distinguish direct effects of cocaine from confounding factors such as concomitant substance use (particularly alcohol, opiates, and tobacco), poor nutrition, maternal age, and lack of appropriate prenatal care. In addition, long follow-up periods are needed to clarify whether these developmental effects of cocaine (both motor and cognitive) are transient or long-lasting (18).

Regular cannabis use during pregnancy has also been associated with obstetric problems (such as abruptio placentae, prematurity, and low birth weight). Long-lasting cognitive abnormalities (particularly attention deficits), impulsivity, and hyperactivity in the offspring have been reported. Being highly lipophilic, tetrahydrocannabinol (THC), the most active ingredient in cannabis, may accumulate in fat tissue for several weeks. Similar to cocaine, the effect of cannabis use during pregnancy is significantly increased by other variables related to the user's social environment (19).

A characteristic withdrawal syndrome is often seen in infants born to mothers who used opiates in the perinatal period. Seizures, sleep abnormalities, feeding difficulties, and weight loss have been reported. Treatment includes administering opiates to the newborn. Other possible approaches are giving sedatives, clonidine, and benzodiazepines. Swaddling these infants is also helpful. During pregnancy, opiate-dependent women should be stabilized with methadone or buprenorphine rather than detoxified. The dose of methadone should be adjusted to the lowest effective dose but may have to be increased later in pregnancy when the woman's body mass has increased. This approach is associated with improved outcomes (20). Treatment with buprenorphine during pregnancy has not been researched extensively, but studies show promising results, with reduced neonatal withdrawal because of the low placental transference of the drug (21).

Tobacco smoking during pregnancy is associated with many different complications. Premature delivery is related to its stimulating effects on oxytocin. Smoking increases the risk of fetal growth retardation, sudden infant death syndrome, low birth weight and height, and hypertension. Also, long-term impairment of lung function has been described even when other confounders are taken into consideration (22).

It is important to evaluate the substance use history of every pregnant woman. Even if she has discontinued use during pregnancy, a woman with an undetected substance use disorder is likely to relapse after delivery, and her disease will significantly interfere with maternal–infant bonding and the woman's ability to be an adequate mother (23).

SOCIOCULTURAL FACTORS

Sociocultural factors, particularly the intense stigma attached to alcoholic and addicted women, show a complex interaction with substance use in women. Although they can prevent girls from starting to use substances, they also have a profound impact on the self-esteem of those women with an already established pattern of substance abuse or dependence and on professionals' ability to detect their problems. Consequently, the same social standards that confer protection to women by deterring them from drinking heavily or using illicit drugs may present a barrier to an addicted woman accessing appropriate care.

Society has always condemned women's drinking more than men's. In fact, men are encouraged to drink socially. Consider, for instance, the fact that the expression "drunk as a lord" has no equivalent, "drunk as a lady." Further, women who drink or use drugs are seen as more sexually available and promiscuous. Even in cases of violence, women victims are seen as having at least "cooperated" or brought about the occurrence if they had been drinking or under the influence of other drugs. Alcohol and other substance use are known to be involved in most cases of violence directed toward women (including domestic violence) (24). Also, substance use in women is associated with victimization; in some a vicious cycle occurs in which trauma leads to the development of a substance use disorder and substance use puts the woman at increased risk of further victimization (25).

Social pressure toward beauty and a slim body influences women's substance use choices. Many substances (such as cocaine, amphetamine, and nicotine) may be used in an attempt to control body weight. A concurrent eating disorder (bulimia or anorexia nervosa) may be present as well (26).

Doctors are also more likely to prescribe tranquilizers for women than for men to treat several symptoms (depression, anxiety, sleep problems, and pain). A proportion of women who take tranquilizers, some of whom may have undiagnosed alcohol dependence, may develop dependence on the prescribed drugs (27). In part because of the guilt and shame experienced by substance-using women and in part because of the lack of proper training of health professionals in detecting these problems, many of these women are incorrectly diagnosed and are treated for concomitant physical or emotional complaints while the substance use continues.

GENETIC FACTORS

It is well known that both genetic and environmental factors contribute to the development of substance use disorders. The impact of these factors is significantly different in women than in men, however. Studies of twins have shown that for alcoholism, the genetic influence is stronger for men than for women, whereas epidemiologic studies estimate a similar heritability across genders, explaining 50% to 60% of overall variance. The sources of the genetic influence, however, may not be the same (10).

Twin studies have also shown that the role of genetics in the development of drug use and drug abuse or dependence may be less significant than in alcohol dependence. Environmental factors seem to play a more important role both in drug use initiation and progression, regardless of gender. However, the genetic influence for drug use and abuse or dependence is larger for men than for women, with estimated heritabilities of 33% for men and 11% for women. There is evidence that genetic factors may have a more significant influence in smoking initiation among women. In women, initiation of illicit drug use (e.g., cannabis and cocaine) is shaped more by environmental than genetic factors, but genetic factors have the strongest impact in the progression from experimental use to patterns of abuse and dependence (8).

PSYCHOLOGICAL FACTORS

Many of the psychological factors involved in substance use among women are the same as discussed in the chapter about substance use in adolescent girls (see Chapter 10 of this book), including the impact of self-esteem and trauma issues.

Rates of psychiatric comorbidity are significantly higher for women than for men with substance use disorders, specifically mood disorders (such as mania and depression), anxiety disorders (such as phobias and post-traumatic stress disorder), and drug use disorders, probably associated to use of tranquilizers. Women with drug use disorders are also at higher risk for dysthymia, obsessive compulsive disorder, and panic disorder, whereas men present higher rates of antisocial personality disorder, pathologic gambling, and attention deficit hyperactivity disorder.

Like adolescent girls, adult women are more likely to have primary psychiatric disorders with secondary substance dependence, whereas in men the substance use disorder is more often primary. When a diagnosis of primary psychiatric disorder (for example, major depression) and secondary substance use disorder is present, the patient should be treated intensively for both disorders. She should also be carefully monitored for recurrent depression during remission from her substance use disorder. When the depression is secondary and a substance use disorder is primary, the depression is more likely to remit spontaneously as recovery is established and less likely to recur in the absence of relapse into substance use.

Psychiatric comorbidity also has an impact on the treatment outcome for women with alcohol dependence. For instance, if both depression and alcohol disorder are treated appropriately, a lifetime diagnosis of depression is associated with a better short-term prognosis of the alcohol disorder in women as opposed to men (28).

TREATMENT

Improving the early detection of substance use problems among women is critical in enhancing treatment effectiveness. Gender-sensitive screening tools, the best example of which is the "TWEAK test," should be part of the general assessment in all primary care settings. The TWEAK (29) consists of one quantity question and four yes/no questions that can easily be incorporated into the assessment interview. A total of two or more points indicates that a drinking problem may be present (see Table 13.1).

TABLE 13.1

TWEAK Screening Tool for Alcohol Use

Do you sometimes drink alcoholic beverages? If you do, please continue this questionnaire.

T	Tolerance: How many drinks does it take before you begin to feel the first effects of the alcohol? (Record number of drinks)
W	Worry: Have close friends or relatives worried or complained about your drinking in the past year?
E	Eye-Opener: Do you sometimes take a drink in the morning when you first get up?
A	Amnesia: Are there times when you drink and afterwards you can't remember what you said or did?
K	Cut-Down: Do you sometimes feel the need to cut down on your drinking?

Scoring key: T: 2 points for 3 or more drinks; W: 2 points for a yes; E, A, K: 1 point for a yes. A total of two or more points indicates that a drinking problem may be present.

Reprinted with permission from: Russell M, Martier SS, Sokol RJ, et al. Screening for pregnancy risk-drinking. Alcohol Clin Exp Res 1994;18:1156–1161.

Treatment modalities for substance use problems involve different levels of intensity, ranging from a brief physician advice for nonpregnant women with risky patterns of ingestion to more specialized approaches for women with abuse or dependence (30). Before developing an individualized treatment plan and obtaining the agreement to it, the health professional should perform an extensive medical and psychiatric assessment of the woman. These are important given women's increased rates of substance-related medical problems, psychiatric comorbidity, and suicidal ideation. The prescription of potentially addictive medications and the supplying of large amounts of medications (particularly antidepressants) should be avoided.

The phases and goals of treatment are similar to those outlined for adolescent girls (see Chapter 10). The adult Patient Placement Criteria published by the American Society of Addiction Medicine are useful in determining the appropriate level of care (31). Detoxification, although not treatment in itself, is a critical first step. For the woman patient, detoxification needs to take in consideration that polydrug use is frequent (particularly concurrent use of prescribed medications). A pregnancy test is useful in defining treatment options in women of childbearing age. During the detoxification period, whether inpatient or outpatient, it is important to educate the patient about her disease and motivate the patient to continue treatment.

Therapeutic strategies for continuing treatment include psychoeducation, individual and group counseling, and psychosocial and pharmacologic interventions. The fact that these are performed in outpatient, inpatient, and residential settings underscores the importance of a multidisciplinary team and network referral systems. Women-only treatment settings may be especially attractive to women with trauma and violence issues. Women who are pregnant should be given priority in admission. Linking them with good obstetric care and dietary counseling will improve the outcome of the pregnancy. Both they and women with children, many of whom are single parents, have a need for child care services and for parenting training. Many of them grew up in chaotic families affected by substance abuse and have poor role models in parenting. Other family members should also be involved in treatment as much as possible, since a woman's substance use is frequently influenced by that of her partner and by the well-being of her children (32).

Mutual help groups, such as Alcoholics Anonymous and Narcotics Anonymous (and Al-Anon and Nar-Anon for family and friends), are important elements of a comprehensive approach. Women-only groups are available in many areas.

Medications such as naltrexone and acamprosate may be helpful in reducing alcohol consumption in individuals with alcohol dependence, as an adjunct to psychosocial strategies (33). Unfortunately, most pharmacologic studies fail to analyze data by gender despite the fact that women and men may respond differently (34,35). Naltrexone, an opiate antagonist that blocks the effects of opiate drugs, is useful in highly motivated opiate-dependent women involved in structured programs with a great deal of support (for example, doctors, nurses, or attorneys in an impaired professionals program), but patients with less monitoring and support often discontinue its use. For other opiate-dependent patients, opiate agonist treatment with methadone or buprenorphine is an option. These long-term treatments are particularly suitable for women who have failed at abstinence-based treatment and are motivated to abstain from all drugs of abuse; the medications block the effects of opiates but do not block the effects of alcohol, sedatives, stimulants, and other drugs. Long-term psychosocial intervention and treatment for comorbid psychiatric disorders are both essential for the success of these treatments.

Pharmacologic treatment is also effective in increasing the rate of smoking cessation. It includes various forms of nicotine replacement therapy (such as patch, gum, or spray) and bupropion (an antidepressant effective in reducing the craving for nicotine). Depressive symptomatology (either current or past) poses a unique challenge to women attempting to quit smoking. Treatment for depression may substantially improve long-term cessation rates. It is also important to time smoking cessation attempts to a woman's menstrual cycle because withdrawal symptoms may be superimposed on premenstrual symptomatology, making quitting smoking more difficult (32).

PREVENTION

Factors useful in preventing substance use disorders in adolescent girls (see Chapter 10 of this book) are also preventive for adult women. In addition, it is important to offer assistance to women who are undergoing stressful life experiences such as separation, divorce, retirement, or widowhood, or who are caring for a disabled child or older relative. Counseling that is combined with education (about the use of substances as a coping mechanism leading to dependence) will prevent later-onset substance dependence. Women in general should also be educated about the correct way to use prescription medications that may be addictive and about women's special sensitivity to alcohol. Strategies aiming to reduce harm are additional public health alternatives to lessen the burden of substance abuse among women. An example of such a strategy is a program designed to reduce illness without necessarily stopping substance use immediately, such as needle and syringe exchange and condom distribution coupled with health information delivery, testing, and referral to specific services.

In sum, this chapter reviews topics of substance abuse as they relate to women. Whereas it is clear that further research is needed in several areas, our current public policies should better reflect the accumulated knowledge of the factors influencing substance use, abuse, and dependence among women.

REFERENCES

1. Kessler R, McGonagle K, Zhao S, et al. Lifetime and 12-month prevalence of DSM-III-R psychiatric disorders in the United States. Arch Gen Psychiatry 1994;51:8–19.
2. Kandall SR. Substance and Shadow: Women and Addiction in the United States. Cambridge, MA: Harvard University Press, 1996.
3. el-Guebaly N, el-Guebaly A. Alcohol abuse in ancient Egypt: the recorded evidence. Int J Addict 1981;16:1207–1221.
4. Smith NT. A review of the published literature into cannabis withdrawal symptoms in human users. Addiction 2002;97:621–632.
5. Lingford-Hughes AR, Davies SJ, McIver S, et al. Addiction. Br Med Bull 2003;65:209–222.
6. Zilberman M, Tavares H, el-Guebaly N. Gender differences and similarities: prevalence and course of alcohol and other substance related disorders. J Addict Dis 2003;22:61–74.
7. Tavares H, Zilberman ML, Beites F, et al. Gender differences in gambling progression. J Gambl Stud 2001;17:151–159.
8. Zilberman ML, Blume SB. Women and drugs. In: Lowinson J, Ruiz P, Millman RB, et al., eds. Substance Abuse: A Comprehensive Textbook, 4th Ed. Philadelphia: Lippincott Williams & Wilkins, 2004:1064–1075.
9. Baraona E, Abittan CS, Dohmen K, et al. Gender differences in pharmacokinetics of alcohol. Alcohol Clin Exp Res 2001;25:502–507.
10. Blume SB, Zilberman ML. Women: Clinical aspects. In: Lowinson J, Ruiz P, Millman RB, et al., eds. Substance Abuse: A Comprehensive Textbook, 4th Ed. Philadelphia: Lippincott Williams & Wilkins, 2004:1049–1064.

11. Greenfield SF, O'Leary G. Gender differences in substance use disorders. In: Lewis-Hall F, Williams TS, Panetta JA, et al., eds. Psychiatric Illness in Women: Emerging Treatments and Research Washington, DC: American Psychiatric Publishing, 2002:467–533.

12. Zeman MV, Hiraki L, Sellers EM. Gender differences in tobacco smoking: higher relative exposure to smoke than nicotine in women. J Womens Health Gend Based Med 2002;11:147–153.

13. National Institute on Alcoholism and Alcohol Abuse (NIAAA). 10th Special Report to the U.S. Congress on Alcohol and Health. Highlights from Current Research. June 2000.

14. Centers for Disease Control and Prevention. Recent trends in mortality rates for four major cancers, by sex and race/ethnicity—United States, 1990–1998. JAMA 2002;287:1391–1392.

15. Sharpe RM, Franks S. Environment, lifestyle and infertility: an inter-generational issue. Nat Cell Biol 2002;4(Suppl):33–40.

16. O'Leary C. Fetal alcohol syndrome: diagnosis, epidemiology, and developmental outcomes. J Paediatr Child Health 2004;40:2–7.

17. Koren G, Nulman I, Chudley AE, et al. Fetal alcohol spectrum disorder. CMAJ 2003;169: 1181–1185.

18. Frank DA, Augustyn M, Knight WG, et al. Growth, development, and behavior in early childhood following prenatal cocaine exposure: a systematic review. JAMA 2001;285:1613–1625.

19. Fergusson DM, Horwood LJ, Northstone K. ALSPAC Study Team. Avon Longitudinal Study of Pregnancy and Childhood. Maternal use of cannabis and pregnancy outcome. BJOG 2002;109: 21–27.

20. Kandall SR, Doberczak TM, Jantunen M, et al. The methadone-maintained pregnancy. Clin Perinatol 1999;26:173–183.

21. Nanovskaya T, Deshmukh S, Brooks M, et al. Transplacental transfer and metabolism of buprenorphine. J Pharmacol Exp Ther 2002;300:26–33.

22. Li YF, Gilliland FD, Berhane K, et al. Effects of in utero and environmental tobacco smoke exposure on lung function in boys and girls with and without asthma. Am J Respir Crit Care Med 2000;162:2097–2104.

23. Center for Substance Abuse Treatment (CSAT). Pregnant, substance-using women: treatment improvement protocol (TIP) series 2. Rockville, MD: U.S. Department of Health and Human Services Publication no (SMA) 95-3056, 1993. Available at: http://hstat.nlm.nih.gov.

24. Sharps PW, Campbell J, Campbell D, et al. The role of alcohol use in intimate partner femicide. Am J Addict 2001;10:122–135.

25. Brady KT, Dansky BS. Effects of victimization and posttraumatic stress disorder on substance use disorders in women. In: Lewis-Hall F, Williams TS, Panetta JA, et al., eds. Psychiatric Illness in Women: Emerging Treatments and Research. Washington, DC: American Psychiatric Publishing, 2002:449–466.

26. Cochrane C, Malcolm R, Brewerton T. The role of weight control as a motivation for cocaine abuse. Addict Behav 1998;23:201–207.

27. Simon GE, VonKorff M, Barlow W, et al. Predictors of chronic benzodiazepine use in a health maintenance organization sample. J Clin Epidemiol 1996;49:1067–1073.

28. Zilberman ML, Tavares H, Blume SB, et al. Substance use disorders: sex differences in psychiatric comorbidities. Can J Psychiatry 2003;48:5–15.

29. Russell M, Martier SS, Sokol RJ, et al. Screening for pregnancy risk-drinking. Alcohol Clin Exp Res 1994;18:1156–1161.

30. Beich A, Thorsen T, Rollnick S. Screening in brief intervention trials targeting excessive drinkers in general practice: systematic review and meta-analysis. Br Med J 2003;327:536–542.

31. American Society of Addiction Medicine. ASAM Patient Placement Criteria for the Treatment of Substance-Related Disorders, 2nd Ed.-Revised. Chevy Chase, MD, 2001.

32. Zilberman ML, Tavares H, Blume S, et al. Towards best practices in the treatment of women with addictive disorders. J Addict Disord Their Treatment 2002;1:39–46.

33. Kranzler HR, Van Kirk J. Efficacy of naltrexone and acamprosate for alcoholism treatment: a meta-analysis. Alcohol Clin Exp Res 2001;25:1335–1341.

34. Naranjo CA, Knoke DM, Bremner KE. Variations in response to citalopram in men and women with alcohol dependence. J Psychiatry Neurosci 2000;25:269–275.

35. Perkins KA. Smoking cessation in women. Special considerations. CNS Drugs 2001;15:391–411.

CHAPTER 14

Psychotic Disorders in Women

Jayashri Kulkarni

HISTORY OF PSYCHOSIS: A FEMALE PERSPECTIVE

Psychiatric history reflects the thoughts and views of philosophers, clerics, and clinicians, predominantly male. The dominant paradigm is male. In order to understand current concepts regarding women and psychosis, it is important to learn about the history of psychiatry from a female perspective. The search for historical contributions from early female thinkers yields little. Interestingly, the famous female patron saint of the mad, St. Dympna, gained her status by mishap. St. Dympna was a seventh-century martyr who fled from Ireland to Belgium to escape the incestuous desire of her father. He caught her and struck off her head in his fury at her rejection. This was observed by several "lunatics," who were immediately shocked into sanity. She then earned the title of "protectress of the mad," and favorable changes in psychosis were attributed to her intercession. This myth contains several messages about the associations between women and madness. Unlike many male saints, St. Dympna was a victim and not a powerful person in her own right. The accidental but beneficial outcome for the mad patients conferred martyr status on St. Dympna but enshrined her role as passive. To this day, many inpatient units around the world are called St. Dympna's Ward.

The twelfth century and other middle ages saw the devastating persecution of women, in particular women with mental illness, through the notorious witch hunts. For women, the consequence of psychotic symptoms was in many instances a painful death. A famous religious visionary in the twelfth century was Hildegard of Bingen. She wrote extensively about gender differences, sexuality, and medicine with a particular regard for women suffering from psychotic disorders. Hildegard claimed her revolutionary treatments for psychosis were transmitted to her in "dreams" and were in fact the ideas of the current pope. In this way she cleverly avoided persecution for witchery, which would have been her fate had she not adopted a passive role. Hildegard of Bingen's theories about mental illness in women actually fit our current thinking in that she advocated a biopsychosocial approach to the etiology and treatment of psychosis.

During the midseventeenth century, rising unemployment and economic crises throughout Europe led to the building of institutions for the poor, the criminal, the alcoholic, and the mad. During this "classical age," madness was seen as a type of moral corruption. Toward the end of the eighteenth century, particularly in France, industry was growing and workers were needed. This led to the release of psychiatric inmates who were capable of working, in particular large numbers of women deemed less severely mad than their male counterparts. Foucault claims that, at this time, when disease spread through French towns, the mad were blamed for the various epidemics and hence doctors became involved with the insane. Initially, doctors acted as moral guardians for the mad, rather than as physicians, but a medical interest in psychosis developed over time. The nineteenth century saw the proliferation of scientific theories about psychosis, coincident with the weakening power of the church and the rising importance of science. In the Victorian era, English psychiatrists theorized that female insanity was largely due to the woman overstepping the boundaries of femininity as determined by Victorian society. By the 1850s, the population of public asylums increased dramatically, with proportionally larger numbers of women than men. The Victorians associated female sexuality, deviancy, and madness. Women who were promiscuous, or who bore an illegitimate child, or those who were sexually assaulted and traumatized as a result, were seen as "mad" because they posed a threat to the view of women as passive and sexually innocent. On frequent occasions, such women were hidden away in asylums. The number of women assumed to be suffering from mental illness in the Victorian era was only partly reflected in the number restrained in asylums, since many were confined to attics or other hiding places. Literary works of the Victorian era, such as Florence Nightingale's *Cassandra,* were to some extent semi-autobiographical accounts, and some portrayed the female perspective about the plight of the mad woman. The madness of Bertha, one of the main characters in "Jane Eyre," was linked to her sexuality, and her worst episodes were related to her menstrual cycle. In the novel, Bertha was managed by confinement to a windowless attic and was treated as a brutish animal. This novel had a profound effect on Victorian readers, including psychiatrists, who subsequently advocated asylum treatment for women in preference to isolation at home.

Darwin's theories of biologic sex differences gave scientific confirmation to the Victorian ideals of femininity. In *The Descent of Man*, Darwin described differences in mental powers of the two sexes. He claimed that, through natural selection, man had become superior to woman in intellect, courage, and inventive genius. Henry Maudsley, a notable Victorian era psychiatrist and the editor of the journal *Mental Science,* was profoundly influenced by Darwin's theories. Maudsley's view was that higher education of women directly contributed to their mental illness.

During the latter part of the nineteenth century, the feminist movement gathered momentum, with women campaigning for access to universities, the professions, and the vote. Many of these women were labeled mentally disturbed, and the diagnosis of hysteria rose in prominence. A strong association was made between rebelliousness and nervous disorders, and there are documented cases of radical women being committed to asylums with symptoms of "overeducation and rebelliousness." One such case was that of Edith Lancaster, described as an honors student at London University working for the Social Democratic Federation in 1895, who was committed to a private London asylum by her father after she began to live with a young railway clerk. The doctor involved explained that her opposition to conventional matrimony and her overeducation were the causes of her insanity. The diagnosis of hysteria, known as the "daughter's disease" was also understood as a mode of expression for women deprived of social and intellectual outlets.

Freud attributed hysterical symptoms to sexual conflicts. Through Freud's work, the female patient's voice became audible. Following World War I, psychiatric attention turned again toward the psychotic disorders—grouped under the heading of "dementia praecox" by Kraepelin in 1896. Kraepelin believed that psychological dysfunction, "a loss of inner unity of intellect, emotion and volition," was secondary to organic brain changes. Kraepelin's theory was modified by Eugene Bleuler, who suggested the term "schizophrenia" in 1908. Bleuler believed the primary problem was an organic loosening of associations, which was the substrate for subsequent psychological mechanisms resulting in delusions and hallucinations. During the 1920s and 1930s, the concept of schizophrenia became much looser and acquired a strong social component that included adolescent turmoil, cultural maladjustment, and political deviation. In this era, the woman with schizophrenia became a central cultural figure, a symbol of linguistic, religious, and sexual breakdown. Yeats's poem "Crazy Jane" in the 1930s and other literature such as "The Mad Woman of Chaillot" in 1945 depicted psychotic women as symbols of repression by society. Women were overrepresented in the number of asylum inpatients in the 1940s and received the majority of organic treatments (insulin and shock therapies). Since 1941, most of the 15,000 leucotomies and lobotomies performed have been on women.

By the 1960s, the feminist movement had grown and found favor with antipsychiatry groups (e.g., R. D. Laing). By the early 1970s, feminists became disenchanted with the antipsychiatry movement, and the early 80s saw the beginning of deinstitutionalization, a worldwide phenomenon of downsizing mental hospitals. The deinstitutionalization process has meant that many psychiatric patients in previous long-stay hospitals are now treated in general hospital units with an emphasis on community-based treatment. This has no doubt improved the quality of life of a significant proportion of patients with mental illness but has raised another issue for women in general—the burden of care. Sedgwick described women as being tied to "traditional servicing roles for their disabled kinfolk . . . the reinforcing of an archaic sexual division of labour"(1). The 1990s and onward have seen the further growth of neuroscience technologies. This has, in turn, impacted on psychiatric research and, in particular, on schizophrenia research. Newer treatments have been developed, and there is greater understanding of brain impairment in psychosis. The consideration of differences between the sexes in schizophrenia has also received new attention. Sex differences in brain development, organization, and, eventually, degeneration are relevant to understanding sex differences in schizophrenia. Understanding sex differences in the experience of schizophrenia becomes increasingly important as the efficacy of newer treatments is being assessed.

EPIDEMIOLOGY OF FEMALE SCHIZOPHRENIA

It is almost universally accepted that schizophrenia first manifests at a later mean age in females than males. Most of the epidemiologic findings come from the Danish Case Register and the Central Institute of Mental Health, Mannheim, Germany (2–4). The mean age of onset of schizophrenia in women is now established as being between 5 and 10 years later than in men. Another well-documented sex difference is in the course and outcome of schizophrenia. Many studies report that women have a more benign course of illness than men (5). Overall, women show fewer negative symptoms, better social adaptation, and treatment response at relatively lower dosages of antipsychotic drug (6). However, social stressors such as homelessness, poverty, and victimization can create a very poor quality of life for women with psychotic illness (7).

THEORIES OF ETIOLOGY: A SEX-BASED APPROACH

NEURODEVELOPMENTAL THEORIES

Normal sexual dimorphisms in brain structures have been demonstrated in many animals, including humans (8). The male preoptic nucleus is larger than the female's, with more cells and larger cells. There is a higher density of neurons in the orbital area of females than in males and the planum temporale shows more right/left shape asymmetry in males.

The question of whether structural cerebral changes are pathognomonic of schizophrenia and inevitably progressive remains controversial. Many studies suggest that the extent of these structural changes differs widely depending on the imaging methods employed, individual characteristics, and the size of the sample studied. A variety of cerebral structures have been investigated, including the hippocampal formation, the cerebellum, and the basal ganglia. A majority of studies have focused on the frontal and temporal lobes. Some find no significant prefrontal cortex gray matter, white matter, or total volume changes in persons with schizophrenia compared to controls, but Bachmann et al. found a decrease of frontal lobe volume in people with first-episode schizophrenia (9). In other work, such as that by Pantelis et al., significant changes relative to controls have been found in the hippocampal volume of prepsychotic persons (10). An important variable that is often overlooked in structural cerebral imaging studies is the need to compare male patients with male controls and female patients with female controls.

The volume of the caudate nucleus increases over time in first-episode patients who receive treatment with conventional antipsychotic medication. This effect is dose dependent and associated with younger age at the beginning of the illness (11). Moreover, a direct effect of conventional antipsychotics on the D_2 dopamine receptor system, with receptor up-regulation has also been described in functional imaging studies (12). Treatment with atypical antipsychotics does not cause volume increases in the caudate (13).

The main conclusion is that there is no convincing evidence that schizophrenia in either sex is accompanied by a progressive loss of global cerebral tissue. Regional changes of frontal and temporal lobe volumes may occur in subgroups of patients and may be related to certain stages of the disease (14).

GENETICS OF SCHIZOPHRENIA AND RELATED DISORDERS

The clinical phenotype of schizophrenia is a highly complex entity with multiple neurochemical, physiologic, and psychological features. Different brain pathways may be under the influence of different susceptibility genes or environmental factors. The investigation of the expression of thousands of genes in mRNA tissue has recently become feasible (15). Illness can be caused by specific sequence anomalies in the DNA (genetics) or by heritable changes in gene expression occurring without necessarily altering DNA sequence (epigenetics) (16). The main known epigenetic mechanisms are inactivation of genes via methylation or acetylation. It has been suggested that schizophrenia has an epigenetic basis (17). The systematic search for vulnerability genes offers strategies for disease–gene identification in schizophrenia.

HORMONAL ASPECTS OF THE ETIOLOGY OF SCHIZOPHRENIA

By and large, it is agreed that schizophrenia is a postpubertal disorder in both males and females. Thus, it is important to understand the effect of the HPG axis hormones, particularly estrogen and testosterone, on neurotransmitter systems involved in schizophrenia. In neonatal and adult rats, Behrens et al. studied the effects of estradiol and testosterone on cataplexy induced by the dopamine antagonist, haloperidol (18). Ferretti et al. found that estrogen administration had little effect on dopamine D_1 receptors but that D_2 receptor density fell in response to low-dose estradiol (19). Fink and colleagues have also shown that estrogen induces a significant increase in 5-HT$_2$A receptors and the serotonin transporter (SERT) in regions in the rat forebrain that mediate mental state, mood, cognition, memory, emotion, and neuroendocrine control (20). Estrogen may protect against psychotic symptoms by way of its actions on the 5-HT$_2$A receptor, SERT, and the D_2 receptor.

SCHIZOPHRENIA IN WOMEN: A LIFE-CYLE APPROACH

EARLY PSYCHOSIS IN WOMEN: POSTPUBERTY TO LATE ADOLESCENCE

During class, in the quiet of the work period, I could hear the street noises . . . each detached, immovable, separated from its source, without meaning. Around me, the other children . . . were robots or puppets, moved by an invisible mechanism. On the platform, the teacher, too, talking, gesticulating, rising to write on the blackboard, was a grotesque jack-in-the-box. . . . An awful terror bound me; I wanted to scream. (21)

This is an excerpt from an autobiography of a girl with schizophrenia during what we would now call the early psychosis phase.

The peak period of onset for men with schizophrenia is 18 to 25 years of age and, for women, 25 to midthirties (3). The size of the age difference depends on the strictness of the criteria for defining the case (2). In early adolescence, the male:female onset ratio is generally 2:1 (22). Approximately 3% to 10% of women have an age of onset greater than 45 years (rare for males) (22). Using an admixture analysis technique, Castle et al. re-analyzed the Camberwell data set; their main findings were that the early-onset peaks showed a marked excess of males, the middle-onset peak was female preponderant, and the very-late-onset peak was exclusively female (22). Although the mean is later age of onset of psychosis in women, this does not exclude first-time presentation of psychosis in adolescent girls. Special care must be taken not to overlook the illness unexpectedly presenting for the first time in very young women.

In considering differences between the sexes at first presentation of psychosis, it has been shown that males are more likely than females to show cognitive deficits. (See Addington and Schultze-Lutter, Chapter 9 of this book.) Females in the general population are more likely than males to show depression, and this sex difference becomes more pronounced in the pre-adolescent and adolescent period. Affective symptoms, particularly depression, are associated with a better prognosis for schizophrenia and psychotic disorders in general (23). This link is consistent with the findings of a more favorable prognosis for women with schizophrenia (24). At the same time, it appears that depressive symptoms in schizophrenia are at least partially genetically determined. Subotnik found that depressive symptoms in patients experiencing first-episode schizophrenia were predicted by the rate of affective disorder in biologic relatives (25). For a number of different reasons, the premorbid functioning of young women has been shown to be superior to that of young men in domains of social functioning and cognitive functioning and academic and work achievement (26).

The early detection of schizophrenia in women poses specific problems for the clinician. The early presentations by women with psychosis can be commonly misdiagnosed as depression, and, often, women are treated with antidepressant medications before psychosis symptoms are recognized. Young women who are inappropriately treated at the start of illness may not have as good an outcome from the treatment. In recent years, evidence has increasingly emerged that delay in starting treatment with antipsychotic drugs is associated with a poorer outcome in a large number of domains (27). Some of the factors that contribute to the difficulties in the early diagnosis of schizophrenia or psychosis in female patients include the relative lack of classical positive symptoms, the expectation of a later age of onset, the prominence of affective symptoms, sheltering by protective families, infrequent exposure to routine screening (as in military settings), and, often, the clinician's lack of appreciation of atypical presentations (28). Assessment strategies outlined by Power and McGorry for all first-episode psychosis patients include taking a careful history, assessing the patient's risk, and performing a physical assessment (29).

BIOLOGIC TREATMENTS AND PSYCHOSOCIAL ISSUES

With the advent of the newer or atypical antipsychotic drugs, the number of significant side effects has lessened, particularly female-specific endocrine side effects. However, there are some special dose and adverse event profiles that need to be considered. Currently, many new drug trials do not include equal numbers of females because of researchers' realistic concerns about the potential teratogenicity of a new drug. As a result, once a new antipsychotic medication has been approved, it could be prescribed in wrong dosages for women. In addition, the concomitant use of sex steroids for contraception is often overlooked in preclinical drug trials. Estrogen and progesterone affect drug kinetics as well as affecting multiple domains of mental function (30). Several studies now suggest that young women require lower dosages of antipsychotic medication than do men and older women (31). In a study of first-episode patients, 87% of the women but only 55% of men achieved remission of symptoms with a standard dosage of fluphenazine hydrochloride (32). The sex difference in response to atypical antipsychotics is yet to be clarified. For both men and women, evidence has shown superior efficacy of clozapine, risperidone, and olanzapine over the older drugs, particularly for negative symptoms but also for positive symptoms, as well as a lower risk of extrapyramidal side effects (33). The new antipsychotic medications are now considered first-line therapy in all phases of schizophrenia for both men and women.

The safety of the new antipsychotics in early pregnancy is still unknown. Side effect profiles of the novel antipsychotics may include hyperprolactinemia, weight gain, and an increased propensity for diabetes. Many women treated with antipsychotic drugs experience sexual problems. The young adolescent female may be especially reluctant to reveal sexual difficulties. Concerns about fertility are widespread among women taking antipsychotic medications, particularly the younger female patients, and this concern may also be difficult to report. Since a young woman may well be prescribed antipsychotic medication for a considerable length of time, it is vital that the choice of medication be as free of side effects as possible. Every effort is required to prescribe the correct type of drug at the correct dosage in order to ensure the best outcomes, including remission of symptoms and promotion of general health.

Psychosocial issues should be addressed in the treatment of young women with first or early episodes of psychosis by means of discussions about contraception, relationship counseling, and assessment of the woman's safety (e.g., the risk of domestic violence, sexual harassment, assault, or rape). Safety and privacy issues in the treatment setting and also in the usual social milieu of the patient need to be addressed. Ongoing education or work rehabilitation as well as financial counseling are important foci of therapy. Good general medical health care is also vital, including routine Pap smears, mammograms, and blood pressure checks.

The location of optimal treatment is an important consideration. In many countries today, the preferred location for treatment is the patient's own home, with continued follow-up from treatment teams (34). If an inpatient stay is necessary due to the severity of the patient's illness or the lack of suitable caregivers, it is important to minimize potential trauma by avoiding forced treatments or seclusion. Such interventions often create secondary morbidity such as post-traumatic stress disorder or depression. Clearly, educating both the patient and family about the illness in its early stages is critical.

Substance abuse is one of the most common associated problems in first-episode psychosis and, although male patients appear to be more at risk, substance use is also common in females (35) Self-medication to cope with distressing psychotic symptoms is one explanation for the substance use, but the onset of psychosis itself may be precipitated by substance misuse. One motivation for on-going substance use is peer group pressure, a potent factor for the young woman suffering from early psychosis. A detailed examination of the reasons for substance misuse and the type of substance involved needs to be addressed in order to optimize a woman's recovery. Activities of leisure and vocational rehabilitation are extremely important factors in the maintenance of recovery and the prevention of deterioration (27). Unfortunately, gender-specific rehabilitation is rare, but every attempt must be made by the clinician to understand the young woman's particular needs in rehabilitation compared to those of her male counterpart.

POSTPARTUM PSYCHOSIS AND ISSUES FOR MOTHERS WITH SCHIZOPHRENIA

Motherhood is a highly valued role in most human societies, and women have a basic right to bear children and parent them. However, for some women, motherhood results in a first episode of psychosis during the postpartum period; for others who already have serious mental illness, motherhood can exacerbate the illness though pregnancy can improve symptoms (36). Bearing children raises many dilemmas that are exacerbated in the case of women with serious mental illness.

POSTPARTUM PSYCHOSIS

The relationship between postpartum psychosis and schizophrenia is still somewhat complex.

> I couldn't hold my baby girl, the voices told me to strangle her . . . they then gave me mind draining drugs that took away the voices, but sucked out my soul. I was a walking corpse. . . . How could I be normal with my baby, when that social worker was watching me, checking if I was a good mother? Could you be normal knowing she could take away your baby? (37)

Postpartum psychosis is the most severe postpartum mood disorder. It is relatively rare and reported to occur in only one or two of every 1,000 women (38). The main feature of the psychotic episode is that it appears within a few days after birth or, at most, within three weeks. The majority of postpartum psychoses fall into the category of major depression with psychotic features or bipolar disorder. Brief reactive psychoses and schizophrenia also occur but are less common. Postpartum psychosis symptoms include hallucinations, altered reality, delusions, rapid mood swings, insomnia, and, often, abnormal thoughts about harming the newborn child. Postpartum psychosis is associated with a 4% rate of infanticide and 5% rate of suicide (39). The outcome for women suffering postpartum psychosis varies, but most researchers agree that approximately 65% of women subsequently experience psychotic episodes not related to further pregnancies and deliveries (40). Benvenuti et al. have reported that up to two thirds of women with one episode of postpartum psychosis experience symptom relapse in subsequent pregnancies (41).

MOTHERS WITH SCHIZOPHRENIA

In a recent survey of women with schizophrenia undertaken by Hearle et al., 59% of the women (i.e., 65 of 110 women surveyed) were mothers (42). The 110 women had had a total of 257 pregnancies, resulting in 198 live births. A total of 134 of the pregnancies (52%) had been unplanned. Of the unplanned pregnancies, 25% had ended in termination. None of the planned pregnancies had been terminated. Sixteen percent of the mothers reported that at least one of their psychiatric admissions had occurred within six months of the birth of one of their children. This study highlights the many special issues concerning reproduction for women with schizophrenia. It is an understudied area with few clinical guidelines. It has been suggested that the rate of pregnancy among women with schizophrenia has increased since deinstitutionalization (43). Fertility rates may have improved with the advent of the newer antipsychotic medications that do not impact on the hypothalamic gonadal axis in the same way as some of the older drugs did.

As a consequence, it becomes increasingly important to consider the special needs of women with schizophrenia: preparing for pregnancy, antenatal care, the postpartum period, and motherhood. Given that good antenatal care is an important primary preventive approach to most neurodevelopmental illnesses, it is especially important for the pregnant woman with schizophrenia to receive optimal antenatal care. Fetuses genetically predisposed to schizophrenia have a special vulnerability to antenatal or perinatal brain damage (44). Women with schizophrenia require good advice about nutrition, stopping smoking, and receiving regular medical checkups throughout the pregnancy. It has been shown that women with schizophrenia tend to have poor attendance records at antenatal visits (45). Good follow-up for pregnant women with schizophrenia remains a special need.

Mental health clinicians lack good-quality data on the use of antipsychotic medications in pregnant women. In particular, data on the use and outcomes for women who have been treated with novel antipsychotic medications are unclear, and the concerned clinician may often cease treating a woman with an effective antipsychotic because of fear of teratogenicity. Because of this, and despite the putatively positive effects of estrogens during pregnancy, the patient may be at risk of relapse during pregnancy and, in particular, during the postpartum period. There is an urgent need for guidelines for preconception counseling and for management and care during pregnancy and lactation. Contraceptive issues need to be addressed with women with schizophrenia who seek assistance in avoiding unwanted pregnancies. Those who do become pregnant require optimal support to ensure safe delivery of a healthy child and optimal mental health in the patient herself (46).

Parenting Assistance for Mothers with Schizophrenia

In the study conducted by Hearle et al., questions about child care were asked of parents with severe mental illness (42). Of the sample of 97 parents, 87% said they relied on relatives for assistance; 24% relied on friends. What emerged was that a very small percentage received assistance or interventions specifically related to child care from government and nongovernment agencies. While it is clear that the needs of mothers with schizophrenia had much in common with those of mothers in general, there were specific areas that required special attention.

One such area was an inability of mothers with schizophrenia to care for their children when they were acutely unwell. Other areas included the difficulty of explaining mental illness to children, respite care, and supportive practical in-home care (47). Further special issues for mothers with schizophrenia include the need for optimizing the woman's quality of life in terms of emotive and cognitive functioning so that she is able to carry out the demands of the parenting role—a role that can be both stressful and satisfying. A common complaint expressed by mothers with schizophrenia is that the antipsychotic medications they are prescribed cause emotional numbing, decreasing their ability to bond with their children. Clinicians need to ensure that mothers with schizophrenia are able to experience the normal range of emotions involved with a parenting role.

Child safety issues need to be considered but balanced against the stigma and stresses that the mothers face in their often unexpressed but deeply felt fears about losing custody of their children. Clinicians have the difficult task of trying, on one hand, to ensure the safety of the child or children while, on the other hand, developing a therapeutic relationship with the mother. These mothers may refuse help from a mental health worker, fearing the child will be taken away. Clinicians need to be sensitive to these complex conflicts in managing a mother with schizophrenia. A study conducted by McGrath et al. found that, for the mentally ill, parenthood can be associated with grief, loss, and frustration (48). Only 17% of offspring in the study resided with their index parents, and many of the parents expressed a desire for more contact with their children. Ten percent of the parents reported past interventions related to the care of the child that were implemented against their will, and nearly one third of the parents said they were reluctant to seek help with child care because they feared that their children would be removed from them. It is very clear that service providers need to address these factors because they impede access to optimal child care. Consumer involvement in service development may assist in building trust between parents and service providers.

PSYCHOTIC ILLNESS AT PERIMENOPAUSE AND MENOPAUSE

> *"No spring, nor summer beauty hath such grace,*
> *As I have seen in one autumnal face."*
>
> —John Donne

Healthy women seem to become generally more action-oriented, confident, and assertive in middle age, a constellation of characteristics termed "peaceful potency" by Germaine Greer (49). As the average life expectancy in the Western world increases, more women will spend longer in the perimenopausal and postmenopausal period. However, for women with established psychosis or predisposing vulnerabilities, the autumn years are not kind.

There is international consensus that a small peak of incidence of schizophrenia in women occurs after menopause (2). To explain this, researchers such as Häfner and Seeman suggested that estrogen protects women against schizophrenia (50, 51). These two researchers used clinical data and animal studies to support their hypothesis. With women who have an ongoing established illness, there is consistent evidence of exacerbation during the perimenopausal time (52). First-episode late-onset schizophrenia is unquestionably more common in women than in men, a finding that has frequently been replicated (53). Although the late onset has not been definitely linked to estrogen withdrawal, there is a striking correlation between waning estrogen levels in the fourth decade and the exacerbation of existing illness or the presentation of new illness.

As women with schizophrenia approach menopause, existing medical conditions may be exacerbated, sometimes because of lengthy treatment with antipsychotic drugs. Hence, it is vital to assess women with schizophrenia carefully as they enter menopause and consider the use of hormone therapy or estrogen treatment for perimenopausal physical symptoms as well as mental state. The current debate about the use of hormone replacement therapy has focused primarily on its use to alleviate troubling symptoms of perimenopause or to help prevent osteoporosis. However, as women with schizophrenia approach menopause, there seems to be an exacerbation of their particular psychotic symptomatology, including an increase in cognitive decline. During the perimenopause, short-term estrogen treatment may have benefits for the woman with schizophrenia. A careful medical assessment is needed to weigh the potential improvements in mental state against the woman's increased risk of breast, ovarian, or uterine cancers due to estrogen therapy. Ongoing medical follow-up is vital for all women but particularly for women with schizophrenia who are receiving hormone therapy. The symptoms of the perimenopause include hot flashes, reduced libido, changes in vaginal lubrication, anorgasmia, and deterioration in working memory and visual memory. Such symptoms along with menstrual irregularities and deterioration in mental state with exacerbation of hallucinations, delusions, and depressed mood may impair the woman's quality of life significantly. Women with schizophrenia often suffer iatrogenic early menopause due to a lifetime of taking antipsychotic medications. The older class of antipsychotic medications led to hyperprolactinemia with secondary estrogen deficiency. Smoking, a sedentary lifestyle, poor nutrition, and obesity have further complicated the health of women with long-standing schizophrenia.

In recent years, researchers and clinicians have become increasingly aware of the importance of cognitive deficits in the poor outcomes for people with schizophrenia. For women with schizophrenia entering the perimenopause, a decline in cognition is a very serious deficit and one that significantly impairs the woman's quality of life. Cognition is a general term that describes human information processing. It includes higher intellect, psychomotor skills, pattern recognition, learning, memory, and abstract reasoning as well as language. In women with schizophrenia in midlife and later life, changes to working memory, long-term memory, and short-term memory are incapacitating in both social and work settings. Antipsychotic medications cannot completely or reliably reverse cognitive disturbances in schizophrenia. Women with schizophrenia often have widespread gaps in cognitive functioning, but the deficits can be highly variable and individual. Many women with schizophrenia in midlife describe serious problems arising from the loss of working memory.

In women who are experiencing severe cognitive decline, perimenopausal physical symptoms, or deterioration in mental state with either an exacerbation of psychosis or an increase in affective symptoms, estrogen therapy may produce significant improvement in mental health and general health domains. We have demonstrated significant improvement for women with schizophrenia with the addition of 100 mcg of transdermal estradiol to standard antipsychotic drug treatment (54). In our more recent work, we are also showing improvements in global cognition with the addition of 100 mcg of transdermal estradiol (55).

When treating any woman with schizophrenia, it is important to carefully consider estrogens and the gonadal axis, particularly during perimenopause and menopause. To date, mental health professionals have been rather remiss in their history taking of menstrual irregularities, amenorrhea, galactorrhea, and symptoms of menopause in women with schizophrenia, often to the woman's detriment. Clearly, there are both general health issues and mental health issues for the woman experiencing perimenopause and menopause. The possibility of brain-specific hormonal manipulation to assist in improving the patient's mental state is an exciting proposition and the advent of selective estrogen receptor modulators is a new and welcome development.

CONCLUSION

Schizophrenia is a multifaceted and devastating illness that can substantially diminish a person's quality of life. In past centuries, the treatment of women suffering from schizophrenia and related psychotic illnesses was marked by tragic episodes from which we need to learn and move forward to gender-sensitive practices. The use of biologic treatments in women with schizophrenia needs to rest on an underpinning of good biologic research in female patients. New directions such as brain-specific hormonal manipulation may be welcomed by a significant proportion of women who suffer from severe psychotic illness. Interventions for women with schizophrenia need to address psychosocial aspects as well as biologic issues in a meaningful manner. Service provision in schizophrenia must take into account the special needs of women such as privacy, safety, and accessibility to outreach care, especially for mothers with dependent children. There are gaps in service provision, particularly in the care of pregnant women with schizophrenia and in the provision of adequate child care and support for mothers with schizophrenia.

Overall, the best way to obtain good results in the treatment of anyone with severe mental illness is to tailor the treatment to the individual. The sex of a person is a very significant individual variable that influences outcome.

REFERENCES

1. Sedgwick T. Psychopolitics. London: Pluto, 1982:241.
2. Castle DJ, Wessely S, Murray RM. Sex and schizophrenia: effects of diagnostic stringency, and associations with premorbid variables. Br J Psychiatry 1993;162:658–664.
3. Häfner H, Riecher A, Maurer K, et al. How does gender influence age at first hospitalization for schizophrenia? A transnational case register study. Psychol Med 1989;19:903–918.
4. Angermeyer MC, Kuhn L, Goldstein JM. Gender and the course of schizophrenia: differences in treated outcomes. Schizophr Bull 1990;16:293–307.
5. Goldstein JM, Santangelo SL, Simpson JC, et al. The role of gender in identifying subtypes of schizophrenia: a latent class analytic approach. Schizophr Bull 1990;16:263–275.
6. Childers SE, Harding CM. Gender, premorbid social functioning and long-term outcome in DSM III schizophrenia. Schizophr Bull 1990;16:309–318.
7. Milburn N, D'Ercole A. Homeless women. Moving towards a comprehensive model. Am Psychol 1991;46:1161–1169.
8. Swaab DF, Fliers E. A sexually dimorphic nucleus in the human brain. Science 1985;228:1112–1115.
9. Bachmann S, Bottmer C, Pantel J, et al. MRI-morphometric changes in first episode schizophrenic patients at 14 months follow-up. Schizophr Res 2004;67:301–303.
10. Pantelis C, Velakoulis D, Suckling J, et al. Left medial temporal volume reduction occurs during the transition from high risk to first episode psychosis. Schizophr Res 2000;41:35.
11. Chakos MH, Lieberman JA, Bilder RM, et al. Increase in caudate nuclei volumes of first episode schizophrenic patients taking antipsychotic drugs. Am J Psychiatry 1994;151:1430–1436.

12. Schröder J, Silvestri S, Bubeck B, et al. D_2 dopamine receptor up-regulation, treatment response, neurological soft signs and extrapyramidal side effects in schizophrenia: a follow up study with ^{123}I-iodobenzamide single photon emission computed tomography in the drug naïve state and after neuroleptic treatment. Biol Psychiatry 1998;43:660–665.
13. Lang DJ, Kopala LC, Vandorpe RA, et al. An MRI study of basal ganglia volumes in first-episode schizophrenia patients treated with risperidone. Am J Psychiatry 2001;158:625–631.
14. Schröder J, Bottmer C, Pantel J. Are structural cerebral changes progressive in schizophrenia? In: Häfner H, ed. Risk and Protective Factors in Schizophrenia. Darmstadt, Germany: Springer, Steinkopff, 2002:83–98.
15. Watson SJ, Akil H. Gene chips and arrays revealed: a primer on their power and their uses. Biol Psychiatry 1999;45:533–543.
16. Wolffe AP, Matzke MA. Epigenetics: regulation through repression. Science 1999;286(5439): 481–486.
17. Maier W, Rietschel M, Linz M, et al. Genetics of schizophrenia and related disorders In: Häfner H, ed. Risk and Protective Factors in Schizophrenia. Darmstadt, Germany: Springer, Steinkopff, 2002:9–28.
18. Behrens S, Häfner H, DeVry J, et al. Estradiol attenuates dopamine-mediated behaviour in rats: implications for sex differences in schizophrenia. Schizophr Res 1992;6:114.
19. Ferretti C, Blengio M, Vigna I, et al. Effects of estradiol on the ontogenesis of striatal dopamine D1 and D2 receptor sites in male and female rats. Brain Res 1992;571:212–217.
20. Fink G, Sumner B, Rosie R, et al. Androgen actions on central serotonin neurotransmission: relevance for mood, mental state and memory. Behav Brain Res 1999;105:53–68.
21. "Renee": autobiography of a schizophrenic girl. In: Shannonhouse R, ed. Out of Her Mind. New York: Random House, 2000:70–76.
22. Castle DJ. Women and schizophrenia: an epidemiological perspective. In: Castle DJ, McGrath J, Kulkarni J, eds. Women and Schizophrenia. Cambridge: Cambridge University Press, 2000:19–34.
23. Tsuang G, Coryell W. An 8-year follow-up of patients with DSM-III-R psychotic depression, schizoaffective disorder and schizophrenia. Am J Psychiatry 1993;150:1182–1188.
24. Lewine RRJ. Gender and schizophrenia. In: Tsuang MT, Simpson JT, eds. Handbook of Schizophrenia. Amsterdam: Elsevier Science, 1988:379–397.
25. Subotnik KL, Nuechterlein KH, Asarnow RF, et al. Depressive symptoms in the early course of schizophrenia: relationship to familial psychiatric illness. Am J Psychiatry 1997;154(11): 1551–1556.
26. Mueser KT, Bellack AS, Morrison RL, et al. Social competence in schizophrenia: premorbid adjustment, social skill and domains of functioning. J Psychiatr Res 1990;24:51–63.
27. Edwards J, McGorry P. Implementing Early Intervention in Psychosis. London: Martin Dunitz, 2002:31–46.
28. Seeman MV, Fitzgerald P. Women and schizophrenia clinical aspects. In: Castle D, McGrath J, Kulkarni J, eds. Women and Schizophrenia. Cambridge: Cambridge University Press, 2000:95–110.
29. Power P, McGorry PD. Initial assessment of first-episode psychosis. In: McGorry PD, Jackson HJ, eds. Recognition and Management of Early Psychosis: A Preventive Approach. Cambridge: Cambridge University Press, 1999:155–183.
30. McEwen BS. Ovarian steroids in the brain: implications for cognition and ageing. Neurology 1997;65:353–359.
31. Kulkarni J. Women and schizophrenia: a review. Aust NZ J Psychiatry 1997;31:46–56.
32. Szymanski S, Lieberman JA, Alvir JM, et al. Gender differences in onset of illness, treatment response, course, and biologic indexes in first-episode schizophrenic patients. Am J Psychiatry 1995;152:698–703.
33. Marder SR, Davis JM, Chouinard G. The effects of risperidone on the five dimensions of schizophrenia derived by factor analysis: combined results of the North American trials. J Clin Psychiatry 1997;58:538–546.
34. Kulkarni J: Home based treatment of first episode psychosis. In: McGorry PD, Jackson HK, eds. Recognition and Management of Early Psychosis: A Preventive Approach. Cambridge: Cambridge University Press, 1999:206–225.
35. Hambrecht M, Häfner H. Substance abuse and the onset of schizophrenia. Biol Psychiatry 1996;40:1155–1163.
36. Hearle J, McGrath J. Motherhood and schizophrenia. In: Castle DJ, McGrath J, Kulkarni J, eds. Women and Schizophrenia. Cambridge: Cambridge University Press, 2000:79–94.
37. Kulkarni J. Thesis for Ph.D; "Jenny"—a mother with schizophrenia. Melbourne, Australia: Monash University, 1997:30–35.
38. Kendell RE, Chalmers JC, Platz C. Epidemiology of puerperal psychosis. Br J Psychiatry 1987;150:662–673.
39. Knopps G. Post partum mood disorders, a startling contrast to the joy of birth. Postgrad Med 1993;93:103–116.

40. Videbech P, Gouliaev G. First admission with puerperal psychosis: 7–14 years of follow-up. Acta Psychiatr Scand 1995;91:167–173.
41. Benvenuti P, Cabras PL, Servi P, et al. Puerperal psychosis; a clinical case study with follow up. J Affect Disord 1992;26:25–30.
42. Hearle J, Plant K, Jenner L, et al. A survey of contact with offspring and assistance with child care among parents with psychotic disorders. Psychiatr Serv 1999;50:1354–1356.
43. Miller LJ. Psychotic denial of pregnancy: phenomenology and clinical management. Hosp Commun Psychiatry 1990;41:1233–1237.
44. Mednick SA, Parnas J Schulsinger F. The Copenhagen High-Risk Project. 1962–86. Schizophr Bull 1987;13:485–495.
45. Miller WH, Bloom JD, Resnick MP. Prenatal care for pregnant chronic mentally ill patients. Hosp Community Psychiatry 1992;43:942–943.
46. Barkla J, McGrath J. Reproductive, preconceptual and antenatal needs of women with schizophrenia. In: Castle DJ, McGrath J, Kulkarni J, eds. Women and Schizophrenia, Cambridge: Cambridge University Press, 2000:67–78.
47. Cowling V. Meeting the support needs of families with dependent children where a parent has a mental illness. Fam Matters 1996;45:22–25.
48. McGrath JJ, Hearle J, Jenner L, et al. The fertility and fecundity of patients with psychoses. Acta Psychiatr Scand 1999;99:441–446.
49. Germaine Greer. The Whole Woman. London: Doubleday, 1999:135–147.
50. Häfner H, Gattaz WF, Janzarik W. Search for the causes of schizophrenia. Berlin: Springer-Verlag, 1987:8–10.
51. Seeman MV. Gender differences in schizophrenia. Can J Psychiatry 1982;27:107–112.
52. Seeman MV. Sex differences in predicting neuroleptic response. In: Gaebel W, Awad AG, eds. The Prediction of Neuroleptic Response. Vienna: Springer-Verlag, 1995:51–64.
53. Faraone SV, Chen WJ, Goldstein JM, et al. Gender differences in age of onset of schizophrenia. Br J Psychiatry 1994;164:625–629.
54. Kulkarni J, de Castella AR, Riedel A, et al. Estrogen: a potential treatment for schizophrenia. Schizophr Res 2001;48:137–144.
55. Kulkarni J, de Castella A, Downey M, et al. Results of two controlled studies on estrogen: avenue to neuroprotection in schizophrenia. In: Häfner H, ed. Risk and Protective Factors in Schizophrenia. Darmstadt, Germany: Springer, Steinkopff, 2002:271–282.

CHAPTER 15

Sexuality and Sexual Disorders in Women

Rosemary Basson

Incultureswhere women's sexual pleasure and wish to engage sexually are endorsed, there are increasing data on the nature of their sexuality, sexual function, sexual problems and dysfunction, and the prevalence of genital pain with sexual activity. However, in cultures where sex is considered from the perspective of the man's pleasure only and the woman's need, preferences, function, enjoyment, and orientation are ignored, we clearly remain ignorant. The picture presented in this chapter is, therefore, far from complete. Seventy-six percent of 3,300 recently surveyed North American women considered sex moderately or very important; Caucasian, African American, and Hispanic women were more likely to deem sex intensely important than were women from China or Japan (1). Of another 987 North American women recently surveyed, 24% reported marked distress about their sexual relationship or their own sexuality or both (2). Thus problems that interfere with this important aspect of women's lives warrant careful assessment and management.

CHARACTERISTICS OF WOMEN'S SEXUALITY

THE SUBJECTIVE EXPERIENCE IS PARAMOUNT

Determinants of women's distress about their sexual relationships and about their own sexuality have recently been studied (2). The subjective response, defined as feeling emotionally close to her partner, feeling pleasure, not feeling displeasure, or feeling indifferent, had the most significant effect of a number of variables. This applied to women's distress regarding both their sexual relationships and their own sexuality. Interestingly, distress about their physical sexual response had a weaker effect on distress about their relationship and no significant effect on distress about their own sexuality. It is therefore possible that relationship problems themselves impair physical response. It was apparent that younger women were more likely to be distressed if they had problems responding physically, but this still only caused distress about their respective sexual relationships—not about their own sexuality.

Emotions during sexual engagement strongly impact women's overall subjective sexual experience, including the composite entity of sexual arousal. Sexually healthy women show highly variable correlation between their subjective arousal and psychophysiologic measures of genital congestion. Such testing involves the woman watching an erotic movie in a private room, while a tamponlike device she has inserted into her vagina records physiologic increase in congestion of blood around her vagina as she views the film. Both sexually healthy women and women reporting chronic low sexual arousal can show prompt genital congestion in response to the erotic video even if they report minimal subjective arousal. In women with chronically low arousal, the video may produce negative affect such as anxiety. Paradoxically, the intensity of this negative affect correlates with the degree of genital congestion. Figure 15.1 is a model of subjective sexual arousal.

Thus, for many women complaining of lack of sexual arousal, there is an apparent "disconnection" between the genital response (prompt and physiologic) and subjective excitement/arousal (absent). The degree to which such women are aware of the genital changes resulting from sexual stimulation varies. Thus some are well aware of an increase in vaginal lubrication despite the absence of any sexual excitement.

For sexually healthy women, marked lubrication may well excite a male partner and indeed may reassure the woman that her response is healthy, but of itself, lubrication rarely affords excitement to the woman. Indeed, in many sexually healthy women, their arousal is more strongly modulated by emotions than by genital feedback. Sometimes physicians see women who complain of excessive lubrication with stimulation, something that causes them embarrassment and displeasure.

Brain studies by functional magnetic resonance imaging of women during sexual arousal show activation of areas involved in cognitive appraisal and areas involved in emotional response as well as areas involved in the organization and perception of genital reflexes. In contrast to findings in similar studies in men, the uptake in the latter areas (including the posterior hypothalamus and rostral

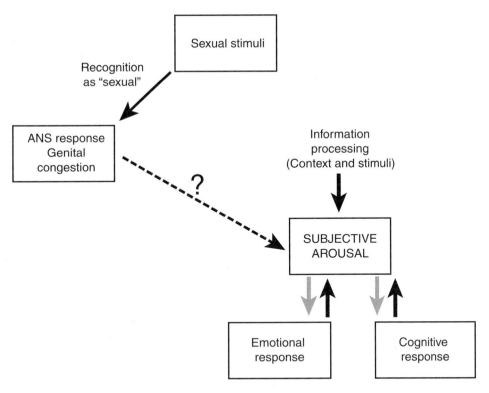

FIGURE 15.1 ● Model of sexual arousal. Adapted from Basson R. Obstet Gynocol 2001; 98:350–353. Used with permission from Elsevier.

anterior cingulate) does not correlate closely with the woman's subjective arousal (4).

WOMEN HAVE MANY REASONS FOR ENGAGING IN SEX

Most studies of women's sexual motivation have been of women in established relationships. Interestingly, for the majority of these women, sexual desire itself is not a frequent reason to initiate or agree to partnered sexual activity (5–7). Frequently cited reasons include increasing her emotional closeness with her partner and enhancing the woman's own sense of well-being as well as avoiding negative consequences of lack of sexual activity in the relationship. Initially she is sexually neutral but willing to become imminently aroused, but only well into the experience does she sense sexual desire. This type of response appears familiar to women. It is clear that providing the experience is enjoyable and the outcome rewarding, women find the experience entirely satisfactory (Figure 15.2).

Sometimes response is augmented or overshadowed by a sense of apparently spontaneous desire, as shown in Figure 15.3. This progression from desire to arousal to orgasm and resolution reflects the original model by Kaplan, Masters, and Johnson.

Cross-cultural study is needed to substantiate the clinical impression that women from some cultures focus strongly on a wish to please the partner as their major motivation. Baseline data from the Study of Women's Health Across the

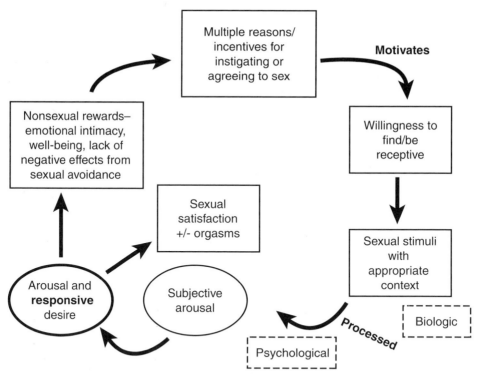

FIGURE 15.2 ● Sex response cycle initiated for reasons other than desire. Adapted from Basson R. Obstet Gynocol 2001; 98:350–353. Used with permission from Elsevier.

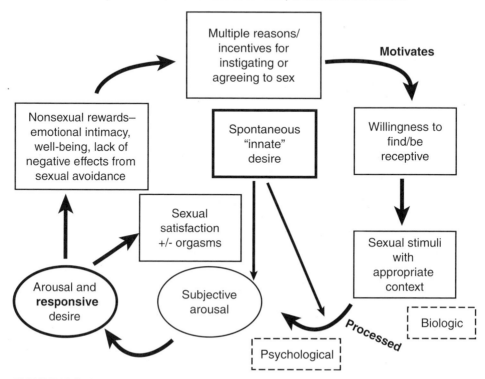

FIGURE 15.3 ● Spontaneous desire augments cycle based on other motivations. Adapted from Basson R. Obstet Gynocol 2001; 98:350–353. Used with permission from Elsevier.

Nation (SWAN) (1) show no marked cultural differences in the percentages of women choosing among three sexual motivations in response to a question on reasons for engaging in sex: expressing love, meeting the partner's sexual needs, lessening their own tension and stress. There are minimal data on lesbian women's reasons or incentives for sexual activity in long-term relationships, where sexual frequency is known to be generally lower than for women in heterosexual relationships. The clinical impression is that as both partners have relatively infrequent spontaneous sexual desire (compared to most men), there is no need for either woman's sexual motivation to be based solely on wanting to meet the sexual needs of the partner.

THE PHASES OF SEXUAL RESPONSE ARE NOT DISCRETE

The models of women's sexual response mentioned above illustrate the overlap of desire and arousal and the lack of any one linear sequence of phases. Additionally, women report merging of the phases of arousal and orgasm. Indeed, orgasm can be multiple and experienced at different levels of intensity of arousal. Orgasms themselves can be discrete events of a few seconds or a prolonged plateau of intense orgasmic excitement lasting more than 30 seconds as originally described by Masters and Johnson. The lack of a refractory period in women allows the potential for prolonged sexual activity in overlapping phases of varying sequence.

WOMEN'S SEXUALITY IS DISCONTINUOUS

Normally during pregnancy, there is reduced sexual desire and infrequent sexual intercourse. These reductions have been related to women's fears about causing miscarriage earlier in the pregnancy or harm to the fetus from intercourse or orgasm at any stage in the pregnancy. Other reasons women cite are physical discomfort, fatigue, or feeling less physically attractive or less sexually desirable than before pregnancy.

A recent survey of 570 women and 550 of their partners showed that an average couple resumed intercourse and nonpenetrative sex by about the seventh week postpartum (9). Women who were breast-feeding reported less sexual activity and less satisfaction. There were no marked differences according to method of delivery, although women who delivered a child by cesarean section were more likely to have resumed intercourse at one month postpartum than were women who had delivered vaginally. Presence or absence of episiotomy or tear was not recorded in the study.

A modest gradual decline in sexual desire, interest, and responsivity occurs with menopause and aging (10). Frequency of partnered sexual activity may or may not decrease given that women have many reasons to engage in sex other than desire. Increased desire and interest are consistently reported with new relationships even many years after the menopause (10).

WOMEN'S SEXUALITY IS CONTEXTUAL AND MAY BE ADAPTIVE

As reflected in the model of women's sex response (Figure 15.2), motivation to be sexual and the mental processing of sexual stimuli are affected by both the larger context of the woman's life and the immediate context of the potential sexual experience. Longitudinal (10) and cross-sectional (11) menopausal studies have confirmed the importance of a woman's feelings for her partner in determining her sexual appetite and responsivity. Her relationship with others, the demands of those relationships, and her positive or negative feelings about them, as well as societal standards and the influence of poverty (12,13), can affect both her motivation and sexual arousability. Specifically, feelings for her partner at the time of sexual interaction and her present stated emotional well-being were the strongest predictors of sexual distress in the recent North American National Probability Sample (2). It has been noted how relatively infrequently women engage in sex for reasons of desire; rather, the stimuli and an appropriate context of the occasion can move the woman from sexual neutrality to sexual responsiveness. Women's lack of sexual responsiveness in problematic contexts may be considered a normative adaptive response that can be construed as healthy rather than unhealthy; to consider this as a dysfunction or disorder may well be inappropriate (2). However, the woman may report that she is experiencing lack of sexual pleasure, dyspareunia, or is disinterested in engaging in sex. Labeling such problems "dysfunction" need not imply something intrinsically wrong with the woman's sex response system. Analogously, a woman with tension headaches due to an ergonomic problem with her chair and computer desk need have no intrinsic musculoskeletal abnormality of her neck but will receive a medical diagnosis nevertheless.

This concept that the environment affects function is basic to the understanding of sexual physiology as well as nonsexual physiology. The tendency in the past to consider etiologies of dysfunction as either biologic or psychological has little scientific foundation. Rather, there are numerous examples of environmental stresses interacting with physiology, as with the immune and hormonal systems, and even areas of the brain—in particular the hippocampus, which can change in volume according to stress levels. Interestingly in female oophorectomized rodents, environmental influences (a male animal in adjacent cage) and past experiences, including conditioned responses, can cause the same increase in sexual behavior afforded by the administration of sex hormones (14).

Physical health and physical well-being also have an impact on sexuality. Disease processes (e.g., spinal cord injury) may directly interfere with sexual response, but many other connected factors are involved as shown in Table 15.1.

TABLE 15.1

Areas of Chronic Illness Potentially Impacting on Sexual Health

1. Biologic disruption of the sexual response
2. Psychological consequences of the illness affecting the sexual response
3. Fatigue, chronic pain
4. Depression
5. Sexual response disruption from treatment of chronic illness
6. Limited mobility necessary for caressing, self-stimulating, or engaging in intercourse
7. Cardiovascular or respiratory compromise such that orgasm or movements of intercourse might be dangerous
8. Associated incontinence or stomas

Specific studies focused on women receiving radical hysterectomy for cancer of the cervix have found a definite possibility of autonomic nerve damage affecting vaginal and vulval sexual response. Some prospective studies failed to confirm the results of a previous retrospective cross-sectional study that reported reduced vaginal lubrication and elasticity after hysterectomy (15). A recent prospective study of 173 women with early-stage cancer of the cervix treated by radical hysterectomy involved surgeries where the incisions in the uterosacral and cardinal ligaments were deliberately placed to spare traversing autonomic nerves that supply the vagina and vulva (16). Problems with sexual response were common in the first few months postoperatively but, nevertheless, sexual interest remained. By two years, sexual response had definitely improved, but both the women and their partners reported lessening of sexual interest. Only 10% of the women complained of significant lubrication difficulties at the two-year mark. The study did not inquire into congestion and pleasurable sensitivity of the vulval structures. Women with cancer of the cervix may also be subjected to marked hormonal changes from surgical oophorectomy or radiation damage to the ovaries. They may or may not receive estrogen therapy. In addition, there are many nonmedical factors involved, given that these women face a potentially life-threatening illness, which perhaps explains the lack of a simple correlation between sexual difficulties and treatment-induced changes whether hormonal, neurologic, or structural.

Diabetes, with its potential to impair endothelial function and autonomic nerve conduction, might be expected to directly affect genital sex response through lack of genital engorgement and lubrication and through anorgasmia. These outcomes have not been found in studies to date. Except for the entity of vaginal lubrication in one large outpatient study (17), psychological rather than somatic factors have largely accounted for women's sexual complaints across studies.

Certain medical factors are very pertinent to breast cancer survivors. In particular, chemotherapy-induced ovarian failure is highly correlated with reports of sexual dysfunction. A predictive model arising out of two large series of women suggested that the most important predictors of sexual health were absence of vaginal dryness, emotional well-being, positive body image, quality of relationship with the partner, and absence of sexual problems in the partner (18).

A male partner's sexual dysfunction (e.g., premature ejaculation or erectile dysfunction) can certainly have a negative impact on women's sex response (19). There has been far less study in lesbian women. This too is a complex area. When sexual activity is simply less frequent because of a male partner's physical sexual difficulty, but sex nevertheless occurs, women's sexual desire can actually increase (10,11).

Acquisition of a new partner has been found to increase women's sexual desire and responsivity (10). This is not surprising, given the likelihood that at this time both partners put significant effort into being close emotionally and providing a romantically erotic context. That women's sexuality is contextual is endorsed in a study of lesbian and bisexual women, more than half of whom, when followed over a course of eight years, changed their sexual identity labels at least once after first "coming out" as nonheterosexual. Often this was because they found themselves in unexpected relationships that contradicted their perceptions of typical lesbian or bisexual behavior. Some even preferred eventually to assume an unlabeled identity. No one label could fully represent the diversity of sexual feelings they experienced with different female and male partners under different circumstances (20).

WOMEN'S SEXUAL RESPONSIVITY AND DESIRE ARE LINKED TO THEIR GENERAL EMOTIONAL WELL-BEING

Women's lack of emotional well-being was one of the stronger predictors of sexual distress in the recent North American National Probability Sample (2). In a similar vein, it has been shown that lack of mental well-being, even if the psychological difficulties do not meet the criteria for clinical diagnosis of a mental disorder, is strongly linked to women's complaints of low desire (21). Specifically, the study compared 50 women with low sexual desire to a group of 100 without complaints about desire and found that the former showed mood instability and fragile self-regulation and self-esteem, and they tended to be more worried, anxious, and introverted, with feelings of guilt. Emotional stability was a robust predictor of women's sexual desire and responsivity in the menopausal studies, both longitudinal and cross-sectional (10,11).

WOMEN'S SEXUAL DYSFUNCTIONS ARE LINKED TO MOOD DISORDER

Complaints of impaired sexual desire have been noted in the majority of studies of women with depression (22). Other studies have shown that compared to controls, women presenting with impaired desire were twice as likely to have a history of major depressive disorder. In one study of 126 women seeking help for sexual dysfunction of various types, a full 50% were assigned a psychiatric diagnosis (23). Paradoxically, one study has suggested that depressed women masturbate more frequently than nondepressed women despite their problems with pain, sexual arousal, and orgasm. Thus a lack of desire for partnered sexual activity should not necessarily be assumed to mean a total lack of sexual appetite. There clearly exists a need to address these issues, including the negative sexual effects of medication given for depression.

Clinically and historically, chronic anxiety states have been linked with impaired sexual function, particularly low desire. It is interesting to find that laboratory-induced anxiety enhances physical genital responding but not subjective arousal (24).

Antidepressant-Associated Sexual Dysfunction

Open-label trials and case series have suggested a number of pharmacologic agents that might improve or reverse the loss of arousal, desire, and orgasm commonly associated with serotonergic antidepressants. These trials have minimal substantiation to date in randomized placebo-controlled studies in women (25,26). It is important to take note of the high placebo response in such studies. When women and their partners expect there might be a better sexual outcome, their expectation encourages them to greater effort.

Newer antidepressants that avoid activating certain subtypes of serotonin receptors thought to mediate sexual dysfunction and that have central noradrenergic action may prove to have fewer negative sexual effects. Recently available mirtazepine may be useful despite its tendency to promote weight gain and possible impairment of sexual self-image. Future medications having dopaminergic and noradrenergic action comparable to bupropion but with different mechanisms of action may also support sexual function. An area in need of research is the high dosages of serotonergic drugs needed to control generalized anxiety and its toll on the woman's sexuality. Despite their risk of delaying orgasms and lessening desire, prescribing a selective serotonin reuptake inhibitor (SSRI) often benefits the woman whose need for control and obsessive thinking preclude her ability to be sexually aroused.

DIFFERENCES BETWEEN MEN'S AND WOMEN'S SEXUALITY

Reconceptualization of the human sex response cycle as in Figures 15.1 and 15.2 has led to widespread acceptance that this is an accurate reflection of heterosexual and lesbian women's sexual response, but there is less acceptance of the accuracy of this cycle for men. Although, perhaps for a majority of men, there is usually awareness of sexual desire at the outset of a sexual experience, men too can begin from a sexually neutral state expecting to very promptly become aroused by the partner or other stimulation. So, it may well be that the context, including the quality of the relationship and the larger social environment, is relatively more important for women's sexual function than for men's.

IMPORTANCE OF EXPECTED DURATION OF RELATIONSHIP AND OF SEXUAL EXCLUSIVITY

Some empirical studies have focused on differences between men's and women's sexuality (13). Detailed analysis of the data from the 1992 National Health and Social Life Survey (NHSLS) has focused on the effect of expected length of a relationship on emotional and physical sexual pleasure. For both women and men, the expectation of a long-term relationship with sexual exclusivity for both partners was strongly tied to emotional satisfaction as much as to physical pleasure from sex. However, interesting gender differences were noted. Whereas men who reported that their partners had an affair in the last year were less satisfied emotionally than those who did not report this behavior, women's sexual emotional satisfaction appeared not to be significantly affected by such behavior in their partner. Both sexes reported that their own lack of exclusivity resulted in less emotional sexual satisfaction. A further difference was that women who expected the relationship to last indefinitely (they were married or engaged) reported more emotional satisfaction with sex. Men who were married, engaged, or in relationships that were expected to last just a year or so all reported similar degrees of emotional satisfaction. Concerning physical sexual pleasure, women reported reduced pleasure if either they or their partner was not sexually exclusive in the previous year. Among men, however, physical pleasure was not related to either the man's or his partner's affair.

IMPORTANCE AND NATURE OF WOMEN'S ORGASMS

The foregoing analysis of the 1992 NHSLS data confirms that the reliability of woman's orgasms was important for both sexes, whereas the reliability of the man's orgasm had rather minimal effect (13). This applied to both emotional satisfaction and physical pleasure. Both sexes typically report that their partner's sexual excitement and arousal are very important to them. It may be that the man's erection is taken as confirmation of his arousal, whereas the lack of physical confirmation of the woman's genital or subjective arousal leads to a focus on her orgasm to confirm that she was aroused and excited.

Moreover, women's orgasms are rather different from men's in that women are very capable of multiple and very prolonged orgasms and the refractory period may be delayed until a number of orgasms have occurred. Women are less likely to separate orgasm and arousal as they describe their experience. Time needed to attain orgasm is often claimed to be considerably longer in women than in men. However, this is usually in the context of partnered sex and, in fact, women can often self-stimulate to orgasm within one or two minutes. Finally, there is clear evidence that orgasm will occur in women despite complete spinal cord transection, which insulates the genitalia from all known sources of somatic and autonomic innervation except possibly a contribution from the vagus nerve to the cervix.

IMPORTANCE OF PHYSICAL ATTRACTION OF THE PARTNER

Physical attraction may be more important for men than women, as reflected by the greater ease of sexual arousal to visual cues in the laboratory shown by men. Empirical studies have shown the relative importance of implied societal status over physical attraction of potential sexual partners for women and the opposite for men (27). In societies where adulation of female beauty is shunned and wealth is devalued, the reasons men and women give for choosing their mates are revealing. These were reported in a group of Chinese immigrants (28). For women, partner's "good looks" was at the bottom of their list, whereas income, job, and socioeconomic class label were at the top. For men, although class label was very important, so too, were the partner's good looks.

EXPERIENCE OF CASUAL SEX

Empirical evidence exists of differences in men and women's interest in and experience of casual sex. Men and women were asked how likely they would be to agree to be sexual with a partner they had known for an hour, a day, a week, a month, six months, a year, two years, or five years. The responses from men and women for the five-year option were similar but, for all other intervals, men were more likely to agree they would have sex under these circumstances. Also, it is possible that when women do engage in casual sex, their motives may differ from those of men. Data suggest women more often report they feel "used" in casual encounters, this being on an emotional rather than a logical basis. They also reported feeling emotionally vulnerable during such liaisons, and the more casual relationships they had, the more frequent the negative thoughts and emotions they experienced. In contrast, the more partners men had, the less anxious they felt (28).

EFFECT OF AGING ON SEXUAL DESIRE AND RESPONSE

Although there is a definite increase in erectile dysfunction as men age, there is no such clear correlation with any sexual dysfunction in women as they age. There is evidence, however, to support a subtle lessening of desire with both age and menopause (10) and conflicting results of desire and age generally (29). It is unlikely that the cavernosal tissues of women's genitalia escape the age-related endothelial dysfunction and loss of vascularity of the counterpart in men's genitalia. However, despite documented reduced volume of clitoral tissue and loss of vulval and vaginal vascularity, which can be obvious on simple physical examination, these changes do not necessarily correlate with sexual symptoms. Interestingly, the percentage increase in congestion around the vagina in response to erotic stimulation is similar in women with estrogen depletion and in those replete with estrogen (30).

CORRELATION OF PHYSICAL GENITAL AROUSAL AND SUBJECTIVE GENITAL AROUSAL

Noted previously in this chapter were the findings of psychophysiologic studies that monitored the increase in congestion around the vagina of sexually healthy female subjects asked to view an erotic stimulus: these studies showed variable and often poor correlation between the subjective experience and increases in congestion. However, studies of penile erection and men's subjective arousal show close correlation. Similarly, functional magnetic resonance imaging during sexual arousal shows brain activation in the posterior hypothalamus organizing and receiving afferent feedback from the genitalia that correlates subjective experience in men but not in women (4).

IMPORTANCE OF THE ACT OF PENILE VAGINAL INTERCOURSE

The genital anatomy of women is such that "efficient" sexual stimulation of the most sexually responsive areas is not afforded by intercourse. The location of the extensive cavernosal tissue within the rami, shaft, head of the clitoris, the bulbs surrounding the anterior vagina, and the urethra is such that orgasm is more easily reached through direct vulval stimulation than by intercourse. Many women are particularly dependent on sufficient nonpenetrative sexual stimulation in order to enjoy the penile vaginal stimulation. The neuroanatomy of men's genitalia is such that the act of intercourse is a very efficient means of stimulating the vast network of sensory nerves around the corona of the glans penis.

Sexual Consequences for Women from Medical Management of Their Male Partners' Erectile Dysfunction

Erectile dysfunction is understood to be a problem that affects both partners of a couple, with interpersonal issues and sexual concerns of the partner interplaying with a variable degree of biologic deficit, particularly that of endothelial dysfunction in the specialized vasculature of the penis. However, with the advent of effective and generally safe medical therapies, there is an increasing tendency for clinicians to consider only the man, assessing the man, prescribing medication, and measuring the outcome in terms of penile firmness, the man's ability to have intercourse, and his overall sexual satisfaction. There are reasons to question whether women's sexual enjoyment and satisfaction will necessarily follow. When asked what is their most enjoyable part of sexual activity, the majority of women whose partners have erectile dysfunction state "foreplay" as opposed to sexual intercourse (31). Similarly, on survey questionnaires women in sexually and generally healthy marriages report foreplay as the most satisfying component of partnered sex; only 11% of responses report sexual intercourse as the most satisfying component (32). Whether men's enthusiasm to caress and pleasure their partners with various forms of nonpenetrative sex increases with their renewed sexual self-confidence and increased sexual excitement in response to their own firm erections requires investigation. Typically women whose partners have erectile dysfunction are older, likely to have evidence of genital atrophy (33), and therefore require more varied and more prolonged nonpenetrative sexual stimulation prior to any intercourse. Across studies men do report high satisfaction with the phosphodiesterase inhibitors, the first of which was sildenafil. One study has shown almost one third of their female partners were not satisfied with the sexual outcome (34). Limited study of the quality of the general relationship—measuring domains such as "tenderness" and "togetherness"—suggests that the partners of men who are highly responsive to sildenafil do report higher scores in these domains than a comparison group of women with as yet untreated partners with similar degrees of erectile dysfunction (35). Both the phosphodiesterase inhibitors and the newer treatment, apomorphine (centrally acting dopaminergic drugs), can only be effective when the man is subjectively sexually excited. This subjective arousal is, for the majority of men, in the longer term dependent on their partner's sexual excitement and enjoyment. Thus, it is hoped that erectile dysfunction will again be seen as a couple entity whereby women's sexual concerns predating or associated with the erectile dysfunction and its treatment will also be addressed.

EMERGING CONCEPTS

Acceptance of the contextual nature of the women's sexual function, the lack of one linear sequence of events or one invariant order of phases, the overlap of phases, and the comorbidity of dysfunction have all led to revision of definitions of dysfunction. It is hoped these expansions and revisions of dysfunction (36) will influence the Committees of the International Statistical Classification of Disease and Related Health Problems (ICD-10) and the American Psychiatric Association's *Diagnostic and Statistical Manual of Mental Disorders,* 4th edition (DSM-IV-TR) to consider much-needed revisions of their official definitions. It is known that distress from any given dysfunction is highly variable. Therefore, in addition to descriptors of lifelong or acquired, situational or generalized, a distress descriptor is recommended for the various dysfunctions that are diagnosed. Given the importance of contextual factors, it is also recommended that these too be incorporated into the diagnosis. The following categories of etiologic descriptors are advocated:

1. Factors to do with the woman's past that may have affected her psychosexual development
2. Factors associated with the current context
3. Medical/surgical/psychiatric factors

These contextual descriptors are felt to be extremely important given the need for scientific study of nonpharmacologic and pharmacologic treatment of women's sexual dysfunction and the pressing need to have more precise definitions in order to show benefit over placebo.

DEFINITIONS OF DISORDERS

The following definitions have been agreed upon by an International Committee organized by the American Foundation of Urological Disease as a result of meetings and extensive electronic communication over 24 months with piloting and further revisions prior to publication. Ongoing use and validation of these definitions are encouraged to allow estimation of their accuracy, reliability, and validity.

Women's Sexual Interest/Desire Disorder

There are absent or diminished feelings of sexual interest or desire, absent sexual thoughts or fantasies, and a lack of responsive desire. Motivations (here defined as reasons/incentives), for attempting to become sexually aroused are scarce or absent. The lack of interest is considered to be beyond a normative lessening with life cycle and relationship duration. (36)

Of note, the intended focus is the many reasons the women may have for instigating or agreeing to sexual activity. The lack of responsive desire triggered during the sexual experience is essential for a diagnosis of interest/desire disorder. In other words, the lack of spontaneous desire per se is not dysfunctional in women.

Subjective Sexual Arousal Disorder

Absence of or markedly diminished feelings of sexual arousal (sexual excitement and sexual pleasure) from any type of sexual stimulation. Vaginal lubrication or other signs of physical response still occur. (36)

As noted, the majority of women complaining of absent subjective sexual arousal do show vaginal vasocongestion in response to an erotic stimulus that is comparable to that of sexually healthy women. Those that report awareness of some physiologic genital responding, usually lubrication, are given the diagnosis of subjective sexual arousal disorder.

Genital Sexual Arousal Disorder

Complaints of absent or impaired genital sexual arousal. Self-report may include minimal vulval swelling or vaginal lubrication from any type of sexual stimulation and reduced sexual sensations from caressing genitalia. Subjective sexual excitement still occurs from nongenital sexual stimuli. (36)

The important point about women receiving this diagnosis are that they are still subjectively sexually excited by a number of stimuli, including reading an erotic book, watching something erotic, caressing the partner, receiving breast stimulation, or kissing. They specifically report a lack of genital response, often using the term "genital deadness." Frequently, these women find great difficulty in reaching orgasm.

Combined Genital and Subjective Arousal Disorder

Absence of or markedly diminished feelings of sexual arousal (sexual excitement and sexual pleasure), from any type of sexual stimulation as well as complaints of absent or impaired genital sexual arousal (vulval swelling, lubrication). (36)

This is commonly a lifelong complaint. Again, studies of women presenting in this manner indicate that despite their symptoms, erotic stimuli cause reflex genital vasocongestion comparable to that of control women under laboratory conditions. Of note, it is the absence of subjective sexual excitement from any type of sexual stimulation in their lives that distinguishes this subgroup of women from those diagnosed with genital arousal disorder.

Some women with sudden premature loss of ovarian androgen have similar complaints and will be diagnosed with combined genital and subjective arousal disorder, and usually with loss of sexual desire/interest, all concurrent with the hormonal loss. As yet, there are no published psychophysiologic studies on this group of women.

Women's Orgasmic Disorder

Despite the self-report of high sexual arousal/excitement, there is either lack of orgasm, markedly diminished intensity of orgasmic sensations, or marked delay of orgasm from any kind of stimulation. (36)

Dyspareunia

Persistent or recurrent pain with attempted or complete vaginal entry and/or penile vaginal intercourse. (36)

Vaginismus

The persistent or recurrent difficulties of the woman to allow vaginal entry of a penis, a finger, and/or any object, despite the woman's expressed wish to do so. There is variable involuntary pelvic muscle contraction, (phobic) avoidance, and anticipation/fear/experience of pain. Structural or other vulval pathology must be ruled out/addressed. (36)

Researchers no longer refer to a presumed "vaginal spasm," since this has never been scientifically verified. Clinically there is much overlap between vaginismus and dyspareunia.

Sexual Aversion Disorder

Extreme anxiety and/or disgust at the anticipation of or attempt to have any sexual activity. (36)

Persistent Sexual Arousal Disorder

Spontaneous, intrusive, and unwanted genital arousal (e.g., tingling, throbbing, pulsating) in the absence of sexual interest and desire. Any awareness of subjective arousal is typically but not invariably unpleasant. The arousal is unrelieved by one or more orgasms and the feelings of arousal persist for hours or days. (36)

Currently, this is simply a provisional definition that may allow further investigation of the prevalence and etiology of this poorly understood syndrome.

FUTURE DIRECTIONS: A BIOPSYCHOSOCIAL APPROACH

Data are increasing on the close link between women's sexual function and their mental well-being. The latter strongly influences motivation to begin a sexual experience, willingness to find or request potentially useful sexual stimuli, and the ease with which the woman becomes subjectively aroused by those stimuli. The larger context of her life as well as the immediate context of the sexual experience have major impact on her subjective sexual experience. The latter correlates more closely with her emotions and thoughts during the experience than with the degree of genital congestion. Feelings for her partner generally and specifically at the time of sexual interaction are strong predictors of a woman's sexual response and satisfaction. Appreciating the many reasons women engage sexually, the overlapping of the phases of their sexual response and, therefore, the usual occurrence of two or more dysfunctions in women with sexual complaints, further facilitates the assessment of women's sexual dysfunction. The revised definitions of dysfunction contain descriptors relating to developmental history and to current sexual context, as well as medical entities as integral parts of the diagnostic framework. Randomized controlled trials for pharmacologic and nonpharmacologic management of sexual dysfunction will be aided by these more precise definitions, but scientifically based individualized treatment is the challenging but preferred future goal.[a]

REFERENCES

1. Cain VS, Johannes CB, Avis NE, et al. Sexual functioning and practices in a multi-ethnic study of midlife women: baseline results from SWAN. J Sex Res 2003;40(3):266–276.
2. Bancroft J, Loftus J, Long JS. Distress about sex: a national survey of women in heterosexual relationships. Arch Sex Behav 2003;32:193–211.
3. Basson RJ. A model of women's sexual arousal. J Sex Marital Ther 2002;28:1–10.
4. Karama S, Lecours AR, Leroux JM, et al. Areas of brain activation in males and females during viewing of erotic film excerpts. Hum Brain Mapp 2002;16:1–13.
5. Hill CA, Preston LK. Individual differences in the experience of sexual motivation: theory and measurement of dispositional sexual motives. J Sex Res 1996;33(1):27–45.
6. Galyer KT, Conaglen HM, Hare A, et al. The effect of gynecological surgery on sexual desire. J Sex Marital Ther 1999;25:81–88.
7. Weijmar Schultz WCM, Van De Wiel HBM, Hahn DEE. Psychosexual functioning after treatment for gynecological cancer and integrated model, review of determinant factors and clinical guidelines. Int J Gynecol Cancer 1992;2:281–290.
8. Basson R. Female sexual response: the role of drugs in the management of sexual dysfunction. Obstet Gynecol 2001;98:350–353.
9. Hyde JS, deLamater JD, Plant EA, et al. Sexuality during pregnancy and the year postpartum. J Sex Res 1996;33(2):143–151.
10. Dennerstein L, Lehert P, Burger H, et al. Factors affecting sexual functioning of women in the midlife years. Climacteric 1999;2:254–262.
11. Avis NE, Stellato R, Crawford S, et al. Is there an association between menopause status and sexual functioning? Menopause 2000;7:297–309.
12. Laumann EL, Paik A, Rosen RC. Sexual dysfunction in United States: prevalence and predictors. JAMA 1999;10:537–545.
13. Waite LJ, Joiner K. Emotional satisfaction and physical pleasure in sexual unions: time horizon, sexual behavior, and sexual exclusivity. J Marriage Fam 2001;63:247–264.
14. Blaustein JD. Progestin receptors: neuronal integrators of hormonal and environmental stimulation. Ann NY Acad Sci 2003;1007:238–250.
15. Bergmark K, Avall-Lundqvist E, Dickman PW, et al. Vaginal changes and sexuality in women with a history of cervical cancer. N Engl J Med 1999;340:1383–1389.
16. Jensen PT, Groenvold M, Klee MC. Early stage cervical carcinoma, radical hysterectomy, and sexual function: a longitudinal study. Cancer 2004;100:97–106.
17. Enzlin P, Mathieu C, van DenBruel A, et al. Sexual dysfunction in women with type 1 diabetes. Diabetes Care 2002;25(4):672–677.
18. Ganz PA, Desmond KA, Bellin TR, et al. Predictors of sexual health in women after breast cancer diagnosis. J Clin Oncol 1999;17:2371–2380.
19. Sjögren Fugl-Meyer K, Fugl-Meyer AR. Sexual disabilities are not singularities. Int J Impot Res 2002;14:487–493.
20. Diamond LM. What we got wrong about sexual identity development: unexpected findings from a longitudinal study of young women. In: Omoto A, Kurtzman H, eds. Recent Research on Sexual Orientation. Washington, DC: American Psychological Association Press (in press).
21. Hartmann U, Heiser K, Rüffer-Hesse C, et al. Female sexual desire disorders: subtypes, classification, personality factors and new directions for treatment. World J Urol 2002;20:79–88.
22. Kennedy SH, Dickens SE, Eisfeld BS, et al. Sexual dysfunction before antidepressant therapy in major depression. J Affect Disord 1999;56:201–208.
23. Derogatis LR, Meyer JK, King KM. Psychopathology in individuals with sexual dysfunction. Am J Psychiatry 1981;138:757–763.

[a]*My sincere thanks to Dr. Peter Rees for his helpful review of the manuscript and to Mrs. Maureen Piper for her excellent secretarial skills.*

24. Palace EM, Gorzalka BB. The enhancing effects of anxiety on arousal in sexually dysfunctional and functional women. J Abnorm Psychol 1990;99:403–411.

25. Michelson D, Bancroft J, Targum S, et al. Female sexual dysfunction associated with antidepressant administration: a randomized, placebo controlled study of pharmacologic intervention. Am J Psychiatry 2000;157:239–243.

26. Clayton AH, Warnock JK, Kornstein SG, et al. A placebo-controlled trial of buproprion SR as an antidote for selective serotonin reuptake inhibitor-induced sexual dysfunction. J Clin Psychiatry 2004;65:62–67.

27. Townsend JM, Levy GD. Effects of potential partner's physical attractiveness and socioeconomic status on sexuality and partner selection: sex differences in reported preferences of university students. Arch Sex Behav 1990;19:149–160.

28. Townsend JM. Sex without emotional involvement: an evolutionary interpretation of sex differences. Arch Sex Behav 1995;24:171–204.

29. Basson R, Weijmar Schultz WCM, Brotto L, et al. Women's sexual dysfunction. In: Khouri S, Rosen R, Basson R, et al., eds. Second International Consultation on Sexual Medicine: Men and Women's Sexual Dysfunction. Paris: Health Publications, 2004.

30. Laan E, van Lunsen RHW. Hormones and sexuality in postmenopausal women: A psychophysiological study. J. Psychom Obstet Gynaecol 1997;18:126–133.

31. Carroll JL, Bagley DH. Evaluation of sexual satisfaction in partners of men experiencing erectile failure. J Sex Marital Ther 1990;16:70–78.

32. Hurlbert DF, Apt C, Rabehl SM. Key variables to understanding female sexual satisfaction: an examination of women in nondistressed marriages. J Sex Marital Ther 1993;19:154–165.

33. Riley A, Riley E. Behavioural and clinical findings in couples where the man presents with erectile disorder: a retrospective study. Int J Clin Pract 2000;54:220–224.

34. Salonia A, Montorsi F, Maga T, et al. Patient–partner satisfaction of sildenafil treatment in evidence-based organic erectile dysfunction. J Urol 2000;161(Suppl 4):abstract 817.

35. Müller MJ. Ruof J, Graf-Morgenstern G, et al. Quality of partnership in patients with erectile dysfunction after sildenafil treatment. Pharmacopsychiatry 2001;34:91–95.

36. Basson R, Leiblum S, Brotto L, et al. Definitions of women's sexual dysfunction reconsidered: advocating expansion and revision. J Psychosom Obstet Gynaecol 2003;24:221–220.

CHAPTER 16

Post-Traumatic Stress Disorder

Debra Kaminer, Soraya Seedat

Since the early 1980s, the impact of trauma on psychological and biologic functioning has been conceptualized in the diagnosis of post-traumatic stress disorder (PTSD). More recently, it has become apparent that PTSD describes only a limited aspect of post-traumatic adaptation. The PTSD diagnosis does not adequately capture the sequelae associated with the types of traumatization most commonly experienced by women, that is, early childhood trauma (particularly sexual abuse) and repeated, chronic trauma (such as domestic violence). This chapter reviews the current state of knowledge regarding the diagnosis, epidemiology, biology, and treatment of both PTSD and "complex PTSD" among women and offers some guidelines to mental health practitioners for assessing and treating female trauma survivors.

HISTORY OF THE PTSD DIAGNOSIS

Although post-traumatic stress has long been recognized in psychiatry, this recognition has tended to focus exclusively on either women or men at different historical junctures. It is only in recent decades that the attention of both clinicians and researchers to post-traumatic stress has encompassed both genders.

In Europe in the latter 1800s, Freud and his colleagues identified psychological trauma (particularly, sexual abuse) as the root cause of hysteria, a condition characterized by somatic symptoms without any medical basis with which many of their female patients presented (1,2). For several decades, as the origins of hysteria were examined through published clinical case studies, women were at the center of the study of psychological trauma. However, by the end of the nineteenth century, Freud had recanted his original theory on the origins of hysteria, arguing that its roots lay in intrapsychic conflict rather than real traumatic experiences, and interest in the traumatic histories of female patients gradually waned.

Indeed, through most of the twentieth century, studies of trauma focused almost exclusively on males, particularly combat survivors. The syndromes of *battle fatigue* and *shell shock* emerged from clinical observations of soldiers in the two world wars, although both public and clinical interest in these phenomena was seldom sustained enough to elicit substantial investigation. It was the Vietnam War and its impact on male American veterans that gave rise to the systematic study of combat-related post-traumatic responses during the1970s. Veterans' organizations initiated both comprehensive reviews of the existing trauma literature and large-scale investigations of the current functioning of Vietnam veterans. Findings strongly supported the existence of a post-traumatic syndrome linked to combat exposure (3), and veterans' organizations pressed the psychiatric community to develop a diagnostic category for this syndrome. Legitimization of this diagnosis provided veterans with both recognition for their suffering and access to treatment resources.

The 1970s also saw the emergence of a complementary popular political movement that, for the first time in decades, brought the traumatic experiences of women to both public and clinical attention. Within the context of the feminist movement, research on the prevalence and impact of rape, domestic violence, and sexual abuse began to enter the psychiatric literature. These studies demonstrated the endemic nature of gender-based violence and identified both a "rape trauma syndrome" and a "battered woman syndrome," which included many of the symptoms reported in studies of combat veterans as well as a range of other symptoms (1,2).

When the American Psychiatric Association (APA) met in the late 1970s to consider a post-trauma diagnosis for inclusion in the third edition of the *Diagnostic and Statistical Manual of Mental Disorders* (DSM-III) (4), advocates of both male Vietnam veterans and female survivors of male-perpetrated violence pressed for recognition of the syndromes documented among their populations of interest. The diagnosis post-traumatic stress disorder (PTSD), when it was included in DSM III in 1980, was something of a compromise that attempted to subsume under a single diagnostic category the varied post-trauma syndromes that had been reported among these diverse populations of trauma survivors (2).

Subsequent empirical data have confirmed that the PTSD diagnosis accurately describes the responses of many women who have survived a single traumatic event. However, it has become increasingly apparent that the diagnosis fails to capture adequately the complex adaptations of survivors of early and prolonged trauma, particularly of female survivors of childhood sexual abuse (1,5), who make up 17% of adult women in the general population (6). The following section discusses the diagnostic criteria for PTSD, as well as recent attempts to formally categorize the complexity of post-traumatic responses typical of female survivors of chronic violence.

DIAGNOSTIC ISSUES

DIAGNOSTIC CRITERIA FOR PTSD

The diagnostic criteria for PTSD, as conceptualized in the current editions of the DSM (DSM IV-TR, 7) and the World Health Organization's International Classification of Diseases (ICD-10, 8), include a stressor dimension, three core symptom clusters, and duration and disability specifications.

The first criterion for the PTSD diagnosis relates to the nature of traumatic exposure. DSM IV-TR specifies that the person should have directly experienced or witnessed an event involving actual or threatened death, serious injury, or threat to physical integrity or learned about unexpected or violent death, serious harm, or threat to physical safety experienced by a loved one (criterion A1). Furthermore, the person's response to this event should have involved intense fear, helplessness, or horror (criterion A2). ICD-10 also delineates the nature of the stressor; however, like earlier versions of the DSM, it describes these events as exceptionally threatening or catastrophic and likely to cause distress to almost anyone.

The three core symptom clusters of PTSD capture the dialectic between hyperremembering and forgetting that characterizes the daily experience of many survivors of extreme trauma. The first cluster specifies that the traumatic event should intrude into the person's present functioning, causing the person to reexperience the event constantly. Reexperiencing or intrusive symptoms include distressing memories (thoughts, images, or perceptions), recurring dreams about the event, and a physiologic fear reaction or intense psychological distress when exposed to reminders of the trauma. Although less common, dissociative flashback experiences in which the trauma survivor actually relives aspects of the trauma in the here and now, in vivid sensory detail, are often considered to be the hallmark symptom of PTSD. The second symptom cluster requires that the person, *in addition* to having vivid remembrances of the event, also avoids reexperiencing the event. Avoidance symptoms may involve active efforts to avoid thoughts, feelings, and conversations about the trauma and activities, people, and places that are reminders of the trauma. Although avoidance may initially focus on direct reminders of the trauma (e.g., the actual place where it occurred), through a process of behavioral conditioning it may eventually generalize to a broad range of stimuli associated with these reminders (e.g., places similar to that where the trauma occurred and any stimuli that come to be associated with these places) (9). Avoidance symptoms may also include amnesia for important aspects of the trauma and emotional numbing that results in an inability to experience either painful or pleasant feelings. Also categorized under avoidance symptoms are a reduced interest in significant activities, feelings of detachment or estrangement from others, and a sense of a foreshortened future. The final symptom cluster specifies that the person should be in a state of persistent physiologic hyperarousal (as if permanently poised for fight or flight), as indicated by difficulty falling asleep, impaired concentration, hypervigilance to threat, an exaggerated startle response to loud noises or sudden movements, and irritability or outbursts of anger. ICD-10 requires intrusive symptoms to be present in order to make the diagnosis, but avoidance and hyperarousal symptoms are not required.

Since many of these symptoms are commonly experienced by trauma survivors in the days and weeks following the event, a diagnosis of the disorder according to DSM IV-TR further requires that the three symptom clusters should be present for longer than one month following the trauma and should cause clinically significant distress or impairment in social, occupational, or other important areas of functioning. Both DSM IV-TR and ICD-10 also provide for a diagnosis of acute stress disorder (ASD), in which PTSD symptoms are present for less than one month following the trauma. According to DSM IV-TR, the person must have experienced a number of dissociative phenomena during the traumatic event in order to meet this diagnosis, whereas ICD-10 emphasizes the depressive and anxiety components of ASD and the mixed and labile nature of the symptoms.

COMORBIDITY

Among both men and women, PTSD is seldom the sole diagnosis; comorbid diagnoses are common. The following comorbid disorders are highly prevalent among women in the general population who also meet diagnostic criteria for PTSD (10,11): major depressive disorder (17%–23% of women with PTSD), panic disorder (13%), specific phobia (36%), generalized anxiety disorder (GAD) (38%), and substance abuse (28% for alcohol abuse and 27% for drug abuse).

A perusal of the three symptom clusters of PTSD reveals a substantial degree of overlap with the symptoms of these comorbid disorders, including the withdrawal, emotional numbing, and vegetative symptoms of depression; the physiologic reactivity and behavioral avoidance that characterize panic disorder and specific phobia; the physiologic hyperarousal of generalized anxiety disorder; and the obsessive ruminations of obsessive compulsive disorder (OCD). These diagnostic overlaps present several pitfalls for accurate diagnosis and treatment of female trauma survivors. Upon assessment, the presence of comorbid disorders may mask the presence of PTSD, resulting in a failure to diagnose and treat the latter (12); alternatively, when the person being examined has a known history of trauma, the clinician may be too quick to attribute all reported symptoms to PTSD, thus failing to assess the person for other comorbid conditions that may require treatment.

The relationship between the core symptoms of PTSD and the manifold comorbid symptoms that frequently accompany these in female trauma survivors is unclear. Two possibilities are that comorbid disorders such as depression and substance abuse may predate and create a vulnerability for trauma exposure and PTSD and that PTSD may enhance the risk of developing secondary disorders (e.g., women may develop major depression or substance abuse in response to the impairment and distress caused by PTSD). However, prospective studies are needed in order to establish the order of onset of PTSD and comorbid disorders (10).

COMPLEX ADAPTATIONS TO TRAUMA

Clinicians working with female survivors of child sexual abuse have long noted a range of presenting symptoms that are not captured by the criteria for PTSD diagnostic or those disorders commonly found to be comorbid with PTSD (1). In the past decade, there have been some attempts to include these phenomena in the psychiatric nomenclature. The DSM IV field trials found that people who had experienced childhood trauma and chronic traumatization in childhood or adulthood reported a disparate range of symptoms and psychological adjustments that are distinct from the symptoms of PTSD (5). These symptoms include impairments in affect regulation, alterations in attention and consciousness, somatization, characterologic changes, and alterations in systems of meaning (see Table 16.1). Consequently, a diagnostic category of "disorders of extreme stress not otherwise specified" (DESNOS; 5), also referred to as complex PTSD (1), was proposed for inclusion in the fourth edition of DSM. The DESNOS symptoms were eventually incorporated into DSM-IV (13) in the section "Associated Features and Disorders" under PTSD rather than as a separate diagnostic category. A subsequent study of combat veterans (14) found DESNOS and PTSD to be distinct disorders that are often comorbid, but this finding awaits replication with female samples.

ICD-10 has captured many of the DESNOS symptoms in a diagnostic category for enduring personality changes after catastrophic experience, which includes permanent hostility and distrust, social withdrawal, feelings of emptiness and hopelessness, increased dependency, and problems with modulation of aggression, hypervigilance and irritability, and feelings of alienation.

What happens to female patients with a history of early or repeated abuse who present to the mental health system with the confusing array of symptoms described by the DESNOS criteria? Frequently, clinicians have diagnosed these patients with a mixed bag of borderline personality disorder (BPD), dissociative

---

TABLE 16.1

Proposed Criteria for Disorders of Extreme Stress Not Otherwise Specified (DESNOS)

A. Alterations in regulating affective arousal
   1. Chronic affect dysregulation
   2. Difficulty modulating anger
   3. Self-destructive and suicidal behavior
   4. Difficulty modulating sexual involvement
   5. Impulsive and risk-taking behaviors
B. Alterations in attention and consciousness
   1. Amnesia
   2. Dissociation
C. Somatization
D. Chronic characterologic changes
   1. Alterations in self-perception: chronic guilt and shame; feelings of self-blame, of ineffectiveness, and of being permanently damaged
   2. Alterations in perception of perpetrator: adopting distorted beliefs and idealizing the perpetrator
   3. Alterations in relationships with others
      a. Inability to trust or maintain relationships with others
      b. Tendency to be revictimized
      c. Tendency to victimize others
E. Alterations in systems of meaning
   1. Despair and hopelessness
   2. Loss of previously sustaining beliefs

Reprinted from van der Kolk BA. The complexity of adaptation to trauma. In: van der Kolk BA, McFarlane AC, Weisaeth L, eds. Traumatic Stress: The Effects of Overwhelming Experience on Mind, Body, and Society. New York: Guilford, 1996:203.

identity disorder (DID), and somatization disorder, because the criteria for each of these disorders focus on some aspects of complex PTSD (DESNOS criterion A, criterion B, and criterion C, respectively), while de-emphasizing others (1).

The fact that there is no unitary diagnostic category that encompasses all the DESNOS symptoms has significant implications for diagnosis and treatment. There is the danger of misdiagnosis. For example, a recent study (15) found that while BPD may sometimes be a distinct comorbid diagnosis among sexual abuse survivors with complex PTSD symptoms, other survivors diagnosed with BPD could more appropriately be diagnosed with complex PTSD. Additionally, patients with DESNOS symptoms may find themselves labeled with a different diagnosis by different clinicians at different times.

The treatment implications of this diagnostic confusion are manifold. First, the link between the symptoms of disorder and their traumatogenic roots becomes obscured. Whereas a diagnosis of PTSD automatically identifies a traumatic experience as the central cause and an important focus for treatment, multiple non-PTSD diagnoses disguise the causal role of previous trauma. Without the recognition of a common etiologic root for the varied symptoms with which the patient presents, intervention becomes fragmented and unfocused and is unlikely to effect therapeutic change. Second, mental health practitioners and organizations are often reluctant to invest time, energy, and other resources in treating patients with diagnoses such as somatization disorders, BPD, and DID, which have notoriously poor prognoses, and may try to refer them elsewhere. Even when they attempt treatment, the association of these disorders with unstable and manipulative behavior on the part of the patient tends to impair the degree of empathy with which clinicians relate to such patients (1,5).

Because of the accumulation of these processes, it is common for clinicians to respond with wariness, frustration, and anger toward female patients with this diagnostic profile, which results in patients being medicated against their will, placed in seclusion, or transferred without warning to another facility (5). This retraumatization of the patient can partly be understood as an unconscious process in which the clinician or clinical team is drawn into the patient's compulsion to recreate the original abusive relationship in the therapeutic relationship. However, the absence of an appropriate post-traumatic diagnosis precludes accurate recognition of this abusive reenactment and limits the possibility of establishing an empathic therapeutic relationship with the patient that acknowledges her past experiences of abuse and the ways in which her adaptations to this abuse impair her present functioning (1).

EPIDEMIOLOGY

Epidemiologic studies have revealed three gender patterns in traumatic exposure and PTSD prevalence that are consistent across the countries and age groups sampled. First, exposure to at least one trauma and cumulative exposure to trauma are significantly higher among men than women (see Table 16.2). Second, women and men are exposed to very different types of trauma: women are far more likely than men to be exposed to rape or sexual abuse, while men are more likely to be exposed to physical assault, military combat, or accidents (11,16–18).

Although seldom specifically assessed in epidemiologic surveys of trauma exposure, recent studies indicate that PTSD can develop as the result of medical experiences unique to women, in particular childbirth trauma (19) and breast cancer

TABLE 16.2

Gender Differences in Trauma Exposure, Prevalence of PTSD, and Conditional Risk for PTSD: Epidemiologic Findings

Study	Country	n	Age Range (years)	Lifetime Trauma Exposure (%)		PTSD Prevalence (%)		Lifetime Conditional Risk for PTSD (%)	
				Men	Women	Men	Women	Men	Women
National Comorbidity Survey, 1995 (11)	United States	5,877	15–44	60.7	51.2	5	10.4	8.2	20.4
Detroit Area Survey of Trauma, 1998 (16)	United States	2,181	18–45	92.2	87.1	10.2	18.3	9.5	17.7
South German Survey on Early Developmental Stages of Psychopathology, 1999 (17)	Germany	3,021	14–24	18.6	15.5	0.4	2.2	2.2	14.5
Norris, Foster, Weisshaar, 2002 (18)	Mexico	1,289	18–92	83	74	9	16	8	20

diagnosis and treatment (20). Third, despite the higher rates of overall trauma exposure among men, prevalence rates of PTSD in the general population, as well as the conditional risk of developing PTSD after exposure, are higher in both girls and women (see Table 16.2). It also appears that PTSD symptoms are more chronic in women than in men (averaging four years from onset to remission, compared with one year for men; 16).

Several explanations for these findings have been advanced. First, aspects of traumatic exposure may play a role. Women are more vulnerable to physical injury during trauma exposure than men, and a greater degree of perceived life threat and actual injury have been found to discriminate PTSD status in women (21,22). Additionally, for both genders sexual violence is associated with the highest conditional risk for PTSD of all forms of trauma exposure (11,16). Since rates of exposure to sexual violence are far higher in women than in men, increased exposure to this most noxious form of trauma may account for the sex difference (18). Second, as with other disorders, the gender difference in PTSD may be influenced by social factors. It has been proposed that women may report post-traumatic symptoms such as fearfulness (criterion A2) and avoidance behavior more readily than men due to social role expectations that encourage expressions of vulnerability, helplessness, and passivity in women but discourage them in men (18). Indeed, recent data confirm that the higher rate of post-traumatic symptoms reported by women as compared to men is more pronounced in societies that hold traditional views of masculinity and femininity, and (although present) less pronounced in societies with less clearly delineated sex role expectations (23). Since women in many societies are more disempowered than men politically, economically, and educationally, it has also been suggested that women's heightened vulnerability to PTSD after trauma may stem from ongoing experiences of poverty, discrimination, and oppression, which reduce women's capacity to cope (18). Biologic factors may also contribute to women's increased vulnerability to PTSD; these are discussed in the following section.

To date, there are no epidemiologic data on the general population prevalence of either DESNOS or ICD-10's category for enduring personality changes after catastrophic experience.

NEUROBIOLOGIC AND NEUROANATOMICAL CORRELATES OF PTSD

Over the past decade, improved tools have permitted investigation of the complex interplay between traumatic exposure and the structural and functional neuroanatomy and neurochemistry of PTSD. Neurobiologic systems that appear to be altered by trauma and that may underlie the symptom formation in PTSD include neuroendocrine (hypothalamic-pituitary-adrenal axis), sympathetic, serotonergic, noradrenergic, glutamatergic, opioid, and GABAergic pathways (24). While the normal stress response is characterized by increase in cortisol and catecholamine levels in dose-dependent fashion, individuals with PTSD have paradoxically low circulating levels of cortisol. Gender and reproductive status may affect the pattern of hypothalamic-pituitary-adrenal (HPA) axis adaptation to stress. Studies in premenopausal women with PTSD have consistently documented high 24-hour urinary cortisol levels or a trend toward high levels, which indicates increased cortisol output (25).

Serum cortisol levels are also lower in the acute post-trauma period in those who subsequently develop PTSD than in those who do not. For example, cortisol levels were lower in women with a history of previous assault in the immediate aftermath of rape than in women with no prior assault history. Perhaps not surprising, prior assault was associated with a higher risk of PTSD regardless of rape severity (26). These findings suggest that the HPA axis may be permanently sensitized after exposure to early life stress such that subsequent responses to stress are affected. Therefore, HPA axis adaptation may partly account for why only a subset of trauma-exposed individuals develops PTSD. In one study, women who were currently depressed and had a history of childhood abuse had significantly greater pituitary-adrenal and heart rate responses to stress compared with control subjects (27). Furthermore, 85% of abused, depressed women in the sample met criteria for PTSD compared with 36% abused, nondepressed women.

In terms of structural abnormalities, a growing literature indicates that the hippocampus, which plays a critical role in learning and memory, is abnormal in PTSD. A variety of mechanisms have been proposed: Sapolsky (28) has shown in animal studies that high levels of cortisol released during stress can cause neurotoxic damage to hippocampal neurons. Of note, several magnetic resonance imaging (MRI) studies have demonstrated smaller hippocampal volumes in both men and women with PTSD. The findings are suggestive of more pronounced left-sided deficits in women and right-sided deficits in men. A quantitative MRI study of women with severe childhood sexual abuse (71% of whom fulfilled criteria for PTSD), found reductions in left hippocampal volume (5%) in abused women compared with nonabused women (29). Left hippocampal volume reduction correlated highly with dissociative symptoms. In contrast, Bremner et al. (30) found reductions in right hippocampal volume (8%) in male combat veterans with PTSD (n = 26) compared with healthy veterans without the disorder who were matched for age, drug and alcohol abuse, and combat experience.

Bilateral hippocampal volume reductions have also been observed in women with and without early childhood abuse (with and without PTSD) (31) and in men with combat-related PTSD (31). Bremner and colleagues (32) were the first to provide converging evidence of structural and functional hippocampal disturbance in PTSD. Abused women with PTSD had significantly lower volumes of the hippocampus (left and right) compared with either abused women without PTSD or healthy controls. In women with PTSD, the left hippocampus was not activated during a verbal memory task. Partially consistent with findings by Stein et al. (29), smaller left hippocampal volumes correlate with dissociative symptoms while smaller right hippocampal volumes correlate with PTSD symptoms. Moreover, deficits in hippocampal structure and function in women with PTSD were specific to a PTSD diagnosis and not a specific outcome of child abuse exposure. It should be noted that studies of women with intimate partner violence and PTSD and maltreated children and adolescents with PTSD have not found smaller hippocampal volumes. Other sex differences have been noted in pediatric PTSD, with maltreated boys showing more evidence of global adverse brain development than girls (33).

Findings from functional imaging studies (positron emission tomography) in women with childhood sexual abuse and PTSD have consistently implicated the hippocampus, amygdala (important for fear responses and emotional salience), medial prefrontal cortex, and anterior cingulate (responsible for modulation of emotional responses). For example, in studies asking women to perform emotionally valenced declarative memory tasks, greater activation was seen in this brain network in abused women with PTSD than in either women with abuse without PTSD or nonabused women (34).

In summary, a number of studies have demonstrated PTSD-specific gender differences; however, similarities far outweigh differences in men and women with the disorder. It should be noted that in traumatized children with PTSD, sex differences are small relative to the developmental variability in the volume of brain structures (33). To answer the question of whether sex differences in neurobiologic abnormalities are a consequence of trauma exposure or a preexisting risk factor for PTSD, future investigations will need to focus on the longitudinal course of the relationship between neurobiology, gender, and trauma outcome.

TREATMENT

PHARMACOTHERAPY

Trials of various antidepressant agents in treatment of PTSD have documented the efficacy of selective serotonin reuptake inhibitors (SSRIs), monoamine oxidase inhibitors (MAOIs), and tricyclic antidepressants (TCAs). In view of their ease of use, lower risk of overdose, and superior tolerability, SSRIs are currently advocated as first-line treatment. SSRIs are broad-spectrum agents that, in addition to reducing core PTSD symptoms, have documented efficacy in disorders that are often comorbid with PTSD, such as major depression and panic disorder (35).

Hormonal fluctuations (associated with menses, menopause, oral contraceptive use, or hormone replacement therapy) may have an impact on the pharmacokinetics and pharmacodynamics of drug therapy, and this needs to be borne in mind when treating women. Many of the major neurotransmitter systems implicated (e.g., serotonin, noradrenaline, dopamine, GABA) are subject to modulation by female sex hormones and are, therefore, potential targets for pharmacologic interventions. For example, gender-related metabolic factors may affect SSRI metabolism through various cytochrome P450 enzymes resulting in clinically relevant alterations in plasma concentrations. Some data suggest that women may respond more favorably to SSRIs and men more favorably to TCAs (36).

Randomized, controlled investigation of the SSRIs sertraline (37), paroxetine (38), and fluoxetine (39) have demonstrated efficacy in large samples of women with chronic PTSD secondary to rape or physical assault. In one mixed-sex study (40), long-term (9–12 months) paroxetine treatment was associated not only with significant improvement in PTSD symptoms but also with an increase in hippocampal volumes, although no gender differences were noted. These findings suggest that SSRIs may also be effective in reversing stress-induced hippocampal damage in PTSD. The Food and Drug Administration has approved both sertraline and paroxetine for treatment of PTSD.

Some of the newer antidepressants also show promise. In male combat veterans with PTSD, open-label studies of the serotonergic agents trazodone and nefazodone have shown benefits in treating sleep, nightmares, agitation, and other intrusive and hyperarousal symptoms of PTSD (35). Mirtazapine, a drug with dual noradrenergic and serotonergic effects, was superior to placebo in a small randomized trial of chronic PTSD patients (58% female) (41). This drug may be useful either as monotherapy or an adjunct to SSRIs in partial responders.

Several open trials have suggested the efficacy of TCAs in treating the intrusive but not avoidant or numbing symptoms of PTSD. Additionally, two 8-week randomized, controlled trials have demonstrated the efficacy of imipramine and amitriptyline (35). However, these trials were conducted in combat veterans and did not include women. The high incidence of adverse effects and risk of over-dose do not make these first-line agents in PTSD.

Monoamine oxidase inhibitors (MAOIs) have been mainly investigated in controlled studies of male combat veterans. Four placebo-controlled trials (two of phenelzine and two of brofaromine, an MAO-A plus serotonin reuptake inhibitor) have produced mixed findings (35). The side-effect profile (risk of hypertensive crisis) along with dietary and drug restrictions preclude the use of these drugs as first-line or second-line agents. Moclobemide, a reversible MAO-A inhibitor that is relatively free of the limitations of the conventional MAOIs, was shown in a 12-week open-label study to improve all three PTSD symptom clusters (42).

Buspirone, a 5-HT$_1$A partial agonist with a low potential for abuse and with-drawal, has also shown efficacy in dosages ranging from 5 mg/day to 60 mg/day. Anticonvulsants and mood stabilizers (e.g., carbamazepine, valproate, lithium, gabapentin, vigabatrin, lamotrigine, and topiramate) have been shown to be effective in PTSD either as monotherapy or as an add-on or for chronic PTSD (35). In addition, atypical antipsychotic drugs (e.g., risperidone, olanzapine) may be useful in patients whose symptoms do not respond to treatment (35). Benzodi-azepines are commonly prescribed in clinical practice for PTSD because of their proven efficacy as anxiolytics. In view of their abuse potential and the risks of rebound anxiety and withdrawal (which may exacerbate PTSD symptoms), these agents should be used with caution.

Few trials have explored the efficacy and safety of long-term treatment in PTSD. To date, sertraline is the only SSRI investigated both in 24-week open-label continuation and 28-week relapse-prevention trials (43). Continued treatment with sertraline was effective in reducing relapse and sustaining improvements in quality of life and psychosocial functioning.

PSYCHOTHERAPEUTIC MANAGEMENT

An important initial concern in the psychotherapeutic management of trauma survivors is establishing both their physical safety (this is particularly important if the woman is living in a context of ongoing abuse) and a sense of emotional safety in the therapeutic relationship before proceeding with intervention (1). Thereafter, a number of psychotherapeutic techniques have demonstrated efficacy in reducing the symptoms of PTSD.

Using behavior therapy techniques, exposure therapies for PTSD aim to habit-uate the anxiety related to the traumatic event through repeated exposure to both traumatic memories and external traumatic reminders (44). The therapist trains the client in breathing and muscle relaxation strategies, which the client employs at each stage of exposure in order to manage anxiety. Additionally, maladaptive cognitive appraisals that arise during exposure may be identified and modified. Exposure therapy continues until the client is able to think about the trauma and to encounter real-life traumatic reminders without feeling intense anxiety or engaging in avoidance strategies.

Exposure may take the form of systematic desensitization, where the therapist together with the client constructs a graded hierarchy of feared cues associated with the traumatic event; once the client has mastered exposure to the least feared cue (using relaxation and cognitive strategies), exposure to the next cue on the hi-erarchy graded exposure can proceed (45). A more recent development in expo-sure therapy for trauma survivors is prolonged exposure (PE), which consists of repeated exposure to the entire traumatic memory over several sessions, again in combination with cognitive modification, as well as gradual exposure to external traumatic reminders (46). The efficacy of these relatively short-term (9–20 sessions) cognitive-behavior therapies for PTSD and for some comorbid disorders such as depression has been demonstrated repeatedly with female survivors of both childhood and adult abuse and, furthermore, these PTSD interventions appear to benefit women even more than men (47). This suggests that cognitive-behavior therapy (CBT) is the psychotherapeutic intervention of choice for women with PTSD. While short-term CBT techniques are clearly effective in reducing PTSD among women who have experienced both single traumatic episodes and repeated abuse, the effect of CBT techniques on more complex post-traumatic adaptations such as DESNOS symptoms is still unclear, since outcome studies have seldom measured changes in these symptoms.

In recent years, researchers have also examined the efficacy of eye-movement desensitization and reprocessing (EMDR). This technique combines exposure and cognitive modification with lateral eye movements that are theorized to accelerate the processing of trauma-related information (48). It has been proposed that the constant reorienting of attention in EMDR activates those areas of the brain (anterior cingulate, amygdala, hippocampus, orbital frontal cortex, and visual cortex) that are also activated (a) in patients with PTSD exposed to script-driven imagery and (b) in REM (Rapid Eye Movement) sleep. Activation of these brain areas during EMDR is thought to produce shifts in memory processing similar to that of REM sleep. Thus, the REM-like state induced by EMDR might facilitate the integration of traumatic memories seen in PTSD (49). Although many controlled studies of EMDR have used samples of male combat veterans, the efficacy of this treatment has also been established with some female samples (50). However, the benefits of EMDR for survivors of prolonged and repeated trauma, rather than a single trauma, are yet to be established.

RECOMMENDATIONS FOR ASSESSMENT AND TREATMENT

A central challenge for mental health professionals lies in correctly identifying female survivors of prolonged and repeated trauma, who may not present with "pure" PTSD or disclose previous traumatization unless asked about it specifically. Sensitive and thorough assessment is necessary in order to explore the trauma histories of all female patients presenting with a mixed bag of diagnoses. Additionally, the high prevalence of comorbid disorders among women with PTSD and the overlap of these comorbid disorders with DESNOS symptoms require clinicians to conduct a careful and thorough differential diagnosis with all female patients who have a known history of trauma. Assessment of DESNOS criteria may be facilitated by the Structured Interview for Disorders of Extreme Stress (SIDES; 51).

With regard to choice of treatment, the following guidelines are offered. Psychotherapy should be the treatment of choice when PTSD symptoms are mild, but psychotherapy in combination with medication may be used for more severe symptoms. With regard to the psychotherapy component, exploration of the trauma in the context of an empathic therapeutic relationship should form an essential part of the treatment plan for women with pure PTSD, PTSD with comorbid disorders, or complex post-traumatic adaptations. The efficacy of trauma exploration through exposure therapy has been demonstrated repeatedly among women with PTSD. However, for women with complex PTSD, the exploration and integration of traumatic memories may be a long and gradual process and should include explorations of the ways in which current stressors are experienced as the return of past traumas, careful reconstruction of the trauma narrative in manageable doses, mourning the losses associated with the abuse, and slowly reestablishing trust in others (1,5).

With respect to pharmacotherapy, SSRIs are the first-line treatment and should be started at a low dose with slow up-titration to an average target dose: 20–50 mg for paroxetine and fluoxetine, 50–150 mg for sertraline, 100–250 mg for fluvoxamine, and 20–40 mg for citalopram. Onset of action on core PTSD symptoms is usually two to four weeks (52). In pregnant or breastfeeding women, pharmacotherapy should be avoided as much as possible. In cases of necessity, SSRIs may be administered, because these drugs do not pose an increased risk of major fetal malformation. Sertraline, paroxetine, citalopram, and fluvoxamine all appear to be compatible with breastfeeding.

For patients with severe PTSD symptoms who experience only a partial response to medication, treatment can be augmented with another medication (preferably a mood stabilizer such as divalproex). For patients who fail to respond to initial treatment over 12 weeks or who are unable to tolerate SSRIs, switching to a MAOI, TCA, or venlafaxine may be effective (52). Once patients have been stabilized, medication should be continued for at least 12 months in the case of acute PTSD and at least 24 months in the case of chronic PTSD. In patients whose symptoms are refractory to treatment (i.e., little or no response to multiple adequate trials of medication and psychotherapy), it is important to evaluate for causes of nonresponse to the medication (e.g., substance abuse problems, psychiatric comorbidity) before trying a different medication combination (e.g., antidepressant plus mood stabilizer *or* antidepressant plus antipsychotic *or* two antidepressants) (52).

CONCLUSION

Current research suggests that women are particularly vulnerable to developing PTSD after traumatization and that those who experience early or prolonged abuse may present to mental health settings with symptoms of complex PTSD. Careful assessment is necessary to establish whether female trauma survivors meet criteria for diagnosis of PTSD, PTSD with comorbid disorders, complex PTSD, or a combination of these. Evidence from studies of the outcomes of treatment with psychotherapy and pharmacotherapy indicates that women with PTSD are responsive to a number of intervention strategies. With regard to future research directions, a better understanding of the pathophysiologic mechanisms that underlie both PTSD and complex PTSD in women may ultimately lead to more focused pharmacologic treatments. Inclusion of complex PTSD symptoms in both pharmacotherapy and psychotherapy outcome studies is necessary for the development of effective treatments for survivors of early and prolonged trauma. Until then, clinician awareness of the diverse and multifaceted sequelae of traumatization will facilitate effective and sensitive treatment of female trauma survivors.

REFERENCES

1. Herman J. Trauma and Recovery: From Domestic Abuse to Political Terror. London: Pandora, 1992.
2. Van der Kolk BA, Weisaeth L, van der Hart O. History of trauma in psychiatry. In: van der Kolk BA, McFarlane AC, Weisaeth L, eds. Traumatic Stress: The Effects of Overwhelming Experience on Mind, Body, and Society. New York: Guilford, 1996:47–74.

3. Egendorf A, Kadushin C, Lanfer RS, et al. Legacies of Vietnam, vols. 1–5. Washington, DC: US Government Printing Office, 1981.

4. American Psychiatric Association. Diagnostic and Statistical Manual of Mental Disorders, 3rd Ed. Washington, DC, 1980.

5. van der Kolk BA. The complexity of adaptation to trauma. In: van der Kolk BA, McFarlane AC, Weisaeth L, eds. Traumatic Stress: The Effects of Overwhelming Experience on Mind, Body, and Society. New York: Guilford, 1996:182–213.

6. Putnam F. Ten-year research update review: child sexual abuse. J Am Acad Child Adolesc Psychiatry 2003;42:269–278.

7. American Psychiatric Association. Diagnostic and Statistical Manual of Mental Disorders, 4th Ed., text rev. Washington, DC, 2002.

8. World Health Organization (WHO). International Classification of Diseases, 10th Ed. Geneva, 1992.

9. Keane TM, Zimering RT, Caddell JM. A behavioral formulation of posttraumatic stress disorder in Vietnam veterans. Behav Ther 1985;8:9–12.

10. Orsillo SM, Raja S, Hammond C. Gender issues in PTSD with comorbid mental health disorders. In: Kimmerling R, Ouimette P, Wolfe J, eds. Gender and PTSD. New York: Guilford, 2002:207–231.

11. Kessler R, Sonnega A, Bromet E, et al. Posttraumatic stress disorder in the National Comorbidity Survey. Arch Gen Psychiatry 1995;52:1048–1060.

12. Zimmerman M, Mattia JI. Psychiatric diagnosis in clinical practice: is comorbidity being missed? Compr Psychiatry 1999;40:182–191.

13. American Psychiatric Association. Diagnostic and Statistical Manual of Mental Disorders, 4th Ed. Washington, DC, 1994.

14. Ford JD. Disorders of extreme stress following war-zone military trauma: associated features of posttraumatic stress disorder or comorbid but distinct syndromes? J Cons Clin Psychol 1999;67:3–12.

15. McClean LM, Gallop R. Implications of childhood sexual abuse for adult borderline personality disorder and complex posttraumatic stress disorder. Am J Psychiatry 2003;160:369–371.

16. Breslau N, Kessler R, Chilcoat H, et al. Trauma and posttraumatic stress disorder in the community: the 1996 Detroit Area Survey of Trauma. Arch Gen Psychiatry 1998;55:627–632.

17. Perkonnig A, Wittchen H. Prevalence and comorbidity of traumatic events and posttraumatic stress disorder in adolescents and young adults. In: Maercker A, Schutzwohl M, Solomon Z, eds. Post-Traumatic Stress Disorder: A Lifespan Developmental Perspective. Kirkland, WA: Hogrefe and Huber, 1999:113–133.

18. Norris FH, Foster JD, Weisshaar DL. The epidemiology of sex differences in PTSD across developmental, societal and research contexts. In: Kimerling R, Ouimette P, Wolfe J, eds. Gender and PTSD. New York: Guilford, 2002:3–42.

19. Ayers S, Pickering AD. Do women get posttraumatic stress disorder as a result of childbirth? A prospective study of incidence. Birth 2001;28:111–118.

20. Andrykowski MA, Cordova MJ, Studts JL, et al. Posttraumatic stress disorder after treatment for breast cancer: prevalence of diagnosis and use of the PTSD Checklist-Civilian Version (PCL-C) as a screening instrument. J Cons Clin Psychol 1998;66:586–590.

21. Resnick HS, Kilpatrick DG, Best CL, et al. Vulnerability-stress factors in development of posttraumatic stress disorder. J Nerv Ment Dis 1992;180:424–430.

22. Epstein JN, Saunders BE, Kilpatrick DG. Predicting PTSD in women with a history of childhood rape. J Traumatic Stress 1997;10:573–588.

23. Norris F, Perilla J, Ibañez G, et al. Sex differences in symptoms of post-traumatic stress: does culture play a role? J Traumatic Stress 2001;14:7–28.

24. Vermetten E, Bremner JD. Circuits and systems in stress. II. Applications to neurobiology and treatment in posttraumatic stress disorder. Depress Anxiety 2002;16:14–38.

25. Rasmusson AM, Vythilingam M, Morgan CA. The neuroendocrinology of posttraumatic stress disorder: new directions. CNS Spectr 2003;8:651–656, 665–667.

26. Resnick HS, Yehuda R, Pitman RK, et al. Effect of previous trauma on acute plasma cortisol level following rape. Am J Psychiatry 1995;152:1675–1677.

27. Heim C, Newport DJ, Heit S, et al. Pituitary-adrenal and autonomic responses to stress in women after sexual and physical abuse in childhood. JAMA 2000;284:592–597.

28. Sapolsky RM. Glucocorticoids and hippocampal atrophy in neuropsychiatric disorders. Arch Gen Psychiatry 2000;57:925–935.

29. Stein MB, Koverola C, Hanna C, et al. Hippocampal volume in women victimized by childhood sexual abuse. Psychol Med 1997;27:951–959.

30. Bremner JD, Randall P, Scott TM, et al. MRI-based measurement of hippocampal volume in patients with combat-related posttraumatic stress disorder. Am J Psychiatry 1995;152:973–981.

31. Gurvits TV, Shenton ME, Hokama C, et al. Magnetic resonance imaging study of hippocampal volume in chronic, combat-related posttraumatic stress disorder. Biol Psychiatry 1996;40:1091–1099.

32. Bremner JD, Vythilingam M, Vermetten E, et al. MRI and PET study of deficits in hippocampal structure and function in women with childhood sexual abuse and posttraumatic stress disorder. Am J Psychiatry 2003a;160:924–932.

33. De Bellis MD, Keshavan MS. Sex differences in brain maturation in maltreatment-related pediatric posttraumatic stress disorder. Neurosci Biobehav Rev 2003;27:103–117.

34. Bremner JD, Vythilingam M, Vermetten E, et al. Neural correlates of declarative memory for emotionally valenced words in women with posttraumatic stress disorder related to early childhood abuse. Biol Psychiatry 2003b;53:879–889.

35. Albucher RC, Liberzon I. Psychopharmacological treatment in PTSD: a critical review. J Psychiatr Res 2002;36:355–367.

36. Kornstein SG, Schatzberg AF, Thase ME, et al. Gender differences in treatment response to sertraline versus imipramine in chronic depression. Am J Psychiatry 2000;157:1445–1452.

37. Brady KT, Pearlstein T, Asnis GM, et al. Efficacy and safety of sertraline treatment of posttraumatic stress disorder. JAMA 2000;283:1837–1844.

38. Stein DJ, Davidson J, Seedat S, et al. Paroxetine in the treatment of post–traumatic stress disorder: pooled analysis of placebo-controlled studies. Expert Opin Pharmacother 2003;4: 1829–1838.

39. Connor KM, Sutherland SM, Tupler LA, et al. Fluoxetine in post-traumatic stress disorder. Br J Psychiatry 1999;175:17–22.

40. Vermetten E, Vythilingam M, Southwick SM, et al. Long-term treatment with paroxetine increases verbal declarative memory and hippocampal volume in posttraumatic stress disorder. Biol Psychiatry 2003;54:693–702.

41. Davidson JRT, Weisler RH, Butterfield MI, et al. Mirtazapine vs placebo in posttraumatic stress disorder: a pilot trial. Biol Psychiatry 2003;53:188–191.

42. Neal LA, Shapland W, Fox C. An open trial of moclobemide in the treatment of post-traumatic stress disorder. Int Clin Psychopharmacol 1997;12:231–237.

43. Stein DJ, Bandelow B, Hollander E, et al. WCA recommendations for the long-term treatment of posttraumatic stress disorder. CNS Spectr 2003;8 (Suppl 1):31–39.

44. Rothbaum BO, Meadows EA, Resick P, et al. Cognitive-behavioral therapy. In: Foa E, Keane TM, Friedman MJ, eds. Effective Treatments for PTSD. New York: Guilford, 2000:60–83.

45. Brom D, Kleber RJ, Defares PB. Brief psychotherapy for posttraumatic stress disorders. J Cons Clin Psychol 1989;57:607–612.

46. Foa EB, Rothbaum BO. Treating the Trauma of Rape: Cognitive-Behavioral Therapy for PTSD. New York: Guilford, 1998.

47. Cason D, Grubaugh A, Resick P. Gender and PTSD treatment: efficacy and effectiveness. In: Kimerling R, Ouimette P, Wolfe J, eds. Gender and PTSD. New York: Guilford, 2002:305–334.

48. Shapiro F. Eye Movement Desensitization and Reprocessing (EMDR): Basic Principles, Protocols and Procedures. New York: Guilford, 1995.

49. Stickgold R. EMDR: A putative neurobiological mechanism of action. J Clin Psychol 2002;58(1):61–75.

50. Chemtob CM, Tolin DF, van der Kolk BA, et al. Eye movement desensitization and reprocessing. In: Foa E, Keane TM, Friedman MJ, eds. Effective Treatments for PTSD. New York: Guilford, 2000:139–154.

51. Pelcovitz D, van der Kolk BA, Roth SH, et al. Development of a criteria set and a structured interview for disorders of extreme stress (SIDES). J Traum Stress 1997;10:3–16.

52. Foa EB, Davidson JRT, Frances A. The expert consensus guidelines series: treatment of posttraumatic stress disorder. J Clin Psychiatry 1999;60:1–76.

SUGGESTED READINGS

Foa EB, Keane TM, Friedman MJ. Effective Treatments for PTSD. New York: Guilford, 2000.

Foa EB, Rothbaum BO. Treating the Trauma of Rape. New York: Guilford, 1998.

Herman, J. Trauma and Recovery. New York: Pandora, 1992.

van der Kolk B, McFarlane A, Weiseath L. Traumatic Stress. New York: Guilford, 1996.

CHAPTER 17

Living with Intellectual Disability

Elspeth A. Bradley, Yona Lunsky, Marika Korossy

Women with intellectual disabilities are the children, adolescents, and adults described in other chapters of this book; they have the same concerns and challenges daily and over the life span. They often need support in understanding and meeting these challenges and may not always be able to articulate or communicate their concerns. Cognitive and communicative challenges can silence the voice of such women as they negotiate equal rights as citizens and try to live dignified, fulfilled lives in which they feel understood and respected. As a society, we tend to dehumanize, neglect, or reject persons who do not communicate with us on our terms and whose worlds, therefore, we do not fully understand. Misinformation, stereotyping, and myths give rise to negative attitudes and exert a negative impact on the mental health of these women. This chapter describes a range of abilities of a diverse population of women and shows their influence on several life span issues. Persons with intellectual disabilities have higher rates of health and mental health problems than the general population. In the final section we will explore why this is so, focusing specifically on the issues for women.

CATEGORIZATION AND TERMINOLOGY

Typically, intellectual disability is categorized as a childhood disorder, but, in reality, it is a lifelong disability; increasing numbers of persons with intellectual disabilities now live until old age. Conceptualizing the disability only from the childhood perspective perpetuates the myth that older persons with intellectual disabilities are childlike, thus ignoring or minimizing their adult status and adult concerns (e.g., struggle for autonomy, sexuality, need for intimacy). For this reason, our chapter is included in the section of this book that addresses adult issues. "Intellectual disability" is one of many terms used to describe persons who, because of limitations in cognitive, communicative, and adaptive functioning presumed present from birth or developing during childhood, require extra assistance in everyday living. Flight from negative societal attitudes has led parent organizations and policy makers alike to periodic revision of diagnostic terms. Developmental disability gradually supplanted the term "mental retardation" during the last 30 years, although the latter term is still retained in both the American Psychiatric Association's *Diagnostic and Statistical Manual of Mental Disorders*, 4th edition, Text Revision (DSM-IV-TR, 1) and the World Health Organization's *ICD-10 Classification of Mental and Behavioural Disorders* (2), as well as a substantial proportion of clinical and research publications in North America. Interestingly, when the term "mental retardation" was adopted in the 1960s, it was viewed as a progressive new alternative to the early twentieth-century designations "feeble minded," "moron," "idiot," and "imbecile." In the UK, the term "learning disabilities" has replaced "mental handicap." This has resulted in some confusion because, in other parts of the world "learning disabilities" is used for persons with specific problems in learning (e.g., disorders of memory or auditory or visual perception of language) but with otherwise normal cognitive and adaptive functioning. Most recently, Canada and, in some contexts, the US, have been phasing in the term "intellectual disability," a term that has been used in Australia since 1986. Around the world, persons with disabilities prefer "people-first language" in which the person always precedes the disability or description of what the person has (3). "People with learning difficulties" is a frequently preferred collective term in this context.

Inconsistencies in terminology are accompanied by considerable variability in diagnostic criteria. For example, DSM-IV-TR (1) continues to rely on a statistical model that measures the severity of mental retardation by standardized tests expressed as an intelligence quotient (IQ) with a cutoff point at 70 or below. The American Association on Mental Retardation (AAMR), in both its 1992 (4) and 2002 (5) classification system revisions, has emphasized supports required rather than level of IQ. This focuses attention on the reality that disability is a consequence of the extent of available supports in a person's environment. Also see World Health Organization publications for eloquent descriptions of impairments, disabilities, handicaps (6), activity and activity limitations, and participation and participation restrictions (7).

Discussing terminology immediately takes us to the heart of a dilemma for workers in this area: clinical research mandates definition and case identification of particular persons and populations in order to study, understand, and provide for their special needs. However, in applying our clinical methods to identify this population, we risk running counter to the sensitivities of persons with these disabilities who tell us they want to be included and integrated into the mainstream, not isolated from it. Among the many perspectives in the area of intellectual disabilities (educational, social, political, economic, clinical, experiential), each has its own language. These tensions not infrequently raise obstacles to sound, evidence-based practice with this population.

Our perspective is one that acknowledges the vulnerabilities of women with intellectual disabilities and considers that these vulnerabilities need to be studied and understood in order to promote full integration and inclusion into the women's specific cultures and local communities.

EPIDEMIOLOGY

MILD AND SEVERE INTELLECTUAL DISABILITY

Epidemiologic research has identified women with mild intellectual disability (IQ, 50 to 70 range) and those with severe intellectual disability (IQ, less than 50). The latter are easiest to recognize in most cultures because the severity of their disabilities necessitates special supports and services. The identification of women with mild intellectual disability is associated with life span landmarks (e.g., educational, marital, occupational, parental) because it is at these times that women with intellectual disabilities require adequate support in order to fulfill specific expectations. Identification of the woman with mild intellectual disability is therefore likely to fluctuate. For example, the highest prevalence of women with mild intellectual disability is found in the school years. After they finish school, such women may be able to hold down a job or get married and may no longer need support services. Persons with mild intellectual disabilities predominate in the total population, constituting 75% to 89% of all persons with intellectual disabilities, compared to 11% to 25% with severe intellectual disabilities.

A dramatic change in recent years for women (and men) with intellectual disabilities has been the greatly increased life expectancy, particularly for some etiologic groups. For example, for women with Down syndrome, the most common recognized cause of intellectual disability, life expectancy is now into the fourth and fifth decade, compared to age 12 in the early part of the 1940s. Curiously, females with Down syndrome may have a significant survival disadvantage compared to males with Down syndrome (8).

There are differences between the sexes in prevalence of intellectual disabilities, with greater numbers of men overall. In the severe range, the difference tends to even out; some studies show greater numbers of women. The implications of these sex differences in terms of required supports have so far not been explored.

BORDERLINE INTELLECTUAL DISABILITY

Women with borderline intellectual disability form an invisible but very large group, poorly understood by both researchers and clinicians. Their IQs range from 70 to 85; they tend to have difficulties managing money; they have social skills deficits and difficulties solving problems; they may be illiterate. Earlier definitions of intellectual disabilities often included these persons but, with a growing emphasis on inclusion along with attempts to reduce services, they have been forgotten (9). The current trend, if indeed their special needs are identified (10), is to label such individuals, while in the school system, as having a learning disability. Prevalence rates based on service use tend to underestimate the size of this population and may underestimate girls more than boys. This is because persons with borderline IQ (and sometimes those with mild intellectual disabilities as well) are typically not identified in school unless they exhibit behavior problems. Behavior problems are more common in boys than girls. As adults, these women may not come to the attention of services unless they have trouble caring for their children or unless they develop major psychiatric difficulties.

AUTISM AND INTELLECTUAL DISABILITY

Autism is the most severe form of a spectrum of related disorders referred to as the pervasive developmental disorders. These disorders are defined behaviorally by impairments in socialization and communication and by a lack of behavioral flexibility (and are sometimes referred to as autism spectrum disorders). It is estimated that about 75% of persons with autism have IQ scores in the intellectual disability range and even those with higher IQs often have relatively lower levels of adaptive functioning and are referred to the intellectual disability sector for services. Evidence suggests that a substantial proportion (one quarter to one third) of persons with intellectual disabilities also have autism; the greater the cognitive impairment, the greater the prevalence (11,12). While the male:female ratio is 3–4:1 in autism without intellectual disability or with mild intellectual disability, the gender difference diminishes with increasing intellectual disability. Some evidence suggests that, when girls are affected, they are likely to be more severely disabled (13). Conversely, some girls with autism who have mild or no intellectual disability have been reported to have fewer social and communication deficits than their male peers. Some investigators have found undiagnosed autism spectrum disorders in girls diagnosed with anxiety disorders, selective mutism, and anorexia nervosa (14,15). Taken together, these findings suggest that girls with autism may have a different phenotype than boys and, in milder cases, may not be recognized as having an autism spectrum disorder (16). Persons with intellectual disabilities and comorbid autism, because of the severity of these disabilities, have historically been the focus of institutional scandal, and with the move toward deinstitutionalization, have been among the last to be reintegrated into community life (17). These persons remain a very vulnerable group requiring considerable care and supervision throughout their lives.

ETIOLOGY

It is very important to investigate the etiology of the intellectual disability because associated health disorders may be present that might otherwise escape detection or be misdiagnosed and fail to receive appropriate treatment.

MILD AND SEVERE INTELLECTUAL DISABILITY

While a biologic etiology can be identified in 60% to 75% of persons with severe intellectual disabilities, it remains obscure for around 25% to 40% of those with mild intellectual disabilities. (In light of diagnostic advances during the past decade, this breakdown, based on earlier epidemiologic data, may no longer be valid. Individuals are increasingly being identified with milder manifestations of established disorders that had previously been recognized only in severely affected persons. New investigative techniques, when applied to persons with mild intellectual disabilities, now detect the underlying cause of previously undiagnosable biologic entities.) However, for all persons with intellectual disabilities, less than optimal health care (e.g., undiagnosed medical disorders such as hypothyroidism or inappropriate use of medication to manage behaviors), and less than optimal support environments (e.g., inappropriate expectations or noisy and disruptive living circumstances, giving rise to stress and anxiety) can contribute to lower levels of functioning. In recent years, recognition has increased that some causes of intellectual disabilities give rise to a characteristic profile of skills, abilities, and emotional responses as well as particular vulnerabilities to other health-related problems. For example, Down syndrome (equally prevalent in males and females) is associated with increased vulnerability to certain comorbid disabilities (e.g., hearing impairment), medical (e.g., thyroid dysfunction), and mental health disorders (e.g., depressive episodes, early onset dementia). Similarly, fragile X syndrome, the most prevalent inherited cause of intellectual disability (women with the fragile X full mutation may or may not have intellectual disability), is associated with a higher than expected prevalence of certain medical disorders (e.g., seizures, mitral valve prolapse, eye problems) and mental health problems (e.g., hyperactivity, social anxiety, obsessive, compulsive, and psychotic behaviors under stress). Other genetic syndromes with documented characteristic behavioral, emotional, and/or psychiatric disturbances include Williams, 22q11.2 deletion, Angelman, Prader-Willi, Smith-Magenis (all of which are equally prevalent in women and men), Rett (almost exclusive to females), and Turner (occurs only in women) syndromes. Recognizing these "behavioral phenotypes" (and their biologic bases) is essential in designing interventions and in providing optimal supports (18).

BORDERLINE INTELLECTUAL DISABILITY

Women (and men) with borderline intellectual disability were once referred to as having "cultural familial" retardation because of the belief that their disability was, in part, due to an impoverished environment; however, this term is less popular now. With recent genetic advances, especially newer diagnostic investigations, such as fluorescence in situ hybridization (FISH), subtelomeric screening, chromosome microdissection, and magnetic resonance spectroscopy (MRS), we now suspect that a large proportion of women in this group also have specific biologic causes to their disability (e.g., 22q11.2 deletion syndrome, fragile X, deletion 1p36.3, treatable metabolic disorders such as Smith-Lemli-Opitz syndrome, or SLOS) (19).

AUTISM AND INTELLECTUAL DISABILITY

The cluster of abnormal patterns of behavior called autism has several different probable etiologies. Autism is associated with a higher than expected prevalence of epilepsy, neurologic symptoms, minor congenital anomalies (birth defects), maternal birth complications, and, as previously stated, intellectual disabilities. Also found in persons with autism are genetic conditions (such as fragile X), metabolic conditions (such as phenylketonuria), viral infections (such as rubella), and congenital anomaly syndromes (such as Möbius syndrome). However, not everyone with autism has these additional diagnoses, and not everyone with these diagnoses develops autism. Autism appears to be the outcome of particular brain damage caused by a variety of biologic insults. A small but significant minority of persons with autism shows deterioration in skills and functioning during adolescence and, for some, seizures may first occur at that time.

LEVELS OF FUNCTIONING

While IQ (and adaptive functioning) may be a guide in supporting women with intellectual disabilities, not all women with the same IQ have the same cognitive or psychological challenges. For example, differences in expressive and receptive language abilities, visual and auditory perceptual processing, memory and learning styles can give rise to hidden challenges. A comprehensive psychological and communication evaluation assists in ensuring that the woman's skills and difficulties are properly understood and that appropriate supports are offered.

Given this caveat, however, it is still helpful clinically to consider the cognitive and adaptive skills of women with intellectual disabilities in the subgroups outlined in DSM-IV-TR, ICD-10, and ICD-10 MR (i.e., mild, moderate, severe, profound levels of functioning). Adaptive functioning, IQ levels, and living circumstances of women in these subgroups and for those with borderline intellectual disabilities and autism are outlined in Table 17.1. Women's issues by subgroup are outlined below.

WOMEN'S ISSUES

Borderline Intellectual Disability

Historically, women in this group were considered either immoral or asexual (20). Many older women in this group were institutionalized and sometimes sterilized without their knowledge or consent because of a false belief that they were promiscuous and would add disproportionately to a defective gene pool. No other information on their sexuality is available except that women with minimal education tend to be misinformed about sexuality and at risk for sexually transmitted diseases and abuse. In this group, even women who appear to be sexually informed may, in fact, not be (21).

Mild Intellectual Disability

Once a trusting relationship has been established, women with mild intellectual disabilities are capable of describing their sexual experiences. The picture that is emerging is that they have negative feelings about their sexual lives and experience very high levels of abuse (22,23). These women are relatively uninformed about safe sex; they often believe that sex revolves around the man's experience and that they are not entitled to sexual satisfaction during sexual relations. Because of a lack of education, combined with highly conservative attitudes, they may feel guilty about enjoying their sexuality (24).

Some women with mild intellectual disabilities are mothers. Given support and guidance in pregnancy and postpartum, these women can successfully rear children (21,25). Child rearing becomes more challenging as their children grow older and advance beyond them cognitively. Parents with mild intellectual disabilities need a large support network of persons who can assist them in raising their children.

TABLE 17.1

Skills, Abilities, and Living Circumstances Associated with Severity of Intellectual Disability

Borderline ID IQ = 70–84 AE* = 11+ years	Living independently Subtle communication difficulties High school dropout or special education Difficulty keeping a job Government assistance At risk for being in an abusive relationship Challenges rearing children, particularly if social and economic resources are inadequate
Mild ID IQ = 55–69 AE = 9–11 years	Relative independence in self-care Can hold a conversation and engage in the clinical interview Information the person provides may not be accurate Varied level of service required May have paid employment
Moderate ID IQ = 40–54 AE = 6–9 years	Has basic communication skills Requires supervision with self-care skills Group home settings Structured day program or workshop setting
Severe ID IQ = 25–39 AE = 3–6 years	Communication difficulties Motor difficulties Requires ongoing supervision Lives with family or in a 24-hour group home or nursing home Alternative day programs with a combination of skills-based and recreational activities
Profound ID IQ < 25 AE = < 3 years	Requires 24-hour supervised care Lives either with family or in group home or nursing home Multiple medical issues Inner world largely unavailable to others because of communication difficulty
Autism and intellectual disability IQ varies AE varies	Four patterns: "aloof," "passive," "active but odd," "overformal, stilted" (43) At higher levels of cognitive functioning: one-sided social and verbal interactions, complex routines, manipulation of objects At lower levels of cognitive functioning: social aloofness, abnormal movements, hypersensitivity to sensory stimuli, confusion and fear of unfamiliar situations or interference with repetitive routines, failure to understand social rules, inappropriate attempts to control events, oversensitivity to sensory input (e.g., noisy environments) can lead to inappropriate and challenging behaviors High levels of support and supervision are generally needed

*Age equivalent

Moderate Intellectual Disability

It is less acceptable for women with moderate intellectual disability to be involved in sexual relationships, although they may have interest in having such relationships. Women in this category may talk about wanting to have a boyfriend or get married, and they may enter into casual or more long-term exclusive relationships. However, their sociosexual knowledge tends to be quite limited and attitudes very conservative (24). These women tend to be sexually sheltered, with limited access to privacy. A common concern is that they can be abused, so caregivers take extra care to protect them and they are, therefore, denied sexual freedoms. For this reason, sexual abuse, when it does happen, tends to be perpetrated by persons close to the woman (relatives, care providers, or others with intellectual disabilities).

Parents may be more prone to seek out sterilization for these women (its availability varies from country to country, but generally sterilization is now much less available than previously) or request birth control to prevent potential pregnancies. These women are unlikely to be parents, and when they are, tend to have difficulties raising children.

Severe Intellectual Disability

Women with severe intellectual disability may have sexual needs or desires but tend to be restricted from sexual relationships. They are, however, still vulnerable to abuse from those close to them. It is important to remember that even if the woman cannot consent to a sexual relationship, she can still have her need for intimacy met in other ways (e.g., sitting close to a friend, hugging, massage, grooming, having a pet). These women tend to have difficulties with hygiene (e.g., toileting, menstrual hygiene). Behavior issues may occur at certain times of their menstrual cycle. In some situations, women with severe to profound intellectual disabilities may be prescribed birth control pills or undergo surgical management to reduce menstrual problems (26–28).

Profound Intellectual Disability

In women with profound intellectual disability, women's issues tend to be ignored. These women are at risk for abuse and have hygiene concerns. Like other women, they benefit from sensory stimulation, which can include touch from others; they may attempt to masturbate. They require hands-on assistance with all aspects of self-care, including toileting and menstrual hygiene.

Autism and Intellectual Disability

Very little is known about women's issues for those with autism. The capacity to make friends, develop social networks, communicate, and share feelings and needs is a core impairment for these women. It is not that they do not need or want friendships but, rather, their capacity to comprehend the meaning and nature of friendships is often limited. They lack the instinctive knowledge of how to make the first moves in being accepted by others. If a relationship does begin, they are often unable to give or take in the relationship; they may make inappropriate demands on the other person. The relationship becomes one sided, and continuation of the relationship is often a consequence of the accommodations made by the other person. The woman with autism may make inappropriate comments or engage in inappropriate behaviors in social settings, and she is particularly vulnerable to the inappropriate advances of others. This lack of social know-how pervades all aspects of her daily life, school, occupation, and recreational activities. The woman with autism will respond best to basic rules applied in a consistent, structured, and supportive way to help guide her through these social perplexities. Autobiographical accounts by more able women with autism, such as Temple Grandin (29) and Donna Williams (30), alert us to those aspects of living and experiencing that people with autism cannot take for granted.

ASSESSMENT AND TREATMENT IMPLICATIONS

BORDERLINE INTELLECTUAL DISABILITY

Women with borderline intellectual disability are most likely to come to the attention of health professionals for reasons other than their intellectual deficits. Their cognitive difficulties may or may not be recognized as contributing factors to their health problems in the assessment and treatment phase. They also may take on the role of care providers for younger women with disabilities. In such cases, additional support may be required so that they can follow through with health recommendations for themselves and for those under their care.

MILD INTELLECTUAL DISABILITY

Women with mild intellectual disability may appear more able than they are. Apparent noncompliance with treatment and missed appointments can be a result of the intellectual disability and not a lack of interest in receiving help. Women with mild intellectual disabilities may not have the necessary support to fully engage in treatment (e.g., adhere to medication regimens, get to appointments), and where this is the case, such support needs to be built into the treatment plan.

In general, the mental health disturbances, clinical presentation, and treatment needs of women in this group are more similar to those of women in the general population than to the specific problems presented by women with more severe intellectual disabilities. However, the difficulties that even women with milder intellectual disabilities have in communicating their subjective experiences and inner discomforts, particularly where health-care workers are unaware of the accommodations they need to make to assist, can give rise to misdiagnoses and inappropriate treatments.

MODERATE INTELLECTUAL DISABILITY

With greater intellectual disability, behavior disturbances ranging from "annoying" and antisocial behaviors to more destructive behaviors such as self-injurious behaviors (SIB) increasingly are markers for underlying emotional and psychiatric disturbances and disorders. One young woman, Suzanne, was referred to our service because she took hygiene products (e.g., soap, shampoo) belonging to other residents and obsessively washed until her skin was damaged. Suzanne was found to suffer from episodes of depression triggered by staff changes, and the onset of the depressive episodes was heralded by obsessive behaviors involving cleanliness. Another woman was referred because she was observed to be "nasty" and progressively more aggressive toward each of her younger cousins in turn when they grew older and more capable and independent than she was. Unfortunately, from a diagnostic perspective, the same behavior disturbance can be the final common pathway of different underlying etiologies. For example, the differential diagnosis of aggressive behaviors includes the full range of medical, emotional, and psychiatric disorders as well as inappropriate expectations on the person, insufficient daily supports, dental problems, and even ingrown toenails! A mental health assessment therefore should include a thorough review of the myriad possible biologic, psychological, and social circumstances that may be causing distress. This distress is unlikely to be well articulated verbally and may be communicated only through patterns of behavior change.

SEVERE INTELLECTUAL DISABILITY

Women with greater intellectual disability may resort to even less desirable behaviors when trying to communicate their discomforts (e.g., head hitting when suffering earache or following the loss of a friendship). This increases the risk of misdiagnosis and inappropriate treatment by health-care personnel unfamiliar with the communication patterns of such women.

Significant modifications to assessment and treatment procedures must be made for women in this group. Although it is fashionable to use terminology like choice and empowerment, it is a challenge to put such terms into play with these individuals. Focus is needed on working with these women's support network so that the network can help in education and empowerment.

PROFOUND DISABILITY

Women with profound disability experience more comorbid medical disorders (e.g., seizures) and disabilities (e.g., sensory and motor impairments) than their less disabled counterparts and have increased mortality associated with feeding problems, being nonambulant and incontinent. We have little or no access to their subjective experiences. Their sometimes challenging behaviors may be understood as a lack of appropriate supports and services or as unrecognized bodily discomforts and medical and mental health disorders. We need to attend to the behavior in order to identify the underlying problem rather than rush to medicate (which essentially "silences" the woman into quieter suffering).

AUTISM AND INTELLECTUAL DISABILITY

The challenge in working with women with autism and intellectual disabilities is in trying to enter a world where shared intuitive knowing between two persons is no longer a given. Persons with autism are communicating in their own way the nature of their difficulties, but we experience their unusual behaviors from our own "intuitive knowing" perspective. Their attempts to engage socially, for example, are experienced as one-sided and demanding, and descriptions such as "manipulative" and "attention seeking" are not infrequent among care providers unfamiliar with autism. Even a person with the most profound intellectual disability but without autism can elicit an ongoing sense of engagement with others, and care providers feel rewarded in providing care. In contrast, care providers working with persons with autism often feel drained, unrewarded, and perplexed, which in turn can lead to inappropriate support practices. Women with autism across the range of functioning are sometimes described as having alexithymia (a disability in recognizing, experiencing, and describing feelings) and anhedonia (a disability in recognizing, experiencing, and describing pleasurable feelings). However, the authors have observed that higher functioning persons with autism may use idiosyncratic language or copy behaviors of others (e.g., cartoon characters from the TV) to communicate (indirectly) particular feeling states. Lower functioning persons often engage in unusual behaviors the communicative function of which remains unclear, even to those who know the person well.

It is essential that health-care staff involved in the assessment and treatment of persons with autism be knowledgeable about this disability. Otherwise, inappropriate assessments and treatments are the likely outcome.

HEALTH AND MENTAL HEALTH

For biologic, psychological, and social reasons, women with intellectual disabilities across the lifespan have relatively high rates of medical and psychiatric difficulties.

BIOLOGIC FACTORS

Women with intellectual disabilities have high rates of seizures, mobility problems, and sensory impairments. They are more likely than other women to be prescribed psychotropic medications and may be more sensitive to side effects but have problems reporting them. In addition, these women may not understand body changes or know how to cope with them (e.g., puberty, menstruation, sexual excitement, and menopause). Very little time is spent educating women with intellectual disabilities about their bodies. They tend to learn on a need to know basis (e.g., a woman gets her period and is taught how to use a menstrual pad).

PSYCHOLOGICAL FACTORS

Women with intellectual disabilities encounter daily stress in terms of stressful relationships, changes in their routine, difficulties navigating the world independently, and being teased or ridiculed. They also experience stress because of not meeting developmental milestones. For example, girls with intellectual disabilities experience high rates of mood and anxiety disorders in adolescence or young adulthood when they realize that they do not have boyfriends, they do not look like the women on TV, they may not get married, and may not have children (31,32). It can be particularly difficult for women with intellectual disabilities to witness their siblings moving out, getting married, or having children (20).

Adjusting to change is of special concern for women with more severe intellectual disabilities and those with autism. Change such as alterations in staff or roommates or modifications in a day program can cause great distress, which, unfortunately, may not always be recognized.

Women with intellectual disabilities may also experience stress because of their communication impairments. They cannot say they are in pain or give accurate information on when a mood or anxiety problem started. Women with milder disabilities are vulnerable to acquiescence and may deny symptoms if they are trying to please the person asking the questions or if they think their feelings are inappropriate.

SOCIAL FACTORS

Women, more so than their male peers with intellectual disabilities (or women in the general population), are likely to be physically or sexually abused in their lifetime, and limited treatment for abuse is available for them. It was once thought that women with intellectual disabilities were not as affected by such events as women of average intelligence, but recent research suggests otherwise (33). Not only are they more likely to have been abused, but they are also likely to have witnessed violence in their homes or workplaces, which can lead to concerns about personal safety and personal boundaries (34,35).

Caregivers may deny that difficulties exist, may infantilize, or may be overprotective and thus prevent the women from having experiences they are entitled to have. In our efforts to take care of these women, we have learned to make decisions on their behalf, sometimes without their involvement. Professionals, not thinking of individuals with intellectual disabilities as women, may attribute difficulties to the intellectual disability itself (diagnostic overshadowing) and not to other women's issues. These attitudinal barriers are a result of inadequate education of professionals who work with women with intellectual disabilities and essentially collude in silencing the important voices these women can contribute to better services by excluding them from those very discussions.

Women with intellectual disabilities are also at risk for health problems because of barriers they face in accessing appropriate services. Intervention tends to happen in late stages, if at all, because of limited appropriate resources. Poverty is another risk factor for this group. Most of these women do not work and are dependent on government assistance or the generosity of others. Housing may be inadequate, and there may be little or no money for services such as staff support, medication, and transportation to medical and other appointments.

Finally, these women often live in stressful environments. They may live with people not of their choosing; their caregivers may also feel alone and unsupported.

EMOTIONAL DEVELOPMENT

Women with intellectual disabilities, depending on their developmental level, need others to help them modulate their emotions. This need is often not understood, and the woman is either expected to manage on her own or else a solution is imposed; neither outcome helps the woman develop emotionally, the latter would require the presence of a responsive other. Women with intellectual disabilities can suffer several other disadvantages in terms of emotional development. They may be more "needy" early on, may be experienced as difficult babies, may need more structure and consistency throughout the life span, may have few coping strategies in response to adverse circumstances, and may be more vulnerable than others to adverse environments. Sensitive behavioral support (e.g., consistent supportive behaviors from care providers in response to escalating behaviors) tailored to the functioning level of the woman provides emotional containment, while psychotherapy (individual or group) helps the woman to better experience and to better learn to modulate her emotional responses. Either individually or together, both interventions have been found to be effective treatments for many behavior disturbances (36,37) and can prevent the development of psychiatric disorders.

PSYCHIATRIC DISORDERS

While the prevalence of psychiatric and behavior disorders for women (and men) with intellectual disabilities is estimated to be four times as great as that for the general population, the range of psychiatric disorders is thought to be similar. For lower functioning persons, some additional disorders are described (e.g., stereotypies, pica). Some psychiatric disorders may be associated with specific genetic etiologies (e.g., psychotic disorders in deletion 22q11.2 syndrome, and Alzheimer dementia in persons with Down syndrome), and for some diagnostic groups the prevalence of psychiatric and behavioral disorders may be higher (e.g., greater prevalence in persons with autism).

Psychiatric disorders are typically diagnosed at later stages, if at all, and are often misdiagnosed. For example, women with intellectual disabilities are more likely to be diagnosed with a psychotic disorder than with anxiety or depression. Comorbid disabilities (e.g., hearing impairment), medical (e.g., thyroid, gastroesophageal reflux disorder), and emotional disorders (e.g., from early abuse) can add great complexity to the clinical presentation. In some situations, it is helpful to distinguish episodic or new onset disorders (e.g., depressive, hypomanic, psychotic disorders) from background more chronic conditions (e.g., hyperactivity or compulsive behaviors) and disorders (e.g., ADHD, OCD) (38). New onset and more chronic disorders can also coexist (e.g., a pattern of bipolar affective disorder, hyperactivity, and tics and compulsive behaviors is sometimes seen in persons with autism). In such potential complexity, it is essential not only to adopt a systematic assessment approach but also to determine the extent to which medical problems, inappropriate supports, and inappropriate expectations on the woman may be contributing to the "psychiatric" behaviors (39,40). In this way, treatments targeted to the appropriate underlying cause can be offered, resulting in fewer side effects and better outcomes. Unfortunately, the main intervention for behavior and psychiatric disturbance is often pharmacologic (41), with little psychotherapy available (42).

Women with intellectual disabilities tend to be excluded from women's mental health research, so there is little empirical support for any given type of therapy (42). Research is needed on what treatments work with this population and how empirically supported interventions should be modified. We have found that an interdisciplinary approach with a solid understanding of both women's issues and intellectual disabilities is necessary. (See Box 17.1.)

BOX 17.1

Clinical Vignette

(To preserve confidentiality, this vignette is fictitious. It is a composite based on the experiences of many different persons, not of any one individual.)

Crystal has mild intellectual disability, as does her mother. Several years after her birth, her mother moved away, and Crystal was looked after by her maternal grandparents. When Crystal was a teenager, her mother reappeared and, concomitantly, Crystal became increasingly behaviorally disturbed. She had frequent visits to the Emergency Department and short psychiatric admissions. Over the years, many diagnoses have been offered, including depression with suicidal ideation, dysthymia, adjustment disorder, eating disorder, self-mutilating behavior, oppositional defiant disorder, attention deficit disorder, impulsiveness, agitation and violence, and aggressive outbursts. Crystal has been treated with a variety of medications, including benzodiazepines, antidepressants, antipsychotics, and stimulants, with limited evidence of benefit. In her late teens, Crystal had a therapeutic abortion following a visit to her mother's home, where she was raped by a male visitor. Currently, Crystal is living in an apartment supported by workers who visit daily and assist with shopping and household tasks, monitor her medications, and help coordinate her medical and other appointments. On weekdays, she attends a supported work setting. She left her grandparents' home because of her disruptive and aggressive behaviors toward some family members (her mother and younger cousins), for which a court order restricting access to these persons was required. In her teens, Crystal gained an excessive amount of weight and now suffers from significant obesity, which causes her great distress. In the past three years, she has been diagnosed with diabetes, for which she takes medication.

Comment

While, on the surface, this appears to be a case study of Crystal, a young woman with intellectual disabilities, it is actually a case study of Crystal, her mother with intellectual disability, and her grandmother. If each of these women had been given the appropriate supports when needed, the situation would be different.

Crystal's grandmother has the double stress of looking after a daughter with mild intellectual disability, promiscuous behavior, and poor judgment and a granddaughter with mild intellectual disability. Supporting her granddaughter places additional stress on her relationship with her daughter. Allowing her daughter independence results in abuse of her granddaughter. Grandmother never had much help in managing her daughter, and she has even less help now in looking after both Crystal and her mother.

As a woman with mild intellectual disability, Crystal's mother was ignored by the school system and mental health system. As an adult, she tried to achieve as normal a life as possible but, with limited sex education and poor assertiveness skills combined with impaired judgment, she conceived a child for whom she was unable to care. Although becoming pregnant and being a mother gave her a boost of self-confidence and helped establish her identity as a woman (and not just a person with intellectual disability), she suffered a loss of self-esteem when she could not cope with motherhood. She finds spending time with her daughter sometimes rewarding but often stressful, particularly

(continued)

BOX 17.1 *(Continued)*

as her daughter matures and can do some things better than her mother. Crystal's mother wants desperately to be loved by a man and taken care of, and to try to achieve this, she often puts herself into compromising and dangerous situations.

Crystal has significant issues with safety and trust. She wants to love her mother but is also very stressed in her presence. Unable to verbalize her frustration and fear, she acts aggressively when anxious, which has led to numerous medications, a resultant excessive weight gain, and restricted visits with family. Crystal has watched her younger cousins achieve milestones that she cannot (e.g., driving, dating) and, when with them, she is prone to explosive outbursts. She now also has a serious medical condition (diabetes), which, if not managed carefully, is likely to lead to further medical complications that will add to her disabilities.

Following an interdisciplinary assessment (involving psychiatrist, psychologist, communication therapist, behavior therapist) and a meeting with her community supports (social worker, grandparents, manager at workplace, community nurse) and a review of all previous hospital visits and admissions, Crystal's mental health issues were reconceptualized within a developmental and biopsychosocial perspective. Crystal was seen as a young woman with mild intellectual disability (with implications for optimal supports) who suffered significant deprivation and abuse during her childhood and who now had difficulties modulating her affect, particularly in the presence of significant triggers (e.g., biologic mother and younger cousins). All previous psychiatric diagnoses could be understood in this context, and the new framework provided opportunities for prevention and rehabilitation. Crystal was recognized as being a very resilient young person (as evidenced by her response to therapy—see below) who, with supports appropriate for someone with mild intellectual disability, can be assisted in finding ways to overcome the impact of early traumas and current social and emotional disadvantage and in managing her emotional responses.

Progress

Crystal has done remarkably well with individual psychotherapy, behavioral support, and systems meetings. Psychotherapy provides her a safe, reliable place where she can identify whatever feeling states arise and learn how to manage these. Behavioral support is the structure and routine in her home and at work that make sure the tasks are appropriate to her abilities, help her to recognize when she needs help and how to ask for it, help her recognize healthy eating and how to manage this, and supports her in a weight reduction program and in linking with the community nurse. Systems meetings include Crystal and everyone involved in her support to ensure follow-through and consistency. Working with her psychotherapist, Crystal has developed a shared language with which to describe her subjective experience, and through this shared language, she has developed self-soothing strategies. In addition, through this shared language with her psychotherapist and psychiatrist, she is now able to provide feedback about her medication experience. This has allowed changes in her medications so that these are more closely attuned to her bodily experiences and feeling states, which in turn has resulted in better compliance with treatment.

CONCLUSION

In this chapter we have tried to outline issues in daily living that impact on the mental health of women with intellectual disabilities. Undoubtedly, as a society, we have come a long way in recognizing the experiences and special needs of these women. It is likely that further progress will be made by focusing on the universality of certain issues for all women and by exploring how these are experienced through the lives of women with disabilities.

REFERENCES

1. American Psychiatric Association, Diagnostic and Statistical Manual of Mental Disorders, 4th Ed., text rev. Washington, DC, 2000.
2. World Health Organization. The ICD-10 Classification of Mental and Behavioral Disorders: Clinical Descriptions and Diagnostic Guidelines. Geneva, 1992.
3. Snow K. People first language [web page]. 2003. Available at: http://www.disabilityisnatural.com/peoplefirstlanguage.htm. Accessed January 28, 2004.
4. American Association on Mental Retardation. Mental Retardation: Definition, Classification, and Systems of Supports. 9th Ed. Washington, DC, 1992.
5. American Association on Mental Retardation. Mental Retardation: Definition, Classification, and Systems of Supports. 10th Ed. Washington, DC, 2002.
6. World Health Organization. International Classification of Impairments, Disabilities, and Handicaps: A Manual of Classification Relating to the Consequences of Disease. Geneva, 1980.
7. World Health Organization. International Classification of Functioning, Disability, and Health: ICF Short Version. Geneva, 2001.
8. Glasson EJ, Sullivan SG, Hussain R, et al. Comparative survival advantage of males with Down syndrome. Am J Hum Biol 2003;15:192–195.
9. Tymchuk AJ, Lakin KC, Luckasson R, eds. The Forgotten Generation: The Status and Challenges of Adults with Mild Cognitive Limitations. Baltimore: Brookes, 2001.
10. MacMillan DL, Gresham FM, Bocian KM, et al. Current plight of borderline students: where do they belong? Educ Train Ment Retard Dev Disabil 1998;33:83–94.
11. Shah A, Holmes N, Wing L. Autism and related conditions in adults in a mental handicap hospital. Appl Res Ment Handicap 1982;3:303–317.
12. Nordin V, Gillberg C. Autism spectrum disorders in children with physical or mental disability or both. I: clinical and epidemiological aspects. Dev Med Child Neurol 1996;38:297–313.
13. Wing L. Sex ratios in early childhood autism and related conditions. Psychiatry Res 1981;5:129–137.
14. Kopp S, Gillberg C. Selective mutism: a population-based study: a research note. J Child Psychol Psychiatry 1997;38:257–262.
15. Nilsson EW, Gillberg C, Gillberg IC, et al. Ten-year follow-up of adolescent-onset anorexia nervosa: personality disorders. J Am Acad Child Adolesc Psychiatry 1999;38:1389–1395.
16. Thompson T, Caruso M, Ellerbeck K. Sex matters in autism and other developmental disabilities. J Learn Disabil 2003;7:345–362.
17. Wing L. Hospital Closure and the Resettlement of Residents. The Case of Darenth Park Mental Handicap Hospital. Aldershott, UK: Avebury, 1989.
18. Dykens EM, Hodapp RM, Finucane BM. Genetics and Mental Retardation Syndromes: A New Look at Behavior and Interventions. Baltimore: Brookes, 2000.
19. Battaglia A, Carey JC. Diagnostic evaluation of developmental delay/mental retardation: an overview. Am J Med Genet 2003;117C:3–14.
20. Scior K. Women with disabilities: gendered subjects after all? Clin Psychol Forum 2000;137:6–10.
21. Finucane BM. Working with Women Who Have Mental Retardation: A Genetic Counselor's Guide. Elwyn, PA: Elwyn, 1998.
22. McCarthy M. Sexuality and Women with Learning Disabilities. London: Kingsley, 1999.
23. McCarthy M. Going through the menopause: perceptions and experiences of women with intellectual disability. J Intellect Dev Disabil 2002;27:281–295.
24. Lunsky Y, Konstantareas MM. The attitudes of persons with autism and mental retardation towards sexuality. Educ Train Ment Retard Dev Disabil 1998;33:24–33.
25. Booth T, Booth W. Unto us a child is born: the trials and rewards of parenthood for people with learning difficulties. Aust NZ J Dev Disabil 1995;20:25–39.
26. Elkins TE, Anderson HF. Sterilization of persons with mental retardation. J Assoc Pers Sev Handicaps 1992;17:19–26.
27. Grover SR. Menstrual and contraceptive management in women with an intellectual disability. Med J Australia 2002;176:108–110.

28. Servais L, Jacques D, Leach R, et al. Contraception of women with intellectual disability: prevalence and determinants. J Intellect Disabil Res 2002;46:108–119.
29. Grandin T, Scariano M. Emergence: Labeled Autistic. Novato, CA: Arena, 1986.
30. Williams D. Nobody Nowhere. New York: Avon, 1994.
31. Heiman T, Margalit M. Loneliness, depression, and social skills among students with mild mental retardation in different educational settings. J Spec Educ 1998;32:154–163.
32. Reynolds WM, Miller KL. Depression and learned helplessness in mentally retarded and nonmentally retarded adolescents: an initial investigation. Appl Res Ment Retard 1985;6: 295–306.
33. Ryan R. Posttraumatic stress disorder in persons with developmental disabilities. Community Ment Health J 1994;30:45–54.
34. Carlson BE. Mental retardation and domestic violence: an ecological approach to intervention. Soc Work 1997;42:79–89.
35. Sobsey D. Faces of violence against women with developmental disabilities. Impact [Feature Issue on Violence and Women With Developmental and Other Disabilities] 2000;13:2–3, 25.
36. Hollins S, Sinason V. Psychotherapy, learning disabilities and trauma: new perspectives. Br J Psychiatry 2000;176:32–36.
37. Gardner WI, Sovner R. Self-injurious Behaviors. Diagnosis and Treatment. Willow Street, PA: VIDA, 1994.
38. Bradley EA, Bolton PF, Bryson SE. Psychiatric comorbidity in persons with intellectual disability with and without autism. J Intellect Disabil Res (in press).
39. Bradley EA, Summers J. Developmental disability and behavioral, emotional and psychiatric disturbances. In: Brown I, Percy ME, eds. Developmental Disabilities in Ontario. 2nd Ed. Toronto: Ontario Association on Developmental Disabilities 2003:751–774.
40. Bradley EA, Hollins S. Assessment of persons with intellectual disabilities. In: Goldbloom D, ed. Psychiatric Clinical Skills. New York: Elsevier (in press).
41. Reiss S, Aman MG. Psychotropic Medications and Developmental Disabilities: The International Consensus Handbook. [Columbus, OH]: Ohio State University Nisonger Center, 1998.
42. Lunsky Y, Havercamp SM. Women's mental health. In: Walsh PN, Heller T, eds. Health of Women with Intellectual Disabilities. Oxford: Blackwell, 2002:59–75.
43. Wing L. The Autistic Spectrum: A Guide for Parents and Professionals. London: Constable, 1996.

SUGGESTED READINGS

Brown I, Percy ME, eds. Developmental Disabilities in Ontario. 2nd Ed. Toronto: Ontario Association on Developmental Disabilities, 2003.
Howlin P. Autism: Preparing for Adulthood. London: Routledge, 1997.
Prasher VP, Janicki MP, eds. Physical Health of Adults with Intellectual Disabilities. Oxford: Blackwell, 2002.
Schwier KM, Hingsburger D. Sexuality: Your Sons and Daughters with Intellectual Disabilities. Baltimore: Brookes, 2000.
Traustadóttir R, Johnson K. Women with Intellectual Disabilities Finding a Place in the World. Philadelphia: Kingsley, 2000.
Walsh PN, Heller T, eds. Health of Women with Intellectual Disabilities. Oxford: Blackwell, 2002.
Walsh PN, LeRoy B. Women with Disabilities Aging Well: A Global View. Baltimore: Brookes, 2004.

WEBSITES

The International Association for the Scientific Study of Intellectual Disabilities. http://www.iassid.org/
Learning About Intellectual Disabilities and Health. http://www.intellectualdisability.info/home.htm
University of Western Ontario Developmental Disabilities Program. www.psychiatry.med.uwo.ca/ddp/

Reproduction

Section V Summary
Commentary from Scandanavia
Berit Schei, Marsha M. Cohen

THE NORDIC COUNTRIES' APPROACH TO PSYCHOSOCIAL ISSUES IN REPRODUCTIVE HEALTH

The Nordic countries referred to in this commentary include Denmark, Finland, Iceland, Norway, and Sweden, a total population of over 20 million people. One aspect that the Nordic countries share is a universal public health care system. Women have access to treatment and services equally, regardless of their social position or economic status. Traditionally, changes in the service provision for women have come from within the public health care system. In the areas of psychiatry or mental health, approaches to psychosocial issues in reproductive health have generally been initiated by gynecologist/obstetricians rather than health care professionals.

The papers included in this section are written by authors from Australia, Canada, and the United States. They address psychological conditions related to pregnancy and delivery, menstrual patterns and cyclical changes in menstruating women, hormonal changes related to the menopause, and depression during motherhood. There are certain facets of these conditions where comparisons with the Nordic countries might be informative. These include a comparison of the prevalence of postpartum depression with Nordic countries where postpartum depression has been well researched (1-5). In contrast to Nordic countries, all the papers are written from the viewpoint of mental health professionals who tend to treat the more extreme end of a spectrum of women's reproductive mental health.

FEAR OF CHILDBIRTH—EXAMPLE OF AN IMPORTANT ISSUE ADDRESSED IN THE NORDIC COUNTRIES

For example, one issue that has not been discussed by the authors in this section on reproductive mental health is fear of childbirth, called tokophobia (6). Another is whether women who request a caesarean section should be granted one. The two questions are linked. On one hand, the debate assumes that a maternal request for a CS is always caused by fear of childbirth. A request for CS might be unrelated to actual fear but related to other factors in women's lives. On the other hand, the current clinical guidelines around indications for CS might not be taking into consideration the relationship between fear of delivery and maternal request for CS. CS is not benign; CS may have a serious impact on delivery as it has been shown to be associated to various complications. Rates of CS are increasing in western countries, and fear of childbirth may be having a still unappreciated impact on the risk for emergency caesarean section (7).

CONCLUDING REMARKS

The papers on reproduction and mental health in this book highlight important issues for bridging the gap between somatic and psychological aspects on reproductive health. This link with somatic health care has been a long tradition in the Nordic countries. Models of good practice in the field in Nordic countries include bringing psychosocial services within the framework of general reproductive health services. This tradition has expanded our understanding of the complex issues of reproductive health care and women's mental health based on empirical research.

REFERENCES

1. Eberhard-Gran M, Tambs K, Opjordsmoen S, Skrondal A, Eskild A. Depression during pregnancy and after delivery: a repeated measurement study. J Psychosom Obstet Gynaecol 2004;25:15–21.
2. Eberhard-Gran M, Tambs K, Opjordsmoen S, Skrondal A, Eskild A. A comparison of anxiety and depressive symptomatology in postpartum and non-postpartum mothers. Soc Psychiatry Psychiatr Epidemiol 2003;38:551–556.
3. Eberhard-Gran M, Eskild A, Tambs K, Samuelsen SO, Opjordsmoen S. Depression in postpartum and non-postpartum women: prevalence and risk factors. Acta Psychiatr Scand 2002;106:426–433.
4. Eberhard-Gran M, Eskild A, Tambs K, Schei B, Opjordsmoen S. The Edinburgh postnatal depression scale: validation in a Norwegian community sample. Nord J Psychiatry 2001; 55:113–117.
5. Eberhard-Gran M, Eskild A, Tambs K, Opjordsmoen S, Samuelsen SO. Review of validation studies of the Edinburgh postnatal depression scale. Acta Psychiatr Scand 2001;104:243–249.
6. Hofberg K., Brockington I. Tokophobia: an unreasoning dread of childbirth. A series of 26 cases. Br J Psychiatry 2000;176:83–85.
7. Ryding EL, Wijma B, Wijma K, Rydhström H. Fear of childbirth during pregnancy may increase the risk for emergency caesarian section. Acta Obste Gynecol Scand 1998;77:542–547.

CHAPTER 18

Menstrual Cycles and Mental Health

Judith H. Gold

Menstruation marks the beginning of fertility and of womanhood. At the same time, it is an event surrounded by myth, ceremony, and controversy. Over the ages, menstruating women have been viewed as unclean in many cultures and religions. Taboos and rituals still exist in some societies, and papers continue to be published that explore the topic of menstrual meaning within a society (1,2). Since the middle of the 1900s, researchers have also been interested in the factors related to the complaints of some women of negative symptoms in conjunction with the menstrual cycle. Concepts such as premenstrual tension (PMT), premenstrual syndrome (PMS), premenstrual exacerbation of preexisting mental and physical disorders, and premenstrual dysphoric disorder (PMDD) have engendered considerable research and, in some instances, controversy. This chapter discusses these concepts.

This chapter is a revised, expanded, and updated version of a paper "Premenstrual dysphoric disorder: an update" published in the Journal of Practical Psychiatry and Behavioral Health *1999;July:1–7. (permission from Lippincott Williams & Wilkins, publishers of JPPBH)*
The author is in private practice, and was the Chair of the LLPDD work group of the American Psychiatric Association Task Force for DSM-IV.

PREMENSTRUAL DISORDERS

First, it is important to outline the events of the menstrual cycle. Beginning with the onset of menstruation, during the follicular phase the gonadotropins, follicle-stimulating hormone and luteinizing hormone (FSH and LH), stimulate the ovarian follicle. This phase lasts approximately 14 days until ovulation occurs. Progesterone and estrogen are produced in the second phase of the cycle, the luteal phase. If the egg is not fertilized, estrogen and progesterone levels fall and menses begins. The cycle then repeats every 28 to 30 days unless pregnancy ensues. Research into the chemistry of this cycle and into biochemical, social, and psychological factors affecting it is discussed below.

The psychosocial meaning of menstruation and the changes that occur in a woman's body have imposed limitations upon women throughout the ages. Many see the woman as unclean during menstruation, and, in some societies, she is then segregated. In Western countries, comments and jokes about a woman's expected premenstrual behavior are commonplace. Discussion about the association of premenstrually attributed behaviors includes social constructs about a woman's place in society and in a culture and her emotional expressiveness. Anger and irritability are the emotions usually associated negatively with the premenstrual period. As noted in the *DSM-IV Sourcebook,* a woman's expression of anger is often "blamed" on premenstrual hormonal changes rather than on the social circumstances in which she exists (3). For some women, the premenstrual period becomes, therefore, a safe time to show anger and dissatisfaction because then, as at no other time, she may be excused for so doing. Instead of examining and rectifying the social practices that forbid women to protest their circumstances, describing anger as pathologic reinforces its proscription. However, for a significant number of women, cyclical symptoms appear to be mediated not by sociocultural influences but by biochemical changes beyond the woman's control. (See Box 18.1.) The debate about such cyclical symptoms being a medical concern and a possible mental disorder continues among those involved with women's health and women's studies (4).

Medical interest in premenstrual disorders was stimulated by the work in the 1930s of R. T. Frank, who began exploring the role of estrogen on women's mood changes. Later, Dalton popularized the use of progesterone to treat premenstrual negative behaviors (5). As debate about the validity of premenstrual disorders grew, clinicians and researchers struggled to find treatments for the women who complained of such symptoms. Many of these symptoms centered on anger, but symptoms also included cyclic depression (even, at times, suicidal thoughts) and marked loss of functioning in daily life.

The course of menstrual cycle symptomatology is not clearly defined by research to date but, clinically, it appears to begin in adolescence, increase in the late twenties to early thirties, and disappear with menopause, whether menopause is induced or naturally occurring (3,5). It has been noted by many that a woman's experience of menstrual symptoms is related to that of her mother and culture. An increasing number of studies from diverse cultures continue to investigate this theory, with some finding a genetic rather than a social influence (1–3,5).

In an attempt to stimulate research into the menstrual cycle and associated (disabling) psychological changes, *The Diagnostic and Statistical Manual of Mental Disorders,* 3rd edition, Revised (DSM-III-R) included a proposed new diagnosis in an appendix for further research: late luteal phase dysphoric disorder (LLPDD) (6).

BOX 18.1

Case Example

A 35-year-old woman was asked by her supervisor if she was having problems at home because she was frequently irritable or absent from the workplace and her behavior seemed to change unpredictably. She noted that her husband and young daughter had made similar observations on many occasions over the past few years. Concerned about the number of sick days she was taking from the workplace and about her interpersonal relationships at home, she consulted her family physician. An additional history of appetite change, sleep disturbance, and suicidal ideation led to a psychiatric referral. The sporadic and unpredictable course of her symptoms led to further questioning. It appeared that she felt sad and angry around the time of her menstrual period; this was confirmed by charting the symptoms over several months. Discussion meanwhile explored her marital relationship, her feelings about her job, and her personal and family background. When symptom free, she was productive, known for her humor, and enjoyed her family and her work. She noted upon reflection that the symptoms had started during her late adolescence but had not affected her life and functioning until recent years. She would be feeling well and would awaken one morning and have difficulty getting out of bed. For the next eight to ten days she would be tearful, have difficulty concentrating, feel irritable, awaken early, have a great desire for chocolate and other sweets, lose interest in her usual activities, argue with her husband, and struggle with hopelessness and thoughts of self-harm. Then her menses would start, her mood would lift, and she would feel renewed energy and pleasure in life.

LLPDD was defined as a dysphoric disorder associated with the menstrual cycle that caused significant impairment in a woman's social and occupational functioning. It was, thus, distinguished from the more common minor premenstrual symptoms experienced by many women and from variously, often imprecisely, defined premenstrual syndromes (PMS) (5). The premenstrual syndromes consist of a variety of both physical and behavioral symptoms showing varying degrees of severity; the 1983 guidelines from the National Institute of Mental Health required a 30% increase in the intensity of symptoms for six days prior to the onset of menses before a diagnosis of PMS could be made. The mainly dysphoric disorder causing severe impairment (LLPDD) was seen as a distinct, severe, psychological, and far less frequent, premenstrual disorder. This chapter focuses on that disorder rather than on the less severe premenstrual disorders (PMS).

The decision to introduce a description of a mental disorder that could occur only in women was controversial. However, it was hoped that research using the LLPDD criteria would resolve the arguments for and against such a diagnosis. In 1992, the World Health Organization (WHO) published the tenth edition of the *International Classification of Diseases* (ICD-10). In the ICD-10, premenstrual disorders were listed only as "premenstrual tension" under "Diseases of the Genitourinary System (N00–N99): N94, Pain and other conditions associated with female genital organs and menstrual cycle" (7). In contrast, the LLPDD criteria did not include pain or dysmenorrhea, nor were physical symptoms required for the diagnosis to be made. In 1994, the DSM-IV was published. Here, the proposed diagnosis of LLPDD was renamed premenstrual dysphoric disorder (PMDD) and was described in Appendix B, "Criteria Sets and Axes Provided for Further Study." PMDD was also listed as a differential diagnosis under Depression Not Otherwise Specified (8). The new name, premenstrual dysphoric disorder, reflected the fact that this dysphoria seemed to be linked to the menstrual cycle since it appeared in the late luteal phase and disappeared with the onset of menses. Placing it as a differential diagnosis for depression emphasized the predominant mood disorder component, reflecting etiologic research that implicated the serotonergic system, as in other mood disorders (9).

The criteria for this research diagnosis require that the symptoms be present during the last week of the cycle, remit with the beginning of the follicular phase, and be absent in the postmenses week. The symptoms must include either depressed mood, marked anxiety, marked lability of mood, or marked anger or irritability or increased interpersonal conflicts. In addition, at least four more symptoms are necessary. These can be symptoms such as decreased interest, poor concentration, fatigue, appetite changes, feeling out of control, and somatic symptoms. In addition, there must be marked interference with work, school, and social interactions. The symptoms must not be an exacerbation of a preexisting illness. Finally, the criteria must be confirmed by prospective daily ratings for at least two cycles.

The literature review, published in 1994 by the DSM-IV work group, noted that a small but significant number of women (4.6%) met the criteria for PMDD but did not meet the criteria for other concurrent mental disorders (10). The symptoms of PMDD in women responded most consistently to medications affecting serotonin pathways and also to ovarian suppression. No other medications or supplements were found to be effective in alleviating symptoms of PMDD. A database reanalysis conducted for the Work Group clarified the set of symptomatic criteria for this proposed diagnosis (11).

Among the important questions requiring answers was why only about 5% of women develop the severe symptoms of PMDD while the vast majority of women do not. Was PMDD indeed a distinct, cyclical mood disorder or a dysphoric variant of PMS? The actual prevalence of PMDD was not known; neither was the familial pattern nor the course of the disorder over a woman's lifetime. What was the biologic basis of the disorder, given that effective treatments for PMDD were medications that either suppressed ovulation or affected the serotonergic system? What were the interactions or links between events of the ovulatory cycle and serotonin? Were the symptoms of PMDD due to abnormalities triggered by the hormonal changes of the menstrual cycle? And if so, were they linked to estrogen or progesterone or both? Did women with PMDD have a biologic trait abnormality that was present constantly, or was the abnormality specific to the luteal state (12)?

REVIEW OF THE LITERATURE SINCE DSM-IV

A search of the literature from 1994 to 2004, using Medline and the Cochrane Library, revealed numerous publications of research studies employing the DSM-IV definition of PMDD.

PREVALENCE

One prospective community study of young women and adolescents over 48 months found a 5.8% baseline prevalence of PMDD, or 5.3% when concurrent major depressive disorder was excluded. The diagnosis remained stable over the 48 months' duration of the study. A further 18.5% had premenstrual symptoms that did not meet PMDD impairment criteria (13). In another small study, women with prospectively diagnosed PMS or retrospectively confirmed PMDD were followed for 5 to 12 years and, in this small group, the PMS symptoms were stable over time (14). Data from many countries and cultures now support the existence of negative premenstrual symptoms, including PMDD (15,16). One such study, of women aged 15 to 52, found significant somatic and psychological premenstrual symptomatology in 52% of the women sampled with no difference between age groups except for the greater frequency of pain in adolescents (17).

Another study examining symptom stability across cycles in women with prospectively confirmed PMDD, during symptomatic cycles only, concluded that mood symptoms, including irritability, anxiety, and affective lability, showed the most stability, and that somatic symptoms, while also stable, were not associated with functional impairment (18). The authors stated that their data supported PMDD as a mood disorder and suggested further that, because of the stability of its symptoms, PMDD might prove to be a model for the study of mood disorders in general.

CRITERIA

Somatic symptoms discriminated the least between women who met PMDD criteria and those who did not, while anger, irritability, and conflict; a sense of being out of control; markedly depressed mood; and decreased interest in usual activities were the most discriminating symptoms (19). Tension, being on edge, and increased interpersonal conflict were also important.

Problems with concentration and memory are frequent complaints both in those with major depression and in women with PMDD. A small study that assessed psychomotor speed, attention, and verbal learning and memory reported that women with PMDD demonstrated psychomotor slowing in the luteal, as compared to the follicular, phase and also compared to women whose symptoms did not meet PMDD criteria. But the PMDD women's scores were still within the normal range despite psychomotor slowing and were independent of measures for depression. Thus, the authors concluded that cognitive changes during the luteal phase are minor and do not cause impaired functioning (20).

Another study examined the degree of symptom severity needed for the diagnosis using daily ratings, as required by the DSM-IV criteria (21). These authors suggested that all studies of PMDD should describe the process of determining how the severity criteria were met. However, it should be noted that studies of no other mental disorder diagnosis require demonstrable measurement of severity of symptoms.

A panel of experts in 1999 evaluated all of the PMDD research data and concluded that PMDD was a distinct clinical entity and was distinguishable from mood and anxiety disorders (22).

ASSOCIATION WITH MOOD DISORDERS

Studies of women who meet PMDD criteria have shown abnormalities in serotonin binding (23,24). These changes were seen independent of the phase of the menstrual cycle, indicating a trait susceptibility in this subgroup of women, rather than a state-specific abnormality. In subjects with PMDD, the most significant complaints in the luteal phase were of anxiety, not depression, but these complaints of anxiety were not matched by the increases in autonomic activity that are usually associated with anxiety. The authors state that these findings further differentiate PMDD from both anxiety and depressive disorders (23,24). However, another explanation could be that the complaints of "anxiety" are an expression of the tension and irritability that accompany depression and form part of the PMDD criteria rather than classical anxiety disorder symptoms. Data also point to abnormal beta-2 adrenergic receptor density as a trait in some women with PMDD (25). The authors speculate that the variable response to antidepressant medications among women with PMDD may mean that this receptor abnormality does not occur in all PMDD women. However, the studies had small numbers of subjects and replication and amplification of these results are needed (25). Others continue to investigate the possibility of comorbidity of PMDD with PTSD, mood and anxiety disorders (26,27).

1,312 twins completed a questionnaire that included four questions concerning premenstrual tiredness, sadness, and irritability on two separate occasions six years apart (28). The results discount the influence of family and environment on the occurrence of premenstrual symptoms but show a marked heritable influence. The data indicate that the biologic relationship of premenstrual symptoms and lifetime major depression is weak in terms of genetics and environmental risk factors. A prospective twin study using the PMDD criteria would be of great value here. The indication that environmental and familial factors are not important in the expression of premenstrual symptoms is contrary to the views of many (29). The absence of a strong association between premenstrual symptoms and mood disorder also needs elaboration. While the twin study is interesting, the use of only a few questions relating to premenstrual experiences limits its usefulness in understanding the origins of severe premenstrual distress.

TWO OTHER AREAS REQUIRING MORE RESEARCH

Links between mood disorder and PMDD have also been studied by looking at circadian rhythm dysregulation as well as seasonal affective disorder (30,31). These small studies found lower, shorter, and advanced nocturnal melatonin secretion in women with PMDD, and they conclude that such blunted circadian rhythms may make such women vulnerable to endogenous and environmental influences that can result in PMDD symptomatology. While there were no differences in the actual levels of progesterone or estrogen between the women with PMDD and the normal controls, the studies' authors suggest that the circadian rhythm clock in those meeting PMDD criteria is influenced by the hormonal changes of the menstrual cycle. These studies are especially interesting since melatonin is synthesized from serotonin (32).

Results from several studies of plasma gamma-aminobutyric acid (GABA) levels have had equivocal results (33,34). A relationship has been mooted between PMDD symptoms and cortical GABA neuronal functioning. More research is needed in this area.

In summary, evidence to date concerning the association of PMDD and mood disorders is tentative but suggestive. The serotonergic basis of both PMDD and mood disorders is reflected in the medications that are often effective for both, although the exact mechanism responsible is as yet unknown. It could be that the same medications are often effective for both because the two disorders have a similar etiologic basis. Or the medications may affect a common final biologic pathway, such as altered serotonergic receptors—that is, different biologic abnormalities may lead to a similar end point, altered serotonin pharmacodynamics. However, such abnormalities have yet to be discerned. Another study followed women with PMDD on either placebo or L-tryptophan for three cycles (35). Those receiving tryptophan had a significant diminution in mood symptoms, suggesting a therapeutic effect of increased serotonin synthesis in the late luteal phase of the cycle.

ENDOCRINE STUDIES

Studies investigating a possible endocrine/ovarian or neurobiologic etiology for PMDD have continued; however, no abnormalities have been found in estrogen or progesterone levels in women with premenstrual symptoms (36). One important study concluded that normal cyclical changes in these hormones resulted in the abnormal expression of severe mood disturbances premenstrually in some women (37). In this placebo-controlled study, normal ovarian function was suppressed by leuprolide (a gonadotropin-releasing hormone [GnRH] agonist) and the hormones were then replaced separately. Once replacement occurred, only women with premenstrual symptoms had a return of symptoms, including sadness, anxiety, irritability, bloating, and impaired functioning. The return of symptoms was related to either estrogen or progesterone and was greatest in the week or two after the hormones were administered, decreasing in the last week of administration. This increase in symptoms did not occur in those women previously diagnosed with premenstrual syndrome who were given leuprolide plus placebo instead of the hormones. Interestingly, not all of the symptomatic women were relieved of their symptoms by the GnRH agonist. The study's authors did not note whether the symptoms in the women studied met the criteria for PMDD. Thus, it is not clear if this finding is applicable to women with the severe symptoms of PMDD. Nor is it known why only some women are susceptible. However, this study effectively summarizes the findings to date regarding possible hormonal influences on the development of PMDD.

Norepinephrine

The results of one study of a small sample showed that women with PMDD had significantly elevated norepinephrine levels both at rest and when under mental stress when compared to controls (38). These women also exhibited greater ratios of norepinephrine to cortisol at rest and when stressed. However, the women with PMDD also reported more current life stressors than did the controls, leading the authors to conclude that a subgroup of women with PMDD, with a history of past and current stressors, have a dysregulation of the stress response. As mentioned above, another study suggests a relationship between childhood abuse and other traumatic events and the later development of PMDD (27). Again, these findings require replication.

Obviously, a probable connection among the hypothalamus, pituitary, and gonadal hormones, and the neurotransmitters will continue to be the subject of future research.

EFFECTIVE TREATMENTS

Inherent problems in regulating neurotransmitters could result in a susceptibility to the normal hormonal changes of the menstrual cycle, the result being the symptoms associated with PMDD. However, why women with PMDD (or women and men with depression) show abnormalities in serotonin pathways is still not known. What has been demonstrated is the effectiveness of several of the SSRIs (selective serotonin reuptake inhibitors) in treating the symptoms of depressive mood disorder and of PMDD. Treatments for PMDD that have demonstrated efficacy in studies done after the publication of DSM-IV include ovariectomy, gonadal hormone–releasing agonists, several of the SSRIs, and clomipramine. Multisite studies of fluoxetine (39) and of sertraline (40) administered for the entire cycle demonstrated effective symptomatic relief in women with PMDD. Other studies have examined the effectiveness of giving the medication *only* in the luteal period (41,42), and have found that the intermittent dosing was effective.

However, fluoxetine has a long-lasting metabolite that would remain active in the follicular phase and this might account for its efficacy when given only in the luteal phase. In contrast, sertraline is short acting but also effective when given intermittently. Thus, the reason for the effectiveness of these SSRIs is unclear. Nevertheless, in both cases, the advantage of intermittent dosing is the short period during which a medication has to be taken and the resultant diminution in side effects. Fluvoxamine and paroxetine have also been shown to relieve PMDD symptoms (43). A meta-analysis concluded that of the SSRIs, fluoxetine was more effective than sertraline (44). The SSRIs have been shown to be effective at relatively low dosages compared to those required in major depression (45). Similarly, the onset of effectiveness is more rapid in PMDD cases than in major depression. Recent studies have demonstrated the role of serotonin neurotransmission in those cases where SSRIs are effective (46).

In all of the studies cited above, the majority, *but not all,* of the women with PMDD were relieved of their symptoms and had few side effects from the medications. As mentioned in the discussion of hormonal influences on the occurrence of premenstrual dysphoria, this finding again points to a varying etiology for PMDD, with some cases not responding to serotonin agonism. Future studies should focus on women who do not respond to SSRI treatments, on women who drop out of treatment due to the side effects of the SSRIs, and on women who do not experience symptomatic relief following ovarian suppression.

CLINICAL IMPLICATIONS

The literature reviewed here indicates that PMDD must be considered as a differential diagnosis in all women with dysphoric mood complaints. However, premenstrual exacerbation of a preexisting mood disorder must not be confused with PMDD, nor should the mood and behavioral effects of concurrent psychosocial stressors. *Importantly, the diagnosis of PMDD should be made only if the research criteria are met.*

Once such a diagnosis is confirmed, the indicated treatment appears to be pharmacologic. An SSRI can be prescribed from midcycle to the onset of menses. Some women, however, find it easier to remember to take the medication if it is given throughout the month. The effective dosage will probably be lower than that needed for depressive disorders. Clinical experience has shown that, as with the use of SSRIs for depressive disorders, the effectiveness of the medication may diminish after a number of months. An increase in the dosage usually brings relief once again. When this occurs, women should be reevaluated and other diagnoses, including acute stress responses, ruled out before the medication is increased or changed.

It is not clear if women who do not respond to treatment with one SSRI will respond to other SSRIs or to ovarian suppression. Therefore, a variety of SSRIs should be tried before declaring them ineffective. Because of the side effects of ovarian suppression, most clinicians prefer to use this treatment only when SSRIs have failed.

In addition, as with PMS, it is recommended that women with symptoms meeting PMDD criteria limit their intake of salt and caffeine and increase exercise (47). Recently, researchers have been studying the effectiveness of new oral contraceptive agents containing low-dose estrogen and a spironolactone analog, drospirenone, in treating PMDD (48). Also, at least one study has demonstrated improvement of symptoms in women with PMDD after six months' treatment with cognitive-behavioral therapy (CBT) equal to the effects of fluoxetine (49). This work deserves replication and indicates a treatment approach that appears to assist some women with their negative perceptions of menstruation and its psychological consequences.

As noted at the beginning of this chapter, fears remain that women's symptoms will be medicalized and treatments given to remove symptoms while ignoring the social realities of women's lives. Attribution of a woman's expression of anger, unhappiness, or anxiety to her menstrual cycle is often a convenient and socially accepted excuse or a way of denigrating her feelings and thoughts. However, this sociologic fact cannot be used alone to dismiss the research findings summarized above. Women and men do live in societies and cultures that have differing gender expectations and rules, just as there are biologic differences between men and women. Exploring the latter does not mean ignoring or minimizing the former. Rather, finding biologic explanations and treatments for gender-specific disorders should assist, not harm, women.

OTHER RESEARCH

In addition to the research areas noted above in this chapter, the literature is sparse about premenstrual exacerbation of medical and psychiatric disorders. There is a well-established clinical literature and impression that a number of disorders grow worse in the immediate premenstrual period, but research data are difficult to find (50–52). Nevertheless, clinicians must be aware of the possibility of premenstrual exacerbation of symptoms of physical and mental disorders. This is important in the management of women with disorders and symptoms, especially when medication is prescribed. Increasing the dose of medication according to symptom worsening in the premenstruum may result in severe side effects during the rest of the cycle. As well, both the woman and the clinician may decide that the disorder is not responding to appropriate treatments for the disorder and lose hope for recovery or stabilization, instead of considering the possibility of a premenstrual exacerbation. Similarly, treatment of premenstrual symptoms may be ineffective if underlying medical or mental disorders are not treated adequately (53,54).

CONCLUSION

Since 1994, researchers into the etiology and treatment of PMDD have been using the criteria for PMDD as listed in the DSM-IV appendix for proposed disorders. The availability of these research criteria has standardized the definition of the type of cases studied and made replication attempts possible, unlike in prior years when studies confused a variety of definitions of PMS. This has enabled investigators to distinguish this severe dysphoric disorder more carefully from more common premenstrual symptoms. Nevertheless, the links between PMDD, major depression, and anxiety disorders require more clarification.

Treatment studies have demonstrated the efficacy of the SSRIs in treating PMDD, while oblating the ovarian hormones by chemical or surgical means is also effective. Hormonal menstrual cycles do not seem to cause the symptoms of PMDD, but rather, the normal hormonal surges appear to precipitate dysphoric symptoms in susceptible women. Why these women are susceptible is still unknown, but twin studies discount familial and environmental factors, pointing instead to inherited factors. However, not all women who meet the PMDD criteria are relieved of their symptoms by the SSRIs or by ovarian suppression. Thus, it appears that different etiologic factors may result in the symptoms of PMDD, and these remain to be elucidated.

The complex endocrine-pituitary-hypothalamic axis remains the focus of biologic investigations. The social, personal, and occupational benefits of the development of treatments for this severely disabling disorder have been substantial (55). While the etiologic basis for PMDD requires further research, a similar conclusion can be stated about most other mental disorders. Finally, as when diagnosing and treating all mental disorders, consideration must be given to the psychosocial and cultural aspects of the lives of women who complain of premenstrual symptoms. This, too, remains an area requiring further research.

REFERENCES

1. Moawed S. Indigenous practices of Saudi girls in Riyadh during their menstrual period. East Mediterr Health J 2001;7:197–203.
2. Dan AJ, Monagle L. Sociocultural influences on women's experiences of perimenstrual symptoms. In: Gold JH, Severino SK, eds. Premenstrual Dysphorias: Myths and Realities. Washington, DC: American Psychiatric Press, 1994:201–211.
3. Gold JH, Endicott J, Parry B, et al. Late luteal phase dysphoric disorder. In: Widiger TA, Frances AJ, Pincus HA, et al, eds. DSM-IV Sourcebook, vol 2. Washington, DC: American Psychiatric Association, 1996:317–394.
4. Chrisler JC, Caplan P. The strange case of Dr Jekyll and Ms Hyde: how PMS became a cultural phenomenon and a psychiatric disorder. Annu Rev Sex Res 2002;13:274–306.
5. Gold JH. Historical perspectives of premenstrual syndrome. In: Gold JH, Severino SK, eds. Premenstrual Dysphorias: Myths and Realities. Washington, DC: American Psychiatric Press, 1994:174–177.
6. American Psychiatric Association. Diagnostic and Statistical Manual of Mental Disorders. 3rd Ed., rev. Washington, DC, 1987.
7. World Health Organization. International Classification of Diseases and Behavioral Disorders. 10th Ed. Geneva, 1992.
8. American Psychiatric Association. Diagnostic and Statistical Manual of Mental Disorders. 4th Ed. Washington, DC, 1994.
9. Gold JH. Late luteal phase dysphoric disorder: final overview. In: Widiger TA, Frances AJ, Pincus HA, et al. eds. DSM-IV Sourcebook, vol 4. Washington, DC: American Psychiatric Association, 1998:1035–1045.
10. Rivera-Tovar AD, Frank E. Late luteal phase dysphoric disorder in young women. Am J Psychiatry 1990;147:1634–1636.
11. Hurt SW, Schnurr PP, Severino SK, et al. Late luteal phase dysphoric disorder in 670 women evaluated for premenstrual complaints. Am J Psychiatry 1992;149:525–530.

12. Kouri EM, Halbreich U. State and trait abnormalities in women with dysphoric premenstrual syndromes. Psychopharmacol Bull 1997;33:767–770.
13. Wittchen HU, Becjer E, Lieb R, et al. Prevalence, incidence and stability of premenstrual dysphoric disorder in the community. Psychol Med 2002;32:119–132.
14. Roca CA, Schmidt PJ, Rubinow DR. A follow-up study of premenstrual syndrome. J Clin Psychiatry 1999;11:763–766.
15. Gold JH. Premenstrual dysphoric disorder: what's that? JAMA 1997;278:1024–1025.
16. Banerjee N, Roy KK, Takkar D. Premenstrual dysphoric disorder: a study from India. Int J Fertil Womens Med 2000;45:342–344.
17. Sinanovic O, Subasic A, Bacaj D. Psychological disorders in women in Bosnia and Herzegovina associated with menstruation. Med Arh 2003;57(5–6 Suppl 1):17–18.
18. Bloch M, Schmidt PJ, Rubinow DR. Premenstrual syndrome: evidence for symptom stability across cycles. Am J Psychiatry 1997;154:1741–1746.
19. Gehlert S, Chang C-H, Hartlage S. Establishing the validity of premenstrual dysphoric disorder using Rausch analysis. J Outcome Meas 1997;1:2–18.
20. Resnick A, Perry W, Parry B, et al. Neuropsychological performance across the menstrual cycle in women with and without premenstrual dysphoric disorder. Psychiatry Res 1998;77:147–158.
21. Smith MJ, Schmidt PJ, Rubinow DR. Operationalizing DSM IV criteria for PMDD: selecting symptomatic and asymptomatic cycles for research. J Psychiatr Res 2003;37:75–83.
22. Endicott J, Amsterdam J, Eriksson E, et al. Is premenstrual dysphoric disorder a distinct clinical entity? J Womens Health Gend Based Med 1999;8:663–679.
23. Gurguis GNM, Yonkers KA, Phan SP, et al. Adrenergic receptors in premenstrual dysphoric disorder: I. Platelet alpha2 receptors: Gi protein coupling, phase of menstrual cycle, and prediction of luteal phase symptom severity. Biol Psychiatry 1998;44:600–609.
24. Gurguis GNM, Yonkers KA, Blakeley JE, et al. Adrenergic receptors in premenstrual dysphoric disorder. II: Neutrophil beta2-adrenergic receptors: Gs protein coupling, phase of menstrual cycle and prediction of luteal phase severity. Psychiatry Res 1998;70:31–42.
25. Bixo M, Allard P, Backstrom T, et al. Binding of [3H] paroxetine to serotonin uptake sites and of [3H] lysergic acid diethylamide to 5-HT2A receptors in platelets from women with premenstrual dysphoric disorder during gonadotropin releasing hormone treatment. Psychoneuroendocrinology 2001;6:551–564.
26. Kim DR, Gyulai L, Freeman EW, et al. Premenstrual dysphoric disorder and psychiatric co-morbidity. Arch Women Ment Health 2004;7:37–47.
27. Wittchen HU, Perkonigg A, Pfister H. Trauma and PTSD: an overlooked pathogenic pathway for premenstrual dysphoric disorder? Arch Women Ment Health 2003;6:293–297.
28. Kendler KS, Karkowski LM, Corey LA, et al. Longitudinal population-based twin study of retrospectively reported premenstrual symptoms and lifetime major depression. Am J Psychiatry 1998;155:1234–1240.
29. Dan AJ, Monagle L. Sociocultural influences on women's experiences of perimenstrual symptoms. In: Gold JH, Severino SK, eds. Premenstrual Dysphorias: Myths and Realities. Washington, DC: American Psychiatric Press, 1994:201–211.
30. Praschak-Rieder N, Willeit M, Neumeister A, et al. Prevalence of premenstrual dysphoric disorder in female patients with seasonal affective disorder. J Affect Disord 2001;63:239–242.
31. Parry BL, Berga SL, Mostofi N, et al. Plasma melatonin circadian rhythms during the menstrual cycle and after light therapy in premenstrual dysphoric disorder and normal control subjects. J Biol Rhythms 1997;12:47–64.
32. Walther DJ, Bader M. A unique central tryptophan hydroxylase isoform. Biochem Pharmacol 2003;66:1673–1680.
33. Backstrom T, Anderson A, Andree L, et al. Pathogenesis in menstrual cycle-linked CNS disorders. Ann NY Acad Sci 2003;1007:42–53.
34. Epperson CN, Haga K, Mason GF, et al. Cortical gamma-aminobutyric acid levels across the menstrual cycle in healthy women and those with premenstrual dysphoric disorder: a proton magnetic resonance spectroscopy study. Arch Gen Psychiatry 2002;59:851–858.
35. Steinberg S, Annable L, Young SN, et al. A placebo-controlled study of the effects of L-tryptophan in patients with premenstrual dysphoria. Adv Exp Med Biol 1999;467:85–88.
36. Rubinow DR, Schmidt PJ. The treatment of premenstrual syndrome: forward into the past. N Engl J Med 1995;332:1574–1575.
37. Schmidt PJ, Nieman LK, Danaceau MA, et al. Differential behavioral effects of gonadal steroids in women with and in those without premenstrual syndrome. N Engl J Med 1998;338:209–216.
38. Girdler SS, Pedersen CA, Straneva PA, et al. Dysregulation of cardiovascular and neuroendocrine responses to stress in premenstrual dysphoric disorder. Psychiatry Res 1998;81:163–178.
39. Luisi AF, Pawasauskas JE.Treatment of premenstrual dysphoric disorder with selective serotonin reuptake inhibitors. Pharmacotherapy 2003;23:1131–1140.
40. Yonkers KA, Halbreich U, Freeman E, et al: Symptomatic improvement of premenstrual dysphoric disorder with sertraline treatment: a randomized controlled trial. JAMA 1997;278:983–988.

41. Freeman EW, Rickels K, Sondheimer SJ, et al. Continuous or intermittent dosing with sertraline for patients with severe premenstrual syndrome or premenstrual dysphoric disorder. Am J Psychiatry 2004;161:343–351.
42 Halbreich U, Kahn LS. Treatment of premenstrual dysphoric disorder with luteal phase dosing of sertraline. Expert Opin Pharmacother 2003;4:2065–2078.
43. Steiner M, Judge R, Kumar R. Serotonin re-uptake inhibitors in the treatment of premenstrual dysphoria: current state of knowledge. Int J Psychiatry Clin Prac 1997;1:241–247.
44. Dimmock PW, Wyatt KM, Jones PW, et al. Efficacy of selective serotonin-reuptake inhibitors in premenstrual syndrome: a systematic review. Lancet 2000;356:1131–1136.
45. Yonkers KA, Brown WA. Pharmacologic treatments for premenstrual dysphoric disorder. Psychiatric Ann 1996;26:586–589.
46. Roca C, Schmidt PJ, Smith MJ, et al. Effects of metergoline on symptoms in women with premenstrual dysphoric disorder. Am J Psychiatry 2002;159:1876–1881.
47. Bianchi-Demicheli F, Ludicke F, et al. Premenstrual dysphoric disorder: current status of treatment. Swiss Med Wkly 2002;132:574–578.
48. Rapkin A. A review of treatment of premenstrual syndrome and premenstrual dysphoric disorder. Psychoneuroendocrinology 2003;28 (Suppl 3):39–53.
49. Hunter MS, Ussher JM, Cariss M, et al. Medical (fluoxetine) and psychological (cognitive-behavioral therapy) treatment for premenstrual dysphoric disorder: a study of treatment processes. J Psychosom Res 2002;53:811–817.
50. Case AM, Reid RL. Menstrual cycle effects on common medical conditions. Compr Ther 2001;27:65–71.
51. Hsiao MC, Hsiao CC, Liu CY. Premenstrual symptoms and premenstrual exacerbation in patients with psychiatric disorders. Psychiatry Clin Neurosci 2004;58:186–190.
52. Dzolijic E, Sipetic S, Vlajinac H, et al. Prevalence of menstrually related migraine and nonmigraine primary headache in female students of Belgrade University. Headache 2002; 42:185–193.
53. Pearlstein T, Stone AB. Premenstrual syndrome. Psychiatr Clin North Am 1998;21:577–590.
54. Basoglu C, Cetin M, Semiz UB, Agargun MY, et al. Premenstrual exacerbation and suicidal behavior in patients with panic disorder. Compr Psychiatry 2000;41:103–105.
55. Halbreich U, Borenstein J, Pearlstein T, et al. The prevalence, impairment, impact, and burden of premenstrual dysphoric disorder (PMS/PMDD). Psychoneuroendocrinology 2003;28 (Suppl).

SUGGESTED READINGS

Grahn J. Blood, Bread and Roses: How Menstruation Created the World. Boston. Beacon Press, 1994 (reprinted).
Gold JH, Severino SK, eds. Premenstrual Dysphorias: Myths and Realities. Washington, DC: American Psychiatric Press, 1994.

Pregnancy and Mental Health

Anne Buist

Pregnancy is a unique developmental transition resulting in a woman being no longer responsible just for herself but also for another. (See also Chapter 13.) Because of the enormous physical and mental changes that must occur in the transition, it is a time of particular vulnerability, both physically and mentally. Mental health is influenced by multiple factors from the woman's earlier life and own development, current relationships and support, and the cultural context in which the pregnancy occurs.

Different theoretical models influence the understanding of both motherhood and mental illness in the perinatal period; the medical model emphasizes the role of hormones, sleep deprivation, and early influences on biologic responses to stress; feminist theories look at the influence of the medicalization of childbirth reinforcing feminine helplessness as a cause of difficulties, while attachment and interpersonal theories emphasize the importance of changing relationships at this time of developmental change (1). Theorists in evolutionary psychology emphasize the role of depression as a response to inadequate support, in order to ensure their partner, in particular, increases his investment in the child (2). These theories all provide valid views and are not necessarily at odds with one another.

How the mother adapts to these changes as she prepares for motherhood will depend on multiple factors. (See also Chapter 20.) This will include her own theoretical perspective, biology, personality, background, general health, current supports, and whether this child was planned and wanted. This chapter examines the psychosocial and physical aspects of pregnancy that have been seen to influence mental health, and then looks at screening for mental health issues in health care. It finally outlines what our current understanding is of depression, anxiety, and psychosis in pregnancy and their effects on both mother and infant. The aim is to improve understanding of mental health issues in pregnant women for all health professionals in order to enhance prevention, early identification, and assertive management and, thus, improved outcome for this and future generations.

PSYCHOSOCIAL FACTORS AND MENTAL HEALTH

DEVELOPMENTAL PHASE

Erikson's theory of life stages describes the parent as one who has a firm sense of self both within and separate from the relationship with a partner, and that from this position, parents are able to develop and see their child as a separate individual who is dependent on them and whose needs are placed first. For teenagers, many single parents, and those whose childhoods were emotionally deprived, such developmental tasks have often not been mastered prior to parenthood.

Teenage pregnancies have reduced considerably in some Western countries, by more than two thirds in the last 30 years in Australia, for example. They now constitute 18 per 1,000 pregnancies (3). This compares to the United States at 51.5 per 1,000 and the United Kingdom at 29 per 1,000 (the highest in Europe) and is six times the rate in the Netherlands (4). Differences in the prevalence are likely to relate to different cultural and religious attitudes in these countries, which influence sex education, availability of contraception, and financial supports for teenagers. The experience of pregnancy when it does occur in this setting will affect the transition to motherhood (Table 19.1) and may have unrealis-

TABLE 19.1

Factors Influencing Transition to Motherhood

Age
Physical health
Cultural beliefs
Poverty
Relationship difficulties or no relationship
Domestic violence
Psychiatric diagnosis
Financial security
Education
Life stresses

tic expectations attached, such as "My child will be the one person who will love me unconditionally" or "This is the one job I will do well."

Older mothers—particularly first-time mothers and those who have become mothers as a result of in vitro fertilization (IVF)—present with different psychological conflicts. Delaying the age of first-time motherhood has been a universal trend, with the average age 29 years in Australia up from 25.8 years in 1991 (3). For those mothers who delay longer (1 in 35 wait until 35 or older for their first child), reduced fertility has become an increasing concern, balanced, though not evenly, by improved reproductive technology. If there have been difficulties in conceiving, the woman may have difficulty believing she will have a healthy child and may be anxious about the viability of the infant. This can be heightened by any physical difficulties experienced during pregnancy. Idealization of mothering may produce a flurry of activity in preparing the nursery but often also widens the divide between what motherhood is thought to be about and the reality of the experience in the postpartum period. These expectations may contribute to a negative transition. Improved obstetric care has meant better maternal and child outcomes but also shorter hospital stays and a high dissatisfaction with postnatal supports (5).

THE MEANING AND EXPERIENCE OF PREGNANCY

Historically, society has viewed motherhood as a natural and sacred role, but the epitome of fulfillment and bliss that radiates from women on the covers of mother and baby magazines is for many women an elusive myth. In order to continue the species, it is in society's interests to promote such views. Rapid change in technology, however, has meant a marked change in women's roles. With reliable contraception available in the Western world, motherhood is now viewed as a choice.

For many women, the desire to have an infant is a complex one. The motivations are not always conscious, and the woman's ability to see her infant as separate depends on her ability to understand, to some degree at least, these motivations. In some cases, the pregnancy will be unplanned or unwanted. Studies have varyingly associated this circumstance with an increased risk of depression, although it appears that the "unwanted" carries a greater risk, given that the definition of unplanned varies from a failure of contraception to participation in an active sexual relationship with a steady partner where neither is taking precautions to prohibit pregnancy. These unwanted pregnancies may also include both first pregnancies, where the risk of depression is highest, and grandmultiparity with short interpregnancy breaks, where the risk has also been noted to be increased (6).

Where a woman elects to terminate a pregnancy, as some 1.5 million women do each year (7), there is debate and controversy regarding potential psychological sequelae. Researchers such as Reardon et al. (8) have concluded that there is an increased risk of psychiatric admission following abortion, and pro-life organizations support this association with testimonies of grief and regret. The research, however, has been significantly hampered by methodologic flaws such as not assessing the woman's mental state at the time of her decision, no controls, and the impossible scenario of how she would have been had she not had the termination. Major (9) noted Reardon et al.'s (8) conclusions to be misleading; indeed women with a mental illness have been noted to be more likely to have unwanted pregnancies rather than the termination itself necessarily leading to mental illness.

It is not uncommon for women to experience some sadness or guilt from a termination, either at the time or after subsequent children, but this is usually transient and does not warrant a psychiatric diagnosis (7).

The experience of a completed pregnancy may have particular relevance to mental health after birth. In Gross et al.'s (10) study, women who reported their pregnancy as being very hard or one of the worst times of their life were at least 4.6 times more likely than comparison women to be depressed postpartum.

PERSONALITY

Emotionally deprived and abusive or chaotic backgrounds are more likely to be associated with development of personality styles that pose challenges to parenthood. Factors that influence personality development are summarized in Table 19.2. Personality, in turn, will affect how women respond to pregnancy and motherhood and the circumstances in which they conceive.

Individuals diagnosed with borderline personalities have many unmet emotional needs. The vulnerability in their infant is likely to awaken these needs and put them in competition with their infant, more as a sibling than as a mother. In pregnancy, this may manifest as the inability to consider the needs of the fetus. The use of drugs, smoking, and poor obstetric care are likely results. In the setting of becoming mothers, childhood traumas and their own vulnerability are likely to surface—with potential for negative mental health outcomes for both the woman and her child (11).

Temperament and childhood experiences that have shaped the woman's personality will influence coping strategies during a considerably heightened level of physical and emotional change. Avoidance strategies have been associated with more negative outcomes of fertility and pregnancy, including depression and failed in vitro fertilizaton. High self-esteem is associated with a smoother transition to motherhood. Huizink et al. (12) looked at coping strategies in normal-risk nulliparous pregnant women and identified two key strategies that were used: emotional-focused and problem-focused coping. The former was associated with more distress and pregnancy complaints.

Women's relationship to their bodies and the feeling of control—or need for control—are likely to influence attitudes. Women with perfectionistic personality styles are at greater risk of postnatal depression (13); the idealization of motherhood most likely begins in childhood but becomes a focus during pregnancy. Women with eating disorders may have particular difficulties of control with respect to body image disturbance and intake. Although researchers have found that

TABLE 19.2

Factors Influencing Personality Development

Genetic (including temperament, intellect)
Fetal exposure to drugs or illness
Availability and appropriateness of attachment figure—"the good enough" mother
Role model
Early childhood experiences (e.g., abuse, trauma)

there is a reduction in anxiety about weight and body image in pregnancy, this nevertheless remains the most significant concern (14).

SOCIAL FACTORS

Lower socioeconomic status and education, poor social supports, and poor marital relationship as well as an increased number of life stresses come up consistently as being linked with an increased risk of perinatal depression (Table 19.1; 10–16). Teenage pregnancies have a high rate of each of these factors (4). The practicalities of caring for a child (or more than one) physically and emotionally, especially when there are financial difficulties and no child care support, put a burden on a mother who may already be vulnerable to depression and poor coping due to a variety of factors: genetic loading, poor role models, and stress in her childhood (11). Such stresses may also be correlated to difficulties in the pregnancy. Morten et al. (17) found stress increased the risk for preterm delivery at 30 weeks, the risk increasing with the level of psychological distress. Such stresses then add further pressure on the transition to motherhood.

RELATIONSHIP ISSUES

In the setting of pregnancy, the role of the partner becomes crucial. The relationship, whether stressful or abusive, can add its own independent risk (10) to the woman's mental health. Domestic violence is underreported and underrecorded, with an estimated 1 in 3 to 4 women between 16 and 59 experiencing domestic violence and one woman dying every three days as a result in the United Kingdom and the United States (18,19). In Australia, 23% of women report lifetime partner abuse; 61% of these women had children in their care, and 42% were abused when they were pregnant (20). For 20% to 30% of women, the abuse happened for the first time in the course of pregnancy (18,20). Similarly, 1 in 5 women in the United States report domestic violence, with pregnancy rates estimated at between 8% and 26% of pregnant women (21). In this setting, the frequent direction of the physical attack is toward the abdomen, which not only may result in intrauterine damage and prematurity, but also is likely to increase stress on the woman regarding her unborn infant and its viability as part of the family unit.

Partners of women who are depressed are in turn more at risk of depression, and men themselves have particular issues adjusting to the changes in family structure and expectations of fathers, which make them more likely to experience stress (22). Morse et al. (22) noted men to have considerable stress in the gender role, torn between the traditional provider model of husband and father, and the current expectations of attending the birth and participating—potentially equally—in baby and child care. Such confusion is likely to have an impact on the relationship and on the mother's mental health.

CULTURAL FACTORS

Cultural expectations and society's support for parents vary. In Scandinavian countries there have been practical changes with respect to child care and maternity leave, but other countries have been less able or willing to consider such changes. In non-Western countries such as India, economic hardship and sex of the infant are cited as major factors in maternal depression (23).

Women whose beliefs mean that birth control is not an option may find themselves at odds within their culture if the child is not wanted, although they may find more social recognition of the importance of motherhood and support from within this same culture.

PHYSICAL FACTORS AND MENTAL HEALTH ISSUES

HORMONAL BASIS OF MOOD DISORDERS RELATED TO PREGNANCY

During pregnancy, there are dramatic increases in plasma progesterone (10-fold to 18-fold) and estrogens (up to 1,000-fold). Significant changes are also observed in several other steroid and peptide hormones, including corticotrophin-releasing hormone, prolactin, and oxytocin (24). However, attempts to identify a consistent relationship between one or more of these hormones and symptoms of depression and anxiety have been contradictory and inconsistent. Moreover, studies have looked primarily at postnatal mood changes rather than antenatal ones. Some hormonal studies suggest possible mechanisms for the early onset of symptoms postnatally but not for the increase in mood symptoms that appear to occur in the second and third trimesters and continue, for some women, after they give birth (25).

Studies that have evaluated hormonal therapies have not implicated progesterone as having a potential role in increasing depression in those at risk (26). This may be of relevance to women considering the "minipill" (progesterone only) postpartum.

Studies that have been more pregnancy focused have postulated a dysregulation of the maternal-placental-fetal axis secondary to depression, possibly involving placental blood flow, as a cause for the association between depression, anxiety, and stress and preterm birth, as well as increased risk for operative deliveries (17,27,28). Studies have been inconsistent, with small numbers, and the meaning of the complex interplay of hormonal changes—potentially only in genetically vulnerable women—remains unclear.

INFERTILITY

A number of studies are now investigating psychological issues in women who conceived a child (or children) through assisted technology. There were early suggestions that women on IVF programs were more likely to be anxious, particularly while waiting to conceive, and stress may be a factor in causing infertility. At such times there are added pressures on the relationship, changing the sexual relationship from one of intimacy to goal-driven necessity. Women on fertility drugs must deal with side effects such as nausea and vomiting as well as uncertainties about the safety of metformin hydrochloride in the first trimester and the small but serious risk of ovarian hyperstimulation syndrome. This is more likely to occur when fertilization has occurred, so the woman faces both the loss of the fetus and a risk to her own life.

Recent studies suggest that the progression to parenthood after conception is not more troubled than for other mothers. Women on IVF appear similar to naturally conceiving women on measures of anxiety, depression, self-esteem, and marital satisfaction, both antenatally and postnatally. There are possible differences in infant temperament (IVF infants being less easy to soothe) and parenting characteristics: IVF mothers are less positive about breastfeeding, less concerned about the sexual relationship and the husband's sharing of duties, as well as less concerned about decreased attractiveness and restriction of independence (29,30).These differences are largely in keeping with the nature of the pregnancy being very wanted and waited for, with increased emphasis on the mothering role and less on the relationship with the partner.

POOR SELF-CARE

Women with a serious mental illness are significantly less likely to seek and receive adequate antenatal care, often delaying visits and not adhering to dietary suggestions. In addition, they have higher rates of smoking. As a consequence, there is a significantly higher risk of prematurity, intrauterine growth retardation, and low-birth-weight babies. These have been linked with maternal depression, but the evidence is contradictory (27,28).

If women are on psychotropic medication, there are the potential risks to the infant from medication they are receiving and risks to both mother and child if the medication is ceased. Illicit drug use poses a further hazard. These risks are discussed in subsequent sections.

SUBSTANCE USE

Substance use through pregnancy has potentially long-lasting effects on the infant; prescription medications contain warnings of risks, and women are generally resistant to use of medications because of this. However, a significant number of women continue to smoke through pregnancy. In the United Kingdom one study in 2000 reported a rate of 19% in mothers aged 25 to 29 years, increasing to 29% in the 20 to 24 year old age group, and 39% in teenage mothers whose fetuses also have a higher exposure to alcohol and a range of illicit substances. (30A). An estimate of antenatal alcohol use in the United States is around 17%, and illicit drugs 3% (31). These women, with comorbid mental health (depression, personality disorders, and schizophrenia) and substance abuse issues, constitute an important and increasing group who are involved postpartum with protective services (32).

Alcohol has been associated with significant birth defects (fetal alcohol syndrome) and intrauterine growth retardation. Illicit drug use and teratogenicity are less clearly related, but there is an increased risk of intrauterine growth retardation, stillbirth, withdrawal, and deaths from sudden infant death syndrome (SIDS) (33).

SCREENING FOR MENTAL HEALTH ISSUES IN PREGNANCY

Although the vast majority of pregnant women in the Western world see a health professional during their pregnancy, for many with mental health issues, those issues go undetected (34). Given the high rate of contact and the potential for early intervention with respect to child outcomes, the concept of screening for both depression and domestic violence has been targeted by a number of countries (34,35).

In both cases, there has been controversy around the introduction of screening programs. The major concern has been lack of studies showing acceptability of the screening and the lack of appropriate treatment or resources (35,36).

In Ramsay's review (35) a majority of women found being asked about domestic violence acceptable, depending on the circumstances. This brings into play the importance of seeing women without their partner, which is not always possible. A postnatal study on depression screening found a higher level of unacceptability (36), but this appears more related to service delivery than the tool itself and has not been replicated by others (37). There is no uniformity about how questions on domestic violence are asked.

The Edinburgh Postnatal Depression Scale (38) has been validated in pregnancy and used widely for screening, though not in a systematic manner. Although it does not include the somatic symptoms of other depression scales that can be misleading at a time of physical change, the high level of anxiety in pregnancy—accounting for 47% of the pregnancy score in Ross et al.'s (39) study—has led to concern about its suitability. Of note, it is of use as a screen for current depression, and not as a predictor of later postnatal depression (PND) although antenatal depression is a key risk factor for PND (40).

Whether screening for depression during pregnancy or postpartum is preferred has not yet been evaluated, though it is currently being assessed by the beyondblue Australian National Postnatal Depression initiative, which found health professionals less able to identify antenatal depression than postnatal depression (34). Adequate access to resources and evidence-based treatment needs to be available before screening is undertaken widely. In pregnancy, there have been no specific treatment trials and the potential ramifications for the fetus should be taken into account when considering treatment using medications in major depression. To date, postnatal treatments aimed at improving infant outcome have been unsuccessful. It is possible that this treatment would be better beginning antenatally before a negative pattern of interaction has been established.

DEPRESSION AND ANXIETY

PREVALENCE

Significant depressive and anxiety symptoms occur in over 20% of pregnant women and, in pregnancy probably more than at any other time, appear interwoven. The actual prevalence of disorders is unclear, depending on whether self-report or structured interview is used, what questionnaires were utilized, as well as the characteristics of the population. It appears, however, that these symptoms are more common antenatally than postnatally, reported in some 25% (25), though more likely to represent a level of 12% from a meta-analysis and are highest in the second and third trimesters (41). This may represent some "normal" pregnancy anxiety but also stress effects on women where there are physical or psychological concerns about continuing with a pregnancy.

Evans et al. (25) in a large study concluded that depressive symptoms were more common antenatally than postnatally, but this was based on one screening tool, the Edinburgh Postnatal Depression Scale (EPDS; 38), which picks up anxiety symptoms (39) and is not diagnostic for depression.

Over one third of women with preexisting panic disorders have been noted to have a reduction in anxiety symptoms in pregnancy, but a small number (20% to 30%) have worsening of symptoms (42).

PRESENTATION

Because anxiety is common in pregnancy, an underlying disorder is frequently missed. Other symptoms such as fatigue and lethargy are also mistakenly attributed to the woman's physical rather than psychological state. Women often downplay their symptoms, but continued (if fluctuating) lowered mood and tearfulness are more suggestive of a mood disorder than a normal transition to motherhood.

Although some mild concern in the pregnant woman for the well-being of the fetus can be beneficial (e.g., ensuring that she reduces or ceases alcohol and smoking), any ongoing concern that is without basis, whether specific or general, is not "normal." Persistent lowered mood and tearfulness are also suggestive of a depressive disorder, not pregnancy. Suicide risk at this time is less than in the nonpregnant population, the exceptions being those who cease preexisting antidepressant medication because they were pregnant and women with bipolar disorder (43).

ANTENATAL PREVENTION

A number of researchers have attempted to improve postnatal outcome through psychological interventions in high-risk populations in pregnancy. These studies have failed to produce conclusive results, largely because of their poor design, inadequate numbers, and high dropout rates (40).

Other researchers have looked at the use of prophylactic medication in those at risk. This strategy is useful only for those women who have previously been treated successfully with medication. Prophylactic treatment of the woman during pregnancy results in fetal exposure to psychotropic medication; an alternative is to commence treatment immediately postpartum. The risks need to be weighed and discussed with the patient. The benefits of mood stabilizers are well documented in women with bipolar disorder. The benefits of antidepressants are less clear, with initial positive findings not replicated in a randomized controlled trial (RCT) and further assessment still pending (44).

TREATMENT ISSUES

One of the key considerations in managing antenatal psychiatric illness is the potential impact of treatment or lack of treatment on the fetus. It is probably for these reasons, as well as society's strong albeit mixed messages about motherhood, that there is a significant underrecognition of mental illness at this time. Whether a woman seeks help and what if any help she receives depend on her own view of motherhood and mental illness, as well as that of her health professional and on the services that are both affordable and accessible.

A recent Australian survey (34) suggests that women have a low likelihood of considering mental illness in pregnancy, and both they and health professionals share a reluctance for biologic treatments, although this is truer for the women. In milder to moderate cases, biologic treatments may be unnecessary; in all cases a holistic approach is needed. Ideally, the approach should be tailored to the woman's needs but should also take into consideration her own perception and concepts of herself as a whole being as well as mother and her construct of mental illness. In a society that is underresourced in the health sector, this is not always possible, but if used as a principle is likely to have better outcomes.

Few studies look specifically at treatment of depression and anxiety in pregnancy, aside from reports on potential effects of drugs on the fetus. Antidepressants have not been shown to be teratogenic and may be used with caution if necessary, but, given potential concerns for subtle neurobehavioral changes in the infant, increased attention to supports and psychological interventions is important to consider. These considerations are reviewed more extensively elsewhere (45) and summarized later in this chapter.

PSYCHOSIS

PREVALENCE

Although postpartum psychosis and relapse of bipolar psychosis postpartum have been long recognized, occurring in 1 in 600 women, much less is known about psychosis in pregnancy. Historically it was thought that women with schizophrenia had low fertility (c.f. high fertility in bipolar illness) but this may at least in part relate to the segregation of the mentally ill into asylums, as well as severe illness preventing relationships, plus medication effects.

Women with an existing psychosis will have an increased risk of relapse if, when trying to conceive or on finding they are pregnant, they cease medication. This is a common response, but many of these women relapse and need to recommence medication (46,47). The pregnancy itself, however, appears not to confer an increased risk of psychotic illness.

PLANNING AND MANAGING A PREGNANCY

For women with a history of psychosis, planning pregnancies in advance is preferable to unplanned pregnancy (46,48). Any woman of reproductive age being treated with a mood stabilizer should be warned of the risks of teratogenicity and relapse. Ideally, her partner should be involved in planning discussions, and the information given should be documented. General principles of planning include encouraging women to be well for at least a year before considering pregnancy and minimizing stresses and maximizing supports. This includes consideration of lifestyle issues that will promote good health both through the pregnancy and into the postpartum period. Each case will be different, and the risk:benefit ratio for decreasing or ceasing medication needs to be considered, but the doctor can only provide the best current evidence; the woman and her partner must ultimately make the decision. It is important also to discuss options if deterioration occurs, regarding medication, hospital admission, and child care for older children. If mood stabilizers must be continued through pregnancy, then close monitoring of blood levels and splitting of doses to prevent peaks of drug concentration may decrease the risk of negative outcomes.

Liaising with the obstetrician is also important, and decreasing medication prior to delivery and/or commencing again after delivery are all issues of which women need to be aware. In addition, good sleep management is important, though the role of sleep deprivation needs further research (48).

EFFECTS OF TREATMENTS ON THE FETUS

While the effects of the illness on the fetus include factors related to poor self-care and changes in hormones and blood flow discussed earlier, treatments may also affect development when medication is used in pregnancy and require careful consideration of the risks and benefits not just to the mother but also to the unborn fetus. These concerns can be divided into three broad areas:

First, the development of the fetus can be adversely affected by the exposure to medication in the first trimester. This is a danger for women who are being treated for mental disorder and then become pregnant. Many will not realize that they are pregnant until five or six weeks' gestation, and much of the damage to the fetus has already occurred by this time. Many women will choose to abruptly discontinue medication on the return of a positive pregnancy test, either because of their own fears of harming the fetus or on the advice of their clinician. In Einarson et al.'s (47) study of 36 women who discontinued medication, 70% of women who did so reported adverse effects—including 11 of 26 women who developed suicidal ideation. Sixty percent of these women subsequently elected to recommence their medications. Three women did not continue with the pregnancy (one abortion, two miscarriages), and the remaining children were well at birth. The authors concluded that discontinuation could have serious adverse effects.

For those women whose infants have been exposed to medication or who develop an illness in the first trimester, *it is important to know which medication is safest.* Dose and peak levels may also be relevant, but less information is available on this.

There are now a number of naturalistic studies on antidepressants. Numbers are adequate to conclude that tricyclic antidepressants appear to be safe, and that the SSRIs, fluoxetine and sertraline are unlikely to be teratogenic. With the SSRIs, however, there have been potential short-term effects noted in the newborn, and use should be cautious. In particular, placental transfer varies among drugs, and one study suggests significant differences, with less fetal exposure to sertraline compared to fluoxetine (49).

Less is known about the antipsychotics, although the old style neuroleptics have been in use for over 50 years with no evidence of teratogenicity. Increasingly available data on olanzapine suggest that it may also be safe (50).

Benzodiazepines conversely have been associated with teratogenic effects; doses of 30 mg/day of valium or equivalent carry an increased risk of cleft palate, and should be avoided in this dose range (46).

Mood stabilizers carry the most risk of teratogenicity. Lithium has been associated with a risk of 0.1% of heart malformations, and anticonvulsants with neural tube defects at a rate more than 5% (46). Valproate risk may be higher.

The second issue for the fetus is the potential for problems at birth. Once the umbilical cord is cut, the infant must metabolize the medication. Infants who are premature, who are unwell, and who continue to be exposed to the drug via breast milk are at particular risk. Where delivery can be planned, decreasing medication briefly can decrease this exposure. This is only applicable to short-acting agents. Particular problems that have been noted at birth include irritability, sedation, floppiness, and cyanosis (the latter two with lithium). These appear to settle, but long-term outcomes are underresearched. Fluoxetine in pregnancy has been associated with a risk of prematurity and given its long half-life, may present particular problems. See review of studies (51).

The final concern is a longer-term developmental issue for infants exposed to these drugs. Short-term studies on tricyclics, sertraline, and citalopram have revealed no current concerns.

Overall, Cohen and Rosenbaum (46) in their review concluded that taking the above information into account, many psychotropics do not appear to have negative effects and this fact needs to be weighed against the potential adverse effects of ceasing medication.

CONCLUSIONS

Pregnancy is a time of enormous change from a biologic, psychological, and social perspective and of immense importance from a political, feminist, and evolutionary perspective. In preparing the woman for motherhood, pregnancy begins a process of development for the woman that continues into the postpartum period. It is a crucial time of biologic development that will impact heavily on the child's future.

Change is often difficult, and for those women whose circumstances—such as current illness or inadequate resources—are such that the pregnancy represents a burden, this time is likely to be particularly arduous and hold significant mental health implications. Risks to the infant may come from a number of avenues: exposure to medication or illicit drugs, inadequate antenatal care, trauma, and altered placental blood flow and hormonal changes.

Mental illness has been thought to be less frequent in pregnancy than at other times, but recent studies suggest a similar prevalence of depression and anxiety to that postpartum, an increase in relation to women without children. In addition, those women with a preexisting illness may be at higher risk of relapse, particularly if medication is ceased abruptly.

Despite this high level of mental illness, women have low likelihood of seeking help, and though health professionals have an increasing awareness of *postnatal* disorders, they are less likely to detect antenatal mental illness. This is largely a question of training and resources. As yet, we do not know how to prevent illness, aside from careful drug monitoring of those with preexisting illness, so the key is identification of those who are unwell or at high risk and the institution of appropriate strategies. Establishing the effectiveness of such supports needs to be a high priority for researchers, with the potential for better outcomes for a large number of children, as well as their mothers, and reduced cost of intergenerational issues at a mental health and economic level.

REFERENCES

1. Beck CT. Theoretical perspectives of postpartum depression and their treatment implications. MCN Am J Matern Child Nurs 2002;27(5):282–287.
2. Hagen EH. The functions of postpartum depression. Evol Hum Behav 1999;20:325–359.
3. Australian Institute of Health and Welfare Perinatal Statistics Unit. Australian Mothers and Babies 2000: Canberra, 2003.
4. Social Exclusion Unit. Teenage Pregnancy. Office of the Deputy Prime Minister, London, UK. Crown 1999; 143–422.
5. Brown S, Darcy M, Bruinsma F. Victorian Survey of Recent Mothers 2000. Centre for Mothers and Babies. Latrobe University, 2001.
6. Gurel SA, Gurel HG. The evaluation of determinants of early postpartum low mood: the importance of parity and inter-pregnancy interval. Eur J Obstet Gynecol 2000;91:21–24.
7. Stotland NL. Psychiatric aspects of induced abortions. Arch Women Ment Health 2001;4(1):27–31.
8. Reardon DC, Cougle JR, Rue VM, et al. Psychiatric admissions of low income women following abortion and childbirth. Can Med Assoc J 2003;169(10).
9. Major B. Abortion Points Debated. Can Med Assoc J 2003;169(2).
10. Gross KH, Wells CS, Radigan-Garcia A, et al. Correlates of self-reports of being very depressed in the months after delivery: results from the pregnancy risk assessment monitoring system. Matern Child Health J 2002;6(4):247–253.
11. Buist A. Childhood abuse, postpartum depression and parenting difficulties: a literature review of associations. Aust NZ J Psychiatry 1998;32:370–378.
12. Huizink AC, de Robles MPG, Mulder JH, et al. Coping in normal pregnancy. Ann Behav Med 2002;24(2):132–140.
13. Boyce P, Parker G, Barnett B, et al. Personality as a vulnerability factor to depression. Br J Psychiatry 1991;159:106–114.

14. Patel P, Wheatcroft R, Park RJ, et al. The children of mothers with eating disorders. Clin Child Fam Rev Psychol Rev 2002;5(1):1–18.

15. Logsdon MC, Usui W. Psychosocial predictors of postpartum depression in diverse groups of women. West J Nurs Res 2001;23(6):563–574.

16. Bergant AM, Heim K, Ulmer H, et al. Early postnatal depressive mood: associations with obstetric and psychosocial factors. J Psychosom Res 1999;46(4):391–394.

17. Morten H, Henriksen TB, Sabroe S, et al. Psychological distress in pregnancy and preterm delivery. Br Med J 1993;307:234–239.

18. Baird K. Domestic violence in pregnancy: a public health concern. MIDIRS Midwife Digest 2002;12(Suppl 1).

19. American Psychological Association. Violence and the Family. Report of the American Psychological Presidential Task Force in Violence and the Family. Washington, DC, 1996:10.

20. Australian Bureau of Statistics. Women's Safety Survey. Catalogue no 4128.0. Canberra, 1996.

21. Family Violence Prevention Fund and the Trauma Foundation. San Francisco. CA 1994.

22. Morse C, Buist A, Durkin S. First time parenthood: influences on pre and postnatal adjustment in fathers and mothers. J Psychosom Obstet Gynaecol 2000;21:109–120.

23. Chandran M, Tharyan P. Post-partum depression in a cohort of women from a rural area of Tamil Nadu, India. Br J Psychiatry 2002;181:499–504.

24. Russell JA, Douglas AJ, Ingram CD. Brain preparations for maternity—adaptive changes in behavioral and neuroendocrine systems during pregnancy and lactation: an overview. Brain Res 2001;133:1–38.

25. Evans J, Heron J, Francomb H, et al. Cohort study of depressed mood during pregnancy and after childbirth. Br Med J 2001;323:257–260.

26. Granger ACP, Underwood MR. Review of the role of progesterone in the management of postnatal mood disorders. J Psychosom Obstet Gyn 2001;22:49–55.

27. Dayan J, Creveuil C, Herlicoviez M, et al. Role of anxiety and depression in the onset of spontaneous preterm labour. Am J Epidemiol 2002;155(4):292–301.

28. Hedegaard M, Henriksen TB, Sabroe S, et al. Psychological distress in pregnancy and preterm delivery. Br Med J 1993;307(6898):234–239.

29. Gibson FL, Ungerer JA, Tennat C, et al. Parental adjustment and attitudes to parenting after in vitro fertilization. Fertil Steril 2000;73:5650–5674.

30. Greenfield D, Klock SC. Transition to parenthood among in vitro fertilization patients at 2 and 9 months. Fertil Steril 2001;76:626–627.

30A. Catherine Dennison. Teenage pregnancy: an overview of the research evidence. Health Development Agency (NHS) 2004; 11.

31. Office of Applied Studies. Results from the 2002 National Survey on Drug Use and Health: National Findings. DHHS Public no SMA 033836. NHSDA Survey H-22. Rockville, MD, 2003.

32. Buist A, Minto B, Szego K, et al. Mother–Baby Psychiatric Units in Australia: The Victorian Experience. Arch Women Ment Health 2004;7(1):81–87.

33. Horrigan TJ, Schroeder AV, Schaffer RM. The triad of substance abuse, violence and depression interrelated in pregnancy. J Subs Abuse 2000;18:55–58.

34. Buist A, Barnett B, Milgrom J, et al.. To screen or not to screen—that is the question in perinatal depression. Med J Aust 2002(7/10/02 Issue):S101–S105.

35. Ramsay J, Richardson J, Carter YH, et al. Should health professionals screen women for domestic violence? Systematic review. Br Med J 2002;325(August 10):1–13.

36. Shakespeare J, Blake F, Garcia J. A qualitative study of the acceptability of routine screening of postnatal women using the Edinburgh Postnatal Depression Scale. Br J Gen Pract 2003;53(493):614–619.

37. Cox J, Holden J. Using the EPDS in clinical settings: research evidence. In: Royal College of Psychiatrists. Perinatal Mental Health: A Guide to the EPDS. Glasgow: Bell & Bain, 2003:26–33.

38. Cox JL, Holden JM, Sagovsky R. Detection of postnatal depression: development of the 10-item Edinburgh Postnatal Depression scale. Br J Psychiatry 1987;150:782–786.

39. Ross LE, Evans G, Sellers EM, et al. Measurement issues in postpartum depression part 1: anxiety as a feature of postpartum depression. Arch Women Ment Health 2003;6:51–57.

40. Austin MP, Lumley J. Antenatal screening for postnatal depression: a systematic review. Acta Psychiatr Scand 2002;106:1–8.

41. Bennett HA, Einarson A, Taddio A, et al. Prevalence of depression during pregnancy: systematic review. Obstet Gyn 2004; 103(4):698–709.

42. Hertzberg T, Wahlbeck K. The impact of pregnancy and puerperium on panic disorder: a review. J Psychosom Obstet Gyn 1999;20(2):59–64.

43. Appleby L, Mortensen PB, Faragher EB. Suicide and other causes of mortality after post-partum psychiatric admission. Br J Psychiatry 1998;173:209–211.

44. Wisner KL, Wheeler SB. Prevention of recurrent postpartum major depression: clinical trial. Hosp Community Psychiatry 1994;45(12):1191–1196.

45. Marcus SM, Barry KL, Flynn HA, et al. Treatment guidelines for depression in pregnancy. Int J Gynaecol Obstet 2001;72:61–70.

46. Cohen LS, Rosenbaum JF. Psychotropic drug use during pregnancy: weighing the risks. J Clin Psychiatry 1998;S9(2):18–28.

47. Einarson A, Selly P, Koren G. Discontinuing antidepressants and benzodiazepines. Can Fam Physician 2001;47:457–672.

48. Yonkers KA, Wisner KL, Stowe Z, et al. Management of bipolar disorder during pregnancy and the postpartum period. Am J Psychiatry 2004;161:608–620.

49. Hendrick V, Stowe ZN, Altshuler LL, et al. Placental passage of antidepressant medication. Am J. Psych 2003; 5:993–996.

50. Gardiner SJ, Kristensen JH, Begg EJ, et al. Transfer of olanzapine into breastmilk, calculation of infant drug dose and effect on breast-fed infants. Am J Psychiatry 2003;160:1428–1431.

51. Buist A. Guidelines for the use of antidepressants in pregnant and lactating women. Psychopharmacology. Submitted 2004.

CHAPTER 20

Postpartum and Its Mental Health Problems

Sophie Grigoriadis

N o time in a women's life is as likely to be filled with as much change as the postpartum period. Changes in all aspects of a woman's life (biologic, psychological, as well as sociocultural) during the first year following childbirth define the postpartum period. Although the addition of a new family member is usually a time of joy and excitement, for many women the postpartum time is not the period of well-being depicted by women's and parenting magazines. Instead, it is a high-risk period for significant psychiatric illness.

Many adaptations need to occur following childbirth. Following labor, the physiologic changes of pregnancy resolve during the early postpartum period. Changes in body shape require increased attention to diet and exercise with consideration for the needs of lactation if nursing. Over and above the medical complications that may occur during the early and late postpartum period, maternal sleep deprivation is common and can lead to exhaustion. The infant is completely dependent on the caregiver around the clock and the immediate postpartum time is centered on the infant's needs, which pose physical as well as psychological demands. Both mother and infant need to learn the skills involved in breast-feeding, an intense physical connection between mother and infant. Pain during feedings (from irritated nipples or mastitis) can create heightened anxiety and interfere with the process and the formation of the maternal–infant bond. Feeding difficulties can heighten insecurities the mother may have regarding the adequacy of care she is providing. Over time, the new mother becomes increasingly attuned to her infant's cues and usually comes to terms with her new maternal role and identity. As her infant develops, the challenge of parental adjustment impacts on both the mother and her relationship with her partner. Although the presence of the child solidifies the family unit, the mother's time for herself is reduced as are time for the couple and for socialization. The many challenges can lead to a resurfacing of old conflicts between partners or to the development of new ones. Housing and economic difficulties can negatively affect the developing relationship with the infant further. Economic necessity or career aspirations may require the mother's return to work and decisions on how to coordinate child care and previous working commitments (1). In Western societies, where women are usually expected to be the primary caregiver for their infants following childbirth, an emotionally and instrumentally supportive relationship between the partners can help moderate stress on the mother. In non-Western societies, traditional rituals enable the mother to receive much needed family and community support following childbirth—a potentially protective factor (2). The physical changes and the combination of new and multiple demands in all aspects of life postpartum can be overwhelming to many women, and some develop psychiatric illness for the first time; others experience a recurrence of illness.

POSTPARTUM PSYCHIATRIC DISORDERS

Postpartum psychiatric disorders are characterized by the onset of emotional symptoms during the weeks or months that follow childbirth. These mood and anxiety disorders have been described since antiquity, but they continue to be poorly recognized, undertreated, and underresearched. Recently, there has been a growth of interest, but the length of time characterizing the postpartum period has not been consistently agreed upon. Although this categorization is not reflected in the nosology of the *Diagnostic and Statistical Manual of Mental Disorders,* 4th edition, Text Revision (DSM-IV-TR), most researchers categorize the mood disturbances of this period into postpartum blues, postpartum depression (PPD), and postpartum psychosis. Panic disorder or postpartum obsessive compulsive disorder typify the anxiety disorders of this period. Debate has ensued over whether the disorders manifesting during the postpartum time are distinct from the mood and anxiety disorders that manifest at other times of the life cycle (3). Given that research in postpartum psychiatric illness has only recently begun to gain momentum, the relationship and potential overlap between the categories remains to be adequately delineated and are still empirical. Moreover, at the early onset of symptoms, many clinicians find it difficult to differentiate between normal postpartum emotional adjustment and postpartum psychiatric illness.

POSTPARTUM MOOD DISORDERS

Etiology

The temporal association between childbirth and psychiatric illness reinforced the hypothesis that the etiology of postpartum disturbance rests in a biologic aberration. Early theories examined the "withdrawal phenomenon" related to the rapid shift in the hormonal environment and the consequences on the activity of neurotransmitter or circadian systems. Gonadal steroids such as estrogen and progesterone, cortisol and the hypothalamic-pituitary-adrenal (HPA) axis, androgens, thyroid hormones, polypeptide hormones, mineralocorticoids, inhibin, β-endorphins, and gonadotropins have been examined as potential etiologic factors in postpartum mood disorders (4). However, studies investigating potential biologic aberrations have been negative, inconsistent, or not replicated. Nonetheless, there may be endocrinologic changes that are causally linked to postpartum mood disorders in a vulnerable subgroup of women who may be specifically sensitive to changing titers of reproductive hormones. In a key biologic study, Bloch and colleagues pharmacologically simulated pregnancy, parturition, and the postpartum period and found that women with a history of PPD developed significant mood symptoms during the hormonal add back and withdrawal periods; none of the control women developed symptoms (5). These investigators suggest that women with a history of PPD are differentially sensitive to the mood-destabilizing effects of the marked changes in gonadal steroid levels. It has also been suggested that estrogen plays a role in the regulation of circadian rhythms and may, in part, contribute to sleep loss. Sleep loss in turn has been suspected to have an etiologic role in the onset of postpartum psychosis in susceptible women (6). The mechanism of these changes remains to be determined.

A positive personal or family history of a mood disorder has been well associated with all types of postpartum psychiatric illness in retrospective, cross-sectional, and prospective studies (7). Recurrence of a postpartum episode is common; rates as high as 70% for postpartum psychosis and up to 50% for postpartum depression have been reported. From 20% to 50% of women with bipolar disorder experience a relapse during the postpartum time. Women with a history of major depression are also at risk for relapse during the postpartum, especially those with severe and recurrent illness, and rates as high as 30% have been reported (8). (See also Chapter 19.) The development of depressive symptoms during pregnancy increases the likelihood of postpartum depression regardless of history for major depression (9). Although there is a subpopulation of women who develop their index episode during the postpartum time (up to 50%) and subsequently experience psychiatric illness only following future childbirths, the majority of women go on to develop nonpuerperal episodes (8).

Attempts to delineate risk factors for vulnerability to psychiatric disturbance during the postpartum time (for example, age, marital status, parity, educational level, and socioeconomic factors) have been inconsistent and weak (8). Primiparous women may be at higher risk for postpartum psychosis than multiparous women, and obstetric complications (cesarean section, perinatal death) may also increase the risk for postpartum psychosis; replication of these findings is needed. Moreover, the impact of psychosocial factors in the development of postpartum psychiatric illness can be significant. High levels of marital conflict or dissatisfaction, low levels of social and spousal support, and increased number of life events during pregnancy have consistently been reported by women with postpartum affective illness (10). Studies attempting to link personality traits and coping styles with the risk of illness during the postpartum have not produced consistent findings. It is likely that many risk factors act synergistically to predispose women to postpartum affective disorders or increase the likelihood of the development of such disorders.

Most of the research in postpartum mood disorders has been done on PPD. Robertson and colleagues identified risk factors for PPD following their comprehensive review of the literature and grouped the factors as strong to moderate, moderate, small, and no effect (11). Strong to moderate risk factors include depression and anxiety during pregnancy, stressful recent life events, lack of social support, and a previous history of depression. Moderate factors include high levels of stress related to child care, low self-esteem, neuroticism, and difficult infant temperament. Small factors include obstetric and pregnancy complications, cognitive attributions, quality of relationship with partner, and socioeconomic status. Ethnicity, maternal age, level of education, parity, and gender of child (within Western societies) were found to have no effect. These authors concluded that the identified risk factors for postpartum depression are methodologically robust, replicated within numerous studies across sample populations, and well established.

Postpartum Blues

Postpartum blues is a mild, transitory mood state characterized by rapid mood shifts, mild depression, irritability, anxiety, tearfulness, fatigue, insomnia, poor appetite, headaches, poor concentration, and confusion (7). Symptoms generally begin within the first week postpartum, last a few hours up to two weeks, and resolve spontaneously without sequelae. The mother's functioning is only minimally affected, and if treatment is necessary, it is limited to support and reassurance. Given that the incidence has been reported to range from 26% to 85% of new mothers, it has been debated whether postpartum blues constitute a normal variant of maternal behavior rather than a psychiatric disorder (7). It may be of value to identify women experiencing these symptoms because as many as 25% will develop PPD during the first postnatal year (9).

Postpartum Depression

Postpartum depression (PPD) is estimated to occur in 10% to 15% of women, and prevalence ranges from 5% to over 20% have been reported (9). This wide variation reflects the fact that the disorder has been poorly characterized and unreliably diagnosed. This is due in part to the poorly defined diagnostic criteria and conflicting definitions of the postpartum period. Most experts currently do not support the notion that PPD is phenomenologically distinct from major depression that occurs at other life stages. PPD is now included in the DSM-IV-TR as a major depressive disorder with postpartum onset, beginning within the first four weeks after delivery. Historically, the clinical course of PPD was not well characterized; it was thought to begin insidiously after the second or third week postpartum, most patients developing symptoms within six weeks. The severity of the disorder is variable, ranging from mild dysphoria to melancholia to psychotic depression. Commonly, women are tearful, report mood lability, obsessional thinking (especially with regard to the infant's health), feelings of hopelessness, somatic complaints (especially fatigue), anorexia, sleep disturbance, poor concentration and memory, and feelings of guilt and inadequacy. Clearly some of the symptoms, such as alterations in sleep pattern, energy, libido, appetite, and body weight, are common during the postpartum period; their overlap with the symptoms of depression as well as with medical disorders common during the postpartum time often renders accurate diagnosis difficult. The duration of postpartum illness is variable, depending on the severity of the illness, with most episodes lasting no more than three months (12); however, some residual depressive symptoms are common up to one year following delivery (13). Women with a previous history of major depression may have more severe and prolonged illness. With treatment, the prognosis is good. The outcome may be better for those women who receive treatment early (8).

Few treatment studies have been conducted in women with PPD. There is one randomized controlled trial (RCT) comparing fluoxetine to a hybrid cognitive-behavioral counseling approach, one open-label trial of sertraline, one open-label trial of venlafaxine, a fluoxetine case series, and one retrospective chart review of several antidepressants and the most recent RCT which compares paroxetine to paroxetine plus cognitive-behavioral therapy combination therapy in postpartum women with depression and comorbid anxiety disorder (14–18A). The limited information about antidepressant treatment for PPD often leads clinicians at present to extrapolate from studies of nonpostpartum samples; such extrapolation may not be appropriate. Many women with PPD breast-feed, and the amount of antidepressant entering breast milk must be given special consideration. Hendrick and colleagues also argue that women with PPD recover more slowly and may not have the same response profile as women with depression not related to childbearing (18). Therefore, not only are trials needed to compare the efficacy of various treatments in postpartum women with special considerations for lactation, but studies addressing response profiles such as rapidity of response in the management of PPD would also advance the field. The evidence for estrogen as a treatment is also still at the initial stages (19,20). Although Gregoire and colleagues demonstrated a positive response to estrogen that was sustained at three-month follow-up and there was no evidence of endometrial hyperplasia, over one third of the women in that study were also using an antidepressant (20). As a result, the evidence from this study may support estrogen as an adjunctive treatment, not necessarily as a primary treatment. Other interventions being investigated for the treatment of PPD include bright light therapy (21) as well as sleep interventions (22). It is difficult to compare the efficacy of these studies because of differing diagnostic criteria, rating scales used, and sample populations. Moreover, many of the results are still preliminary and require replication with larger samples. However, double-blind placebo-controlled crossover trials of pharmacologic interventions cannot be easily designed because postpartum psychiatric illness can be such a risk to the mother, her infant, and the family that it may be unethical to include a placebo arm.

The best evidence for psychotherapy as an effective treatment for postpartum depression is for interpersonal psychotherapy (IPT); the evidence comes from three studies, two open trials, and a wait list controlled trial (23–25). Although IPT reduces depressive symptoms and improves social adjustment, it also involves a time commitment by the new mother and may not be appropriate as stand-alone treatment for women with severe depressive symptoms. Cognitive-behavioral therapy (CBT) (14,18A, 26,27), counseling by health nurses (28) or health visitors (29), peer support (30–32), and partner support (33) have been shown to be helpful, although randomized controlled trials with larger sample sizes need to be conducted. If breast-feeding, some women avoid drugs despite the severity of their depressive symptoms. This is because the long-term effects of antidepressants on breast-fed infants are unknown. Studies comparing different treatment modalities to determine which treatments are most suited to certain clinical presentations would significantly advance the field, because it is unlikely that one treatment would be the first choice for all patients.

Very little published research examines predictors of treatment response in women with postpartum depression. Hendrick and colleagues, in their retrospective chart review, reported that neither symptoms of depression during pregnancy nor the timing of a postpartum depression onset (before or after four weeks postpartum) predicted antidepressant response (18). Subsets of PPD subjects have been reported with psychomotor retardation, symptoms of anxiety, or obsessive thoughts. It is unknown at this time if symptom profiles can mediate or predict response to treatment. Moreover, postpartum depression affects the mother, child, and family unit, and treatment of one in isolation may be insufficient. The treatment of PPD may eventually require a multidimensional model with different interventions targeted at mother, infant, or family unit at different times. Because many disciplines may be involved in the care of a woman with PPD and her family, it is important to acknowledge that clinicians' choice of intervention is affected by the theoretical perspective from which they practice. Although this chapter is written from the medical viewpoint, which is the dominant theoretical perspective currently, a comprehensive treatment plan can include different points of view with a resultant array of interventions (34).

Postpartum Psychosis

Postpartum psychosis is relatively rare, with an incidence in the range of 0.1% to 0.2% (8). It is an agitated highly changeable psychosis that typically occurs within the first two to four weeks postpartum; however, the presentation can be dramatic with symptom onset within the first 48 to 72 hours following delivery. Typically, women first appear restless and irritable and show sleep disturbance. The psychosis evolves rapidly and is characterized by depressed, elated, or labile mood; disorganized behavior; and delusions or hallucinations, all of which cause significant dysfunction. The delusions often include beliefs about the infant; auditory hallucinations instructing the mother to harm or kill herself or her baby have been reported. In contrast to women with nonpsychotic depression, in whom thoughts of harming the infant are also common (35), women with postpartum psychosis are more likely to act on their thoughts (36). Although postpartum psychosis is more commonly associated with delirium and confusion than with affective psychosis, there has been debate about whether postpartum psychosis is a discrete diagnostic entity or a form of bipolar disorder. In a recent review of the literature, it was concluded that not all cases of postpartum psychosis fall into the bipolar spectrum although substantial evidence for a fundamental link between the two exists (37). In the DSM-IV-TR, postpartum psychosis is given as an example of a psychotic disorder not otherwise specified. Given the close relation with affective disorders, the postpartum onset specifier can be applied to major depressive disorder, bipolar disorder, or brief psychotic disorder.

Postpartum psychosis is typically a psychiatric emergency. Aggressive treatment is critical, and hospitalization is usually indicated, especially if there is a risk of suicide or harm to the infant through neglect, abuse, or infanticide. The immediate goals include protecting the infant, stabilizing the mother, and subsequently helping her with the process of maternal role attainment. Systematic and empirically derived guidelines in treating this disorder are lacking. Although treatment is directed at the underlying illness if it is known, short-term treatment typically includes the use of antipsychotic medication for the acute phase. High-potency antipsychotics such as haloperidol are generally preferred over low-potency medication (38). When the psychosis is deemed a manifestation of an underlying bipolar disorder, treatment with a mood stabilizer or treatment with an atypical neuroleptic with antimanic properties are options (37). Lithium has most commonly been used. Prophylactic lithium immediately following delivery has been suggested in women who have experienced a previous episode or are known to have bipolar disorder (39). Prophylactic estrogen treatment has also been found effective in two of three small studies (40–42). Electroconvulsive therapy (ECT) may be the treatment of choice in postpartum psychosis (and severe depression) when rapid restoration of the patient's function is paramount. The appropriate duration of pharmacologic treatment has not been well established. Although evidence for systematic empirically derived psychosocial treatments is also lacking, women often require education about child care as well as instrumental and emotional support from partners, family, friends, and community agencies. Individual or marital therapy may also be indicated. In addition to the issue of infant exposure to medication, breast-feeding may also not be advisable in women with postpartum psychosis because of their need for sleep and reduction of their stress level. Moreover, as described earlier, it has been argued that sleep loss may be causally linked to the development of postpartum psychosis.

POSTPARTUM ANXIETY DISORDERS

Postpartum anxiety disorders have only recently received research attention. It has been suggested that a previous history of an anxiety disorder may be a greater risk factor for a postpartum depression or anxiety than a history of a depressive disorder (43). The postpartum time appears to be a period of increased vulnerability for recurrent panic symptoms, although the extent of risk conferred by the preexisting condition is unknown. Panic disorder can have a variable and complicated course during the postpartum time (44). The symptoms of panic disorder are typical of those experienced during other life stages. Some women can develop symptoms for the first time postpartum; in a small analysis, 11% of women reported experiencing panic symptoms for the first time after childbirth (45). The increased vulnerability to panic symptoms may be related to the abrupt changes in reproductive hormone concentrations on monoaminergic binding sites or rapid decline in progesterone levels following delivery. During pregnancy, the elevated progesterone levels produce hyperventilation and decreased Pco_2 levels. The rise in Pco_2 levels following delivery may correspond to the decrease in progesterone and may thus predispose to panic attacks (46).

Women with obsessive compulsive disorder are also at increased risk for relapse postpartum. Although this area has not received much attention, one retrospective study found up to 29% of women evaluated described symptom worsening following childbirth (47). Postpartum onset of OCD has also been described, and in one study, 8 of 16 patients reported symptom onset following childbirth (48). Features include a rapid escalation of obsessions related to harming the baby and heightened anxiety; mothers typically become avoidant of their infants. Symptom onset is usually within the first six weeks postpartum and women go on to develop panic attacks and depression. A high rate of relapse following subsequent pregnancies has been reported (49).

Recent studies have investigated the possibility of development of post-traumatic stress disorder (PTSD) following traumatic labor; rates ranging from 1.7% to 6% have been reported (50,51). In keeping with the recent emphasis on the presence of postpartum anxiety symptoms, the results of a recent community-based study suggest generalized anxiety disorder is even more prevalent than postpartum depression; the small sample size of this study, however, precludes definitive conclusions (52). No doubt, treatment for anxiety disorders during the postpartum will soon receive more research attention; to date, these disorders are believed to respond to the same interventions used at other life stages.

LACTATION ISSUES

Breast-feeding has been promoted as the best source of infant nutrition and as a result, many pregnant women plan to nurse in North America. However, breast-feeding requires a significant adjustment by the mother in the postpartum period and is a skill that must be acquired. The process can be impeded if the infant has a poor "latch" on the nipple, for example, or by nipple irritation, cracks, or fissures, which can lead to mastitis and further anxiety around feedings. Postpartum psychiatric illness can also impede the process not only because it may be more difficult to acquire the requisite skill but also because of concerns that psychotropic medications may affect the infant through the breast milk. Reviews on this topic have concluded that all psychotropic medications investigated are excreted into breast milk, and thus the infant is always exposed to some amount of the drug the nursing mother is taking (53). Most of the data available are for antidepressants, especially of the selective serotonin reuptake inhibitor (SSRI) class. Drugs that are found in the breast-feeding infant at a concentration of less than 10% of that in mother's plasma generally are felt to be safe for the infant, and most studies have found that most SSRIs meet this criterion. Mood stabilizers and antipsychotics are not as benign. Lithium was contraindicated during lactation, but now the American Academy of Pediatrics has changed its classification to "should be given to nursing mothers with caution" (54). Use of valproic acid and carbamazepine during breast-feeding can be safe, although the data mostly come from the epilepsy literature. The use of lamotrigine is not compatible with breast-feeding (55), and antipsychotic (both typical and atypical) use has not been advised (56). No information is available to date on the use of gabapentin and topiramate. A thorough risk:benefit assessment needs to be conducted for each woman, and her partner should be involved in the decision-making process. The consequences of untreated maternal psychiatric illness, previous psychiatric history, and treatment response also need to be taken into account. Minimizing simultaneous exposure of the infant to maternal mental illness and medication should be a goal. Despite the fact that data with the SSRIs indicate that adverse events are limited in the short term, data on the long-term effects of psychotropic exposure through lactation are lacking.

IMPACT ON CHILD OUTCOME

Maternal psychiatric illness affects not only the mother but also the mother–infant dyad, thus directly affecting both the infant's immediate well-being and longer-term growth and development. Most of the research on maternal mental illness has been conducted on depressed mothers and has demonstrated deleterious effects on mother–infant attachment, infant cognitive competence, and child development and behavior. Depressed mothers perceive their infants more negatively and as more difficult to care for (57). Infants as young as 6 weeks old respond with distress and avoidance to disrupted maternal communication (58). Martins and Gaffin, following a meta-analysis of seven studies on the effects of maternal depression on mother–infant attachment in children less than 3 years old, found the infants of depressed mothers displayed significantly reduced likelihood of secure attachment and increased likelihood of avoidant and disorganized attachment (59). Further, childhood behavioral disturbance has been associated with PPD at five-year follow-up (60). In terms of cognitive effects, 18-month-old infants of mothers who had postpartum depression were found to perform significantly less well on cognitive tasks than infants of mothers in a control group (58). Although preliminary, PPD may also have an impact on child physical development: infants of mothers with PPD were found to be significantly more underweight and shorter than infants of mothers who were controls (61). It is not known if the effects of maternal depression are long-standing, but recently altered cortisol levels have been reported in 13-year-old adolescents whose mothers had PPD (62). The presence of other variables, such as neonatal risk factors, may potentiate the effects of maternal psychiatric illness, but this remains to be investigated.

The research that does exist on the effects of maternal anxiety disorders on infants also supports detrimental developmental effects. Children of mothers with anxiety disorders have been found to have increased rates of psychiatric difficulties, behavioral inhibition, and insecure attachment (63,64). Extended longitudinal studies are needed to confirm these findings.

Most of the studies evaluating the impact of maternal depression and anxiety on infant functioning have not explored the impact of treatment. For example, the chronicity of a mother's depression may determine the effect on the infant. In mothers who recovered within six months postpartum, the depressive behavior in the infants also remitted, and their development was normal at one year (65). However, Murray and colleagues, following their controlled trial comparing routine primary care, nondirective counseling, CBT, or brief psychodynamic therapy, found that although psychological treatments had significant benefit to the mother–infant relationship and infant behavioral problems in the short term, the treatments had no significant impact on infant cognitive development or child outcome at age 5 years and suggest that more prolonged intervention may be needed (66). More research is required to delineate the extent to which treatment can ameliorate the aforementioned effects. Early and prolonged intervention for both the mother and infant may be able to limit or even prevent detrimental effects.

Maternal psychiatric illness not only interferes with optimal mothering and provision of adequate care to the infant, it can lead to neonaticide (murder of the infant within 24 hours following its birth) or filicide (murder of a child after 24 hours following its birth by the parent), especially if left untreated. Psychiatric morbidity is a risk factor for filicide although most women with mental illness do not harm their children. Estimating accurate incidence rates has proven difficult because most cases are purportedly not discovered (67). Regardless, infants of mothers with PPD are at risk through neglect, lack of judgment, accident, or direct homicidal act.

CULTURAL CONSIDERATIONS

It has been hypothesized that PPD may represent a "culture-bound syndrome" found in Western societies, and a number of explanations have been proposed to explain the phenomenon (68). In Canada, mother and infant are discharged very soon after delivery usually to an isolated environment without extended family; typically there is no provision for help at home during the first few weeks after birth. In contrast, cross-cultural studies of non-Western societies found that high levels of community and family support are activated by childbirth (2). In this way, education, social support, child care services, and social recognition of the new life stage are ensured. Cultural patterns may facilitate the prevention or mask the experience of negative emotional states (68), although more research is needed into the relationship of childbearing rituals to postpartum adaptation and its relation to psychiatric illness. The ideology of motherhood in Western society, which idealizes the exclusive care of the infant by the mother, may be important in the development of postpartum psychiatric difficulties. More traditional societies share infant care among relatives. Role conflict has been implicated in the development of postpartum psychiatric difficulties (68). It has also been argued the medicalization of childbirth by Western societies may also be an important factor because it may interfere with individualized sensitive care of the mother (69). Indeed, lower rates of postpartum psychiatric disorders have been reported in non-Western societies, although methodologic issues have hindered the interpretation of accurate incidence rates.

Results from cross-cultural studies comparing postpartum depression, however, have found similar rates across cultures. For example, recently Affonso and colleagues found Asian and South American women to have higher rates of depressive symptoms than European and American women, challenging the notion that PPD is most common among Western women (70). Others have also found similar rates in Western and non-Western countries (71) although what has been labeled PPD in Western society is not always viewed as an illness by non-Western societies (72). More research is needed on the global perspective of postpartum psychiatric disorders. Limiting factors include the cultural differences in the presentation of psychiatric illness, which render common assessment instruments inappropriate. The development of a body of cross-cultural comparative research, however, may rest on the development of uniform diagnostic criteria and diagnostic instruments.

IMPACT OF LIFE-CYCLE STAGE AND CHALLENGES

Robinson and Stewart argue that with the birth of a new child, the family system needs to be reorganized; many couples at this time revert to traditional roles (1). As a result, the woman accepts the larger share of parenting tasks. This transition may be easier for women who decide to have children earlier in life and not work outside the home. Women who have focused on their careers often delay childbearing, and, undoubtedly, the new maternal role impacts on previous career strivings, although to date this notion has not been systematically investigated. Employed mothers have reported stresses such as feelings of inadequate energy, time, and resources; unrealistic expectations; guilt about their infants' needs; anger and resentment; and unmet personal needs (73). Research is needed into the role of such factors in the development of postpartum psychiatric illness. The recruitment of other caregivers either in the home or at a daycare center impacts the mother's adjustment; whether such arrangements mediate the effects of maternal postpartum psychiatric illness on the infant needs study.

Postpartum psychiatric illness can significantly impair the developmental task of parenthood. Mothers may have difficulty attaining the maternal role and caring for the new child. For example, mothers with postpartum depression report difficulties in managing their infant's crying and other demands. Research into the father's role in postpartum psychiatric illness remains rudimentary. Although it is known that marital discord is an important variable in the development of postpartum depression, it is not known if the father can help mitigate the negative impact of maternal postpartum illness on both the mother and infant. Many countries are experimenting with different options for parental leave from work following childbirth. It is not known what impact extended paternity leave will have on maternal psychiatric illness. Although there is some evidence of paternal psychiatric illness in reaction to maternal postpartum depression, it has not been well studied (74). Recruitment of an ill partner in the treatment plan of the mother would be plagued by difficulty at the outset. Undoubtedly, paternal postnatal psychiatric illness would add to the adverse impact of maternal illness on parenting tasks, further stress the family unit, and affect the psychological development of the child, although research into this is lacking.

CONCLUSIONS

The postpartum time is unique, with multiple neuroendocrine and psychosocial challenges for the mother. It is not a period of happiness and satisfaction for all women, and ironically it is at this time, when women suppress their own needs relative to those of the new infant, that they are at special risk for illness. The public health impact of postpartum psychiatric disorders is substantial. Although research in the area has received more attention recently and is evolving rapidly, unfortunate high-profile cases in the media involving filicide or suicide in postpartum depressed mothers have also raised public awareness. Much work needs to be done. This chapter has highlighted emerging concepts that can further advance knowledge and the focus of future investigations. Despite the debate on whether or not postpartum psychiatric disorders are distinct entities, these disorders do need to be investigated separately. Their consequences have a wide impact, and they pose unique challenges such as safety of the infant and mother, the risk of toxicity to the breast-fed infant, and time constraints on the mother's availability for treatment. Research has begun to focus on interventions, and postpartum treatment is an emerging standard of care. Nonetheless, women coming for treatment continue to face the dilemma that there is a serious lack of evidence to guide clinicians on therapies for postpartum disorders. Although beyond the scope of this chapter, work is also needed to accurately identify women at risk for onset or relapse of illness and to identify strategies for prevention. Clearly, attention needs to be paid to all aspects of the postpartum period. This is best addressed by a multidimensional approach to etiology and treatment.

REFERENCES

1. Robinson GE, Stewart DE. Postpartum disorders. In: Stotland NL, Stewart DE, eds. Psychological Aspects of Women's Healthcare. The Interface Between Psychiatry and Obstetrics and Gynecology. 2nd Ed. Washington, DC: American Psychiatric Press, 2001:117–139.
2. Cox JL. Childbirth as a life event: sociocultural aspects of postnatal depression. Acta Psychiatr Scand 1988;344:S75–S83.
3. Whiffen VE. Is postpartum depression a distinctive diagnosis? Clin Psychol Rev 1992;12:485–508.
4. Bloch M, Daly RC, Rubinow DR. Endocrine factors in the etiology of postpartum depression. Compr Psychiatry 2003;44:234–246.
5. Bloch M, Schmidt PJ, Danaceau M, et al. Effects of gonadal steroids in women with a history of postpartum depression. Am J Psychiatry 2000;157:924–930.
6. Sharma V, Mazmanian D. Sleep loss and postpartum psychosis. Bipolar Disord 2003;5:98–105.
7. O'Hara MW, Schlechte JA, Lewis DA, et al. Prospective study of postpartum blues: biologic and psychosocial factors. Arch Gen Psychiatry 1991;48:801–806.
8. Nonacs R, Cohen LS. Postpartum psychiatric syndromes. In: Sadock B, Sadock V, eds. Comprehensive Textbook of Psychiatry. 7th Ed. Philadelphia: Lippincott Williams & Wilkins, 2000: 1276–1283.

9. O'Hara MW, Swain AM. Rates and risk of postpartum depression: a meta-analysis. Int Rev Psychiatry 1996;8:37–54.

10. O'Hara MW. Social support, life events and depression during pregnancy and the puerperium. Arch Gen Psychiatry 1991;43:569–573.

11. Robertson E, Celasun N, Stewart DE. Risk factors for postpartum depression. In: Stewart DE, Robertson E, Dennis CL, et al., eds. Postpartum depression: literature review of risk factors and interventions. Report for Toronto Public Health. Toronto: University Health Network and Toronto Public Health, 2003:9–70.

12. Cox JL, Murray D, Chapman C. A controlled study of the onset duration and prevalence of postnatal depression. Br J Psychiatry 1993;163:27.

13. Cooper PJ, Campbell EA, Day A, et al. Non-psychotic psychiatric disorder after childbirth: a prospective study of prevalence, incidence, course and nature. Br J Psychiatry 1988;152:799–806.

14. Appleby L, Warner R, Whitton A, et al. A controlled study of fluoxetine and cognitive-behavioural counselling in the treatment of postnatal depression. Br Med J 1997;314:932–936.

15. Stowe ZN, Casarella J, Landry J, et al. Sertraline in the treatment of women with postpartum major depression. Depression 1995;3:49–55.

16. Cohen LS, Viguera AC, Bouffard SM, et al. Venlafaxine in the treatment of postpartum depression. J Clin Psychiatry 2001;62:592–596.

17. Roy A, Cole K, Goldman Z, et al. Fluoxetine treatment of postpartum depression. Am J Psychiatry 1993;150:1273.

18. Hendrick V, Altshuler L, Strouse T, et al. Postpartum and nonpostpartum depression: differences in presentation and response to pharmacologic treatment. Depress Anxiety 2000;11:66–72.

18A. Misri S, Reeby P, Corral M, Milis L. The use of paroxetine and cognitive-behaviorial therapy in postpartum depression and anxiety: A randomized controlled trial. J Clin Psychiatry 2004; 65:1236–1241.

19. Ahokas A, Kaukoranta J, Wahlbeck K, et al. Estrogen deficiency in severe postpartum depression: successful treatment with sublingual physiologic 17beta-estradiol: a preliminary study. J Clin Psychiatry 2001;62:332–336.

20. Gregoire AJ, Kumar R, Everitt B, et al. Transdermal oestrogen for treatment of severe postnatal depression. Lancet 1996;347(9006):930–933.

21. Corral M, Kuan A, Kostaras D. Bright light therapy's effect on postpartum depression. Am J Psychiatry 2000;157:303–304.

22. Parry BL, Curran ML, Stuenkel CA, et al. Can critically timed sleep deprivation be useful in pregnancy and postpartum depressions? J Affect Disord 2000;60:201–212.

23. Klier C, Muzik M, Rosenblum KL, et al. Interpersonal psychotherapy adapted for the group setting in the treatment of postpartum depression. J Psychother Prac Res 2001;10:124–131.

24. Stuart S, O'Hara MW. Treatment of postpartum depression with interpersonal psychotherapy. Arch Gen Psychiatry 1995;52:75–76.

25. O'Hara MW, Stuart S, Gorman LL, et al. Efficacy of interpersonal psychotherapy for postpartum depression. Arch Gen Psychiatry 2000;57:1039–1045.

26. Chabrol H, Teissedre F, Saint-Jean M, et al. Prevention and treatment of post-partum depression: a controlled randomized study on women at risk. Psychol Med 2002;32:1039–1047.

27. Meager I, Milgrom J. Group treatment for postpartum depression: a pilot study. Aust NZ J Psychiatry 1996;30:852–860.

28. Wickberg B, Hwang CP. Counselling of postnatal depression: a controlled study on a population based Swedish sample. J Affect Disord 1996;39:209–216.

29. Holden JM, Sagovsky R, Cox JL. Counselling in a general practice setting: controlled study of health visitor intervention in treatment of postnatal depression. Br Med J 1989;298:223–226.

30. Chen CH, Tseng YF, Chou FH, et al. Effects of support group intervention in postnatally distressed women: a controlled study in Taiwan. J Psychosom Res 2000;49:395–399.

31. Morgan M, Matthey S, Barnett B, et al. A group programme for postnatally distressed women and their partners. J Adv Nurs 1997;26:913–920.

32. Dennis CL. The effect of peer support on postpartum depression: a pilot randomized controlled trial. Can J Psychiatry 2003;48:115–124.

33. Misri S, Kostaras X, Fox D, et al. The impact of partner support in the treatment of postpartum depression. Can J Psychiatry 2000;45:554–558.

34. Beck CT. Theoretical perspectives of postpartum depression and their treatment implications. MCN Am J Matern Child Nurs 2002;27:282–287.

35. Jennings KD, Ross R, Popper S, et al. Thoughts of harming infants in depressed and nondepressed mothers. J Affect Disord 1999;54:21–28.

36. Attia E, Downey J, Oberman M. Postpartum psychosis. In: Miller LJ, ed. Postpartum Mood Disorders. Washington, DC: American Psychiatric Press, 1999:99–117.

37. Chaudron LH, Pies RW. The relationship between postpartum psychosis and bipolar disorder: a review. J Clin Psychiatry 2003;64:1284–1292.

38. Altshuler LL, Cohen LS, Moline ML, et al. The Expert Consensus Guideline Series. Treatment of depression in women. Postgrad Med 2001;(Spec No):1–107.

39. Stewart DE, Klompenhouwer JL, Kendell RE, et al. Prophylactic lithium in puerperal psychosis: the experience of three centres. Br J Psychiatry 1991;158:393–397.

40. Ahokas A, Aito M, Rimon R. Positive treatment effect of estradiol in postpartum psychosis: a pilot study. J Clin Psychiatry 2000;61:166–169.

41. Sichel DA, Cohen LS, Robertson LM, et al. Prophylactic estrogen in recurrent postpartum affective disorder. Biol Psychiatry 1995;38:814–818.

42. Kumar C, McIvor RJ, Davies T, et al. Estrogen administration does not reduce the rate of recurrence of affective psychosis after childbirth. J Clin Psychiatry 2003;64:112–118.

43. Matthey S, Barnett B, Howie P, et al. Diagnosing postpartum depression in mothers and fathers: whatever happened to anxiety? J Affect Disord 2003;74:139–147.

44. Cohen LS, Sichel DA, Dimmock JA, et al. Postpartum course in women with preexisting panic disorder. J Clin Psychiatry 1994;55:289–292.

45. Sholomskas DE, Wickamaratne PJ, Dogolo L, et al. Postpartum onset of panic disorder: a coincidental event? J Clin Psychiatry 1993;54:476–480.

46. Klein DF, Skrobala AM, Garfinkel RS. Preliminary look at the effects of pregnancy on the course of panic disorder. Anxiety 1994–1995;1:227–232.

47. Williams KE, Koran LM. Obsessive-compulsive disorder in pregnancy, the puerperium, and the premenstruum. J Clin Psychiatry 1997;58:330–334.

48. Maina G, Albert U, Bogetto F, et al. Recent life events and obsessive-compulsive disorder (OCD): the role of pregnancy/delivery. Psychiatry Res 1999;89:49–58.

49. Sichel DA, Cohen LS, Rosenbaum JF, et al. Postpartum onset of obsessive-compulsive disorder. Psychosomatics 1993;34:277–279.

50. Wijma K, Soderquist J, Wijma B. Posttraumatic stress disorder after childbirth: a cross sectional study. J Anxiety Disord 1997;11:587–597.

51. Creedy DK, Shochet IM, Horsfall J. Childbirth and the development of acute trauma symptoms: incidence and contributing factors. Birth 2000;27:104–111.

52. Wenzel A, Haugen EN, Jackson LC. Prevalence of generalized anxiety at eight weeks postpartum. Arch Women Ment Health 2003;6:43–49.

53. Stowe Z, Llewellyn A, Hostetter A, et al. The use of psychiatric medication during breast-feeding. In: Steiner M, Yonkers KA, Erickson E, eds. Mood Disorders in Women. London: Martin Dunitz, 2000:329–351.

54. American Academy of Pediatrics Committee on Drugs. Transfer of drugs and other chemicals into human milk. Pediatrics 2001;108:776–789.

55. Chaudron LH, Jefferson JW. Mood stabilizers during breastfeeding: a review. J Clin Psychiatry 2000;61:79–90.

56. Patton SW, Misri S, Corral MR, et al. Antipsychotic medication during pregnancy and lactation in women with schizophrenia: evaluating the risk. Can J Psychiatry 2002;7:959–965.

57. Murray L, Cooper PJ. The impact of postpartum depression on child development. Int Rev Psychiatry 1996;8:55–63.

58. Murray L. The impact of postnatal depression in infant development. J Child Psychol Psychiatry 1992;33:543–561.

59. Martins C, Gaffin EA. Effects of early maternal depression on patterns of infant–mother attachment: a meta-analytic investigation. J Child Psychol Psychiatry 2000;41:737–746.

60. Sinclair D, Murray L. Effects of postnatal depression on children's adjustment to school: teacher's reports. Br J Psychiatry 1998;17:58–63.

61. Patel V, DeSouza N, Rodrigues M. Postnatal depression and infant growth and development in low income countries: a cohort study from Goa India. Arch Dis Child 2003;88:34–37.

62. Halligan SL, Herbert J, Goodyer IM, et al. Exposure to postnatal depression predicts elevated cortisol in adolescent offspring. Biol Psychiatry 2004;55:376–381.

63. Weissman MM, Leckman JF, Merikangas KR, et al. Depression and anxiety disorder in parents and children: results from the Yale Family Study. Arch Gen Psychiatry 1984;41:845–852.

64. Manassis K, Bradley S, Goldberg S, et al. Attachment in mothers with anxiety disorders and their children. J Am Acad Child Adolesc Psychiatry 1994;33:1106–1113.

65. Field T. Infants of depressed mothers. Infant Behav Dev 1995;18:1–13.

66. Murray L, Cooper PJ, Wilson A, et al. Controlled trial of the short- and long-term effect of psychological treatment of postpartum depression. Br J Psychiatry 2003;182:420–427.

67. Craig M. Perinatal risk factors for neonaticide and infant homicide: can we identify those at risk? J Roy Soc Med 2004;97:57–61.

68. Stern G, Kruckman L. Multidisciplinary perspective on postpartum depression: an anthropological critique. Soc Sci Med 1983;17:1027–1041.

69. Hayes MJ, Roberts S, Davare A. Transactional conflict between psychology and culture in the etiology of postpartum depression. Med Hypotheses 2000;54:7–17.

70. Affonso DD, De AK, Horowitz JA, et al. An international study exploring levels of postpartum depressive symptomatology. J Psychosom Res 2000;49:207–216.

71. Thorpe KJ, Dragonas T, Golding J, et al. The effects of psychological factors on the mother's emotional well-being during parenthood: a cross sectional study of Britain and Greece. J Reprod Infant Psychol 1992;10:205–217.

72. Oates MR, Cox JL, Neema S, et al. Postnatal depression across countries and cultures: a qualitative study. Br J Psychiatry 2004;184(Suppl 46):s10–16.

73. Hall W. Comparison of the experience of women and men in dual earner families following the birth of their first infant. Image 1992;24:33–38.

74. Zelkowitz P, Milet TH. The course of postpartum psychiatric disorders in women and their partners. J Nerv Ment Dis 2001;189:575–582.

SUGGESTED READINGS

Appleby L, Warner R, Whitton A, et al. A controlled study of fluoxetine and cognitive-behavioural counselling in the treatment of postnatal depression. Br Med J 1997;314:932–936.

Chaudron LH, Pies RW. The relationship between postpartum psychosis and bipolar disorder: a review. J Clin Psychiatry 2003;64:1284–1292.

Martins C, Gaffin EA. Effects of early maternal depression on patterns of infant–mother attachment: a meta-analytic investigation. J Child Psychol Psychiatry 2000;41:737–746.

Murray L, Cooper PJ, Wilson A, et al. Controlled trial of the short- and long-term effect of psychological treatment of postpartum depression. Br J Psychiatry 2003;182:420–427.

Riecher-Rossler A, Hofecker Fallahpour M. Postpartum depression: do we still need this diagnostic term? Acta Psychiatr Scand Suppl 2003;418:51–56.

CHAPTER 21

Menopause and Mental Health

Donna E. Stewart, Mona J. Khalid

"We did not change as we grew older; we just became more clearly ourselves" (1). Menopause is a normal life stage characterized by major changes in hormone secretion, reproductive status, bodily appearance, and sexuality in a psychosocial, cultural, and economic context (2). The transition to menopause happens over a course of several years for most women. The majority experience little or no psychological difficulty, but during this time a small subset of women appear more vulnerable to new or recurrent psychological problems, including depression, anxiety, and psychosis. However, the fact that some women experience difficulties should not overshadow the fact that many women welcome the cessation of menstruation and the end of the risk of unwanted pregnancies. Increasingly, women at midlife enjoy the opportunity to return to education, further establish their careers, or develop new interests.

THE CONTEXT OF LIFE AT MENOPAUSE

For many women, the onset of menopause signals the beginning of aging. It is at this time of life that many women begin to notice changes in their physical appearance and may develop minor health problems. It is also a time when children

297

may be leaving home, partners may be thinking about retirement, and the women's own work situation may be changing. A woman's experience of menopause is shaped by the psychological, social, and cultural context in which she lives (3). The woman whose partner leaves her or who develops health problems during midlife will clearly view the menopause very differently than will the healthy, active woman who gets a job promotion. Women who had hoped for children now realize they will never have any. Many women at midlife also join the "sandwich generation," who are responsible simultaneously for child rearing and for the care of aging parents. Caring for sick relatives may especially burden women at risk for depressive and anxiety symptoms and may rob them of their autonomy and ability to care for themselves (although some women feel enriched and empowered by their caregiving roles) (4). Women also may be affected by the ill health of their spouses or friends, and those women entering retirement may face a marked decrease in standard of living.

In North America and Europe, women are also affected by the substantial difference between the way society views middle-aged women and the way it views middle-aged men. Too often women of this age group are seen as being "over the hill," while men of a similar age are seen as "mature," "experienced," and at the peak of their prowess (5). These perceptions have obvious repercussions in the workplace.

Perceptions and symptoms of women at midlife also vary across cultures. In some cultures women gain respect and support as they age; in others they are marginalized. It is well known that women in Japan experience few menopausal symptoms, while many women in North America experience severe vasomotor symptoms. Body image concerns are common at midlife. New wrinkles appear, abdominal obesity is common, and fitness may decline. Arthritis may appear, and physiologic breast atrophy and hot flashes announce to the woman, and sometimes her associates, that menopause has arrived.

Changes in sexuality also occur at midlife. Reduced libido, thinning and drying of the vaginal lining as a result of decreasing estrogen levels, and societal attitudes toward midlife women's sexuality may all play a role. (See Chapter 15 of this book, on women's sexuality and sexual disorders.) Several studies have found that the partner's sexual health is probably the strongest determinant of women's sexual activity, particularly if sexual activity is solely defined as penetrative vaginal intercourse. It is too easy to attribute all the changes at this time of life to hormonal fluctuations rather than looking at the woman's relationship with her partner and their total life context.

Factors known to influence the health of women as they age include education, socioeconomic status, gender-based division of domestic chores, abuse, violence, access to health care, and paid employment (6). Women more often work in informal sectors, as part-time workers, or in family businesses where they are less likely to be protected by pension plans, health insurance, and other benefits. Cognitive abilities greatly affect women's quality of life. Early symptoms of forgetfulness as a symptom of benign aging may begin in the postmenopausal period and lead to anxieties about incipient Alzheimer disease or other dementias. The fact that most women age well and remain cognitively intact is often overlooked.

During the last five years, public interest in menopause has increased enormously. Wholesale advocacy of hormone replacement therapy was shattered in 2002 when the Women's Health Initiative published the unexpected negative outcomes of its investigations, which threw both women and their physicians into uncertainty about the best medical management of menopause (7).

PHYSIOLOGY OF PERIMENOPAUSE AND MENOPAUSE

The average age of menopause in North American and European women is 51.3 years, but 1% of women have a premature menopause before the age of 40. Women who are smokers and those who have been diagnosed with depression are likely to have an earlier age of onset of menopause (8). Menopause is defined as 12 consecutive months of amenorrhea, and it is diagnosed retrospectively. Well before menopause, however, most women begin to experience symptoms of the transition, a phase termed perimenopause. As ovarian function declines, follicle-stimulating hormone (FSH) concentration rises in an attempt to stimulate resistant ovarian follicles. Luteinizing hormone (LH) and inhibin B also decrease, and when all ovarian follicles have been depleted, the ovary stops producing significant amounts of estrogen. Because there is no further corpus luteum formation, progesterone secretion also stops. Elevated FSH and LH concentrations may be used to confirm the diagnosis of perimenopause, but such measurements are often unreliable because fluctuations are common. Menstrual cycles may become irregular, longer, and often heavier (9). Episodes of amenorrhea and vasomotor symptoms such as hot flashes may be experienced. It is during perimenopause that women experience most of the physiologic symptoms described in the next section and may be more prone to psychological symptoms.

The Massachusetts Women's Health Study and the Study of Women's Health Across the Nation (SWAN) found that the perimenopausal transition usually began about four years before the cessation of menstrual periods. Previous studies have shown that mean serum sex hormone–binding globulin decreases by 43% from four years before and two years after the final menstrual period (10).

With the onset of menopause, the ovarian production of estradiol, progesterone, and testosterone almost ceases. Changes occur in the amount of total estrogen as 17β-estradiol decreases and estrone, a less active form of estrogen (resulting from the conversion of testosterone and androstenedione by the enzyme aromatase), becomes the predominant estrogen after menopause (11). Declining estrogen levels are considered responsible for most of the symptoms discussed in the next section.

SYMPTOMS OF PERIMENOPAUSE

VASOMOTOR SYMPTOMS

Vasomotor symptoms, including hot flashes, night sweats, and sometimes feelings of faintness, accompanied by palpitations and dizziness, are the commonest symptoms experienced in perimenopause. Severe vasomotor symptoms may disrupt sleep and be distracting and a source of embarrassment during waking hours (12).

The etiology of hot flashes is still incompletely understood, but it is likely that changes in the thermoregulatory set points located in the anterior portion of the hypothalamus are most likely responsible (13). A small increase in core body temperature precipitates a hot flash in symptomatic women. Many women experience sweating, which may be profuse, at the start of a hot flash. Heart rate, skin blood flow, and temperature increase during hot flashes, which may last from several seconds to a few minutes. The average hot flash lasts about four minutes (14). Women often respond to the increase in core body temperature by attempting to cool down through sweating, vasodilatation, and behavioral changes (such as removing clothing). Once these cooling mechanisms return the core body temperature to normal, the hot flash terminates. Although the precise role of estrogen in the etiology of hot flashes is unknown, estrogen therapy effectively alleviates them.

The frequency of hot flashes and the way in which they are experienced within and among individual women vary tremendously (15). Although they may occur spontaneously without obvious precipitants, they can also be triggered by stress, heat, exercise, hot drinks, caffeine, and alcohol in some women (15). Approximately 20% of North American menopausal women never experience hot flashes or night sweats (16). Although 20% experience hot flashes for four years or longer, clinical experience suggests that many women have flashes for a longer time. Approximately 70% of women reported that they were not bothered by their hot flashes, while another 30% consulted a physician for treatment, usually because hot flashes or night sweats were frequent, severe, or embarrassing.

The Study of Women's Health Across the Nation (SWAN) investigated many factors associated with menopause in American women. Participating in this study between 1995 and 1997 were 14,906 women between the ages of 40 and 55 from seven regions across the United States. Over 12,000 of these women reported hot flashes and night sweats. Vasomotor symptoms were more frequent among African American women (45.5%), Hispanic women (35.4%), and Caucasian (31.2%) and less common among those of Asian ancestry (20.5%). The duration of the vasomotor symptoms for the majority of women in other studies was less than seven years (60.0%), but 15% reported symptoms for more than 15 years (8). It is vital to understand that more than estrogen levels determine vasomotor phenomena. Stressful contexts, cultural norms, and psychosocial factors appear to moderate both the experience and reporting of hot flashes (17).

Insomnia caused by hot flashes is one of the primary reasons women seek medical care and estrogen therapy during the menopausal transition (15). Estrogen therapy rapidly reduces the frequency and severity of hot flashes, improves sleep, and may reduce the frequency of other perimenopausal symptoms such as joint stiffness and aches, fatigue, and transient memory disturbances.

MENSTRUAL AND BODY CHANGES

Irregular menstrual bleeding is a hallmark of perimenopause. Menstrual periods may become irregular; intramenstrual spotting may occur; menstrual periods may be excessive and prolonged; or there may be intervals without periods. These effects may vary from cycle to cycle and may be unpredictable.

Breast tissue undergoes involution at menopause and becomes less glandular, less dense, and more fatty. This process results in less firmness in the breast and may cause sagging or a change in shape. Some women complain of intermittent breast tenderness during perimenopause.

Skin changes occur primarily in the collagen layer and may result in thinning and more wrinkling. Atrophy of the vaginal mucosa results in less lubrication, which may cause discomfort during intercourse. The labia majora decline in size, and pubic hair may become sparse. Thinning of the urethral and bladder lining may result in more frequent lower urinary tract infections.

Cognitive and affective symptoms may also occur in perimenopause and menopause and will be discussed later following the section on the effect of reproductive hormones on the central nervous system.

EFFECT OF REPRODUCTIVE HORMONES ON THE CNS DURING MENOPAUSE

Estrogen receptors occur in most cells in the body but are particularly numerous in the brain, breast, and the urogenital system. The occurrence of abrupt hormonal changes, especially in estrogen, during the perimenopause has effects on many organ systems. It is not fully understood how estrogen works in the brain, but estrogen α and β receptors are particularly active in the medial amygdala, hippocampus, and limbic systems—the same areas that are so salient for emotions. Estrogens act through nuclear receptors as transcription factors by binding as dimers to specific response elements in DNA and regulating the expression of targeted genes. Estrogens may rapidly up-regulate or down-regulate the excitability of neurons and may exert an agonistic effect on serotonergic activity by increasing the number of serotonergic receptors, the uptake of the neurotransmitter, and the synthesis of serotonin (18). Accordingly, it is not surprising that rapid changes of estrogen during perimenopause may result in affective perturbations in some women.

Progesterone receptors are also found in the limbic system and hypothalamus (19). Progesterones may act as hypnotics and anxiolytics and also may have a negative effect on mood, resulting in dysphoria and irritability (20). Women who are prescribed progesterone (progestins) as a part of hormone therapy to prevent the increased risk of endometrial carcinoma incurred by unopposed estrogen frequently report negative mood symptoms during the interval they are taking progestins.

Testosterone and all other androgens decrease significantly with aging. Produced by the adrenal glands and ovaries, androgens include dehydroepiandrosterone (DHEA) and dehydroepiandrosterone sulfate (DHEAS). Plasma testosterone levels appear to correlate with women's sexual drive, and lower testosterone levels during perimenopause may lead to a lack of sexual desire and interest. Studies have explored the clinical utility of exogenous testosterone in enhancing libido, sexual response, and mood (21). The side effects of this treatment may include acne, hirsutism, and deepening of the voice as well as increased risk of cardiovascular disease. Although exogenous testosterone is currently a popular treatment, the effects of its long-term use in women have not been studied sufficiently.

DHEA and DHEAS may have a positive effect on mood, and women with higher levels may be less likely to experience depressive symptoms (22). Continuing studies are exploring the use of DHEA for depression in menopausal women (23).

Selective estrogen receptor modulators (SERMs) are synthetic compounds that act as estrogen agonists or antagonists on selected organs (24). Although tamoxifen and raloxifene are the only ones currently available for clinical use, numerous SERMs are currently being investigated for their ability to target specific organs and to avoid others. These new chemicals represent an exciting area for future research, but it is not currently possible to determine their full effects on the central nervous system or in the modulation of mood or cognition.

A variety of other substances with potential therapeutic effects are being investigated, including phytoestrogens and herbal preparations. Of the many herbal preparations that have been advocated for the treatment of perimenopausal symptoms, most have been disproved in double-blind, randomized control trials (RCTs) There is however, some continuing interest in use of black cohosh, for which both positive and negative trials have been reported (25,26).

MOOD DISORDERS IN PERIMENOPAUSE AND MENOPAUSE

The psychiatric literature has long included descriptions of mood disorders in perimenopausal and menopausal women. Early investigators (27) described a mixed depressive and anxiety state combined with vasomotor symptoms and other somatic symptoms. Involutional melancholia, a severe form of depressive illness with psychotic features, was described in earlier editions of the *Diagnostic and Statistical Manual of Mental Disorders* (DSM-II and DSM-III). Studies during the 1970s (28,29) disputed the existence of involutional melancholia, and the diagnosis was subsequently dropped from the DSM.

More recently, new evidence is emerging that depression may accompany menopausal transition in some women (30).

Although most longitudinal community-based studies do not show an increase in depressive symptoms or depressive illness in menopausal women, some that have looked specifically at the perimenopausal stage have found a positive association (30–32). However, 45% of perimenopausal women attending gynecologic outpatient clinics have clinically significant scores on depressive rating scales (10,33,34). The SWAN study (35) measured psychological distress; symptoms included sadness, anxiety, and irritability for at least two weeks. The results of this cross-sectional survey found that perimenopausal women had significantly more psychological distress than premenopausal or postmenopausal women. A recent prospective study (30) focused on the increased likelihood of depressive symptoms during transition to menopause and the decreased likelihood after menopause, after adjusting for history of depression, severe premenstrual syndrome, poor sleep, age, race, and employment. Measurements of hormone levels provided corroborating evidence that the changing hormonal milieu contributes to dysphoric mood during transition to menopause.

Anxiety symptoms and irritability have also been described in perimenopausal women (33). The association of anxiety or panic symptoms during perimenopause may be difficult to distinguish from the physiology of hot flashes. This may also explain why estrogen may alleviate these symptoms in some women.

Recent studies, such as the Stages of Reproductive Aging Workshop, or STRAW (36), have examined the relationship between depression and reproductive aging and hormone disturbance, attempting to use more reliable methods such as measurements of hormone levels and structured diagnostic interviews to characterize more carefully the stages of reproductive aging. Recent RCTs employing standardized psychiatric diagnostic interviews have studied the response to estradiol in depression during menopause (37,38). Schmidt et al. (37) found in an RCT that 17β-estradiol effectively treated perimenopausal depression independent of its salutary effects on vasomotor symptoms. In another RCT Soares et al. (38) found that transdermal estradiol was an effective treatment for depressed perimenopausal women and that the antidepressant effects lasted beyond a four-week washout period despite increasing intensity and severity of somatic symptoms.

Animal studies also demonstrate that sex hormones influence several neuroregulatory systems that are involved in the pathophysiology of affective disorders and the action of antidepressant treatments (39–41). Exciting new research with cyclic AMP response element binding protein (CREB) and brain-derived neurotropic factor (BDNF) has begun to explain the therapeutic actions of antidepressants. Interestingly, estradiol is also reported to influence many neuroregulatory processes by increasing CREB activity (42) and BDNF (43).

Various theories have been proposed to explain the occurrence of depression in some perimenopausal women. These include "the hormone withdrawal or deficiency theory," which postulates a correlation between the plasma levels of estrogens or androgens and the severity of depressive symptoms. However, systematic studies have been unable to confirm previous reports of lower basal plasma levels of LH, estrogen, FSH, testosterone, or free testosterone in depressed women compared to nondepressed women (22,44). Interesting hormonal research work in women with a first onset of depression during perimenopause found significantly lower levels of plasma DHEA and DHEAS but not cortisol compared to nondepressed controls (44).

In summary, there seems to be increasing evidence that some perimenopausally depressed women improve with the restoration of ovarian function (45) and that estrogen therapy may improve mood in depressed perimenopausal women (38,44). Interestingly, Morrison et al. (46) have reported that estrogen has no more effect than placebo in postmenopausal depressed women, in contrast to previous studies in perimenopausal women, thereby suggesting that women undergoing menopause are more responsive to estrogen than those in whom hormone status has stabilized.

A "domino" theory of hot flashes and dysphoria has also been proposed in which it is suggested that hot flashes and perimenopausal depression either share the same pathophysiology or that a causal relationship exists between them (for example, hot flashes lead to sleep disruption, which results in dysphoria). However, recent evidence would suggest that hot flashes and depression can occur independently and that women with perimenopausal depression without hot flashes also respond to estrogen treatment (37). Moreover, Soares et al. (38) have shown that in depressed women successfully treated with estrogen, hot flashes may return when the estrogen is withdrawn but the depression may not necessarily recur. In short, hot flashes are not necessary or sufficient to cause depression in perimenopausal women.

Negative life events, psychosocial factors, and attitudes toward aging have also been postulated as etiologic factors in the onset of perimenopausal depression (47,48). Recent work does not support this concept because depressed perimenopausal women do not report more negative events than controls but rather appear to demonstrate an increased vulnerability to the negative impact of these events (49). It may be that genetic predisposition (50,51), self-efficacy (52), health, and social support (53) determine whether negative events trigger depression.

It appears that some women are at increased risk of depression during perimenopause, and these women more often report other hormone-initiated mood disorders (34). The apparent reduction in depression rates after menopause suggests that it is the transitional phase that presents increased risk for some women rather than a stabilized period of lower levels of gonadal hormones (30).

MANAGEMENT OF MOOD DISORDERS IN PERIMENOPAUSAL/MENOPAUSAL WOMEN

Clinical inquiry should include questions about past episodes of depression or bipolar affective disorder and the circumstances under which these appeared. Affective and anxiety symptoms should be elicited as well as their relationship to vasomotor symptoms such as hot flashes. Other symptoms associated with perimenopause and menopause such as vaginal dryness, urinary incontinence, sexual dysfunction, and sleep disturbance should be sought. Any comorbid conditions and their treatment should be assessed in relation to their ability to cause mood disorders (such as the treatment of hypertension). The woman's reaction to her aging and perimenopausal symptoms may be important if these lower her self-esteem. As noted earlier, work, relationships, social, economic, and cultural contexts of a woman's life are vitally important, and queries about these factors should be part of the assessment.

In women whose depressive symptoms appear to be secondary to vasomotor symptoms (hot flashes, insomnia), low doses of estrogen for the shortest time possible may be helpful. In women with a past history of depression and only mild to moderate perimenopausal symptoms, the usual management with antidepressant medication or psychotherapy is most likely to be helpful. As mentioned earlier, hormonal measures such as FSH and LH may fluctuate from cycle to cycle and are not necessarily useful in determining the best course of treatment. For treatment-resistant women, antidepressant medication may be augmented with low doses of estrogen. Any contraindication to estrogen therapy such as a personal history of breast cancer obviously precludes its use. Progestins should be administered sequentially or cyclically with estrogen to women with intact uteri to prevent increased risk of endometrial cancer due to unopposed estrogen. However, progestins may cause depression and other dysphoric states in some women.

Recent research has documented the benefits of venlafaxine and paroxetine in the management of hot flashes, but these medications are not as effective as estrogen. Although estrogen is no longer appropriate for the prophylaxis of cardiovascular, cerebrovascular, or Alzheimer disease, it is still a reasonable choice for the management of acute perimenopausal vasomotor symptoms when used at the lowest effective dose for the shortest time possible.

Newer treatments for depressed perimenopausal women currently under investigation include DHEA, SERMs, and phytoestrogens. As previously mentioned, testosterone has also been used to improve libido, but the long-term effects of its administration in women are unknown. Psychotherapy is useful to treat depression during perimenopause and menopause as at other times of life and may be used either independently or as an adjunct to other forms of treatment.

PSYCHOTIC ILLNESS IN WOMEN AT PERIMENOPAUSE AND MENOPAUSE

As early as 1896, Kraft Ebbing reported that some women became psychotic during low estrogen phases of their menstrual cycle, and in the early 1900s Kraepelin (54,55) reported that schizophrenia stemmed partly from disturbed hormonal balance. Since that time a number of investigators have reported the association of low estrogen with an increase in psychotic symptoms, particularly in women suffering from schizophrenia. Seeman (56) reported that women may be protected against the early onset of schizophrenia and this protective effect wears off in midlife. Although men and women have the same overall incidence and lifetime prevalence of schizophrenia, the onset occurs sooner in men (57). Late-onset schizophrenia is more common in women than in men (58), which supports an estrogen protection hypothesis. This theory is also supported by the observation that psychotic symptoms tend to be low during pregnancy, when estrogen levels are high. Clinical reports indicate that women respond better than men to antipsychotic medication and that women of child bearing age tend to respond better than older postmenopausal women (59).

Late-onset schizophrenia, which predominantly occurs in women, is characterized by a severe symptomatology and course (60). Jeste (61) reported that women with late-onset schizophrenia were more likely to have paranoid delusions but better premorbid adjustment. Moreover, women with schizophrenia appeared to have fewer negative symptoms.

An open-label pilot study by Kulkarni et al. (62) showed more rapid symptom improvement in women who received estrogen augmentation of antipsychotic medication than in women who were treated with antipsychotic medication alone. (See Chapter 14.)

Because many women gain weight around the time of perimenopause and menopause and because antipsychotics also increase weight gain, this may be a major problem in the management of women with psychosis. Antipsychotics may also cause prolactin elevation in women resulting in decreased libido, poor vaginal lubrication, and galactorrhea. Some newer antipsychotics may also increase the risk of diabetes mellitus.

There is controversial evidence on whether estrogen decreases the risks of tardive dyskinesia when administered with antipsychotics (63).

Although bipolar affective disorder shows no overall difference in sex prevalence, women are at increased risk for rapid cycling bipolar disorder (64). Women with bipolar disorder also appear to experience more relapses or exacerbations during low-estrogen phases of the cycle, or perimenopause, similarly to women with schizophrenia (65). Burt et al. (66) and Soares and Almeida (67) have reported increased incidence of depression in bipolar women during perimenopause and advocate comprehensive assessment of somatic symptoms such as vasomotor symptoms and sleep disturbance in developing a management plan.

MEDICAL ASPECTS OF PERIMENOPAUSE AND MENOPAUSE

After menopause, women enter a period of increased risk for a variety of medical conditions including cardiovascular disease, stroke, thyroid diseases, cancer, osteoporosis, arthritis, and dementia. The major causes of morbidity and disability are osteoporotic fractures, arthritis, and dementia (68,69).

WOMEN'S HEALTH INITIATIVE

The Women's Health Initiative (WHI) is a large, multicenter observational and interventional primary prevention study that recruited 161,809 postmenopausal women between 1993 and 1998 (70). One arm of the study, involving 16,608 postmenopausal women with intact uteri in a double blind, placebo-controlled, randomized trial of combined estrogen plus progesterone therapy, was terminated early in May 2002 after an average of 5.2 years (7). The results of this study showed an increase in coronary heart disease events, strokes, thromboemboli, invasive breast cancers, ovarian cancers, and gallbladder disease in women treated with estrogen and progesterone and a decrease in fractures and colorectal cancers. Subsequently, early termination of the estrogen-only arm of this trial in March 2004 revealed an increase in risk for stroke in common with the earlier trial but no increased risk for breast cancer.

Best evidence to date for the effect of gonadal hormones on memory is the Women's Health Initiative Memory Study (WHIMS) (71). This WHI substudy included over 4,000 postmenopausal women who did not have dementia at study initiation. The study showed that combined estrogen and progesterone increased the risk for dementia in postmenopausal women aged 65 or older after an average of four years of follow-up. In addition, hormone therapy did not prevent mild cognitive impairment as had previously been reported in less rigorous studies.

A large primary prevention trial in the United Kingdom, the Women's International Study of Long Duration Estrogen After Menopause (WISDOM) has also recently been stopped (72). As a result of this evidence, the U.S. Preventive Task Force, the North American Menopause Society, the American College of Obstetricians and Gynecologists, and the Food and Drug Administration (FDA) have all recently recommended against using estrogen and progesterone therapy for the prevention of chronic diseases. The FDA has extended the warning to recommend against using estrogen for the prevention of chronic diseases but states that for the acute treatment of perimenopausal symptoms such as vasomotor symptoms and atrophic vaginitis, the lowest dose of estrogen for the shortest duration possible is permissible.

Clinical practice has responded rapidly to recent evidence. Hormone therapy prescriptions declined substantially after July 2002, and many patients have discontinued hormone therapy or are tapering to lower doses. Relative to the period from January to June 2002, prescriptions from January to June 2003 declined by approximately 66% for estrogen and progestin combination therapy and 33% for estrogen-only therapy based on U.S. data from the National Prescription Audit Database (73).

CONCLUSIONS

Most women go through perimenopause and menopause with mild symptoms and inconvenience and do not experience psychological problems. However, a small subset of women, especially those with previous psychiatric illness associated with hormonal changes, may be vulnerable to psychiatric illness in perimenopause. Any assessment of the role of hormonal factors must also include a consideration of the woman's life context and other stressors.

Although early evidence suggests that gonadal hormones (especially estrogen) may be useful in the treatment or augmentation of treatment in selected women with depression or psychosis, adequately powered randomized controlled trials of benefits and risks are urgently needed before this becomes a standard practice.

REFERENCES

1. Hall L. Where Have All the Tigers Gone? New York: Scribner, 1989.
2. Stewart DE. Preface. In: Menopause: A Mental Health Practitioner's Guide. Washington, DC: American Psychiatric Publishing, 2005; pp. ix–xii.
3. Stotland N. The context of midlife in women. In: Stewart DE, ed. Menopause: A Mental Health Practitioner's Guide. Washington, DC: American Psychiatric Publishing, 2005; 1–16.

4. Veltman A, Cameron J, Stewart DE. The experience of providing care to relatives with chronic mental illness. J Nerv Ment Dis 2002;190(2):108–114.
5. Greer G. The Change: Women, Aging, and the Menopause. New York: Ballantine, 1991.
6. Rondon M. Beyond menopause: the psychopathology and psychotherapy of older age women. In: Stewart DE, ed. Menopause: A Mental Health Practitioner's Guide. Washington, DC: American Psychiatric Publishing, 2005; pp. 189–214.
7. The Writing Group for the Women's Health Initiative Investigators. Risks and benefits of estrogen plus progestin in healthy postmenopausal women: principal results for the Women's Health Initiative Randomized Control Trial. JAMA 2002;288(3):321–333.
8. Santoro N. What a SWAN can teach us about menopause. Contemp Ob/Gyn 2004;49:69–79.
9. Baram D. Physiology and symptoms of menopause. In: Stewart DE, Robinson GE, eds. A Clinician's Guide to Menopause. Washington, DC: American Psychiatric Publishing, 1997:9–28.
10. Dennerstein L, Smith AMA, Morse C, et al. Menopausal symptoms in Australian women. Med J Aust 1993;159:232–236.
11. Shifren JL, Braunstein GD, Simon JA, et al. Transdermal testosterone treatment in women with impaired sexual function after oophorectomy. N Engl J Med 2000;343:682–688.
12. Avis NE, Stellato R, Crawford S, et al. Is there a menopausal syndrome? Menopausal status and symptoms across racial/ethnic groups. Soc Sci Med 2001;52:345–356.
13. Speroff L. The perimenopause: definitions, demography, and physiology. Obstet Gyn Clin North Am 2002;29:397–410.
14. Speroff L, Glass RH, Kase NG. Clinical Gynecologic Endocrinology and Infertility. 5th Ed. Baltimore: Williams & Wilkins, 1999.
15. Kronenberg F. Hot flashes. In: Lobo RA, ed. Treatment of the Postmenopausal Woman: Basic and Clinical Aspects. New York: Raven, 1994:97–117.
16. Avis NE, McKinlay SM. The Massachusetts Women's Health Study: an epidemiologic investigation of the menopause. J Am Med Womens Assoc 1995;50:45–63.
17. Stearns V, Ullmer L, Lopez JF, et al. Hot flushes. Lancet 2002;360:1851–1861.
18. Soares CN, Steiner M, Prouty J, et al. The effects of reproductive hormones and selective estrogen receptor modulators (SERMS) on the central nervous system during menopause. In: Stewart DE, ed. Menopause: A Mental Health Practitioner's Guide. Washington, DC: American Psychiatric Publishing, 2005; pp. 37–64.
19. Sherwin BB. Can estrogen keep you smart? Evidence from clinical studies. J Psychiatry Neurosci 1999;24:315–321.
20. Lawrie T, Hofmeyer G, de Jager M, et al. A double-blind randomised placebo-controlled trial of postnatal noethisterone enanthate: the effect of postnatal depression and serum hormones. J Obstet Gynaecol 2000;105:1082–1090.
21. Sands R, Studd J. Exogenous androgens in postmenopausal women. Am J Med 1995;98(1A):76S–79S.
22. Barrett-Connor E, von Muhlen D, et al. Endogenous levels of dehydroepiandrosterone sulfate, but not other sex hormones, are associated with depressed mood in older women: the Rancho Bernardo Study. J Am Geriatr Soc 1999;47:685–691.
23. Wolkowitz OM, Reus VI, Keebler A, et al. Double-blind treatment of major depression with dehydroepiandrosterone. Am J Psychiatry 1999;156:646–649.
24. Mayeux R. Can estrogen or selective estrogen-receptor modulators preserve cognitive function in elderly women? N Engl J Med 2001;344:1242–1244.
25. Lichtman R. Perimenopausal and postmenopausal hormone replacement therapy. Part 2, Hormonal regimens and complementary and alternative therapies. J Nurse Midwifery 1996;41(3):195–210.
26. Jacobson JS, Troxel AB, Evans J, et al. Randomized trials of black cohosh for the treatment of hot flashes among women with a history of breast cancer. J Clin Oncol 2001;19:2739–2745.
27. Conklin WJ. Some neuroses of the menopause. Trans Am Assoc Obstet Gynecol 1889;2:301–311.
28. Winokur G, Cadoret R. The irrelevance of the menopause to depressive disease. In: Sachar EJ, ed. Topics in Psychoendocrinology. New York: Grune & Stratton, 1975:59–66.
29. Weissman MM. The myth of involutional melancholia. JAMA 1979;242:742–744.
30. Freeman WE, Sammel MD, Liu L, et al. Hormones and menopausal status as predictors of depression in women in transition to menopause. Arch Gen Psychiatry 2004;61:62–70.
31. Matthews KA. Myths and realities of the menopause. Psychosom Med 1992;54:1–9.
32. Hunter M. The south-east England longitudinal study of the climacteric and postmenopause. Maturitas 1992;14:117–126.
33. Hay AG, Bancroft J, Johnstone EC. Affective symptoms in women attending a menopause clinic. Br J Psychiatry 1994;164:513–516.
34. Stewart DE, Boydell K, Derzko C, et al. Psychologic distress during the menopausal years in women attending a menopause clinic. Int J Psychiatry Med 1992;22:213–220.
35. Bromberger JT, Meyer PM, Kravitz HM, et al. Psychologic distress and natural menopause: a multiethnic community study. Am J Public Health 2001;91:1435–1442.
36. Soules MR, Sherman S, Parrott E, et al. Executive summary: stages of reproductive aging workshop (STRAW). Fertil Steril 2001;76:874–878.

37. Schmidt PJ, Nieman L, Danaceau MA, et al. Estrogen replacement in perimenopause-related depression: a preliminary report. Am J Obstet Gynecol 2000;183:414–420.

38. Soares CD, Almeida OP, Joffe H, et al. Efficacy of estradiol for the treatment of depressive disorders in perimenopausal women: a double-blind, randomized, placebo-controlled trial. Arch Gen Psychiatry 2001;58:529–534.

39. Woolley CS, Schwartzkroin PA. Hormonal effects on the brain. Epilepsia 1998;39:S2–S8.

40. McEwen BS, Alves SE, Bulloch K, et al. Ovarian steroids and the brain: implications for cognition and aging. Neurology 1997;48(Suppl 7):S8–S15.

41. Rachman IM, Unnerstall JR, Pfaff DW, et al. Estrogen alters behavior and forebrain c-fos expression in ovariectomized rats subjected to the forced swim test. Proc Natl Acad Sci USA 1998;95:13941–13946.

42. Zhou Y, Watters JJ, Dorsa DM. Estrogen rapidly induces the phosphorylation of the cAMP response element binding protein in rat brain. Endocrinology 1996;137:2163–2166.

43. Murphy DD, Cole NB, Segal M. Brain-derived neurotrophic factor mediates estradiol-induced dendritic spine formation in hippocampal neurons. Proc Natl Acad Sci USA 1998;95: 11412–11417.

44. Schmidt PJ, Murphy JH, Haq N, et al. Basal plasma hormone levels in depressed perimenopausal women. Psychoneuroendocrinology 2002;27:907–920.

45. Daly RC, Danaceau MA, Rubinow DR, et al. Concordant restoration of ovarian function and mood in perimenopausal depression. Am J Psychiatry 2003;160:1842–1846.

46. Morrison MF, Kallan MJ, Ten Hav T, et al. Lack of efficacy of estradiol for depression in postmenopausal women: a randomized, controlled trial. Biol Psychiatry 2004;55(4):406–412.

47. Deeks A. Psychological aspects of menopause management. Best Pract Res Clin Endocrinol Metab 2003;17(10):17–31.

48. Dennerstein L, Guthrie JR, Clark M, et al. A population-based study of depressed mood in middle-aged, Australian-born women. Menopause 2004;11(5):563–568.

49. Schmidt PJ, Khine K, Luff JA, et al. Mood disorders, midlife and reproductive aging. In: Stewart DE, ed. Menopause: A Mental Health Practitioner's Guide. Washington, DC: American Psychiatric Publishing, 2005; pp. 65–94.

50. Kendler KS, Kessler RC, Walters EE, et al. Stressful life events, genetic liability, and onset of an episode of major depression in women. Am J Psychiatry 1995;152:833–842.

51. Caspi A, Sugden K, Moffitt TE, et al. Influence of life stress on depression: moderation by a polymorphism in the 5-HTT gene. Science 2003;301:291–293.

52. Maciejewski PK, Prigerson HG, Mazure CM. Sex differences in event-related risk for major depression. Psychol Med 2001;31:593–604.

53. Seeman TE, Crimmins E. Social environment effects on health and aging: integrating epidemiologic and demographic approaches and perspectives. Ann NY Acad Sci 2001;954:88–117.

54. Krafft-Ebbing G von. Untersuchungen uber Irresein zur Zeit der Menstruation: Ein Klinischer Beilrag zur Lehne von periodischen Irresein. Arch Psychiatrie 1896;8:65–107.

55. Kraepelin E. Psychiatrie. bd 1–4. Leipzig: Barth, 1909–1915.

56. Seeman MV. Gender differences in schizophrenia. Can J Psychiatry 1982;27:107–112.

57. Hafner H, an der Heiden W. Epidemiology of schizophrenia. Can J Psychiatry 1997;42:139–151.

58. Faraone SV, Chen WJ, Goldstein JM, et al. Gender differences in age of onset of schizophrenia. Br J Psychiatry 1994;164:625–629.

59. Seeman MV. Sex differences in predicting neuroleptic response. In: Gaebel W, Awad AG, eds. The Prediction of Neuroleptic Response. Vienna: Springer-Verlag, 1995:51–64.

60. Riecher-Rossler A, Loffler W, Munk-Jorgensen P. What do we really know about late onset schizophrenia? Eur Arch Psychiatry Clin Neurosci 1997;247:195–208.

61. Jeste DV, Harris M, Krull A. Clinical and neuropsychological characteristics of patients with late onset schizophrenia. Am J Psychiatry 1995;152:722–730.

62. Kulkarni J, Riedel A, de Castella A, et al. Estrogen: a potential treatment for schizophrenia. Schizophr Res 2001;48:137–144.

63. Kulkarni J. Psychotic illness in women at perimenopause and menopause. In: Stewart DE, ed. Menopause: A Mental Health Practitioner's Guide. Washington, DC: American Psychiatric Publishing, 2005; pp. 95–116.

64. Leibenluft E. Women with bipolar illness: clinical and research issues. Am J Psychiatry 1996;153:163–173.

65. Hendrick V, Altshuler LL, Burt VK. Course of psychiatric disorders across the menstrual cycle. Harvard Rev Psychiatry 1996;4:200–207.

66. Burt VK, Altshuler LL, Rasgon N. Depressive symptoms in the perimenopause: prevalence, assessment and guidelines for treatment. Harvard Rev Psychiatry 1998;6:121–132.

67. Soares CN, Almeida OP. Depression during the perimenopause (letter). Arch Gen Psychiatry 2001;58(3):306.

68. Chaudhry R, Cheung AM. Postmenopausal/senior women. In: Stewart DE, Cheung AM, Ferris LE, et al., eds. Ontario women's health status report. Toronto: Ontario Women's Health Council, 2002:314–337.

69. Cheung AM, Chaudhry R, Kapral M, et al. Perimenopausal and postmenopausal health. In: DesMeules et al., eds. Women's health surveillance report: a multidimensional look at the health of Canadian women. Toronto: Canadian Institute for Health Information, 2003.

70. The Women's Health Initiative Study Group. Design of the Women's Health Initiative clinical trial and observational study. Control Clin Trials 1998;1:61–109.

71. Shumaker SA, Legault C, Rapp SR, et al. WHIMS Investigators. Estrogen plus progestin and the incidence of dementia and mild cognitive impairment in postmenopausal women: the Women's Health Initiative Memory Study: a randomized controlled trial. JAMA 2003;289(20):2651–2662.

72. Medical Research Council. MRC stops study of long term use of HRT. Press Release, October 23, 2002. Available at: http://www.mrc.ac.uk/prn/index/public-interest/public-press_office/public-press_releases_2002/public-23_october_2002.htm.

73. Hersh AL, Stefanick ML, Stafford RS. National use of postmenopausal hormone therapy. JAMA 2004;291:1:47–53.

SUGGESTED READINGS

Avis NE, Stellato R, Crawford S, et al. Is there a menopausal syndrome? Menopausal status and symptoms across racial/ethnic groups. Soc Sci Med 2001;52:345–356.

Cheung AM, Chaudhry R, Kapral M, et al. Perimenopausal and postmenopausal health. In: DesMeules et al., eds. Women's health surveillance report: a multidimensional look at the health of Canadian women. Toronto: Canadian Institute for Health Information, 2003.

Freeman WE, Sammel MD, Liu L, et al. Hormones and menopausal status as predictors of depression in women in transition to menopause. Arch Gen Psychiatry 2004;61:62–70.

Kronenberg F. Hot flashes. In: Lobo RA, ed. Treatment of the Postmenopausal Woman: Basic and Clinical Aspects. New York: Raven, 1994:97–117.

McEwen BS, Alves SE, Bulloch K, et al. Ovarian steroids and the brain: implications for cognition and aging. Neurology 1997;48(Suppl 7):S8–S15.

Schmidt PJ, Khine K, Luff JA, et al. Mood disorders, midlife and reproductive aging. In: Stewart DE, ed. Menopause: A Mental Health Practitioner's Guide. Washington, DC: American Psychiatric Publishing, 2005; pp. 65–94.

Shumaker SA, Legault C, Rapp SR, et al. WHIMS Investigators. Estrogen plus progestin and the incidence of dementia and mild cognitive impairment in postmenopausal women: the Women's Health Initiative Memory Study: a randomized controlled trial. JAMA 2003;289(20):2651–2662.

Soules MR, Sherman S, Parrott E, et al. Executive summary: Stages of Reproductive Aging Workshop (STRAW). Fertil Steril 2001;76:874–878.

The Writing Group for the Women's Health Initiative Investigators. Risks and benefits of estrogen plus progestin in healthy postmenopausal women. JAMA 2002;288(3):321–333.

Mothering and Depression

Sydney L. Hans

Lifetime rates of depression are higher in women than in men, with nearly one in five women experiencing a clinically significant episode of depression at some time during their lives (1). Many women experience more than one episode (2), and many suffer from subclinical levels of depression for prolonged periods (3). Moreover, major depression often first occurs during the childbearing years and remains high throughout early adulthood (4). Between 8% and 15% of women experience clinical depression during the postnatal period (5). Taken together, these statistics suggest that many women are struggling with depression and the demands of motherhood at the same time (6).

A large and growing body of literature suggests that children with depressed mothers, although a heterogeneous group, are at risk for a variety of mental health and developmental problems. Children of depressed parents have high rates of depression themselves when compared to children with parents who have never had psychiatric illness (7–9). However, children whose mothers suffer from depression are at risk for other mental health problems as well, including disruptive behavior disorders, anxiety psychiatric disorders, and alcohol use/abuse during adolescence. Onset of disorders may be earlier and more impairing in young people with depressed parents.

Children with depressed mothers have been reported to have a variety of other problem behaviors that do not qualify as mental disorders or psychiatric syndromes. For example, infants with depressed mothers are more likely to be irritable and negative than other infants (10,11), even during the newborn period (12,13), and to show delays in cognitive development (14). Toddlers whose mothers are depressed react to stress with greater negativity and have more difficulty regulating their negative emotions (15). School-age children with depressed mothers may be less socially competent, have lower self-esteem, and display more behavior problems at home and in school (16–18).

A variety of mechanisms have been proposed to explain the associations between parents' depression and the behavior or developmental problems of their offspring (8). It is possible that genetic factors are involved in the intergenerational transmission of depression itself or in the transmission of neuroregulatory processes related to stress re-activity or modulation of negative emotion (19,20). Claims have also been made that children with depressed mothers may be at risk because they are exposed prenatally to a neuroendocrine environment that interferes in the development of the hypothalamic-pituitary-adrenal axis (21,22). This hypothesis is supported by documented high levels of stress hormones in pregnant women and in their newborns (23). The most frequently invoked explanation for the increased incidence of problems in children with depressed mothers is that children are exposed to patterns of parenting that place them at risk. This chapter provides an overview of what is known about how depression affects parenting. The chapter also considers ways in which parenting may affect women's mental health.

INTERACTIONS BETWEEN DEPRESSED MOTHERS AND THEIR CHILDREN

Since depression is an affective disorder whose symptoms include sadness, diminished pleasure in activities, and a certain amount of self-absorption, one might expect that depressed mothers would differ from other women in their display of positive affect and energy with their children. Emotional communication may be particularly central to the development well-being of very young children (24), and many studies have examined the emotional communication between depressed mothers and their infants. These studies typically involve careful and detailed observations of facial expressions and vocalizations from videotapes made of mothers and children in structured settings, including during face-to-face interaction. These reports do, in fact, suggest that depressed mothers have fewer positive exchanges with their infants (25–28). Their interactions include less talking and play and more silence and social withdrawal (29,30). Similar findings come from studies of older children in which depressed mothers are less warm and positive with their children (31–33). In a study of a nationally representative sample, Lyons-Ruth and colleagues (34) examined the impact of maternal depression on whether women engaged in positive routines with their children such as reading books to them or playing with them. For each symptom of depression endorsed, the odds that mothers would engage in such activities decreased substantially.

Not only is parental interactive behavior less positive when women are depressed, but it may be less responsive to their children's signals and less contingently related to children's behavior (25,35). A lack of experience with coordinated interactions with their mothers may deprive infants of important opportunities to learn to regulate their own physiologic states and emotions or to develop a sense of efficacy in communication with others.

Although one tends to think of the core feature of depression as reduced positive affect, mood disorder can manifest itself through irritability and displays of negative affect (36,37). Many studies of mother–child interaction have shown high rates of display of negative affect by depressed mothers (28,38,39). Especially as their children get older, depressed mothers may be more likely to show impatience (40), to criticize their children (16,41,42), and to have flare-ups of anger (31,42,43).

A meta-analysis (44) reviewing approximately 30 studies of maternal depression summarized the results with respect to three categories of parenting behavior: negative, disengaged, positive. The meta-analysis suggested effects of maternal depression on each of these categories of parental behavior. Depression had a small inverse effect on mothers' display of positive affect. Depression had a larger, moderate effect on mothers' disengagement from children and negativity.

Some investigators have suggested that there may be two different types of depressed mothers—those who typically are more withdrawn and those who typically are more intrusive (26,45). Withdrawn mothers are affectively disengaged from their infants, verbalizing less, and relatively expressionless in face and voice. Intrusive mothers are overstimulating and interfering, poking and jabbing their babies, talking loudly, and exhibiting annoyance. The developmental course for children of these two parenting experiences could be quite different. One might expect that infants with withdrawn mothers would learn from their mothers a sense of helplessness, ineffectiveness, and passivity in social relationships. Infants of intrusive mothers on the other hand might learn to avoid interaction to protect themselves from intrusion or to protest and fend off their mothers' unwanted actions by angry displays.

Other investigators have written about ways in which parents combine disengagement and anger into their interactions with their children. Studies of children with behavior problems have shown that they and their parents engage in patterns of "coercive" interactions (46). Coercive interactions begin when parents passively tolerate children's noncompliance. Children often escalate their negative behavior in efforts to seek parental attention, and parents eventually respond with anger. Thus parents and children get caught up in cycles of interaction in which children escalate their angry displays, and parents vacillate between disengagement and angry outbursts. Studies of depressed mothers suggest patterns of interaction with coercive features. Depressed mothers, when faced with children's noncompliance, may alternate between dropping their demands or persisting uncompromisingly (47). Depressed mothers of older children and adolescents may be generally lax in monitoring, guiding, and disciplining their children but punctuate their relationship with episodes of anger and harsh punitive discipline (28,33,48–50).

A different line of research suggests that, when guiding their children, depressed mothers are less likely than other mothers to give positive feedback to children (40) and may be especially likely to use child management strategies that involve guilt and anxiety induction (51,52). By shaming children, parents may be making children feel a greater burden of personal responsibility and helplessness. Moreover, induction of guilt makes children feel responsible for parents' emotional states. Several studies of depressed mothers suggest that their young children may feel the need to care for their parents emotionally. In both laboratory-based and home-based studies, children exposed to elevated expression of parental sadness have shown an increased tendency to comfort and care for their parents (53,54).

FACTORS AFFECTING THE PARENTING OF DEPRESSED WOMEN

Although the literature strongly associates depression with problematic parenting, there is a great deal of variability in parenting among depressed parents, and much remains to be learned about which depressed parents are at greatest risk.

Women who have participated in studies of depressed mothers have been an extremely varied group from a clinical perspective. In some studies women reach diagnostic criteria for syndromal depression, and in others they report elevated depressive symptoms that could be more transient and less impairing. In some studies, women meet current diagnostic criteria for depression, whereas in other studies, women have lifetime but not current mood disorders. Studies relying on diagnostic criteria might not make distinctions between single and recurrent major depressive episodes and the more prolonged, but less severe, symptoms of dysthymia. Although the findings of problematic parenting in depressed women have been fairly robust across these great differences in levels of severity, chronicity, and syndrome in depressed mothers, there likely are important differences in the parenting of women with different clinical experiences. For example, Lovejoy and colleagues (44), in their meta-analysis of parenting in depressed mothers, found that maternal negativity was typically observed in samples of women with current depression but not those where mothers have lifetime, but not current depression. Lack of positive affect was found in women who met lifetime criteria for depression, regardless of whether the disorder was current.

Inadequate attention has been given to a host of factors associated with maternal depression, including father's mental health problems as well as comorbid mental health and substance abuse problems in mothers themselves. Many depressed women have comorbid personality disorders that could also have strong impacts on their parenting (55–57).

Rates of depression are higher in women living in stressed circumstances. Inadequate attention has been given to whether the relation between maternal depression and parenting difficulties might be a reflection of those more general stressors rather than simply maternal depression. For example, marital difficulties in families affected by depression are common (58,59), and a large body of literature finds links between couple difficulties, including both amount and style of conflict and problematic parenting (60). Also, women experiencing economic stresses are especially likely to become depressed. In Lovejoy et al.'s meta-analysis (44), positive maternal behavior was found to be reduced in depressed mothers only in those studies conducted with low-income samples.

Increasingly, research attention has been devoted to whether depressed women's parenting may be affected by characteristics of their children. It is too often assumed that parent–child interaction operates in a "top-down" fashion, with the primary direction of influence being the parent shaping the behavior of the child. However, developmental theory and research suggest that parent–child effects are bidirectional, with children affecting parenting behavior just as parenting influences child behavior (61,62).

A growing literature suggests that children born to depressed mothers, beginning from the first days of life, may be more difficult to care for than other children. Depressed women have, in many studies, reported their children as displaying more challenging or "difficult" behavioral characteristics (63–65). Compared to other women, depressed mothers are more likely to report that their children are stressed (66), irritable (67), negative (39,68), and vulnerable (69). For example, in a study of Finnish mothers (70), depressed women saw their 2-month-olds as prone to crying, unsoothable, and difficult, and their 2-year-olds as unadaptable and dependent.

One could argue that infants of depressed mothers are not necessarily more difficult, but that their mothers only perceive them that way. However, other studies, not affected by the potential biases of maternal report, also suggest that children with depressed mothers have more difficult temperamental characteristics and more frequent displays of negative emotionality (71,72). For example, newborns of women who were depressed during pregnancy were more likely to be assessed by blind observers as prone to crying and inconsolability during the neonatal period (12,13). Data to date do not demonstrate whether such early infant regulatory problems are associated with later parenting difficulties. However, one provocative study illustrating the potential control of infants over adult behavior showed that nondepressed strangers interacting with children of depressed mothers become less positive and expressive than when interacting with children of nondepressed mothers (73).

PARENTING AS A RISK FACTOR FOR WOMEN'S DEPRESSION

A great deal of public and research concern has focused on the risks for depression during the first months of motherhood. It is often assumed that motherhood leads to increased risk for depression. A voluminous literature exists on depression during pregnancy and the postpartum period. Although there is a brief period after giving birth that many women experience "the blues," possibly related to rapid changes in hormonal levels, data do not suggest that rates of major depression during the months following childbirth are especially elevated compared to those for young women who have not given birth (5), and links between hormonal status to major depressive disorders have not been clearly shown (74).

The physical and social stresses of parenting, however, may be linked to depression in mothers. The transition to parenthood is a stressful period for most women, involving increased work burdens, deprivation of sleep, and rearrangement of relationships with other family members (75). Some evidence suggests that women's depression is related to the amount of burden from childrearing, including the number of young children in the home (76). Data suggest that mothers whose children are more difficult to care for are more likely to experience depressive symptoms. Using maternal reports and objective assessments, infant difficult behavior accounted for 30% of the variance in maternal depressive symptoms in one sample of new mothers (63). The authors suggested that parenting difficult infants led women to perceive themselves as low in self-efficacy, which in turn contributed to depression. Other parents report that caring for difficult children contributes to a sense of loss of control in their lives (77). In one longitudinal study in which infants' behavior was evaluated by an examiner at three days of age, infants who were less alert and adept at social orientation were more likely to have mothers who reported postnatal depression six weeks later (78).

When children are older, parenting stress is clearly linked to women's mental health. Mothers whose children have chronic diseases are more likely to experience depression (79). Increased rates of depression are observed among women whose children are referred to clinics for mental health services. For example, Civic and Holt (80) report that women whose children had multiple adjustment problems, including tantrums and unhappiness, were more than three times as likely to have elevated rates of depression than other mothers. Similarly, Harrison and Sofronoff (81) found that child hyperactivity accounted for 21% of variance in maternal depression, and that parent perception of low levels of control contributed to this relation. Hammen found that children's psychiatric problems tend to occur close in time to onset of maternal major depression, with child problems often preceding mothers' depression (82). Similarly, Feske et al. (83) observed that before onset of major depression, women often report an increase in "entrapping" difficulties, generally difficulties related to child psychological and behavioral problems that mothers feel they cannot manage.

INTERVENTION FOR DEPRESSED MOTHERS

The often close interconnections between depression and the maternal role require that these issues be considered together in terms of mental health practice. When mothers are depressed, parenting is likely compromised, and children in the family are often also stressed. When children are experiencing physical or mental health problems, their mothers are likely at risk for depression. Mothers' and children's senses of well-being are so mutually dependent that treatment will likely be most effective if the needs of mothers and children are approached simultaneously. Mental health interventions for women need to target reduction of women's symptoms directly with pharmacologic and individual psychotherapeutic approaches but will be limited in their effectiveness unless efforts are also made at reducing the enduring social challenges that place women at risk. Pharmacologic treatment alone is not likely to be effective in terms of supporting mothers as parents. Treatment modalities, such as family therapy, are well suited to the systemic nature of women's depression.

Direct efforts to help women to be efficacious in their roles as parents seem an important strategy not only for improving parenting but also for treating symptoms of depression. Women need to understand how their parenting behavior affects their children and makes them feel as mothers. A number of programs that were designed to help parents better care for their children have the secondary impact of reducing maternal depressive symptoms. For example, the Webster-Stratton program uses behavioral techniques to help parents manage children's disruptive behavior, including breaking cycles of coercive interactions. The program not only reduces child behavior problems but reduces maternal depressive symptoms (84).

Other interventions focused on younger children are also promising. One intervention study contrasted two alternative models of mother–infant psychotherapy for clinic-referred infants (85). The Watch, Wait, and Wonder (WWW) program is an infant psychotherapy model in which mothers are encouraged to follow their children's lead during play interactions supervised by a psychotherapist. A more traditional infant psychodynamic model included the infants in the therapy sessions but focused more at the level of the mothers' thoughts and feelings about their children and parenting. Both treatment models showed positive effects in reducing infant symptoms and reducing mother stress and depression, with the results emerging more quickly for the WWW program.

Other interventions have been tested where the entry into treatment is the mother's depression rather than the child's behavioral problems. Cicchetti, Rogosch, and Toth (14) developed a model of toddler–parent psychotherapy in which children participated in the treatment. The model emphasized improving mothers' communication with their children, fostering positive communication, helping mothers understand and respond to their children's cues, and exploring mothers' feelings about their children. This intervention shows promising results with respect to preventing developmental delays in children of depressed mothers

The programs reported in these studies, however, only demonstrate the potential of therapeutic models addressing the mental health and parenting needs of women as well as the developmental needs of their children. Much work remains to be done at the level of program development, as well as health care, educational, and child welfare policy, before programs such as these will be widely available and accessible to families in greatest need. Moreover, intervention needs to be implemented preventively through mental health screening during pregnancy as well as parent support and education programs during pregnancy and the transition to parenthood. However, the message for program developers and policy makers must be that women's mental health and parenting are a transactional system in which maternal mental health affects parenting behavior and child development and in which women's success in the parenting role has an impact on the mother's mental health.*

REFERENCES

1. Kessler RC. The epidemiology of depression. In: Gotlib IH, Hammen CL, eds. Handbook of Depression: Research and Treatment. New York: Guilford, 2002:23–42.
2. Belsher G, Costello CG. Relapse after recovery from unipolar depression: a critical review. Psychol Rev 1998;104:84–96.
3. Boland RJ, Keller MB. Course and outcome of depression. In: Gotlib IH, Hammen CL, eds. Handbook of Depression: Research and Treatment. New York: Guilford, 2002:43–60.
4. Weissman MM, Jensen P. What research suggests for depressed women with children. J Clin Psychiatry 2002;63:641–647.
5. O'Hara MW. The nature of postpartum depressive disorders. In: Murray L, Cooper PJ, eds. Postpartum Depression and Child Development. New York: Guilford, 1997:3–31.
6. Hammen C. Children of depressed parents: the stress context. In: Wolchik SA, Sandler IN, eds. Handbook of Children's Coping: Linking Theory and Intervention. New York: Plenum, 1997: 131–137.
7. Beardslee WR, Versage EM, Gladstone TRG. Children of affectively ill parents: a review of the past 10 years. J Am Acad Child Adolesc Psychiatry 1998;37:1134–1141.
8. Goodman SH, Gotlib IH. Risk for psychopathology in the children of depressed mothers: a developmental model for understanding mechanisms of transmission. Psychol Rev 1999; 106:458–490.
9. Weissman MM, Warner V, Wickramaratne P, et al. Offspring of depressed parents. Arch Gen Psychiatry 1997;54:932–940.
10. Cohn JF, Matias R, Tronick EZ, et al. Face-to-face interactions of depressed mothers and their infants. In: Tronick EZ, Field T, eds. Maternal Depression and Infant Disturbance. San Francisco: Jossey-Bass, 1986:31–45.
11. Martinez A, Malphurs J, Field T, et al. Depressed mothers' and their infants' interactions with nondepressed partners. Infant Ment Health J 1996;17:74–80.
12. Abrams SM, Field T, Scafidi F, et al. Newborns of depressed mothers. Infant Ment Health J 1995;16:233–239.
13. Zuckerman B, Bauchner H, Parker S, et al. Maternal depressive symptoms during pregnancy and newborn irritability. J Dev Behav Pediatr 1990;11:190–194.
14. Cicchetti D, Rogosch FA, Toth SL. The efficacy of toddler–parent psychotherapy for fostering cognitive development in offspring of depressed mothers. J Abnorm Child Psych 2000; 8:135–148.
15. Radke-Yarrow M, Klimes-Dougan B. Parental depression and offspring disorders: a developmental perspective. In: Goodman SH, Gotlib IH, eds. Children of Depressed Parents:

This paper was written while the author was being supported by research grant R40 MC 00203 from the U.S. Maternal and Child Health Bureau. The author expresses her gratitude to Linda Henson for her support and feedback.

Mechanisms of Risk and Implications for Treatment. Washington, DC: American Psychological Association, 2002:155–173.

16. Cummings EM, Davies PT Maternal depression and child development. J Child Psychol Psychiatry 1994;35:73–112.

17. Gotlib IH, Goodman SH. Children of parents with depression. In: Silverman WK, Ollendick TH, eds. Developmental Issues in the Clinical Treatment of Children. Boston: Allyn & Bacon, 1999:415–432.

18. Gotlib IH, Lee CM. Impact of parental depression on young children and infants. In: Mundt C, Goldstein MJ, Hahlweg K, et al., eds. Interpersonal Factors in the Origin and Course of Affective Disorders. London: Royal College of Psychiatrists, 1996:218–239.

19. Silberg J, Rutter M. Nature–nurture interplay in the risks associated with parental depression. In: Goodman SH, Gotlib IH, eds. Children of Depressed Parents: Mechanisms of Risk and Implications for Treatment. Washington, DC: American Psychological Association, 2002:13–36.

20. Sullivan PF, Neale MC, Kendler KS. Genetic epidemiology of major depression: review and meta-analysis. Am J Psychiatry 2000;157:1552–1562.

21. Field TM. Prenatal effects of maternal depression. In: Goodman SH, Gotlib IH, eds. Children of Depressed Parents: Mechanisms of Risk and Implications for Treatment. Washington, DC: American Psychological Association, 2002:59–88.

22. Glover V. Maternal stress or anxiety in pregnancy and emotional development of the child. Br J Psychiatry 1997;71:105–106.

23. Dawson G, Frey K, Panagiotides H, et al. Infants of depressed mothers exhibit atypical frontal brain activity: a replication and extension of previous findings. J Child Psych Psychiatry 1997;38:179–186.

24. Tronick EZ. Emotions and emotional communication in infants. Am Psychol 1989;44:112–119.

25. Cohn JE, Campbell SB, Matias R, et al. Face-to-face interactions of postpartum depressed and nondepressed mother–infant pairs at 2 months. Dev Psychol 1990;26:15–23.

26. Field T, Healy B, Goldstein S, et al. Behavior-state matching and synchrony in mother–infant interactions of nondepressed versus depressed dyads. Dev Psychol 1990;26:7–14.

27. Forbes EE, Cohn JF, Allen NB, et al. Infant affect during parent–infant interaction at 3 and 6 months: differences between mothers and fathers and influence of parent history of depression. Infancy 2004;51:61–84.

28. Goodman SH, Brumley HE. Schizophrenic and depressed mothers: relational deficits in parenting. Dev Psychol 1990;26:31–39.

29. Downey G, Coyne JC. Children of depressed parents: an integrative review. Psychol Bull 1990;108:50–76.

30. Pound A, Abel K. Motherhood and mental illness. In: Abel K, Buszewicz M, Davison S, et al., eds. Planning Community Mental Health Services for Women: A Multiprofessional Handbook. Florence, KY: Taylor & Francis/Routledge, 1996:20–35.

31. Conger RD, Patterson GR, Ge X. It takes two to replicate: a mediational model for the impact of parents' stress on adolescent adjustment. Child Dev 1995;66:80–97.

32. Gelfand DM, Teti DM, Seiner SA, et al. Helping mothers fight depression: evaluation of a home-based intervention program for depressed mothers and their infants. J Clin Child Psychol 1996;25:406–422.

33. Hops H. Parental depression and child behavior problems: implications for behavioural family intervention. Behav Change 1992;9:126–138.

34. Lyons-Ruth K, Wolfe R, Lyubchik A, et al. Depressive symptoms in parents of children under age 3: sociodemographic predictors, current correlates, and associated parenting behaviors. In: Halfon N, McLearn KT, Schuster MA, eds. Child Rearing in America: Challenges Facing Parents with Young Children. New York: Cambridge University Press, 2002:217–259.

35. Stanley C, Murray L, Stein A. The effect of postnatal depression on mother–infant interaction infant response to the still-face perturbation and performance on an instrumental learning task. Dev Psychopathol 2004;16:1–18.

36. Born L, Steiner M. Irritability: the forgotten dimension of female-specific mood disorders. Arch Women Ment Health 1999;24:153–167.

37. Pasquini M, Picardi A, Biondi M, et al. Relevance of anger and irritability in outpatients with major depressive disorder. Psychopathology 2004;374:155–160.

38. Gordon D, Burge D, Hammen C, et al. Observations of interactions of depressed women with their children. Am J Psychiatry 1999;146:50–55.

39. Lovejoy MC. Maternal depression: effects on social cognition and behavior in parent–child interactions. J Abnorm Child Psychol 1991;19:693–706.

40. Forehand R, Lautenschlager GJ, Faust J, et al. Parent perceptions and parent–child interactions in clinic-referred children: a preliminary investigation of the effects of maternal depressive moods. Behav Res Ther 1986;24:73–75.

41. Hammen C, Adrian C, Hiroto D. A longitudinal test of the attributional vulnerability model in children at risk for depression. Br J Clin Psychol 1988;27:37–46.

42. Nolen-Hoeksema S, Wolfson A, Mumme D, et al. Helplessness in children of depressed and nondepressed mothers. Dev Psychol 1995;31:377–387.

43. Larson R, Richards MH. Divergent Realities: The Emotional Lives of Mothers, Fathers and Adolescents. New York: Basic, 1994.

44. Lovejoy MC, Graczyk PA, O'Hare E, et al. Maternal depression and parenting behavior: a meta-analytic review. Clin Psychol Rev 2000;20:561–592.

45. Tronick EZ, Weinberg MK. Depressed mothers and infants: failure to form dyadic states of consciousness. In: Murray L, Cooper PJ, eds. Postpartum Depression and Child Development. New York: Guilford, 1997:54–81.

46. Patterson GR, DeBaryshe BD, Ramsey E. A developmental perspective on antisocial behavior. Am Psychol 1989;44:329–335.

47. Kochanska G, Kuczynski L, Radke-Yarrow M, et al. Resolutions of control episodes between well and affectively ill mothers and their young children. J Abnorm Child Psychol 1987;15:441–456.

48. Dumas JE, Gibson JA, Albin JB. Behavioral correlates of maternal depressive symptomatology in conduct-disorder children. J Cons Clin Psych 1989;57:516–521.

49. Ghodsian M, Zajicek E, Wolkind S. A longitudinal study of maternal depression and child behavior problems. J Child Psych Psychiatry 1984;25:91–109.

50. Kaslow NJ, Deering CG, Racusin GR. Depressed children and their families. Clin Psychol Rev 1994;14:39–59.

51. Radke-Yarrow M, Sherman T. Hard growing: children who survive. In: Rolf JE, Masten AS, Cicchetti D, et al, eds. Risk and Protective Factors in the Development of Psychopathology. Cambridge, UK: Cambridge University Press, 1990:97–119.

52. Zahn-Waxler C, Kochanska G, Krupnick J, et al. Patterns of guilt in children of depressed and well mothers. Dev Psychol 1990;26:51–59.

53. Cummings EM, Davies PT. Maternal depression and child development. J Child Psych Psychiatry 1994;35:73–112.

54. El-Sheikh M, Cummings EM, Reiter S. Preschoolers' responses to interadult conflict: the role of experimentally manipulated exposure to resolved and unresolved arguments. J Abnorm Child Psychol 1996;24:665–679.

55. Carter AS, Garrity-Rokous FE, Chazan-Cohen R, et al. Maternal depression and comorbidity: predicting early parenting attachment security and toddler social-emotional problems and competencies. J Am Acad Child Adolesc Psychiatry 2001;40:18–26.

56. Hans SL, Bernstein VJ, Henson LG. The role of psychopathology in the parenting of drug-dependent women. Dev Psychopathol 1999;11:957–977.

57. Rutter M, Quinton D. Parental psychiatric disturbance: effects on children. Psychol Med 1984;14:853–880.

58. Cummings EM, Davies PT. Depressed parents and family functioning: interpersonal effects and children's functioning and development. In: Joiner T, Coyne JC, eds. The Interactional Nature of Depression. Washington, DC: American Psychological Association, 1999:299–327.

59. Sarigiani PA, Heath PA, Camarena PM. The significance of parental depressed mood for young adolescents' emotional and family experiences. J Early Adolescence 2003;233:241–267.

60. Cummings EM, Graham M. Couples' and children's functioning in families: toward a family perspective on relationship maintenance and enhancement. In: Harvey JA, Wenzel A, eds. A Clinician's Guide to Maintaining and Enhancing Close Relationships. Mahwah, NJ: Erlbaum, 2002:81–193.

61. Bell RQ. Socialization findings reexamined. In: Bell RQ, Harper R, eds. Child Effects on Adults. Hillsdale, NJ: Erlbaum, 1977.

62. Sameroff AJ, Chandler MJ. Reproductive risk and the continuum of caretaking casualty. In: Horowitz FD, Hetherington M, Scarr-Salapatek S, et al., eds. Review of Child Development Research, vol. 4. Chicago: University of Chicago Press, 1975:187–245.

63. Cutrona CE, Troutman BR. Social support infant temperament and parenting self-efficacy: a mediational model of postpartum depression. Child Dev 1986;576:1507–1518.

64. Gotlib IH, Whiffen VE, Wallace P, et al. A prospective investigation of postpartum depression: factors involved in onset and recovery. J Abnorm Psychol 1991;100:122–132.

65. Whiffen VE. Maternal depressed mood and perceptions of child temperament. J Genet Psychol 1990;151:329–339.

66. Frankel KA, Harmon RJ. Depressed mothers: they don't always look as bad as they feel. J Am Acad Child Adolesc Psychiatry 1996;35:289–298.

67. Edhborg M, Seimyr L, Lundh W, et al. Fussy child—difficult parenthood? Comparison between families with a "depressed" mother and non-depressed mother 2 months postpartum. J Reprod Infant Psychol 2000;18:225–238.

68. Galler JR, Harrison RH, Ramsey F, et al. Postpartum maternal mood feeding practices and infant temperament in Barbados. Infant Behav Dev 2004;27:267–287.

69. Field T, Estroff DB, Yando R, et al. "Depressed" mothers' perceptions of infant vulnerability are related to later development. Child Psychiatry Hum Dev 1996;27:43–53.

70. Pesonen A-K, Raikkonen K, Strandberg T, et al. Insecure adult attachment style and depressive symptoms: implications for parental perceptions of infant temperament. Infant Ment Health J 2004;25:99 116.

71. Fox CR, Gelfand DM. Maternal depressed mood and stress as related to vigilance self-efficacy and mother–child interactions. Early Dev Parenting 1994;3:233–243.

72. Whiffen V, Gotlib IH. Infants of postpartum depressed mothers: temperament and cognitive status. J Abnorm Psychol 1989;3:274–279.

73. Field T, Healy B, Goldstein S, et al. Infants of depressed mothers show "depressed" behavior even with non-depressed adults. Child Dev 1988;59:1569–1579.

74. Glover V, Kammerer M. The biology and pathophysiology of peripartum psychiatric disorders. Primary Psychiatry 2004;113:37–41.

75. Cowan P, Cowan CP. Normative family transitions: normal family processes and healthy child development. In: Walsh F, ed. Normal Family Process. 3rd Ed. New York: Guilford, 2003: 424–459.

76. Brown GW, Harris T. Social Origins of Depression: A Study of Psychiatric Disorder in Women. New York: Free, 1978.

77. Sirignano SW, Lachman ME. Personality change during the transition to parenthood: the role of perceived infant temperament. Dev Psychol 1985;21:558–567.

78. Sutter-Dallay A-L, Murray L, Glatigny-Dallay E. Newborn behavior and risk of postnatal depression in the mother. Infancy 2003;44:589–602.

79. Breslau N, Davis GC. Chronic stress and major depression. Arch Gen Psychiatry 1986; 43:309–314.

80. Civic E, Holt VL. Maternal depressive symptoms and child behavior problems in a nationally representative normal birthweight sample. Matern Child Health J 2000;4:215–221.

81. Harrison C, Sofronoff K, ADHD and parental psychological distress: role of demographics child behavioral characteristics and parental cognitions. J Am Acad Child Adolesc Psychiatry 2002;41:703–711.

82. Hammen C, Burge D, Adrian C. Timing of mother and child depression in a longitudinal study of children at risk. J Cons Clin Psychol 1991;59:341–345.

83. Feske U, Shear MK, Anderson B. et al. Comparison of severe life stress in depressed mothers and non-mothers: do children matter? Depress Anxiety 2001;14:109–117.

84. Taylor TK, Schmidt F, Pepler D, et al. A comparison of eclectic treatment with Webster-Stratton's parents and children series in a children's mental health center: a randomized controlled trial. Behav Ther 1998;29:221–240.

85. Cohen NJ, Lojkasek M, Muir E, et al. Six-month follow-up of two mother–infant psychotherapies: convergence of therapeutic outcomes. Infant Ment Health J 2002;234:361–380.

Aging

Section VI Summary
Commentary from China

Helen F. K. Chiu

The three chapters of this section, by Hassett, Perkins, and Melding, eloquently explore the topics of psychosocial challenges, cognitive challenges, and physical health challenges in older women. As Hassett pointsed out in the introduction to Chapter 23, "Age and gender hierarchies shape female lives across the life course in specific social and historical contexts" (1). I agree. Socio-cultural factors are very important in determining some of the challenges involved. Previous research work about older women has been mostly carried out in developed countries. Relatively few studies have examined the challenges experienced by older women in non-Western cultures. It is likely that these issues differ in diverse cultures, and I would like to illustrate this from a Chinese perspective using suicide as an example.

There are interesting differences in the sex ratio in suicide rates in older people across countries. In most Western countries, the male:female ratio of completed suicide is around 3 to 1. In China, this ratio is 0.8 to 1 (2). China is one of the few countries where the suicide rate of females is higher than that of males. In the Chinese elderly, the male: to female ratio is 1.1 to 1. In addition, there is a striking difference in the rates of suicide between the urban and rural areas in China, with the rural rate three times that of the urban rate (2). If one looks at the actual suicide rates in older women in various countries, the differences are even more striking. In 1999, suicide rates of older women aged 75 or above in Australia, the United Kingdom, the United States, and rural China were 3.4, 5.1, 4.6, and 102.2 per 100,000, respectively (3). Clearly, older women are at considerably higher risk of suicide in China than in many Western countries.

Another interesting phenomenon concerns the relationship between marital status and suicide. Being widowed or divorced is a risk factor for suicide in Western countries. In contrast, in older women in Hong Kong (a special administrative region in China), being married is associated with a higher risk of suicide, compared with the risk associated with status of being single, widowed, or divorced (4). The reasons for this intriguing finding are still unclear.

Although there are few studies have examined the psychosocial stress and challenges for older Chinese women, it is likely that China's changing family structure and social attitudes play a significant role. In parallel with its change from a planned to a market economy, China has undergone tremendous social changes in recent years. In the past, Chinese culture placed a great emphasis on the family, and adult children had the responsibility to look after their elderly parents at home. Furthermore, status and authority increased with age. Close family ties and intimacy acted as buffers against life stresses. In recent years, the extended family structure has been replaced by the smaller nuclear family. This may be partly explained by the one-child policy in China. In addition, young people in rural areas tend to move away from their parents' home to big cities to seek jobs (5). Apart from the decreasing family support, there has been a gradual attrition of the traditional respect for the elderly. The situation is worse for women in rural areas, where the status of females is still very low. Other important factors include poor health care services in rural areas and the stigma of mental illness, which are all barriers to accessing health care. All the above factors are challenges for the older persons in China and may also be relevant in explaining the high suicide rate in the elderly.

The population is aging in many countries in Asia and elsewhere in developing countries. For instance, the population in China is now 1.3 billion, with 7% aged 65 or above. This will increase to 13% by 2025; that is, almost 168 million people will be aged 65 or above. These numbers are enormous. There is, thus, a pressing need for more research into the challenges experienced by older women in China and other developing countries, to better delineate potential sources of resilience for older women in non-Western countries.

REFERENCES

Markson E. Communities of resistance: older women in a gendered world: facing the mirror. Gerontologist, 1999; 4:495-502.

Phillips MR, Li XY, Zhang YP. Suicide rates in China, 1995-99. Lancet 2002; 359:835-840.

Chiu HFK, Chan SSM, Lam LCW. Suicide in the elderly. Curr Opin in Psychiatry 2001; 14:395-399.

World Health Organization. World Health Report 2002. Geneva. 2002.

Yu X, Shen YC. Epidemiology of vascular dementia in China. In: O'Brien J, Ames D, Gustafson L, et al., eds. Cerebrovascular Disease and Dementia. 2nd Ed. CRC Press, 2003:75-83.

CHAPTER 23

The Psychosocial Challenge for Older Women

Anne Hassett

"Age and gender hierarchies shape female lives across the life course in specific social and historical contexts" (1). Why devote a chapter in a book on women's mental health specifically to the psychosocial challenges facing older women? With increasing life expectancy in developed countries there is a burgeoning literature on adaptive processes in later life, but until recently this research has lacked a gender-specific focus. And yet, women dominate the population of older people, are known to suffer from greater psychological morbidity in later life, and are more likely than men to spend their later years living alone, and with less financial security (2). Much has been written about sexism and ageism as forms of societal oppression; older women are vulnerable to a double jeopardy in this regard. For women of minority ethnic groups, racism can be a further compounding factor, which contributes to their marginalization and disempowerment (3). It is not surprising then that gender and age politics have been powerful forces shaping a widespread negative perception of aging womanhood. This is not to deny that ageist practices do not impact on men, but they are to an extent buffered by the power relations implicit in the gender hierarchy.

The recognition that later life is a developmental stage in its own right has greatly expanded the theoretical discourse on aging, so that the focus is no longer solely on issues of loss and decline. Erik Erikson's epigenetic theory of human development has been seminal in this regard. He describes the psychosocial challenges that characterize the sequential stages of the life span, continuing to shape later life with the potential for mature creativity and the attainment of wisdom (4). Fundamentally, according to

Erikson's model, the successful negotiation of the challenges of each life stage is dependent on the maturational building blocks of previous life stages. For example, adolescents' specific developmental task is defining their individual identities so as to achieve healthy separateness from their families of origin. This is not simply about moving away from the parental home but requires the adolescent to identify with and internalize positive childhood role models. The person who fails to achieve this maturational task will inevitably struggle with subsequent adult developmental challenges. These include forming intimate relationships, creating a satisfying role in society, and maintaining a sense of meaning in their later years. However, while this theoretical framework has been heuristic in its depiction of a more positive culture of aging, overly simplistic interpretation of Erikson's later life-stage developmental tasks has resulted in a tendency to homogenize the experience of aging.

More recent writers have expanded the focus in social gerontology to include an exploration of the importance of gender, time, and place in shaping an individual's later years. In particular, the far-reaching historical events and societal changes during the course of the twentieth century have necessitated a closer examination of the impact of these factors on individual development. In Western societies, increased longevity and pluralization of lifestyle options have resulted in greater personal choice and responsibility for the individual in determining their own future. And yet, are older women today better able to actualize their developmental potential than their mothers and grandmothers? Their life expectancy is now twice as long as for women in the late nineteenth century, when less than 50% of the population survived beyond adolescence (5). But what about the quality of these additional years, which, pessimistically, could be regarded as just lengthening the time that women have to endure ageist and sexist societal attitudes? For example, the association of female worth and attractiveness with youthfulness is a prominent ageist stereotype in Western culture. This pervasive social myth powerfully reinforces women's preoccupation with the physical signs of aging long before they need to be concerned about other aging-related issues, such as functional decline and loss of independence. Now that Western women can reasonably expect to live into their late 70s or early 80s, they are likely to be subjected to socially sanctioned negative images of female aging over many decades. As a consequence, aging women are vulnerable to feeling marginalized as they struggle with the populist notion that their attractiveness, and by implication also their worth, is dependent on maintaining a youthful appearance (1).

If Western women are growing old in a cultural paradigm characterized by negative representations of their physical maturation, from where do they draw their resilience? Will the vocal generation of baby boomer women challenge these entrenched female stereotypes? In order to answer these questions, we need to look beyond the one-dimensional portrayal of aging as physical and mental decline. We need to examine the resources that enable older women to maintain a coherent, unified sense of self and identity in the face of adversity. The following sections examine the themes of older women's roles in family life, the workforce, and the broader community. The term "being older" will not be specifically defined in terms of chronologic age because of the subjectivity and diversity with which women view themselves, and others view them, with regard to the aging process. As a consequence the discussion will include women from more than one generation—older female baby boomers, their mothers, and their grandmothers, who are now the very old. Only now, with an increased life span for women in developed countries, can this transgenerational appraisal of aging be undertaken and cohort-specific issues examined. What is most striking when the three generations of women who might now be considered older are compared as separate cohorts is that their early developmental paths were intersected by very different major historical events. These included world wars and dramatic sociodemographic shifts in the structure of the family unit and women's involvement in the workforce.

Today's very old women were born in the early years of the twentieth century, were adolescents during the First World War, young homemakers during the years of the Great Depression, and then had to endure another world war. Their lives have spanned a century of remarkable change, and to have survived and adapted must say a great deal about the resilience of their psychosocial resources. They are truly the experts on aging as society has decreed them as being old for the greater proportion of their adult lives. The next broad cohort of older women comprises those who would generally regard themselves as now being in the phase of later life, but perhaps are still struggling with this adjustment. This cohort were young women during the Second World War, and like their mothers, were subjected to the untimely deaths of brothers, fiancés, and husbands. They also experienced the emancipation and responsibility that went with maintaining a male-depleted workforce. However, after the war, they were expected to return quietly to the traditional role of homemaker. They received little recognition for their wartime achievements and sacrifices, and regardless of their aspirations, they were expected to relinquish paid employment to the returning men. In contrast, their baby boomer daughters grew up during postwar economic prosperity. This was also a time when new patterns of family life were emerging, and female participation in the labor force became acceptable once again and not just as a wartime measure. Although all three cohorts had exposure to the turbulence of the women's liberation movement of the 1960s, this occurred during the late adolescence and early adulthood of the early female baby boomers. This cohort would have been most impressionable and likely to embrace a philosophy of radical change in the way women perceived their role in society and their sense of control over their own destinies.

These three successive generations of women all share the experience today of being categorized as older women. However, very different sociohistorical contexts have shaped each generation's collective developmental trajectory. One consequence may be that the older generations' practical knowledge and accumulated wisdom have become less relevant for subsequent generations (5). Examining this issue, Grob et al. (5) compared the biographical narratives of three cohorts of Swiss women—a group born between the world wars (1920–1925), a group who were early baby boomers (1945–1950), and a group from "Generation X" (1970–1975). They found that the three generations of women shared traditional developmental concerns and were similar in the broad construction of the chronology of their lives. The three groups differed in that, although the Generation X cohort mostly expected to have children, only a minority expected to marry. In contrast, most of the early baby boomer participants in the study had married and borne children. Subsequently though, about half divorced, highlighting the increasingly transitory phase that marriage appears to occupy in women's lives today. Overall, there was a progressive shift for younger participants to be more preoccupied with issues of lifestyle, relationships, and personal freedom. They expected to be able to exert more control over their destinies but were also more uncertain about being able to achieve happiness because of the range of choices to be made. The older subjects were profoundly affected by their experiences during the Second World War, whereas no single historical event had shaped the lives of the two younger cohorts. The authors of this study suggest that their findings illustrate the importance of examining developmental issues within a sociohistorical context. They conclude that aging is not simply a matter of advancing chronologic age, but the aging process for women is greatly influenced by cohort-specific differences that shift the social context of role definitions and norms from generation to generation.

SELF-IDENTITY

Although an illusive concept, a sense of continuity is fundamental to a person's construction of an individual identity and its preservation over time and into later life. Characteristics such as age, gender, ethnicity, and class define an external form of continuity that embeds the person in a particular social role and status. Internal continuity is more related to self-esteem and personality style, which influence quality of relationships and the capacity for positive maturation. From middle age onward, evidence suggests significant continuity in the global aspects of self and identity, despite aging adults perceiving substantial changes in the ebb and flow of their lives. This is achieved through the consolidation of personal experiences and their transformation into life themes, which serve to refine and give meaning to a sense of self and identity (6). This focus on individualistic themes advances and complements adult developmental theories, which emphasize the commonality of experiences in the attainment of psychosocial maturation. As a consequence, aging can be conceived as a continual creation of the self through the ongoing interpretation of past experiences and their incorporation into a person's current emotional and social context. However, anthropologist Barbara Myerhoff notes that continuity in life does not arise spontaneously but must be "achieved;" that is, the individual needs to actively seek continuity as she or he goes through ordinary daily existence interpreting, and ultimately finding meaning in, their life circumstances (7).

Maintaining a degree of continuity in relationships is a major goal for most older people, enhancing their sense of identity and facilitating adaptation to the aging process. For older women who have been traditional homemakers, identity has always been inextricably linked with their role in the family. A century ago shorter life expectancies and relatively high infant mortality rates meant that, within the family unit, women had a well-defined and crucial role in maximizing their children's chances of surviving to adulthood. In traditional societies particularly, if they survived beyond these childbearing and child-rearing years, their sense of identity was maintained by their continued role within the family as "cultural expert" instructing and advising children and grandchildren (1). Today, as the links between generations of aging women appear to be becoming more tenuous, a sense of "loss of role" has become an issue for older women. This is most apparent in Western societies, where transformations in the structure of the family have been far reaching. Because of mothers' participation in the labor force, it is now the norm that persons other than parents are involved in raising children. Parenthood is no longer such a defining identity for women, either because they remain childless or because of their participation in work and community contexts outside the home. Further, grandparents are less likely to be geographically close and available for substitute parenting. Nevertheless, today's family is more likely to be multigenerational, even if not within one household, and older women, in particular, can find themselves with multiple responsibilities toward spouse, children, and aging parents (3). These societal trends are challenging for the older woman as social roles are now less prescribed but still powerfully influence her sense of identity and its continuity over time with aging.

PARENTHOOD

Although parenthood continues to be regarded as a major developmental goal for women, childlessness is an increasing social phenomenon. In fact, single, childless women are one of the fastest growing groups in Western societies. Greater career opportunities, increasing divorce rates, and unbalanced gender ratios in middle and later adulthood have been contributing factors to this sociodemographic shift. In particular, highly educated women are the group most likely to remain single or become single through divorce (8). And yet, little empirical literature has explored the developmental consequences for this fast-growing cohort. Traditional theories focus on establishing a nuclear family unit as a fundamental rite of passage for women progressing adaptively through the sequence of life stages. What happens to childless women as they age? Of course, there are diverse reasons why women might remain childless. The majority of today's "oldest old" women who have remained childless did so because of physiologic infertility or because they did not marry rather than because they deliberately chose not to have children. Economic hardship during the Great Depression and early widowhood during World War II were historical factors that have also contributed to childlessness in this group of older women. However, the last few decades have seen the rise of voluntary childlessness rather than childlessness occurring inadvertently (9). More sophisticated birth control, better career opportunities, and the greater acceptability of remaining unmarried have allowed women, both married and single, to exert choice in regard to parenthood. In particular, this social shift has challenged the paternalistic stereotype of the "spinster" with its implication of lack of fulfillment and reduced social credibility. The pathways to childlessness have thus become more diverse, and the psychological consequences for aging women who do not have children are likely to reflect this diversity.

Koropeckyi-Cox (9) examined the issue of incongruence between attitudes and childless status in a sample of women 50 to 89 years. She found that those who considered themselves unfulfilled because of their childlessness described themselves as significantly more lonely and depressed than those who were accepting of their situation. The former group were also more likely to be less educated and have a marital status of separated, divorced, or widowed rather than never married. Comparing these childless women with a group of similar-aged mothers, Koropeckyi-Cox found that the women who were content with being childless were similar in their sense of psychosocial well-being to mothers who described mutually supportive relationships with their children. Interestingly, she found that mothers who had a conflicted or distant relationship with at least one child reported levels of depressive symptomatology similar to those of the women who did not want to be childless. These findings suggest that it is the discrepancy between attitudes or expectations and actual circumstances, not parental status per se, which impact on women's self-identity and sense of contentment as they age. Further, the ability to choose to remain childless rather than have this state imposed is likely to be a crucial factor and one more able to be exercised by better educated women.

OLDER WOMEN WITHOUT A PARTNER

No discussion about the psychosocial challenge for older women can ignore the state of widowhood and increasingly separated status, which is shared by a very large number of women. In modern Western societies loss of a long-term partner has come to be defined more by a collapse of old roles and structural supports than by norms and institutions that can provide new roles and a meaningful sense of social status. In contrast, preindustrial societies had very clear roles for widows, in particular. Some were very extreme, such as the expectation that Brahmin widows in traditional Indian society would throw themselves on their husband's funeral pyre. In many African societies, a widow and her children were "inherited" by a male relative, thereby becoming one of his several wives in a polygamous family. These may not have been particularly desirable options for the recently widowed woman, but her destiny was clearly prescribed for her. In industrial societies, widowhood has evolved into what has been called a roleless role, a social category without a central source of identity and with little social credibility (10). Certainly, today's "old-old" widows were a generation that defined themselves primarily as wife-mother-housewife despite the reality that these roles often occupied a relatively transient period in their life course. As divorce, separation, and choosing to remain single join widowhood as reasons for women of the baby boom generation to age without a partner, will we see a shift away from the negative perceptions associated with this social status?

A well-established finding in the literature is that having a long-term partner (usually a marital partner) is one of the best positive predictors of a person's health status and mortality. This has been noted in the general population, and especially among older adults. However, although older married men generally report higher levels of well-being than older single men, the situation is more complex for older women. In particular, never married older women appear to fare better than divorced or separated older women. Comparing long-term effects for the latter two groups, Choi (11) found that long-term female divorcees were generally better educated and financially more secure than long-term widows. However, they were also more likely to be socially isolated and rely on paid helpers for functional help when they became frail. Of note, these subjects, who were recruited in the late 1980s in their eighth decade, were still part of that generation for which divorce was not a typical life-course transition for many women; that is, it was even less recognized as a credible social status category than widowhood. Further, these women were still a small group in terms of numbers, and the twenty-first century will see a significant increase in the numbers of divorced elderly women who are likely to age alone and have fewer children to provide them with support. Despite better education, these women will remain at risk of social marginalization if societal attitudes do not change.

RETIREMENT

Although women have constituted a steadily increasing component of the workforce over the last five decades, little is known or written about the impact of retirement on them. Much of what is written about retirement concerns men, but are retirement issues different for women? Fundamentally, they must be because women live longer, have more chronic health problems, are generally poorer, and are much more likely to be widowed and living alone in later life. Inevitably, if women outlive their spouses, they must extend smaller incomes over time that may stretch into decades (12). The opportunity for women to enter paid employment exploded during World War II, and this major demographic shift has continued since that time. A driving force has been economic necessity associated with the increasing number of female-headed households. However, despite their gradual inclusion in white-collar occupations, women remain overrepresented in lower paying occupations. As a consequence, they are far more at risk than men of financial insecurity after they leave the workforce. The term "feminization of poverty" is particularly pertinent to older women, especially if they also belong to an ethnic minority group or their earning capacity is compromised because of disability or chronic illness. They are also more likely to have to retire early for health and caregiving reasons. Of note, the majority of women who provide care for frail elderly parents or other family members are middle-aged or older (12). If they have to leave the workforce or reduce their working hours in order to serve as primary caregivers, these women receive minimal financial recognition for the sacrifice they are making. There is also minimal social credibility accorded the demanding work they undertake as caregivers. As well as the increased risk of living in poverty, these caregiving women are susceptible to social isolation, poor self-image, and feelings of uselessness. The implications for the development of mental health problems in these reluctant older women retirees are significant but minimally acknowledged or examined. It is interesting that, although the women's movement has greatly improved younger women's opportunities for choice in employment and lifestyle, the needs of aging women in preparing for security in old age have only been minimally addressed in the feminist agenda.

ABUSE

While women of all ages experience abuse, older women are particularly vulnerable to physical, emotional, and financial exploitation. However, even those who are not physically frail and/or very elderly are a silenced and invisible group. Much of what is known about elder abuse has come from population-based studies in developed countries. The evidence suggests that 4% to 6% of elderly people, mostly women, are subjected to abuse at home (13). In addition, institution-based abuse occurs in hospitals and residential care facilities. In developing countries there is an utter paucity of data on the rates of elder abuse, except for isolated reports such as undertaken by the World Health Organization (WHO) (13). In African and Latin American countries, where civil war and increasing crime have severely strained the fabric of community life, the WHO reports that rape and violence toward older female family members have become alarmingly common. Before any primary or secondary interventions can be undertaken, increasing public and governmental awareness of the problem is necessary. A major difficulty in exposing the extent of the problem is that the abuse of older women mostly occurs within the family, usually by spouses or adult children. As such, it is considered to be a private matter, often by both perpetrator and victim. This perception entrenches and maintains social isolation and dysfunctional power dynamics within the abusive family. Financial dependence, limited social outlets, and ageist community attitudes are further barriers to identifying older abused women and empowering them to change their situation. There is some evidence to suggest that older women from ethnic minority groups with traditional ideas about male dominance in the home are particularly at risk of abuse. The extent of their social isolation is often exacerbated by unfamiliarity with the language, norms, and sources of support in the dominant culture (14).

It is understandable that domestic violence intervention programs predominantly focus on younger women with small children, as they have the highest reported level of abuse. It is now imperative with an aging population that the needs of older abused women are also addressed. One program specifically supporting older abused women, age 53 to 90 years, found no common sociodemographic profile. Similarly, generalizations cannot be made about younger abused women. Their common link was living with an abusive family member. Of the 132 women in this program, 40% were able to free themselves from their abusive situations with assistance. This figure belies the ageist and sexist stereotype of older women being passive and resistant to constructive change in their lives (13). It is hoped that, as the baby boom generation of women age, they will be empowered by their number and expectation of lifestyle quality to challenge the prejudices and ignorance that continue to underpin the neglect of older abused women.

WELL-BEING AND MENTAL ILLNESS

Older women suffer from greater psychiatric morbidity than older men, especially in relation to depression. In developed countries, where the rates of mental illness are well documented, approximately one quarter of all women are estimated to suffer at least one significant depressive episode during their lifetime. This contrasts with half that rate for lifetime prevalence in men. Among the elderly, it is estimated that up to 1 in 5 community-dwelling elderly experience symptoms of depression; once again, the rate for older women is twice as high as for older men (15). The development of depression and other mental health disorders in later life adversely affects quality of life, and has been associated with increased physical illness, such as cardiovascular disease (16). Functional disability, high health care utilization, and increased mortality are other consequences that necessitate prioritizing the mental health needs of an increasing population of aging persons. And yet, misdiagnosis, underdiagnosis, and undertreatment of mental illness in older persons have been well substantiated in the literature (17).

Fiske, Gatz, and Pedersen (18) examined the relationship between health status and depressive symptoms in a large Swedish sample, aged 29–93 years. Participants were asked about 38 medical conditions and completed a self-report measure of depressive symptoms. The study used a longitudinal as well as a cross-sectional design so as to examine if depressive symptoms change with age or whether differences between middle age and old age represent cohort or other selection effects. The findings demonstrated modest increases in depressive symptoms with age for both women and men, particularly for older participants. They also confirmed the higher levels of depressive symptoms among women than men throughout late life. Although the study did not find an interaction between health and aging, current physical illnesses were significantly associated with the level of depressive symptomatology in older female subjects.

Physical disability and resulting functional limitation are prevalent in older women, and increase significantly as they join the ranks of the old-old (19). Estimates suggest that more than one quarter of women over 65 years old report difficulty with activities of daily living (i.e., involving mobility and self-care). This figure rises to nearly half of women over the age of 85 years. Another Swedish study, of male/female twin pairs born between 1905 and 1925, found that the women experienced more total health problems, particularly disabling, nonfatal chronic diseases such as arthritis than their brothers (20). The males, in contrast, had proportionately fewer health problems, but these were mainly potentially life-threatening conditions such as serious cardiovascular disease. In terms of self-rated health, there were no gender differences between the twin pairs.

The authors suggest that the men's fewer but more serious conditions were counterbalanced by the women's more numerous but less life-threatening health problems. This is a research area that has generated conflicting findings. Pinquart and Sorenson (21) found that gender differences in subjective well-being only emerged in very old subjects. They postulated that this age effect may reflect the compounding disadvantages of chronic illness with greater longevity for the oldest women.

Apart from physical illness, other health-related habits, such as alcohol consumption, cigarette smoking, poor diet, and lack of exercise, have also been associated with the psychological distress that predisposes women to becoming depressed. The majority of the research in this area is cross-sectional, and so causal relationships are difficult to establish. Does an unhealthy lifestyle predispose to depression, or do the motivational deficits and low self-esteem associated with depression make women (and men) more vulnerable to unhealthy lifestyles? Lee (22) examined depressive symptoms in relation to smoking, weight, alcohol use, and exercise status in a sample of 612 Australian women from three age groups (18–23 years, 45–50 years, and 70–75 years) . She found that unhealthy lifestyle patterns were associated with psychological distress and depressive symptoms across the three age cohorts. However, overall, the older women consumed alcohol and smoked less than the younger women and reported less psychological distress. The author acknowledged that changes in socially acceptable behavior may have produced cohort effects to explain health-related lifestyle differences. Also, the oldest subjects may have represented a biased group of healthy survivors who had been able to maintain physical and mental well-being into late life. She cites evidence to suggest that later middle age is a time when women are most likely to actively reassess and reorient their values and life goals. These women, if able to make necessary constructive changes, can then adapt and adjust psychologically as they grow older.

Nevertheless, substance abuse is an increasing problem in the older population, has been called the hidden epidemic, and is often comorbid with mood disturbance (23). While excess alcohol consumption remains the major form of substance abuse in older males, misuse of prescription (especially benzodiazepines) and over-the-counter medications is an underrecognized problem in older women. It is estimated that older persons receive approximately 50% of all benzodiazepine prescriptions, and the majority of these recipients are women. The Australian National Drug Strategy Household Survey (24) also found that a surprisingly larger percentage (40%) of older women consumed over-the-counter medications on a daily basis. These included laxatives, vitamins, analgesics, cold and allergy drugs, and antacids. There is minimal literature about the levels of misuse of these substances nor the extent to which they are taken as a form of self-medication to relieve psychological distress as well as physical symptoms.

As well as its association with substance misuse, depression is a strong predictor of suicidality. Because aging women are more vulnerable to mood disturbance, it might be expected that they would attempt suicide more frequently than aging men. After all, they live longer and have higher lifetime rates of depression. They are also more likely to spend a significant period of their later lives with some form of chronic disability or illness. Nevertheless, although older women are more likely to attempt self-harm, their rate of successful suicide is far lower than for older men (25). In Australia, males over 75 years have always had the highest rates of suicide, although this has been surpassed by young adult males in the last few years (26). A greater tendency by young and older males to use more lethal means to harm themselves is one significant factor contributing to this gender difference. By contrast, older women are more likely to take an overdose of prescription medication and are usually not sure about what might constitute a lethal dose.

Several authors have reported that women's suicidal behavior most commonly occurs in the context of relationship problems that generate feelings of helplessness and inadequacy (25). Haight and Hendrix (25) used a life narrative approach to identify themes that differentiated a sample of six older women (mean age 81 years) who rated significantly on the Beck Scale for Suicidal Ideation from six older women (mean age 79 years) who considered themselves satisfied with their lives. The suicidal women reported that their childhoods were unhappy and non-nurturing. Consequently, they had experienced difficulty in establishing intimate relationships and generating love and security in their own lives. They felt intense loneliness and had a pervasive sense of negativity about their capacity to cope. In contrast, the " satisfied" older women experienced a strong social network and described cohesive, caring families of origin. They appeared to have endured as many hardships as the suicidal women but were "better copers" and able to establish satisfying relationships. It is not clear from the reporting of this study to what extent the suicidal women were suffering from an acute relapse of their depressive symptoms, which would have intensified a negative perspective of their life trajectories. Overall, the suicidal women reported a lifelong coping style that seemed to predispose them to impoverished relationships and demoralizing loneliness.

Apart from depression and anxiety, older women are also more vulnerable to developing a psychotic illness in later life. This may be in the context of a depressive or dementing illness, but late-onset schizophrenia is far more common in women than men (unlike early-onset schizophrenia) (26). No satisfactory explanation for this gender disparity has been generated in the literature, but it is certainly a striking reality for those who work in aged mental health. From the few epidemiologic studies undertaken in this area, it is estimated that 4% to 6% of community-dwelling elderly experience psychotic symptoms in the form of delusions or hallucinations; the prevalence is much higher in institutional and residential care settings. One study noted that less than half the elderly psychotic persons surveyed were receiving any treatment (27). This finding is not surprising as the majority are socially isolated elderly women who rarely leave their homes. Their delusional ideas are usually about having "phantom boarders" in their houses, or they develop false persecutory ideas about their neighbors. Generally, it is only when they start to act upon their delusional ideas, which may be years after they first develop symptoms, that they become known to psychiatric services. Calling the police to remove the unwanted "boarder" or to reprimand the neighbors is a common precipitant that brings them to treatment. As these elderly women are usually distressed by their paranoid ideas, it is important that they be treated, even though they are quite resistant because of their lack of insight. However, a neglected area with regard to the psychotic symptoms experienced by these isolated elderly women is that they bring meaning into their otherwise barren lives. Totally removing these elderly women's delusional ideas, which have given them a distorted sense of purpose, often leaves them bereft and vulnerable to depression. This highlights the complexity of adaptation in later life and poses a challenge for mental health clinicians. Simply removing symptoms with pharmacologic interventions does not necessarily improve quality of life if these older women are then left with a sense of meaningless and even greater isolation (28).

RESILIENCE

What determines coping style, and most importantly what are the factors that foster maturation and resilience, enabling the achievement of "integrity" in later life, the final Eriksonian psychosocial challenge? These are particularly pertinent questions for aging women as they struggle to find their place in a changing society. The unresolved nature versus nurture debate suggests that both hereditary and environmental factors influence the development of personality traits and the unconscious defense mechanisms that are needed to manage life's stresses and tribulations. While acknowledging the role of heredity, Vaillant proposes that healthy psychosocial maturation can be attained only if young children are exposed to love and nurturance (29). As well as providing a model for how to connect emotionally with others, this enables the young child to internalize their loved parents. From this bedrock of ego development, empathy, healthy interactional patterns, and the capacity to reciprocate affection can develop. Of course, life is an evolving process and assigning the responsibility for psychosocial maturation solely to childhood experiences does not give much hope to the many who are emotionally deprived and neglected during this stage of their lives. The reality is that childhood is a critical developmental stage and achieving later life satisfaction is more of a struggle if the building blocks of emotional security are not laid down at this time. The suicidal women described above are testament to this tenet of psychological development. However, development is not static, and the adaptability of human nature is such that positive emotional experiences at any time during life's pathway can heal psychological damage wrought by traumatizing childhoods. As Vaillant observes, "At the heart of this recovery from disadvantage is *resilience*." In his book *Wisdom of the Ego* he attempts to deconstruct this concept through illustrative narratives of the participants in three longitudinal studies (29). The lives of these men and women have been followed since adolescence, and those still alive are now in later life. Although intelligence and material affluence were the fortune of many of these subjects, these attributes did not necessarily correlate with their capacity to deal with adversity or to feel contentment in the sunset of their lives. Vaillant postulates that resilience has to be viewed as multidetermined, and is often context-specific. He considers that a "balance sheet" in which protective factors outweigh risk factors is too simplistic to explain the multifarious concept of resilience. A stable sense of self appears to be crucial, but temperament, luck, and coping styles characterized by altruism, humor, and sublimation are other significant factors contributing to the capacity to remain positive and engaged with life despite adversity.

Among the aging subjects described by Vaillant were a group of women recruited as children in 1922 by Lewis Terman at Stanford University for his longitudinal study of gifted children (29). These highly intelligent female children were not a representative sample of their generation, but their life narratives provide us with a snapshot of the opportunities, or lack thereof, that were the lot of intelligent women born into an affluent society in the early years of last century (even though not all the families of the Terman women were financially comfortable). As the course of their adult lives was set long before the women's movement and the rise of feminism, the majority of these women were unable to actualize their potential in terms of career opportunities and public life. They had no female role models to provide guidance and mentoring for the application of their intellectual talents, and consequently their lives were filled with paradox. Vaillant uses the framework of "defense mechanisms," or life's coping strategies, to examine how these remarkable women coped with the constraints imposed upon their lives. One 78-year-old woman who had, at age 14 years, told the Terman study interviewer that she desperately wanted to be a doctor or an astronomer, could rationalize in late life that learning to cook and raise a garden were achievements in life that had given her joy. At some level, this very intelligent older woman had been able to reframe the disappointments in her life so as not to be bitter and resentful. In contrast, another female subject from the Terman study, despite the advantages of having an affluent and academically gifted family, could never rise above the self-doubt, hypochondria, and social isolation that characterized her entire life.

Vaillant and other authors interested in the concept of "successful aging" have concluded that material affluence and genetic attributes, such as intelligence, are helpful but do not necessarily correlate with better coping in later life (30–32). The capacity for creativity, defined in the sense of putting into the world what was not there before, appeared to characterize the Terman women who could still experience enjoyment in later life, have a sense of humor, and accept without bitterness the denied opportunities in their lives. This creativity did not necessarily bring them public acclaim but more often took the form of community work or an absorbing personal activity. They did not differ from the less creative, less contented Terman women in terms of education, social privilege, or even parental support. However, they were more likely to manifest altruism, "playfulness," and emotional connectedness in their coping styles (29). As such, they appeared to have mastered an adaptive maturity, which enabled them to preserve hope despite having to endure significant frustrations and losses.

Hope and meaning appear to be central to the maintenance of the creativity and resilience that characterize "successful aging." Participation in relationships and experiencing personal growth were the most important sources of meaning for a sample of 372 urban Australian women divided into five age cohorts (18–91 years). Interestingly, this was a common finding in both younger and older women, suggesting some continuity in particular aspects of meaning across the lifespan. When other sources of meaning were examined, the youngest group scored highest for participation in pleasurable activities, the middle-aged women scored highest for interest in social causes, and older women rated the preservation of values and ideals most highly (33). This study used the same instrument for measuring sources of personal meaning as undertaken in a previous age-stratified Canadian sample. Reker and Wong (34) found that there was a qualitative shift toward a philosophical orientation and innerdirectedness in later life. This increased "interiority" in older persons is also reflected in the findings of studies that have examined the relevance of spirituality and faith with increasing age. Neill and Kahn (35) found that life satisfaction was greater for older widowed American women who described themselves as "religious." In particular, engaging in organized religious activities provided them with friendships, a sense of community, and a means of contributing to the welfare of others. Reviewing the American literature in this area, Van Ness and Larson (36) found that the hope created by the salutary aspects of "religiousness" was protective for older people in terms of their vulnerability to depression and suicide. They also noted that religious older persons report higher levels of life satisfaction and other subjective measures of well-being. In contrast, the Australian study cited above found that participation in religious activities was not rated highly by older or younger women as an important source of personal meaning. Comparison between studies that have used different constructs of meaning cannot readily be made, but the above findings perhaps highlight the importance of sociocultural contexts for the way in which women make sense of the aging experience.

FUTURE DIRECTIONS

The growing literature on gender and aging is compelling in its elucidation of how much more vulnerable women are than men in later life. They have higher physical and mental morbidity with a longer life expectancy, have disproportionate responsibility for unpaid domestic work and care of dependent family members, and are confronted with persistent gender inequalities in the workforce (37). Ageist, sexist, and racist prejudices, even in developed societies, have greatly hindered macrolevel structural change that would address the needs of disadvantaged aging women. As a consequence, widowhood, childlessness, poverty, and ethnic minority status greatly increase the likelihood that older women will be socially marginalized, and their quality of life severely compromised.

And yet, it is also apparent that some older women can call on extraordinary resilience in facing loss, physical decline, and adversity. Researchers interested in the notion of successful aging have identified personal attributes and environmental circumstances that facilitate positive adaptation to age-related changes, and some of these have been discussed in this chapter. What is missing from this body of knowledge is a gender-specific focus to tease out the differences as well as the commonalities of the aging experience for women and men. Although life-span developmental models have greatly enhanced an appreciation of the positive aspects of aging, there has been a tendency to neglect the heterogeneity of adaptive age-related processes. Aging women require their own psychosocial research agenda that is able to examine their specific issues within a matrix that is focused on the individual within her society, and is multiculturally sensitive. Lessons to be learned from previous generations of aging women can be included only if a sociohistorical context is also considered. Longitudinal prospective studies, such as the Terman study of gifted children, are uniquely suited to exploring the connection between historical and social shifts and individual life courses (29). However, they will always be few in number, given the expense, logistic challenges, and time involved. Identifying and removing negative ageist and sexist stereotypes and the ignorance that underpins and maintains them would at least be a start in empowering and enabling the potential of older women to be expressed. Aging women require younger women from across the ethnic and class spectrum to join them in this struggle, as they will be the recipients of the benefits from more gender-egalitarian societies.

REFERENCES

1. Markson EW. Older women in a gendered world: facing the mirror. Gerontologist 1999; 39:495–503.
2. Ruffing-Rahal MA, Barin LJ, Combs CJ. Gender role orientation as a correlate of perceived health, health behavior, and qualitative well-being in older women. J Women Aging 1998; 10:3–20.
3. Laws G. Understanding ageism: lessons from feminism and postmodernism. Gerontologist 1995; 35:112–119.
4. Erikson EH. The Life Cycle Completed. New York: Norton, 1985
5. Grob A, Krings F, Bangerter A. Life markers in biographical narratives of people from three cohorts: a life span perspective in its historical context. Hum Dev 2001;44:171–191.

6. Atchley RC. A continuity theory of normal aging. In: Gubrium JF, Holstein JA, eds. Aging and Everyday Life. Cambridge, MA: Blackwell, 2000.

7. Kaufman SR. The ageless self. In: Gubrium JF, Holstein JA, eds. Aging and Everyday Life. Cambridge, MA: Blackwell, 2000.

8. Lewis VG, Borders LD. Life satisfaction of single middle-aged professional women. J Couns Dev 1995;75:94–101.

9. Koropeckyi-Cox T. Beyond parental status: psychological well-being in middle and old age. J Marriage Fam 2002;64:957–972.

10. Hiltz SR. Widowhood: a roleless role. Marriage Fam Rev 1978;1:1–14.

11. Choi NG. Long-term elderly widows and divorcees: similarities and differences. J Women Aging 1995;7:69–92.

12. Perkins K. Psychosocial implications of women and retirement. Soc Work 1992;37:526–532.

13. Nelson D. Violence against elderly people: a neglected problem. Lancet 2002;9360:1094.

14. Seaver C. Muted lives: older battered women. J Elder Abuse Neglect 1996;8:3–22.

15. Husaini BA, Cummings S, Kilbourne B, et al. Group therapy for depressed elderly women. Int J Group Psychother 2004;54:295–319.

16. Wasserthiel-Smoller S, Shumaker S, Ockene, J, et al. Depression and cardiovascualar sequelae in postmenopausal women. Arch Intern Med 2004;164:289–298.

17. Hedelin B, Strandmark M. The meaning of mental health form elderly women's perspectives: a basis for health promotion. Perspect Psychiatr Care 2001;37:7–15.

18. Fiske A, Gatz M, Pedersen NL. Depressive symptoms and aging: the effects of illness and non-health-related events. J Gerontol B Psychol Sci Soc Sci 2003;58B:320–329.

19. Simonsick E, Kasper JD, Phillips CL. Physical disability and social interaction: factors associated with low social contact and home confinement in disabled older women. J Gerontol B Psychol Sci Soc Sci 1998;53B:S209–S218.

20. Gold CH, Malmberg B, McGleam GE, et al. Gender and health: a study of older unlike-sex twins. J Gerontol B Psychol Sci Soc Sci 2002;57B:S168–S177.

21. Pinquart M, Sorensen S. Gender differences in self-concept and psychological well-being in old age: a meta-analysis. J Gerontol B Psychol Sci Soc Sci 2001;56B:195–214.

22. Lee C. Health habits and psychological well-being among young, middle-aged and older Australian women. Br J Health Psychol 1999;4:301–315.

23. Whelan G. Alcohol-related health problems in the elderly. Med J Aust 1995;162:325–327.

24. Australian Bureau of Statistics. National Drug Strategy Household Survey 2001. Canberra.

25. Haight BK, Hendrix SA. Suicidal intent/life satisfaction: comparing the life stories of older women. Suicide Life Threat Behav 1998;28:272–285.

26. Australian Bureau of Statistics. Suicides, Australia 1921–1998. Canberra.

27. Christenson T, Blazer CR. Epidemiology of persecutory ideation in an elderly population in the community. Am J Psychiatry 1984;141:1088–1091.

28. Hassett A. A patient who changed my practice: the lady with a plumber in her roof. Int J Psychiatry Clin Prac 1998;2:309–311.

29. Vaillant GE. Aging Well. North Carlton, Victoria: Scribe, 2002.

30. Ranzijn R. Towards a positive psychology of ageing: potentials and barriers. Aust Psychol 2002;37:79–85.

31. Baltes PB. The many faces of human ageing: toward a psychological culture of old age. Psychol Med 1991;21:837–854.

32. Schulz R, Heckhausen J. A life span model of successful aging. Am Psychol 1996;51:702–714.

33. Edward P. Sources of personal meaning in life for a sample of younger and older urban Australian women. J Women Aging 1997;9:47–64.

34. Reker GT, Wong PTP. Aging as an individual process: Toward a theory of personal meaning. In: Birren J, Bengston VL, eds. Emergent Theories of Aging. New York: Springer, 1988.

35. Neill CM, Kahn AS. The role of personal spirituality and religious social activity on the life satisfaction of older widowed women. Sex Roles 1999;40:319–329.

36. Van Ness PH, Larson DB. Religion, senescence, and mental health: the end of life is not the end of hope. Am J Ger Psychiatry 2002;10:386–398.

37. Meyer MH. Toward a structural, life course agenda for reducing insecurity among women as the age. Gerontologist 1997;37:833–837.

SUGGESTED READINGS

Arber S, Ginn J, eds. Connecting Gender and Aging: A Sociological Approach. Bristol, PA: Open University Press, 1995.

Barusch AS. Older Women in Poverty: Private Lives and Public Policy. New York: Springer, 1994.

Vaillant G. Ageing Well. North Carlton, Victoria: Scribe, 2002.

van den Hoonard DK. The Widowed Self: The Older Woman's Journey through Widowhood. Waterloo, Ontario: Wilfred Laurier University Press, 2002.

Aging and Cognition in Women

Chris Perkins

Worldwide, more than 470 million women are over 50 years of age and one-third of these will live into their 80s. It is anticipated that nearly two-thirds of the current US population will survive to 85 years or beyond.

Women have a longer life expectancy than men; thus in absolute numbers more women than men suffer from the neurodegenerative disorders that occur in very old age. Dementia is the most prevalent of these disorders, occurring in about 5% of people over 65 years of age and about 20% of those over 80. In 1997, of the 2.32 million people who were affected with Alzheimer's type dementia in the United States, 68% were women (1). Once they develop Alzheimer's disease, women on average live longer than men (2). Dementia is very much a women's health problem.

Dementia is now the third most common neuropsychiatric disorder in high-income countries (3). However, as the population in developing countries ages, dementia is also becoming commoner there. In China, for example, at least 10% of the population are now over 60 years of age. Although that rate of dementia is low compared to the rate for persons of Caucasian ancestry, an estimated 5 million people in China, mostly women, have dementia. Social trends in Asia, such as smaller families and increased opportunity for paid work for women, mean that the family is less able to fulfill the traditional role of caring for aging parents. Currently in China about 1 in 10 older persons live alone (4). In India, women surviving into old age are often vulnerable and disadvantaged and may be the only caregivers for the disabled (5). In Latin America and the Caribbean, where populations are aging rapidly, most of the elderly are women living in urban centers. A lifetime of ill health and poverty makes them vulnerable to the diseases of old age (6).

Women not only make up a high proportion of the people suffering from dementia, but they are also the main caregivers, both as family members and as employees in the aged care sector. Their services are often underrecognized and undervalued. As the "baby boomers" enter old age and life expectancy in developing countries increases, governments and insurers are starting to realize that the support of large numbers of older people with dementing illnesses will become prohibitively expensive. Thus preventive, diagnostic, and treatment strategies for the dementias are now receiving urgent attention. In this chapter we consider the changes in cognition that may occur with age and the diagnosis, prevention, and management of dementia. We discuss caregiving for older people with cognitive impairment and the risks of exploitation and abuse in this very vulnerable population.

"NORMAL" COGNITIVE CHANGES WITH AGE

Older people often report difficulties with cognitive ability, especially memory. It is difficult to determine what changes in cognition can be anticipated with normal aging. People become increasingly different from each other as they age, resulting in increased variability on tests of cognition. Thus, average scores across an age group may be less relevant than for younger people. Unrecognized illness (including dementia) or medication can also affect cognitive ability and confound the results of testing.

Comparing young and old in cross-sectional studies fails to account for generational differences in diet, health care, education, and other experiences between cohorts. These studies may exaggerate the age-related deterioration in cognition. In longitudinal studies that repeatedly test a group over many years, the less healthy subjects tend to drop out, leaving more of the more cognitively able members of the cohort. Such studies minimize the differences in cognition between older and younger people. However, some changes in cognitive function with age are broadly accepted.

LEARNING AND MEMORY

Declarative (or episodic) memory declines over time in longitudinal studies. Declarative memory is the recognition or recall of previously presented information; an example is the free recall of word lists or narrative material. Younger people may have better strategies for remembering over the short term; for example, when memorizing a list of objects they will group them somehow, such as by the first letter of the name. If older people are taught to do this, their recall improves significantly.

Older adults may have more difficulty with working memory, that is, more difficulty simultaneously retaining and processing information. Remote recall for many years past is usually good.

SPEED OF PROCESSING

Perceptual speed is the speed with which simple perceptual comparisons can be performed, as measured, for example, by timed tasks requiring symbol substitution. When age-related differences in perceptual speed are controlled for in some standard psychological tests, some other age-related differences disappear.

The commonly used Weschler Adult Intelligence Scale–Revised (7) has verbal and performance tasks. For older persons taking the test, little change is found on the verbal tasks that reflect a person's accumulated experience, education, and knowledge (crystallized intelligence). The performance tasks, however, begin to decline in midlife. These depend on speed and mental flexibility, which diminish over time. How much these changes actually affect an older person's functioning is unclear.

ATTENTION

The ability to sustain attention does not appear to change with age although it becomes more difficult to ignore extraneous stimuli and perhaps to shift or divide attention.

LANGUAGE

Apart from the well-known difficulty of retrieving names or other words, language does not normally deteriorate (8).

COGNITIVE IMPAIRMENT NO DEMENTIA (CIND)

The boundary between normal aging and pathologic change that would predict likely progression to dementia has yet to be identified. Since the development of the antidementia drugs, it has become important to try to clarify this boundary. If early cognitive impairment can be detected in an elderly person (and has not already resulted in sufficient functional or intellectual decline to merit a diagnosis of dementia), then appropriate treatment may delay or prevent the onset of the dementia.

The focus of investigation in this area has mainly been on age-associated memory impairment (AAMI), also known as amnestic mild cognitive impairment (aMCI). This focus has helped detect decline in people who may go on to develop Alzheimer's disease, memory impairment being an important early symptom. Amnestic MCI is defined as performance at 1.5 SD below age norms on a memory test, subjective memory complaints, intact general cognition, and not meeting criteria for dementia (9). However, non-Alzheimer forms of dementia often show deterioration in other areas of cognitive performance before memory declines. "Cognitive impairment no dementia," or CIND, includes other cognitive deficits as well as memory and may predict other forms of dementia as well as Alzheimer's disease. CIND, not consistently defined as yet, is characterized by difficulty with memory and/or other areas of cognition not sufficiently severe to meet criteria for dementia (10). Various studies show high rates of CIND in the elderly population (10.7% to 23.4% in those over 65), with the rate increasing with the age of the population studied (11,12). Of possible risk factors for CIND, only education has been shown to predict its rate in population studies; people with fewer years of formal education show a greater rate of cognitive decline than more educated persons (12,13). The current cohort of elderly women may show more cognitive deterioration than their better educated male peers. A recent community study of a sample of people 70 to 79 years old showed an insignificant decrease in the number of cognitively normal women compared with the number of cognitively normal men (14).

The annual rates of conversion from aMCI to Alzheimer's disease are between 3.7% and 8.3% (15,16); the conversion rates from CIND to dementia (all types) are 5.8% to 9.4% (17,18).

DEMENTIA

Dementia is defined as the development of multiple cognitive deficits (including memory impairment) due to

- The direct physiological effects of a general medical condition
- The persisting effects of a substance, or
- Multiple etiologies (DSM-IV)

These cognitive deficits are often accompanied by psychological symptoms such as anxiety, delusions, and hallucinations. Personality and behavioral changes occur, and there may be motor disturbances, depending on the type of dementia.

Of the many different types of dementia, the most common are Alzheimer's disease (50%–60% of cases); vascular dementia (15%–20%); mixed Alzheimer's and vascular dementia (10%); and Lewy body dementia (15%). The frontotemporal dementias (about 10%) and subcortical dementias form a heterogeneous group of diseases, often affecting people with movement disorders. The boundaries between the different types of dementia are blurred clinically and neuropathologically. Recent research has shown that vascular risk factors increase the likelihood of Alzheimer's dementia as well as vascular dementia (19,20). Brain infarction, detected on MRI, appears to hasten or precipitate the clinical expression of Alzheimer's disease (21). This suggests that the dementias are not necessarily separate clinical entities.

In some studies the incidence of Alzheimer's disease is higher in women than men. (22). Others (23) find only borderline differences or an increase in the female over male rate after 90 years of age only. However, men have a higher rate of vascular dementia (24), and there is a slight excess of males with Lewy body dementia (25).

The male:female ratio in the frontotemporal and subcortical dementias depends on the etiology. However, given women's longevity and the increased prevalence of dementia in people aged over 80, in absolute numbers many more women than men suffer from dementia.

PREVENTING DEMENTIA

Possible preventive approaches are described in the following paragraphs.

Education and cultural activities. As with CIND, the incidence of dementia is lower in people with more years of education. A study controlled for education found that participation in intellectual and cultural activities after formal education reduced the risk of dementia for women but not for men (27).

Medications. Treatment of hypertension and the use of lipid-lowering agents may prevent both vascular and Alzheimer's dementias (19,20). Good diabetic control, cessation of smoking, the regular use of aspirin, and treatment of extracerebral sources of embolism may help prevent vascular dementia.

Weight. Women who are overweight in old age may be more prone to developing dementia. For every unit of increase in the body mass index score, the risk of developing Alzheimer's disease increased by 36%. These increases were not found in men (27).

Richness of expression in youth. In the Nun study (a longitudinal study of the Sisters of Notre Dame in the United States), those with a wide and expressive writing style in youth were less prone to develop dementia. Low linguistic ability early in life may reflect suboptimal neurologic and cognitive development, which could increase susceptibility to the development of Alzheimer's disease pathology in later life (28).

Antioxidants. Intake of vitamin E and other antioxidants such as beta carotene and flavonoids may prevent Alzheimer's disease (29). Green tea and gingko biloba may lower the risk of Alzheimer's disease or slow its progression.

ESTROGEN

The apparently greater incidence of Alzheimer's disease in postmenopausal women compared to men of the same age led to interest in using exogenous estrogen to prevent the development of the disorder. This had a theoretical basis in that estrogen reduces the formation of beta amyloid (found in plaques in Alzheimer's disease) and affects oxidative stress, inflammation, and cerebral vasculature. Observational studies had also indicated that women who used hormone replacement therapy (HRT) were less likely to develop Alzheimer's disease than those who did not take HRT.

The Women's Health Initiative Memory Study (WHIMS), a randomized, double blind, placebo-controlled trial of estrogen and progestin versus placebo involving over 4,000 women aged 65 to 79 years, ran from May 1996 until July 2002. The study was stopped prematurely because of certain increased health risks (heart disease, stroke, pulmonary embolus, and breast cancer) in the women receiving the combined hormones. The outcome after 4.05 years was an *increased* risk of developing dementia (usually Alzheimer's disease) in the treatment group (hazard ratio 2.05), an increase of 23 cases of dementia per 10,000 women per year. The investigators concluded that combined therapy increased the risk for probable dementia in postmenopausal women 65 years or older. The combined therapy also did not prevent the development of mild cognitive impairment (30). The estrogen-only arm of the trial (in women who have undergone hysterectomy) is continuing.

Other researchers have argued that the timing of HRT administration is important and that its use at the menopause and early postmenopause (rather than in women over 65) might be more effective before the brain is affected by estrogen deficit (31).

DIAGNOSIS

Important differential diagnoses of dementia include delirium, depression, and normal aging. Although investigations for reversible causes of cognitive impairment such as B_{12}/folate and thyroid function tests are recommended (32), it is now rare that a truly reversible condition is found, perhaps because treatable psychiatric and metabolic conditions are less often confused with the primary dementias (33). Routine brain imaging may change diagnosis or management in 10% to 15% of cases. No diagnostic test for Alzheimer's disease exists yet, but clinical diagnosis with laboratory and x-ray investigation is about 80% accurate.

The diagnosis of dementia is often delayed because of its insidious onset, the popular acceptance and expectations of cognitive failure in old age, and the stigma surrounding the disorder. A family member or concerned friend (rather than the person with dementia) usually initiates the assessment visit to the primary care doctor. The information that person offers is vital for both diagnosis and subsequent management.

Family practitioners often fail to make the diagnosis until the disease is moderately advanced. The situation might be improved with better education of general practitioners about the disease and closer liaison with specialist services such as neurology and psychogeriatrics (34).

GENETICS

Half of *early onset* Alzheimer's disease cases appear to be transmitted as an autosomal dominant trait. The three causal genes are beta APP and presenilin 1 and 2, which if present, can help predict the likelihood of early onset dementia. However, these represent only 2% to 3% of people with dementia; for most people, dementia begins after the age of 65. In the older age group, 50% carry the apolipoprotein E epsilon 4 allele. Having this allele may increase the risk of developing Alzheimer's disease and hasten its onset by several years. However, there are clearly other genetic or environmental risk factors. ApoE genotyping cannot be used as a predictive test for late onset Alzheimer's disease and is of only minimal diagnostic value. It may be of use in determining response to treatment, but this needs further investigation.

DISCLOSING THE DIAGNOSIS

Much debate has ensued about the usefulness or harm of telling a person that he or she has a dementing illness. Most psychogeriatricians tell people with mild dementia their diagnosis and prognosis, although they are less likely to be so open with people with more severe disease. Sometimes they use more benign labels like "memory loss" or discuss the situation only with the patient's family. The evidence on the best course for clinicians to follow is inconsistent: the perspective of the people diagnosed with dementia has been largely neglected and needs more good-quality investigation (35). In one study, people who knew they had dementia feared others would find out, that they would be socially embarrassed, have long-term dependency needs, and not be listened to. Common effects of knowing the diagnosis were social withdrawal and hypervigilance for evidence of cognitive failure (36). However, it is important that patients and their caregivers (who may be elderly themselves) know the diagnosis so that they can plan for the future and make informed decisions about treatment. The disclosing physician needs to assess how much information should be given and at what stage. In fact, many people with mild dementia are aware there is something wrong and appreciate the knowledge, however painful. The manner in which people are told is important, ideally gradually, offering hope and ongoing support.

MANAGEMENT

Over the last decade drugs specifically targeting the disease process in dementia have been developed. These include the anticholinesterase inhibitors (ACEIs), which address the cholinergic deficit in Alzheimer's, vascular, and Lewy body dementias, and memantine, which blocks the action of glutamate that causes neuronal damage at N-methyl-D-aspartate (NMDA) receptors. The ACEIs are recommended for mild to moderate dementia, and memantine may be used at any stage by itself or in combination with the ACEIs. Studies have consistently shown modest benefits, with slight improvements in cognitive function and a slowing in the rate of decline compared with placebo.

A recently published study, AD2000 (37) showed no reduction in time to institutionalization, nor any significant change in caregiver stress or use of services in a group given donepezil, an ACEI, compared to a group given a placebo. It concluded that there was no economic advantage in using the ACEIs. AD2000 has been criticized in terms of numbers, diagnostic methods, and study design and because it fails to take into account the individuals who improve significantly. However, it remains the largest and longest independent trial of an ACEI. There is a need for more trials that are not commercially funded to assess fully the long-term usefulness of ACEIs and to define which groups benefit most.

The antidementia drugs are expensive, and not all countries include them in their publicly funded benefit schemes. Thus many women do not have the option of using these medications if they cannot personally afford them.

The mainstay of management remains good medical, psychological, social, and spiritual care over the prolonged course of the illness as the person with dementia becomes increasingly frail and dependent on others. Many different therapies aim at slowing cognitive decline, reducing behavioral disturbance, and improving quality of life. It is usually a matter of trial and error to decide which therapy is most beneficial for each individual.

FAMILY CARE

In the United Kingdom, 5.7 million people are household caregivers. Half of these informal caregivers look after someone over the age of 75. In the United States, an estimated 5 million people are caring for their parents at any one time and a similar number of spouses are looking after an elderly partner (38). Many of those needing care have dementia.

Often, the caregivers are also themselves elderly. In the United Kingdom, 27% of caregivers are over 65 years of age (39). If the dependent person has a spouse, that person, wife or husband, usually provides care.

However, if a single parent needs care, it is likely to be provided by daughters (even if there are sons), or if there are only sons, by daughters-in-law rather than the sons themselves. Daughters often feel a sense of obligation to provide care.

Over one third of those caring for a relative with dementia report a high level of stress, depression, or general psychological morbidity (40). In a 1993 U.K. survey 97% of caregivers were suffering from some form of emotional difficulty: stress, tiredness, depression, or loneliness (41). One third had some form of physical problem, such as back pain, as the result of being a caregiver (39). In contrast, many people take on caregiving with a sense of vocation; despite feeling tired, worried, and frustrated at times, they find that caring is a loving and rewarding task.

The degree of stress is affected by the nature of the relationship before the cared-for person developed dementia. It may be difficult for someone to accept the role of caring for a person the caregiver did not much like even when that person was well. Some spouses feel resentment toward the person, who by becoming ill has prevented fulfillment of their retirement dreams. Caring out of a sense of duty or guilt increases the emotional stress. However, if the relationship has been warm previously, the family may accept the situation and get on with the caring with minimal strain.

Factors affecting stress in a caregiver include *care recipient factors* such as

- High demands or needs on the part of the person with dementia (e.g. incontinence, night-time disturbance, emotional lability)
- Withdrawal, decreased social activity, apathy, and depression in the person with dementia. The reduced response to the caregiver by the person with dementia affects feelings of mutuality and satisfaction (42).

Caregiver factors include

- Relationship to the care-recipient. Spouses may be physically frail and financially poorly off, but they often have a wholehearted commitment to the partner. Daughters usually have responsibilities in paid work or toward other family members and thus experience distressing role conflict and disruption of their lives.
- Living situation. If caregivers live in the same house as the person with dementia, they are likely to notice the strain on the relationship and restriction of social activities.

Wives report greater strain than their husbands, but also greater emotional and behavioral disturbance on the part of their partner (43). Wives appear to be more emotionally involved, compared with husbands, who have a task-oriented approach to giving care. As time goes on, wives learn to distance themselves emotionally. Husbands report satisfaction in caring for their demented wives because they feel they can now repay the care their wives previously gave them.

Useful interventions to reduce caregiver stress include education, group support, practical care, respite care, emotional support, and psychotherapy. There is no one, simple solution to the multiple problems that arise during the long course of the illness. Multicomponent programs are necessary to support caregivers.

COMMUNITY CARE

Many older women live alone and if they develop dementia they are at increased risk of accidents, self-neglect, and exploitation. Balancing the need for choice and independence with the necessity for protection is often very difficult. Despite stereotypes of "sweet little old ladies," many older women are determinedly independent, outspoken, and resistant to interference in their lives. They want to remain living in their own homes and refuse assistance for as long as possible. Not wishing to "be a burden," they minimize their difficulties until later in the dementing process, when they fail to recognize that there are problems at all. These people need careful support from skilled, respectful community workers who attempt to maximize their clients' dignity and independence while minimizing risk.

This job is often done by kindly but untrained women who are paid a pittance. There is a lack of recognition and valuing of the complex nature of their work and its importance to the welfare, both economic and humane, of society in general.

INSTITUTIONAL CARE

People with dementia enter formal care when the risks of remaining in their own homes or the demands on their caregivers are too great or when the caregivers' health or other circumstances change. Incontinence, sleep disruption, marked dependence, behavioral disorders (such as wandering and irritability), or withdrawal are common reasons for institutionalization.

Most (up to 80%) of residents in nursing facilities are women. The prevalence of psychiatric disorders in these institutions is high. In one study 80.2% had some psychiatric disorder; of these, 67.4% had dementia.

Approximately 20% of residents with dementia have delusions or hallucinations, about 10% also have depression, and another 10% have a superimposed delirium. It is possible that if some of these conditions were treated with known effective approaches, cognitive function would improve (44).

Difficult behaviors are common in dementia (up to 90% of persons with dementia manifest some challenging behavior in the course of the dementing illness). Ideally, these should be managed by behavioral or environmental interventions. However, such management is often not the case, and there is a high rate of prescription of neuroleptic drugs in the attempt to control behavior. The rate of prescription of neuroleptics is higher for men than for women, probably because men's behavior is perceived as more dangerous (45). Long-term care providers complain of inadequate advice input from geriatric psychiatry services (46).

Quality of Life in Long-Term Care

The quality of life in long-term care for dementia depends on optimal cognitive functioning, activities of daily living, social interaction, and psychological well-being (47). These requirements often are not met in underfunded, understaffed residential settings. Residents in long-term care need autonomy and choice as much as possible, privacy (if they desire it), dignity, social interaction, meaningful activity, individuality (personal preferences, interests, and backgrounds should be taken into account), enjoyable (rather than aversive) stimulation, safety and security, spiritual well-being, clarity of structure (clearly stated rules and norms governing resident behavior), and functional competence (the staff and environment should contribute to the maintenance of their everyday skills) (48). People with dementia cannot always ask for their needs to be met, though their demeanor and behavior will often signal that something is wrong.

Nonpharmacologic Therapies in Residential Care
Person-centered care

Kitwood, a psychologist who led the Bradford (U.K.) Dementia Group in the 1990s, developed a model of dementia that involves the interaction between neurologic changes affecting the person and her environment (49).

Often, he suggests, professional caregivers of the person with dementia erode her skills, self-esteem, confidence, and social status through the action of "malignant social psychology." Some examples of such behavior are: *disempowerment*, in which a caregiver takes over a task that the person with dementia could have done herself (with adequate time and support) or by ignoring the person, for example by talking as if she were not in the room. Ultimately, the dementia sufferer loses her status as a person, her "personhood." Caregivers do not intend to be malicious but merely lack insight into what it might be like to suffer from dementia.

From this theory, he developed "Dementia Care Mapping," an observational quality assurance tool aimed at providing a person-centered picture of care to enhance the insight of staff in residential settings and bring about positive change (49).

Numerous other approaches to care, including validation therapy, reality orientation, aromatherapy, art, or other cognitive stimulation therapy, aim to improve quality of life, slow the rate of cognitive decline, and prevent behavioral disturbances.

Unfortunately, there are often too few staff to use these methods regularly. Most paid caregivers, either in community roles or as workers in institutions, are women. They are often recent immigrants, perhaps with a poor grasp of the language of their charges, and are poorly paid and poorly educated. Many have to work overtime to earn a reasonable wage, and there is a high rate of staff turnover and burnout. These factors have an impact on the quality of care provided to those at home or in long-term care.

Many residential facilities provide adequate physical care for people with dementia and ensure their physical safety while ignoring their psychological, emotional, and spiritual needs. Legislation governing the residential care sector is often more focused on the adequacy of fire evacuation plans and food preparation than the residents' less tangible needs for stimulation, company, and meaningful activities.

ELDER ABUSE

Elder mistreatment affects 3.2% of the over-65 population in the United States. The rates vary in different countries but are not directly comparable because of differences in definition (e.g., whether or not theft is included). Neglect is frequent. The very frail elderly, especially those with depression or dementia, are likely targets, as are those who need assistance with activities of daily living or those who are socially isolated (50).

As Tomlin states: "American studies have shown the classic victim to be an elderly person over the age of seventy-five, female, role-less, functionally impaired, lonely, fearful and living at home with one child" (51).

People with dementia are very vulnerable to abuse, often physical perhaps related to their own disruptive behavior. With limited memory and communication skills, they may find it difficult to recall or report incidents of abuse. They may not be believed if they do complain, or they may indeed not report accurately (e.g., a woman may recall an abusive incident from the past as if it has just occurred). There is also the possibility that someone with dementia will misinterpret a procedure (e.g., receiving personal care from a male nurse) as abuse. It is very important for caregivers of people with dementia to be alert to the possibility of abuse, but they should also be aware that the person with dementia might misunderstand the situation.

FINANCIAL ABUSE

Theft from elderly persons with dementia is probably widespread, coming in a variety of forms—the neighbor who takes the person with dementia to the bank to withdraw money; the son who, via his power of attorney, uses his mother's money to finance his business; or the unscrupulous secondhand dealer who buys the person's antiques at rock-bottom prices. Money and jewelry disappear so often from residential care that families are usually advised to take all valuables home. Home care workers who help with shopping have to be fastidious about providing receipts for all spending.

Most jurisdictions have provisions for the appointment of a property manager to assist or take over the financial affairs of the person with dementia. It is (of course) possible for such persons to abuse their position, and in many jurisdictions no legislative sanctions on such behavior exist.

More subtle forms of abuse include families not paying for essential care in an attempt to maximize their inheritance, or residential providers charging extra for services that should be included in their basic contract (e.g., asking for payment for basic hygiene products).

PHYSICAL AND PSYCHOLOGICAL ABUSE

People with dementia can be irritating in the extreme, particularly to someone who does not understand the nature of the disorder. If a caregiver, whether family or paid, is stressed, it is not surprising that anger or frustration may boil over at times. The caregiver may yell, handle the person roughly, or hit her. Caregivers also often put up with abuse from the person with dementia.

Tying a person in a chair, locking her up, ridiculing or ignoring her, or refusing to meet her needs is also abusive. Usually the abusive person is not malicious but acting out of ignorance or desperation; he or she may feel guilty. The proper response generally should not be punitive but should inquire into why the abuse has occurred and how repetition of the behavior can be avoided.

Abuse by family members may be precipitated by their mental illness or alcohol abuse. Other caregiver factors include a poor premorbid relationship with the care recipient and previous abuse.

SEXUAL ABUSE

The prevalence of sexual abuse of persons with dementia is unknown, partly because it is difficult to define when it occurs. Complex ethical issues arise. If a husband demands his conjugal rights from a woman who cannot consent, when does this become abuse? Is it only if she seems upset by it? Is sexual contact with a man whom the woman with dementia misidentifies as her husband acceptable? What if he also has dementia, so that neither can truly consent? Who decides whether to "allow" their relationship to develop?

Adult children are often shocked by their mother's involvement with a man who is not their father and say it is out of character and not what she would have wanted if her mind were not impaired. Should their view be considered, especially if their mother seems to be enjoying the relationship? Residential care staff are also often uncomfortable with such "affairs," and there are rarely suitable rooms in which to conduct them.

There is a paucity of intervention studies in elder abuse. The causes of abuse are multifactorial, and therefore the responses need to be equally complex, applying to both caregiver and victim (52).

SUMMARY

Cognitive decline in old age is already a major issue for older women and will become increasingly important as longevity increases in both developing and developed countries. Older women with cognitive decline are often badly off economically. In many countries, they are triply or quadruply stigmatized: they are old, female, cognitively impaired, and poor. They are at high risk for abuse.

Services are frequently inadequate to provide the care that could improve quality of life for persons with dementia. Their caregivers, who are mostly women, suffer from the stigma associated with their clients: they too are at risk of being exploited.

However, the enormous increase in their absolute numbers will mean that people with dementia and their caregivers cannot be ignored indefinitely. There are signs of growing interest in the prevention and treatment of the neurodegenerative disorders, perhaps because everyone, rich or poor, male or female, young or old, knows someone with dementia.

REFERENCES

1. Brokmeyer R, Gray S, Kawas C. Projections of Alzheimer's disease in the United States and the public health impact of delaying disease onset. Am J Pub Health 1998;88:1337–1342.
2. Larsen E, Shadlen M, Wang L, et al. Survival after initial diagnosis of Alzheimer disease. Ann Intern Med 2004;140(7):501–509.
3. Lyon D, McLaughlin D. Recent advances: psychiatry. Br Med J 2001;323(7323):1228–1231.
4. Chiu HF, Zhang M. Dementia research in China. Int J Geriatr Psychiatry 2000;15(10):947–953.
5. Prakash I. Aging, disability, and disabled older people in India. J Aging Soc Policy 2003:15(2/3):85–108.
6. Restrepo H, Rozental M. The social impact of aging populations: some major issues. Soc Sci Med 1994;39(9):1323–1338.
7. Weshler Adult Intelligence Scale–Revised Manual. New York: Psychological Corporation, 1981.
8. Wilson RS, Bennett DA, Swartendruber, A. In: Nussbaum PD, ed. Handbook of Neuropsychology and Aging. New York: Plenium Press, pp. 7–14.
9. Petersen RC, Doody R, Kurz A, et al. Current concepts in mild cognitive impairment. Arch Neurol 2001;58:1985–1992.
10. Ebly EM, Hogan DB, Parhad IM. Cognitive impairment in the nondemented elderly. Arch Neurol 1995;52:1985–1992.
11. Di Carlo A, Baldereschi M, Amaducci L, et al. Cognitive impairment without dementia in older people: prevalence, vascular risk factors, impact on disability: the Italian Longitudinal Study on Aging. J Am Geriatrics Soc 2000;48:775–782.
12. Unverzargt, Gao S, Baiyewu O, et al. Prevalence of cognitive impairment: data from the Indianapolis study of health and aging. Neurology 2001;57:1655–1662.
13. Evans DA, Beckett LA, Albert MS, et al. Level of education and change in cognitive function in a community population of older persons. Ann Epidemiol 1993;3:71–77.
14. Low L-F, Brodarty H, Edwards R, et al. The prevalence of "cognitive impairment no dementia" in community-dwelling elderly: a pilot study. Aust NZ J Psychiatry 2004;38(9):725–731.
15. Ritchie K, Artero S, Touchon J. Classification criteria for mild cognitive impairment: a population-based validation study. Neurology 2001;56:37–42.
16. Larrieu S, Letenneur L, Orgogozo JM, et al. Incidence and outcome of mild cognitive impairment in a population-based prospective cohort. Neurology 2002;59:1594–1599.
17. Waite LM, Broe GA, Grayson DA, et al. Preclinical syndromes predict dementia: the Sydney older persons study. J Neurology, Neurosurgery Psychiatry 2001;71:296–302.
18. Baiyewu O, Unverzargt FW, Ogunniyi A, et al. Cognitive impairment in community-dwelling older Nigerians: clinical correlates and stability of diagnosis. Eur J Neurology 2002;9:573–580.
19. Skoog I, Lernfelt B, Landahl S, et al. A 15-year longitudinal study of blood pressure and dementia. Lancet 1996;347(9009):1141–1145.

20. Rockwood K, Kirkland S, Haogan D, et al. Use of lipid-lowering agents, indication bias, and the risk of dementia in community-dwelling elderly people. Arch Neurol 2002;59:223–227.
21. Snowdon D, Greiner L, Mortimer J, et al. Brain infarction and the clinical expression of Alzheimer disease. JAMA 1997;277:813–817.
22. Copeland JR, McCracken CF, Dewey ME, et al. Undifferentiated dementia, Alzheimer's disease and vascular-dementia: age- and gender- related incidence in Liverpool: the MRC-ALPHA Study. Br J Psychiatry 1999;175:433–438.
23. Fitzpatrick AL, Kuller LH, Ives DG, et al. Incidence and prevalence of dementia in the Cardiovascular Health Study. J Am Geriatrics Soc 2004;52(20)195–204.
24. Ruitenberg A, Otto A, Van Swieten JC, et al. Incidence of dementia: does gender make a difference? Neurobiol Aging 2001;22(4):575–580.
25. McKeith IG. Dementia with Lewy bodies. Br J Psychiatry 2002;180:144–147.
26. Crowe M, Andel R, Pedersen NL, et al. Does participation in leisure activities lead to decreased risk of Alzheimer's disease? A prospective study of Swedish twins. J Gerontology, Series B, Psychological Sci Social Sci 2003;58(5):249–255.
27. Gustafon D, Rothenberg E, Blennow K, et al. An 18 year follow up of overweight and risk of Alzheimer disease. Arch Intern Med 2003;163(13):1524–1528.
28. Snowdon D, Greiner L, Markesbery W. Linguistic ability in early life and the neuropathology of Alzheimer's disease: findings from the Nun Study. Ann NY Acad Sci 2000;903(April):34–38.
29. Engelhart M, Geerlings M, Ritenberg, et al. Dietary intake of antioxidants and risk of Alzheimer disease. JAMA 2002;287(24):3223–3229.
30. Shumaker SA, Lagault C, Rapp S, et al. Estrogen plus progestin and the incidence of dementia and mild cognitive impairment in postmenopausal women. The Women's Health Initiative Memory study: a randomised controlled trial. JAMA 2003;289(20):2651–2662.
31. Resnick SN, Henderson VW. Hormone therapy and risk of Alzheimer's disease: a critical time. JAMA 2002;288:2170–2172.
32. Knopman D, DeKosky S, Cummings J, et al. Practice parameter: diagnosis of dementia (an evidence-based review). Report of the Quality Standards Subcommittee of the American Academy of Neurology. Neurology 2001;56:1143–1153.
33. Clarfield M. The decreasing prevalence of reversible dementias: an updated meta-analysis. Arch Intern Med 2003;163(13):2219–2229.
34. Löppönen M, Räihä I, Isoaho R, et al. Diagnosing cognitive impairment and dementia in primary health care: a more active approach is needed. Age Ageing 2003;33(3):606–612.
35. Bamford C, Laimont S, Eccles M, et al. Disclosing a diagnosis of dementia: a systematic review. Int J Geriatr Psychiatry 2004;19:151–169.
36. Husband HJ. Diagnostic disclosure in dementia: an opportunity for intervention? Int J Geriatr Psychiatry 2000;15(6):544–547.
37. Anonymous. Long-term donepezil treatment in 565 patients with Alzheimer's disease (AD2000): randomised double blind trial. Lancet 2004;363(9427):2105–2116.
38. Zarit S, Edwards A. Family caregiving: research and clinical intervention. In: Woods RT, ed. Psychological Problems of Ageing: Assessment, Treatment and Care. Chichester, UK: Wiley, 1999:153–193.
39. Office of National Statistics.1995 General Household Survey. United Kingdom, 1997.
40. Schultz R, O'Brien AT, Bookwala J, et al. Psychiatric and physical morbidity effects of dementia care giving: prevalence, correlates and causes. Gerontologist 1995;35:771–791.
41. Alzheimer's Disease Society. Deprivation and dementia: a report by the Alzheimer's Disease Society. London, 1993.
42. Oyebode J. Assessment of carer's psychological needs. Adv Psychiatr Treatment 2003;9:45–53.
43. Barusch AS, Spaid WM. Gender differences in care giving: why do wives report greater burden? Gerontologist 1989;29:667–676.
44. Rovner B, German P, Broadhead J, et al. The prevalence and management of dementia and other psychiatric disorders in nursing homes. Int Psychogeriatrics 1990;3:113.
45. Bronskill S, Anderson G, Sykora K, et al. Neuroleptic drug therapy in older adults newly admitted to nursing homes: incidence, dose and specialist contact. J Am Geriatr Soc 2004;52(5):749–755.
46. Moak G, Boorsin S. Mental health services in long-term care: an unmet need. Am J Geriatr Psychiatry 2000;8(May):96–100.
47. Whitehouse P, Orgogozo J, Becker R, et al. Quality of life in dementia drug development. Alzheimer Dis Assoc Disord 1997;11(3):56–60.
48. Noelker L, Harel Z. Linking Quality of Long Term Care and Quality of Life. New York: Springer, 2001.
49. Kitwood T, Bredin K. Towards a theory of dementia care: personhood and well-being. Ageing Soc 1992;10:269–287.
50. Fulmer T. Elder mistreatment. Ann Rev Nurs Res 2002;20:369–395.
51. Tomlin S. The abuse of elderly people: an unnecessary and preventable problem. London: British Geriatric Society, 1989.
52. Lachs M, Pillemer K. Elder abuse. Lancet 2004;364(9441):1263–1272.

CHAPTER 25

Vicissitudes and Disappointments: Loss and Illness in Late Life

Pamela Melding

"Old age is not a disease—it is strength and survivorship, triumph over all kinds of vicissitudes and disappointments, trials and illnesses" in the words of the late Maggie Kuhn, civil rights activist (1). In historical times, longevity was greatly revered. People who attained old age not only had excellent survivorship but also were considered by their social groups to be a source of wisdom and cultural knowledge. Such accolades are not earned simply by reaching old age but accomplished! Old age is a major developmental period of the life cycle and one with more challenges, "vicissitudes and disappointments, trials and illnesses" to confront than at any other stage of life. Among these are changes to the *physical self* as organ systems become vulnerable to disease and decline. Simultaneously, older people have to confront the *relational self* as they retreat from the active world and their roles in the family and society change. Decline of the physical body and retreat from the active world allow time to confront the *psychological self* and bring the need to reminisce and put into perspective all of one's life experiences, their personal value, meaning, and quality, in preparation of the final, ultimate retreat from life itself. Old age itself is certainly not a disease, and persons who successfully negotiate its challenges have the capacity for "strength, survivorship and triumph," as Kuhn asserted. Successfully negotiating the challenges results in resolution of emotional conflict, integration of experiences and achievements, and appreciation of contextual significance and meaning leading to psychological growth—the elements that are integral to "wisdom." The reality for many women is successful aging—living and adapting well despite the problems of old age. But for others, old age can be a time of difficulty, in which triumph and survivorship seem to be an impossible dream. This chapter considers some of the challenges to overcome, the major "vicissitudes and disappointments" that can negatively influence mental health, and it looks at some of the important factors highlighted by aging studies as conducive to the "triumph and survivorship" of successful aging.

DEMOGRAPHY OF LATE LIFE

The changing population demographics around the world is possibly the most important factor influencing both physical and mental health of older women today. Increasing longevity and decreased fertility are the major causes of aging of the populations in most of the developed and developing world. Between 2000 and 2020, the population of people aged 65 and older is projected to rise rapidly in all countries of the world, with the greatest rise in the cohort over 80 years of age (2). The first countries to feel the impact of this change, Japan, the United Kingdom, Germany, and France, already have to deal with the issues as their elderly people now constitute 20% to 25% or more of their total populations. Others, such as Canada, the United States, Australia, and New Zealand, with elderly populations currently about 12% to 13%, have the benefit of a few years grace to observe how other countries deal with the challenges. The small surplus of males at birth is markedly reversed near the end of the life span because total life expectancy for men is several years less than for women. By age 75 years, women outnumber men by 4 to 3, and by age 80, there are twice as many women as men. This trend is more apparent in the most developed countries, where women have an additional 5 to 12 years of life expectancy, but even in less developed countries, women have greater longevity than men. Older women are more likely than men to be the recipients of retirement benefits, geriatric health care, and institutional care (2).

New Zealand is one of the Western countries that has still to see the impact of population aging. Yet in 2001 a New Zealand national census revealed that 3 of every 4 older men lived with others while only 1 of 2 women did. Twenty percent of men lived alone in contrast to 43% of women who did. While the majority of older men were married, fewer than half of older women were, and if both genders reached their 80s, half the men were likely to have still living spouses whereas only about 10% of women would have a partner (3). These demographics are consistent with similar findings for many other developed countries of the world.

VICISSITUDES, TRIALS, AND DISAPPOINTMENTS

POVERTY

A major consequence of being widowed is that income drops. The New Zealand census found that the median income for men over the age of 65 was more than the median income for women of the same age. Studies in other countries find similar trends. A British Household Study found that health in late life was substantially related to socioeconomic group and that elderly widows were disadvantaged economically. Having poorer resources predicted poorer health and mental health (4).

Poverty is a major social determinant of poor physical and mental health. Many women become impoverished for the first time in old age, after the deaths of their husbands. Many of the current generation of older women never worked in paid employment, or if they did, their working life was interrupted by child rearing. Those that had jobs outside the home were less likely to be educated beyond secondary school and more likely to be in low-paying or part-time employment. Consequently, financial security for many women came from being married. Older women are far less likely than older men to have either public or private pensions of their own. Many widows have to survive on the residual benefits of their deceased husbands' pensions. These are often paid at a lower rate for the surviving spouse and rarely support the living standards the women had while their husbands were alive (5). Widows also lose a contribution toward fixed domestic costs such as property taxes, utility standing charges, maintenance, etc., and thus the discrepancies are larger than might be inferred from the statistics. State pensions (equivalent to Social Security benefits in the United States) barely cover living costs for those who have not contributed to private retirement investment funds, and personal savings diminish over time. Diet, heating, and housing resources can suffer, increasing vulnerabilities to health breakdown. In addition, worry over material resources can significantly undermine the psychological coping of the functionally limited disabled older person (6).

LOSS

Loss is the hallmark of late life. While losses can affect both genders, how they do so may be very different experiences for men and women. Many loss events in an older person's life, such as retirements or bereavements are "on-time," normative events that are anticipated and usually taken in their stride. Unanticipated life events, such as unexpected illness in self or spouse, the loss of an adult child, or natural disasters, are "off-time" events and have a more profound psychological impact. When a loss-inducing life event occurs in a person's life, it can cause a change in circumstances, represent a threat, or be regarded as a challenge, and sometimes all three. Krause (7) postulated that the adverse impact of life events is more severe when an event threatens an aspect of self-image that identifies the person's concept of a salient social role, such as spouse, parent, grandparent, friend, or contributor to the community. Older people subjected to several adverse life events in a short period are much more vulnerable to depression and poor psychological adjustment than others (8).

BEREAVEMENTS

Bereavements are common in late life. Indeed, some older people joke about funerals being their most common social experience. While they may take the deaths of friends and even spouses in their stride as normative events, the impact for long-lived females may be greater than just coping with the loss of dear companions. The loss of a male partner not only deprives a woman of a confidant and support but also changes her social and economic status. Although many older women do try to substitute for a lost partner or dear friend, these substitute ties often do not fully compensate (9).

Another consequence of women's surviving longer than their male partners is that each gender has to deal with health problems in different contexts. In contrast to men, most of whom have partners and expect to be taken care of by that partner (10), most women are without partner support when they most need it. Recent widows may have a marked decline in their physical and mental health status (11). Consequently, women often become increasingly reliant on their social support networks as they age.

SOCIAL SUPPORT

The importance of social networks and their impact on health in late life should not be underestimated. A considerable body of research tells us that psychological and physical stressors may be moderated in older people if they feel cared for and esteemed by their social networks. In a classic London study, Murphy (12) found that older people with confiding relationships were less likely to have depressive illness following a threatening life event. Positive social support possibly may also have a direct effect on illness itself by enhancing immunologic function (13). Of course, the deaths of a spouse, siblings, and friends shrink the size and quality of an older person's support network markedly.

A social network is defined as "those within the person's larger social community who regularly provide support in a range of contexts of day to day life" (14). Social networks are a major source of assistance for older people; they may include (a) members of the same household, (b) relatives, (c) confidants, (d) people perceived by the person as able to provide necessary instrumental and emotional support. A social network enables a person to cope with life and its problems and provides access to resources that help from day to day (15).

Not all networks are strong enough to cope with the vicissitudes of old age. The quality of a support network is probably more important than its size, and discrete networks can respond in different ways to the problems of old age. Some are more robust in offering support to older people; others more vulnerable to breakdown under crisis. Wenger (15) argued that social networks have their own special characteristics and can be predictive both of types of health problems and of the response to them. Wenger developed a useful typology of social networks for older people, based on extensive qualitative research in Wales:

1. *The local family dependent support network* focuses on close family ties, often an old person living with an adult son or daughter. There are usually few neighbors and peripheral friends. The persons being cared for are more likely to be the old-old (i.e., over 80 years of age) and in poor health compared with those supported by other types of networks. They are more likely to be widowed and female.

The local family network is associated with older persons with dementia. In the old-old individuals commonly found in such networks, depression and loneliness tend to occur with increasing dependency along with fear of loss of autonomy and of being a burden (16). The caregivers looking after an elderly person may also be more vulnerable to stress and depression due to the increased burden of care.

2. *The locally integrated support network* is usually based on the long-term residence in one area of an elderly person who has maintained active involvement in community and church organizations over many years. The person sup-

ported by this type of network has close relationships with local family, who live nearby, and with friends and neighbors. The network is often large, and because the network members often know each other, it can be very robust in times of crises when the network pulls together in collaborative action.

3. *The local self-contained support network* is one that supports an elderly person who has arm's-length relationships or infrequent contact with at least one relative, often a sibling or a niece or nephew, but relies primarily on neighbors. The elderly persons tend to keep to themselves and ask for help only in an emergency. The relationships are undemanding, the person has lifelong resistance to reliance on others, and dependency is low.

The self-reliant people living in local self-contained networks often deny difficulties. They are often childless, and relatives are not a source of active emotional support (17). As a result of little interaction they may become subject to feelings of isolation and loneliness. They may also suffer from unrecognized physical and mental health problems.

4. *The wider community focused support network* is exemplified by the middle-class network of the retirement migrant. Typically, the elderly person supported by such a network has no relatives nearby but has active relationships with relatives, usually adult children, who live some distance away. Friends have high salience, and the relationships are characterized by a high degree of reciprocity, at least in the short term. People in wider community focused networks are usually educated and assertive, and they like to be their own case managers. They often go into residential care earlier rather than later if they begin to deteriorate.

5. *The private restricted support network* is associated with an absence of local kin, often childlessness, few nearby friends, and low levels of family or community contacts. Consequently, the network is generally very small. Contact with neighbors is minimal, and there is a low level of community contacts. These older people are often suspicious of others and deny any problems. They are more likely than others to resist medical and social interventions and to struggle to maintain independence against increasing odds. People with this type of support network are overrepresented among older persons with mental health and personality difficulties. Depression is often common, unrecognized, and undertreated. These older people may also adapt very poorly to residential care (15).

Poor economic resources, recent bereavements, social isolation, and impoverishment all carry increased risk for physical and mental disorders in late life (18). Deterioration of social resources for the older person or the inability of a social network to respond to a crisis is often the trigger for greater interaction with health care professionals.

PHYSICAL HEALTH

Of all life events, the most common ones to affect older people are illness stressors (19). Several studies of aging also indicate that illness and disability are the most stressful of all loss events. Physical aging can lead to deterioration in health status, often with resulting psychosocial ripple effects that limit independence, reduce self-determination, and induce a loss of self-esteem. Notably, chronic poor physical health and disability are major correlates of depression, prolonged hospitalization, suicide, and poor psychological functioning in old age (20).

Both sexes are, of course, prone to physical health losses. The leading causes of men's earlier deaths are cardiac disease, stroke, chronic obstructive pulmonary disease (COPD), and cancer. However, because of their longevity, women are more prone to disabling diseases such as arthritis, osteoporosis, degenerative diseases of the brain, and hearing and visual impairments (21). Indeed, women have about two years' more disablement than their male counterparts. These disabling diseases can last for many years, decreasing quality of life by causing persistent pain, restricting mobility, and reducing sensory enjoyment. Loss of visual and auditory acuity not only affects older persons' sensory enjoyment of life but also negatively affects their confidence to manage basic activities of daily living and confidence to socialize and be involved in their communities (22).

Older people frequently experience multiple physical comorbidities. One physical disorder may tax an individual, but several comorbidities can be overwhelming (23). While physical debility may result from an acute change in health status, appetite, nutrition, or bodily rhythms may also be adversely affected. A disease may have secondary effects such as dehydration, metabolic or electrolyte upsets, severe pain or constipation, and the disease process may have a cascade effect, with one dysfunctional system putting additional strain on other marginal organ systems. Treatment may compound the patient's problem through sedation or drug interactions.

Illness events have profound psychosocial effects far beyond the immediate physiologic impact. Illness, especially if accompanied by significant chronicity, pain, or disablement, has a major impact on the older person's functioning, social roles, and relationships. A major insult to self-identity can occur when a person is no longer capable of taking care of himself or herself and becomes reliant on adult offspring or other caregivers. The "life of the party" may lose social confidence or suffer agoraphobia following a serious fall. Physical or cognitive impairment can force an elderly person to give up driving, limiting opportunities for social engagement.

PERSISTENT PAIN

More than 40% of older people report problems with pain or discomfort to some degree. The extent to which pain interferes with daily activities increases incrementally with age, women faring much worse than men (24). Many of the diseases affecting older women have disabling, persistent pain as a major feature (21). The list is long and includes arthritis, osteoporosis, vertebral collapse, sensory neuropathies from diabetes or ischemia, heart disease, stroke, trigeminal neuralgia, temporal arteritis, and more. Yet, despite acknowledgments from clinicians that pain is a symptom in all of these conditions, persistent pain in older people and particularly older women is underdetected and, worse, undertreated both in nursing homes and the community (25,26).

McLean and Higginbotham (27) studied cognitively intact residents of nursing homes in New South Wales, Australia, and found the prevalence of persistent pain to be high, particularly in women (31% women compared to 21% men), with a much lower level of treatment recorded. Agreement between the residents' self-report and the nursing record was borderline (kappa 0.24). The findings of this study were similar to those of several other studies in other countries. Fox and colleagues (28), in a systematic review of several international studies, noted a marked discrepancy between prevalence of pain as determined by self-report or chart reviews and pain actually treated.

Why is persistent pain in elders such a neglected issue? There seem to be several reasons, starting with a lack of basic education on the assessment and treatment of chronic pain per se in medical and nursing school curricula (25). A good pain assessment needs to be thorough, but unsurprisingly, assessment of persistent pain is not a priority for the limited time of health practitioners. Sadly, many persistent pain problems in older people remain underrecognized simply because health professionals do not ask or have the time to ask about the problem and its detrimental effect on a person's functioning or quality of life.

Unlike the senses of hearing or vision, which diminish with age, the notion of "presbyalgia" or a lessening of nociception or pain sensation with age has mostly been dismissed in healthy older adults (25). However, Gibson et al. (29) compared acute pain threshold perception in healthy and cognitively impaired older adults and found that, although acute pain perception was not diminished in the Alzheimer patients, these patients were slower at reporting the noxious stimuli and their reports were less reliable. Certainly, a pathologic brain disease may interfere with cognitive or motivational-affective pathways, thus altering pain experience (30), but this does not necessarily mean that discomfort is any less. Indeed, central neuropathic pain following stroke is well known to be one of the most distressingly painful conditions known (31).

Persistent pain in older women appears to be underdetected and undertreated even in those who are able to verbalize and express it. Many are resigned to their pain, believe they should "suffer in silence," or say they "do not want to be a bother" (32). Sometimes, they may fail to report pain to caregivers and health professionals due to mistaken beliefs that pain signals a dread disease or that they might be admitted to the hospital or worse, an institution, if the true nature of their difficulties becomes known (33). Other concerns that fuel the reluctance to communicate pain are notions that analgesics will have bad side effects or will become addictive. Unfortunately, these notions may be also entertained by primary care physicians (25), which may result in inadequate treatment.

Pain is not just a physical sensation of nociception but *suffering* is also involved. Living with a painful condition has deleterious effects on one's quality of life, and persons so affected are often depressed. Indeed, pain and disability are major risk factors for depression in late life (34). Depression also heightens suffering of pain (35). Pain is also a well-recognized major risk factor for late-life suicide (36).

While the underdetection and treatment of pain in cognitively intact older women who are capable of expressing their needs are bad enough, the situation is much worse in cognitively impaired elders in nursing homes (37), most of whom are women. Language is an early domain affected by the dementias, and the inability to convey inner experience is a major factor in the underreporting of pain, especially in advanced disease. However, communication can be also expressed in behavior and body language or be manifest as agitation or challenging behaviors (38). Most nursing home residents with advanced dementia are women who commonly have comorbid painful musculoskeletal conditions. Detection of pain problems in these patients often proves challenging for clinicians involved in their care (39). Careful observation by staff and close knowledge of the patient seem to be important factors in identifying pain in cognitively impaired elders, who have difficulty in communicating. Indicators of pain can be identified; they include specific physical repetitive movements, agitation, vocal repetitive behaviors, physical signs of pain, and changes in behavior from the norm for that person (40). Both inadequate and inappropriate treatment of persistent pain are major issues for these elders. Balfour and O'Rourke (41) in a Canadian study found that patients with dementia and persistent pain were more likely to have been treated with benzodiazepines and antipsychotics than were their patients without dementia, even after taking pain into account.

Detecting and assessing pain in older people lacking communication skills is a challenge and certainly more difficult, but not impossible, than it is for their cognitively intact counterparts. Several pain scales are now available for use with cognitively impaired patients who cannot conceptualize or verbally express their pain experience (37). As a result of more interest in the problems of pain in elders in the last decade, pain assessment and management is increasingly being incorporated into nursing home protocols, prompted by clinical practice guidelines such as those of the American Geriatrics Society (42).

THE SIGNIFICANCE OF ILLNESS IN LATE LIFE

Psychological stress can result from pathologic changes or the person's appraisal of the illness. An illness in late life may have a profound psychological impact, and the person may appraise a personal meaning about the relationship between themselves and the illness. The illness may represent a change, a threat, or a challenge, each view attracting quite different responses (43). Thus, an illness may represent a major life change, perhaps moving in with others, or even institutionalization. It may signify a threat to quality of life, or a loss of independence, mobility, and sometimes life. For some, illness presents the challenge of learning to be one's own care manager or developing new coping styles.

An older person also perceives an illness stressor from a generational or cohort view. People born in the earlier decades of the twentieth century differ in their worldviews from those born in the post–World War II period. It is useful to remember that today's older people have had lives of unprecedentedly rapid social and technologic change that has undoubtedly shaped their view of life and the way they perceive and respond to stressors (44). Many of today's elders are a cohort of people that were discouraged from expressing how they felt and encouraged to adopt a stoic approach to help them cope with global adverse events. Older people who have had particular adverse experiences such as war combat or the Holocaust or are victims of sexual abuse may have had a lifetime of seemingly good adjustment to their traumas. Yet, with the increased vulnerability of aging and physical illness, unresolved painful traumatic memories suppressed for many years may resurface (45).

STIGMA

If an illness makes a person appear to be "different" in any way, then it is stigmatizing. For example, stroke patients with hemiparesis appear physically distinctive, as do patients with abnormal bodily movements, Parkinsonism, or other physical defects (46). Patients may feel humiliated by having to resort to wheelchairs or walking sticks. Sudden reliance on such aids can diminish a person's confidence because they indicate loss of normal adult autonomy and independence to all and sundry.

Many factors influence the impact of stigma on the older person, including the presence of a medical diagnosis. In some cases, observable symptoms or impairments can serve to validate an illness and thus the associated activity restrictions and needs for caregiver assistance. This validation can be perceived in a positive way by some older persons, such as those with dependent personality traits and those seeking release from home or family responsibilities. The absence of a clear medical diagnosis increases the risk of negative effects from stigma, especially if symptoms are viewed as exaggerated or unfounded by medical professionals, family members, or peers. This is a common occurrence in some types of chronic pain conditions, such as myofascial pain syndromes. For older people, another significant source for negative feelings of stigmatization is the presence of mental health problems and involvement in psychiatric treatment (47).

EMOTIONAL RESPONSES TO PHYSICAL HEALTH STATUS

The cumulative effect of several disease states, anatomical deformations, pain, or loss of mobility all can adversely affect mood state (48). Negative mood states (e.g., depression, anger, fear) complicate the person's appraisal of an illness by negatively influencing the person's perception of the problem itself so that it may seem worse than the reality. Illness or disease, especially when unexpected, impacts on the individuals' personal sense of their ability to control what is happening to them. The attribute of "locus of control" is an individuals' perception of what might be happening to them as either significantly influenced by themselves or determined by external sources such as health care professionals, deities/religious/political figures, or chance/fate/luck. The Amsterdam Longitudinal aging study found that a dominant *external* locus of control is a dominant vulnerability factor for anxiety disorders in late life (49) and a strong *internal* locus of control is protective for depression in women (50). A longitudinal study of changes in physical functioning for older adults found that a predominant internal health locus of control was positively related to physical functioning (51) for women at all levels of baseline functioning but for men only with low physical functioning at baseline. Such beliefs are important to identify because of their protective influence on the process of adaptation; they are important in aging well and essential in coping with the vicissitudes and disappointments of late life (see below).

COPING

Folkman and Lazarus (52) define coping as "the variety of cognitive and behavioral efforts used by the individual to manage the specific external and internal demands that are appraised as exceeding the resources of the individual." Coping simply is the thoughts and actions used to restore a person's state of psychological equilibrium. Coping has two main functions. The first is to deal with the person–environmental relationship that is the source of the problem, and the second is to regulate the accompanying emotional response (43). When coping responses fail to do either of these two things, the person cannot maintain a psychological equilibrium and distress follows. If the disequilibrium or distress is severe, subnormal functioning or disability results. Multiple factors impinge upon an older person's perception of his or her ability to cope with or adapt to late life stressors, particularly to illness. Personality, education, cognitive skills, flexibility, resilience, and previous experience are all important elements in adjusting to and coping with an illness stressor. Individuals' sense of control will determine confidence in themselves to adapt and their belief in their self-efficacy to overcome the problem (53). Data from the MacArthur studies of successful aging indicate that strong self-efficacy beliefs have significant positive impact on subjective perception of functional disability, independent of objective physical limitations (54). Conversely, a dominant external locus of control undermines self-efficacy beliefs (53). High internality of control and a positive sense of self-efficacy are insufficient by themselves. Older people need to believe that their actions are safe and will not compromise them, that the expected outcome will be beneficial. If pain or illness affects mobility and activities of daily living, the older person may prefer to accept increased dependence rather than to struggle with difficulty to maintain self-reliance. For older people, maintaining a sense of self-efficacy is often a trade-off between the need for security and the need for preservation of autonomy or independence.

Coping is a dynamic process that aims to modify meaning of events and the accompanying stress response. Strategies can focus on the problem or the emotion the problem engenders or both (43). Problem-focused coping may be directed to the many practical problems faced by the older woman such as difficulties with normal daily activities such as dressing and mobility, or it may be directed to minimizing a health problem by ensuring good nutrition or adherence to treatment plans. People with a dominant internal locus of control and strong beliefs or self-efficacy are likely to use problem-focused strategies as a first-line resource. Emotion-focused coping concentrates on managing the emotional consequences of stressors such as any resulting anxiety, panic, or dysphoria but without changing the realities of the situation. Active, problem-based strategies are considered, in much of the literature, to be healthier than passive, emotion-based coping, which is considered less adaptive. For some people it is important to address both problem and emotion, either sequentially or simultaneously. Often, one or another aspect may predominate in an individual's coping responses. A person's coping styles are usually stable attributes of personality that have developed over a lifetime and they are influenced by the person's goals and situational intentions (43). Some research has shown that matching of interventions with an individual's primary coping style (i.e., problem-focused or emotion-focused) produces better symptom and psychological coping outcomes (55).

Coping strategies have been classified in other ways besides problem-focused versus emotion-focused, such as active (or instrumental) versus passive, behavioral versus cognitive, and illness-focused versus wellness-focused. There is some overlap in these rather artificial dichotomies especially for sick older people whose repertoire of coping responses may be limited. Homebound older people participating in an investigation on death and dying (56) indicated that the problems they considered necessary to cope with most were (a) physical pain and suffering, (b) risk to personal safety, and (c) threat to self-esteem and the uncertainty of life beyond death. Their coping responses were a mixture of active problem-focused strategies based on internal self-control and seeking social support, but also they successfully used more passive emotion-based coping styles of prayer and preoccupation with objects of attachment. Some cognitive and behavioral strategies such as reinterpretation, mental distraction, and meditation and use of relaxation techniques can be viewed as both passive and active. Other adaptive passive strategies commonly used by older people include acceptance, resignation, humor, and prayer.

Religious coping can span many of these categories of coping. Koenig, George, and Peterson (57) studied elderly medically ill patients and found that those with intrinsic religious or spiritual beliefs had more rapid remission of associated depressive symptoms. Adaptive religious coping also predicted a more positive medical outcome in medically ill older people two years later (58). When an individual has to contend with an uncontrollable and extremely threatening stressor such as a terminal illness, or if the more active strategies have failed, such passive and more reflective styles are both effective and beneficial in controlling associated distress and depression (56). Indeed, when conditions of stress are unchangeable, problem-focused coping is associated with poorer outcomes than the more passive emotion-based coping (43).

However, some emotion-focused, passive styles such as "catastrophizing" (i.e., cognitively overestimating the significance and impact of an event or circumstance) can be as much a means of appraising a stressful situation as a way of coping with a problem (59). As a means of coping with the vicissitudes and trials of late life, catastrophizing leads to greater depression, disability, poorer social support, prolonged illness, increased pain, and poorer all round psychological adjustment to adverse events (60). It is important to identify maladaptive coping styles such as catastrophizing, because these may be amenable to interventions such as cognitive-behavioral therapy.

TRIUMPH, STRENGTH, AND SURVIVORSHIP

Although this chapter has, so far, concentrated on the vicissitudes and disappointments that can occur in the lives of older women, it is important to recognize that older women do survive; they do triumph, and many do age well despite them. There are losses and gains, decreases in some skills and optimization of others, with many older people developing the more reflective "wisdom" skills. Several terms are used in an extensive literature to describe "survivorship" such as healthy aging, successful aging, positive aging, or aging well. Rowe and Kahn (61) used rather rigid medically biased criteria to define successful aging, such as (a) absence of disease, disability, and risk factors like high blood pressure, smoking, or obesity; (b) maintaining physical and mental functioning; and (c) active engagement with life. In contrast, Baltes and Carstenson (62) offered a much broader perspective as "doing the best with what one has," a concept more in keeping with a mental health focus. Considerable evidence points out that physical illness, hospitalization, poor vision and hearing, restricted mobility, and restricted social networks are high risk factors for poorer adaptation, negative psychological functioning, and depression, as discussed previously. Subjective well-being often declines as functional limitations increase, and thus older women would certainly seem to be more at risk to less successful aging (63), but this is not the whole story by any means. Older people themselves view successful aging as a complex issue, and several studies indicate that they value the ability to adapt, to be able to focus on gains rather than losses, a sense of psychological well-being, and social engagement far more than maintaining physical or cognitive functioning (64). Even at the very end of life, when a person is dying, these positive attributes of adaptation, focus on gains, hope, and social engagement are important factors in dying well (65). Although personality and personal attributes developed throughout the life cycle, a sense of control and positive self-efficacy contribute hugely to an older person's capacity to adapt, cope, age, and die well, there are still many things that health professionals can do to assist in helping all older people, and especially the majority who are women, deal with the challenges of late life. We can identify which older people are most at risk for mental disorders: the physically ill, the old, the isolated, the recently bereaved, the poor, and the socially restricted (18). For many older people, we can treat symptoms of illness, pain, and depression very successfully assisting greatly with quality of life. We can discourage risky behaviors, and we can target individual and social interventions that encourage social engagement, maintain confidence, foster family relationships, assist with attainment of goals for living, and promote subjective well-being. "Triumph and survivorship," facilitating older women to do the best they can under sometimes difficult circumstances, should be a main aim for mental health care of all older women.

REFERENCES

1. Kuhn M. Quoted in: New Age 1979 (February).
2. Anderson GF, Hussey PS. Population aging: a comparison among industrialized countries. Health Aff 2000;9(3):191–203.
3. New Zealand Ministry of Health. Health of Older People in New Zealand. A Statistical Reference. Wellington, New Zealand: Ministry of Health, 2002:21–22.
4. Arber S, Ginn J. Gender and inequalities in health in later life. Soc Sci Med 1993;36(1):33–46.
5. Butler R. On behalf of older women: another reason to protect Medicare and Medicaid. N Engl J Med 1996;334(12):794–796.
6. Williams K, Kurina L. The social structure, stress, and women's health. Clin Obstet Gynaecol 2002;45(4):1099–1118.
7. Krause N. Stressors in salient social roles and well-being in later life. J Gerontol Psychol Sci 1994;49(3):137–148.
8. Devanand D, Kim M, Paykina N, et al. Adverse life events in elderly patients with major depression or dysthymic disorder and in healthy-control subjects. Am J Geriatr Psychiatry 2002;10:265–274.
9. Zettel L, Rook K. Substitution and compensation in the social networks of older widowed women. Psychol Aging 2004;19(3):433–443.
10. Troll L. Family-embedded vs. family-deprived oldest-old: a study of contrasts. Int J Aging Hum Dev 1994;38(1):51–63.
11. Wilcox S, Evenson K, Aragaki A, et al. The effects of widowhood on physical and mental health, health behaviors, and health outcomes: The Women's Health Initiative. Health Psychol 2003;22(5):513–522.
12. Murphy E. Social origins of depression in old age. Br J Psychiatry 1982;141:135–142.
13. Thomas P, Goodwin J, Goodwin J. Effect of social support and stress related changes in cholesterol, uric acid level and immune function in an elderly sample. Am J Psychiatry 1985;142(6):735–737.
14. Wenger G, Tucker I. Using network variation in practice: identification of support network type. Health Soc Care Commun 2002;10(1):28–35.
15. Wenger GC. Support networks of older people: a guide for practitioners. Bangor: Centre for Social Policy Research and Development, University of Wales, 1994.
16. Smith J, Baltes P. Profiles of psychological functioning in the old and oldest old. Psychol Aging 1997;12(3):458–472.
17. Johnson C, Troll LE. Family functioning in late late life. J Gerontol Nurs 1992;47(2):S66–72.
18. Taylor R. Elderly persons at risk. In: Copeland J, Abou-Saleh M, Blazer D, eds. Principles and Practice of Geriatric Psychiatry. New York: Wiley, 1994:116–122.
19. Davies A. Life events, health, adaptation and social support. In: Woods R, ed. Handbook of the Clinical Psychology of Ageing. New York: Wiley, 1996:115–140.
20. Smith J, Borchelt M, Maier H, et al. Health and well-being in the young old and oldest old. J Soc Issues 2002;58(4):715–732.
21. Roberto K. The study of chronic pain in later life: where are the women? J Women Aging 1994;6(4):1–7.
22. Marsiske M, Klumb P, Baltes M. Everyday activity patterns and sensory functioning in old age. Psychol Aging 1997;12(3):444–457.
23. Farrell M, Gibson S, Helme R. The effect of medical status on the activity level of elderly chronic pain patients. J Am Geriatr Soc 1995;43:102–107.
24. Thomas E, Peat G, Harris L, et al. The prevalence of pain and pain interference in a general population of older adults: cross-sectional findings from the North Staffordshire Osteoarthritis Project (NorStOP). Pain 2004;110(1–2):361–368.

25. Gloth F. Geriatric pain: factors that limit pain relief and increase complications. Geriatrics 2000;55(10):46–48, 51–44.
26. Melding P. Who is losing the language? Persistent pain in home-dwelling elders. Age Ageing 2004;33(5):432–434.
27. McLean W, Higginbotham N. Prevalence of pain among nursing home residents in rural New South Wales. Med J Aust 2002;177(1):17–20.
28. Fox PL, Raina P, Jadad AR. Prevalence and treatment of pain in older adults in nursing homes and other long-term care institutions: a systematic review. CMAJ 1999;160(3):329–333.
29. Gibson S, Voukelatos X, Ames D, et al. An examination of pain perception and cerebral event-related potentials following carbon dioxide laser stimulation in patients with Alzheimer's disease and age-matched control volunteers. Pain Res Manag 2001;6(3):126–132.
30. Scherder E. Low use of analgesics in Alzheimer's disease: possible mechanisms. Psychiatry 2000;63(1):1–12.
31. Widar M, Samuelsson L, Karlsson-Tivenius S, et al. Long term pain conditions after stroke. J Rehab Med 2002;34(4):165–170.
32. Yates P, Dewar A, Fentiman B. Pain: the views of elderly people living in long-term residential care settings. J Adv Nurs 1995;21(4):667–674.
33. Pitkala K, Strandberg TE, Tilvis R. Management of nonmalignant pain in home-dwelling older people: a population-based survey. J Am Geriatr Soc 2002;50(11):1861–1865.
34. Parmelee P. Pain and psychological function in late life. In: Mostofsky D, Lomrantz J, eds. Handbook of Pain and Aging. New York: Plenum, 1997:207–226.
35. Williamson G, Schulz R. Pain, activity restriction and symptoms of depression among community-residing elderly adults. J Gerontol Nurs 1992;46:367–372.
36. Catell H. Elderly suicide in London: an analysis of coroner's inquests. Int J Geriatr Psychiatry 1988;3:251–261.
37. Frampton M. Experience assessment and management of pain in people with dementia. Age Ageing 2003;32:248–251.
38. Buffum MD, Miaskowski C, Sands L, et al. A pilot study of the relationship between discomfort and agitation in patients with dementia. Geriatr Nurs 2001;22(2):80–85.
39. Cohen-Mansfield J, Lipson S. Pain in cognitively impaired nursing home residents: how well are physicians diagnosing it? J Am Geriatr Soc 2002;50(6):1039–1044.
40. Kovach CR, Weissman DE, Griffie J, et al. Assessment and treatment of discomfort for people with late-stage dementia. J Pain Symptom Manage 1999;18(6):412–419.
41. Balfour J, O'Rourke N. Older adults with Alzheimer disease, comorbid arthritis and prescription of psychotropic medications. Pain Res Manag 2003;8(4):198–204.
42. GS Panel on Persistent Pain in Older Persons. The management of persistent pain in older persons. J Am Geriatr Soc 2002;50:205–224.
43. Lazarus R. Coping with aging: individuality as a key to understanding. In: Nordhus I, VanderBos G, Berg S, et al., eds. Clinical Geropsychology. Washington, DC: American Psychological Association, 1998:109–127.
44. Costa P, Yang J, McCrae R. Ageing and personality traits: generalizations and clinical implications. In: Nordhus I, VanderBos G, Berg S, et al., eds. Clinical Geropsychology. Washington, DC: American Psychological Association, 1998:33–48.
45. Clipp E, Elder G. The aging veteran of World War II: psychiatric and life course insights. In: Ruskin P, Talbott J, eds. Aging and Post Traumatic Stress Disorder. Washington, DC: American Psychiatric Press, 1996:19–51.
46. Caap-Ahlgren M, Lannerheim L. Older Swedish women's experiences of living with symptoms related to Parkinson's disease. J Adv Nurs 2002;39(1):87–95.
47. de Mendonça Lima CA, Levav I, Jacobsson L, et al. Stigma and discrimination against older people with mental disorders in Europe. Int J Geriatr Psychiatry 2003;18(8):679–682.
48. Lindesay J. The Guy's/Age Concern survey: physical health and psychiatric disorder in an urban elderly community. Int J Geriatr Psychiatry 1990;5:171–178.
49. Beekman A, Bremmer M, Deeg D, et al. Anxiety disorders in later life: a report from the Longitudinal Aging Study Amsterdam. Int J Geriatr Psychiatry 1998;13(10):717–726.
50. Van den Heuvel N, Smits C, Deeg D, et al. Personality: a moderator of the relation between cognitive functioning and depression in adults aged 55–85. J Affect Disord 1996;41(3):229–240.
51. Wallhagen M, Strawbridge W, Kaplan G, et al. Impact of internal locus of control on health outcomes for older men and women: a longitudinal perspective. Gerontologist 1994;34:299–306.
52. Folkman S, Lazarus R. An analysis of coping in a middle aged sample. J Health Soc Behav 1980; 21:219–239.
53. Williams J, Koocher G. Addressing loss of control in chronic illness: theory and practice. Psychotherapy 1998;35:325–335.
54. Seeman TE, Unger J, McAvay G, et al. Self-efficacy beliefs and perceived declines in functional ability: MacArthur studies of successful aging. J Gerontology. Ser B. Psychol Sci Soc Sci 1999; 54(4):214–222.

55. Fry P, Wong P. Pain management training in the elderly: matching interventions with subjects' coping styles. Stress Med 1991;7:93–98.

56. Fry P. A factor analytic investigation of home-bound elderly individuals' concerns about death and dying, and their coping responses. J Clin Psychol 1990,46(6):737 748.

57. Koenig HG, George LK, Peterson BL. Religiosity and remission of depression in medically ill older patients. Am J Psychiatry 1998;155(4):536–542.

58. Pargament K, Koenig H, Tarakeshwar N, et al. Religious coping methods as predictors of psychological, physical and spiritual outcomes among medically ill elderly patients: a two-year longitudinal study. J Health Psychol 2004;9(6):713–730.

59. Lackner JM, Gurtman MB. Pain catastrophizing and interpersonal problems: a circumplex analysis of the communal coping model. Pain 2004;110(3):597–604.

60. Severeijns R, van den Hout M, Vlaeyen J, et al. Pain catastrophizing and general health status in a large Dutch community sample. Pain 2002;99(1–2):367–376.

61. Rowe JW, Kahn R. Successful aging. New York: Pantheon, 1998.

62. Baltes M, Carstensen L. The process of successful aging. Ageing Soc 1996;16:397–422.

63. Smith J, Baltes P. Trends and profiles of psychological functioning in very old age. In: Baltes PB, Mayer K, eds. The Berlin Aging Study: aging from 70 to 100. 1999:197–226.

64. Phelan E, Anderson L, Lacroix A, et al. Older adults' views of "successful aging": how do they compare with researchers' definitions? J Am Geriatr Soc 2004;52(2):211–216.

65. Sullivan MD. Hope and hopelessness at the end of life. Am J Geriatr Psychiatry 2003;11:393–405.

Health Services for Women

Section VII Summary
An Historical Perspective

Joan Busfield

The idea that a person can become mad or experience some disturbance of mind has a very long history and predates the development of any services for dealing with or helping such individuals. Terms such as "madness" and "mental disturbance" embody the recognition that these conditions constitute a problem either for the persons themselves or for those around them. We can see two historical strands that led to the emergence of services for persons with mental disturbance. On the one hand, persons disturbed in mind, or their families, might seek help for their problems from a range of healers, particularly if they had the resources to do so. People would seek help for a wide spectrum of problems, ranging from the very severe, real madness, to the less severe, being "troubled in mind." Treatments provided also varied widely (1). On the other hand, particularly as urbanization and industrialization spread, separate "madhouses" and asylums for those considered mad were established by private entrepreneurs, charitable groups, or local authorities and soon expanded in size. Initially asylums were for persons with severe disturbances—individuals who were "out of their minds" and either difficult to look after or control, or deemed to represent some form of threat to social order.

The emergence of a specialist grouping of medical practitioners concentrating on the treatment of what came to be called mental illness can be linked to the growing importance of madhouses and asylums in the nineteenth century with the first use of the term "psychiatry" occurring in the middle of that century. These professionals increasingly defined and categorized the terrain of mental illness in order to make sense of the problems with which they were called upon to deal. In the process, the definition of mental illness was broadened, and new categories of mental illness were created. Whereas in the nineteenth century much of the focus was on disorders of thought, by the middle of the twentieth century, there was a growing attention to disorders of affect or emotion, as well as to disorders constructed primarily in terms of behavior rather than thought or emotion (2). Since the mid-twentieth century, there has been a new focus on services that do not involve confinement, legally compulsory or otherwise. There has also been a growing reliance on psychotropic medicines as the solution to problems of mental health. This trend has developed almost regardless of psychiatrists' ideas about causation of mental illness, which are often broader and more eclectic than their treatment practices would suggest.

How have women fared under the emergence of these complex and changing mental health systems of advanced Western societies? Official psychiatric constructions of mental illness, grounded as they are in notions of scientific objectivity, now tend to be largely gender blind. Nonetheless, gender necessarily permeates practice within the mental health services. In the first place, patients or clients are always gendered individuals, and service providers, like other people, necessarily respond to them as gendered individuals in terms of their expectations and understandings. Moreover, the distribution of problems constituted as mental illnesses varies by gender, in part because the factors that can give rise to these disorders are not equally distributed by gender. Simplifying a complex picture, we can say that whereas the levels of thought disorders such as schizophrenia do not vary much by gender (though there are differences in onset—see Kulkarni and Bertrand, Chapter 14 in this volume), disorders of emotion, such as depression, tend to be more common in women (see Rhodes, Chapter 26, and Astbury, Chapter 27, in the present section of this volume). In contrast, many disorders of behavior, such as drug-related disorders and antisocial conduct disorders, tend to occur more frequently in men. This means not only that gendered expectations inform and shape clinicians' work, but also that men and women are differentially represented in the services provided and differentially affected by the treatments offered. Consequently if, as Jill Astbury argues in Chapter 27, we need to look at the social causes of depression and not simply routinely regard psychotropic medication as adequate treatment, then this is more an issue for women than for men because women are more likely to experience depression as the category is currently constituted.

Indeed what is needed above all is greater attention to the reality of women's lives and the difficulties they face. Concentration on changing women's lives for the better is the key project if we are to improve women's mental health.

REFERENCES

1. MacDonald M. Mystical Bedlam, Madness, Anxiety and Healing in Seventeenth Century England. Cambridge: Cambridge University Press, 1981.
2. Busfield J. The archaeology of psychiatric disorder: gender and disorders of thought, emotion and behaviour. In: Bendelor G, Carpenter M, Vautier C, et al. eds. Gender, Health and Healing. London: Routledge, 2002.

CHAPTER 26

Mental Health Services for Women

Anne E. Rhodes

WOMEN'S NEED FOR AND USE OF MENTAL HEALTH SERVICES

The assessment of need for mental health services occurs at multiple and interacting levels of society. While debate continues about how best to define and measure that need for services for the purposes of resource allocation, the consensus seems to be that key dimensions are diagnosis of a mental illness; duration of the illness; disability and distress associated with the illness; and the risk of harm to self and others (1–3). Additional dimensions considered are the proportion of the population affected and likely to benefit (directly or indirectly) from treatment; the monetary costs of providing the treatment; and the risk of adverse outcomes from treatment (4).

This chapter focuses on major (unipolar) depression and mental health services for women. Depression is one of the most common mental disorders in the general population. About 10% of women annually suffer from major depression in what could be the most joyful and productive years of their lives. Depression is one of the most common hospital discharge diagnoses for women aged 18 to 44 years (obstetrical care being the most common discharge diagnosis). Because depression affects women during their childbearing and child-rearing years, untreated depression may also have health consequences for the offspring (5). The functional impairment of depression is comparable to or greater than that of a number of chronic medical conditions (6). It takes a sizable economic toll in the workplace through reduced productivity and absenteeism (7,8). The Global Burden of Disease Study found that in established market economies, depression ranks second in terms of disability-adjusted life years. It is projected to displace ischemic heart disease as the leading source of disease burden over the next 20 years (9). Further studies echo these findings (10). Depression is associated with premature mortality from cardiovascular disease (11) and suicide. Among those diagnosed with depression, case fatality rates of suicide range between 2% and 6% (12), and depression is a factor in at least 60% of suicides (11).

By definition, a clinical diagnosis of a major depressive episode according to the DSM-IV system of classification of mental disorders implies that significant disability and distress are associated with the symptoms. Depending upon severity, an episode is defined as being mild, moderate, or severe (13). The DSM system, necessary for clinical practice, was not originally designed for the broad purpose of describing pathology in the general population. Depression is thought to be a dimensional construct that falls along a severity continuum that can lead to significant distress and disability. Conditions that do not meet diagnostic criteria are more prevalent in the general population than major depression and can be as disabling (14–17).

WOMEN, DEPRESSION, AND THE NEED FOR MENTAL HEALTH SERVICES

One of the most robust findings from surveys conducted internationally is the twofold higher prevalence of major depression in women compared to men. Although prevalence estimates vary widely between countries, the difference between women and men in these estimates does not. This gender difference emerges between the ages of 11 and 13 years. While hormonal factors may play a role, the link is not yet clear at this age, nor is it clear for the transition to menopause (18).

It has been postulated that the reason more women are identified as having depression than men is that women live longer, have longer episodes of depression, and have more frequent episodes than men. Therefore, when data are collected at one point in time, depression appears to be more common in women. Women are more likely to have a first onset of depression than men; however, there is less evidence to conclude whether the course of the depression varies significantly for men and women. In general, it has been difficult to draw firm conclusions about the etiology and natural history of depression due to problems with lifetime recall and the lack of longitudinal data in representative samples (18,19). As well, the course of illness may be affected by variations in the way men and women use mental health services over time.

A further complication is that depression tends to co-occur with other mental illnesses. Persons with depression are more likely to suffer from anxiety disorders, which, like depression, are more common in women than men (20). Indeed, the pathway for depression in women may be through anxiety disorders (18), although these disorders do not seem to account for the greater prevalence of depression in women (21). After anxiety disorders, substance abuse is the most common mental illness to co-occur with depression in women. While women may report that their depression antedates their substance abuse, depression may also be a result of the substance abuse (22).

A core symptom of depression is suicidal ideation. Suicidal ideation, plans, and behaviors may arise from depression or from other conditions (e.g., borderline personality disorder or eating disorder) or life contexts (e.g., a history of physical or sexual abuse) that co-occur with depression. In treatment settings, approximately one third of persons with depression are suicidal (23). Although men are more likely to die from suicide than women, women engage in more suicidal behaviors, putting themselves at risk for physical harm, associated disabilities, and premature mortality.

THE TREATMENT OF DEPRESSION IN WOMEN

Clinical depression is quite treatable with antidepressants or some psychotherapies or a combination of antidepressants and psychotherapy (24–26). The average duration of a depressive episode is about three months (27). For antidepressants to be effective, they need to be taken a minimum of two months (28); therefore, some consistency or continuity of care with a primary care physician or a referral to a psychiatrist is desirable. A minimum of four counseling visits has been defined as appropriate for follow-up and medication monitoring (29–31). While the hormonal links with depression are not well understood, hormonal factors may play a role in treatment response. There is some research to suggest that men and women differ in their response to different classes of antidepressants. Women's response may differ from men's as well depending upon age-related or hormonal factors (32). Current evidence is insufficient to recommend estrogen therapy as a primary treatment for major depression in perimenopausal and menopausal women (33). Nonpharmacologic treatment of depression includes psychotherapy and, in special circumstances, electroconvulsive therapy. Psychotherapy generally requires multiple sessions with experts who have received specialized training. Combining or sequencing pharmacologic and psychotherapy may provide more long-term benefit than any one therapy alone. Combined therapies may be particularly worth pursuing in those who have a past history of depression (34). In women with a concurrent anxiety disorder, treatment for depression should be initiated as it may improve the symptoms of both disorders. Substance abuse is not a contraindication to treatment of depression. Aggressive treatment may reduce the use of these substances (35).

Until recently, there has been a lack of systematic evidence and guidelines about how to treat suicidal individuals, apart from or in addition to their mental illness (36–39). Controversy continues regarding the relative merits of prescribing the newer antidepressants to suicidal individuals. While they are less toxic if taken in overdose, use of these medications in persons under 18 years of age may be related to an increased risk of suicide-related adverse events (40). If that risk is true, young women may be of greatest concern given a greater likelihood of being prescribed these medications.

During pregnancy women are not "protected" from depression. Pregnant women are at a greater risk when there is a past history of depression, younger age, limited social and economic resources, greater number of children, and ambivalence about the pregnancy. Antidepressant treatment during pregnancy is based on the risks of untreated depression for the mother and what is known about the risks of spontaneous pregnancy loss or teratogenicity of specific antidepressant agents. Less is known about the risks of specific antidepressants for infants during lactation. Mothers may wish to pursue nonpharmacologic options or take antidepressants and provide infant formula. Treatment for women with concurrent substance abuse is particularly important during pregnancy and the postpartum, given that the toxic effects of substances may affect fetal development and early attachment to caregivers. Postpartum psychosis is a rare but severe form of depression that occurs within about two weeks of delivery and requires rapid psychiatric treatment (5,41).

WOMEN, DEPRESSION, AND THE USE OF MENTAL HEALTH SERVICES

Over the past two decades, a series of large mental health surveys has been conducted in a number of countries. A consistent finding across countries was that, compared to men, women in their reproductive years were about twice as likely to use mental health services, largely outpatient (3,42,43).

This may be so for a number of reasons. It has been hypothesized that men and women do not really differ in their use of mental health services; rather, they differ in the types of mental illness they have. It is the type of mental illness that determines use of services. Men are more likely to have substance use disorders or antisocial behaviors or both, whereas women are more likely to have mood or anxiety disorders or both. Use of mental health services is more common among persons with mood and anxiety disorders, which do seem to mediate gender differences in service use, but only partially (20). Somatic symptoms may be particularly relevant. Gender differences in use were not found in Puerto Rico (3). In this sample somatization, an anxiety disorder, was as common in men as women, unlike in other countries (44).

Because women tend to have lower socioeconomic status (SES) than men, when measures of need such as type of mental illness are held constant, one might expect women to be *less* likely to use mental health services than men, particularly specialty services, due to greater financial barriers. This does seem to be the case in settings where insurance coverage is uneven or lacking. Nevertheless, the converse does not seem to be true. Although women are more likely to use mental health services than men in Ontario, Canada, where medical and hospital services are covered by national health insurance, these gender differences in use are not higher than those in countries with less coverage (43).

It is often proposed that women are more willing to seek help for mental health problems than men, and this translates into greater use of services. Work by Leaf and Livingston Bruce in the New Haven Epidemiologic Catchment Area (ECA) site in the United States examined the relationships between willingness to seek help, mental disorder, and gender with use (45). While the findings were suggestive, insufficient statistical power to fully test these hypotheses and cross-sectional data limited this investigation. In cross-sectional studies, measures of willingness to seek help may be proxies for past use. In a follow-up study of the Puerto Rico sample, past use was reported more commonly by women than men and was strongly associated with current use. When levels of need and use over time were examined, men were more likely to report use when their level of need was at the highest level (46). Taken together, these findings suggest that even when the effects of disorder and SES are taken into account, men seek help when their illness is more severe.

What happens to depressed men and women when they enter the formal health care system may also be quite different. Few researchers have been able to study the relationships between gender, depression, and the use of different types of providers over time in the general population. Two large surveys examined gender and depression according to the use of primary and specialty care providers. In the ECA survey, among those with new onsets of mental illness, women were more likely than men to report use in the primary care sector (47). In a prospective study of mental health visits to physicians according to claims data in Ontario, women were about twice as likely as men to be seen by primary care physicians, whereas men were about twice as likely to be seen by psychiatrists (48). The preferential use of primary care by women in both studies, regardless of measures of need and SES, is of interest. In light of the fact that the Ontario study was based on insurance claims data, the patterns are not attributable to a reporting bias (49,50). Essentially, women who had depression were more likely than men to be seen by a primary care physician, and women without demonstrable need were also more likely than men to be seen by a primary care physician. In the Ontario study, persons who saw psychiatrists made more visits than those who saw primary care physicians only. For those who saw physicians, very few reported seeing physicians *and* nonmedical providers for mental health reasons (50).

IMPLICATIONS FOR HEALTH CARE PLANNING AND DIRECTIONS FOR FUTURE RESEARCH

The findings from these studies raise two main concerns. First, if women are not in demonstrable need, should they be accessing mental health services? Earlier it was noted that depression is not a rigid category. In primary care settings, there are more persons whose illness is subthreshold or minor in nature. Some may remit, some may become worse, and some may be recovering from a previous episode of depression. While ongoing treatment may be indicated in the latter scenario, supportive care and monitoring may be as effective in the other scenarios (35). An argument has been made that mild cases in treatment consist of high proportions of older, well-educated females who are at low risk of progressing to serious mental illness (42). Moral hazard is said to occur when patients or clinicians demand payment for care that is not needed.

The second issue pertains to whether women with depression are receiving adequate treatment for their depression in the primary care sector. Concerns about the detection and treatment of depression in primary care are long-standing (51,52). Although trials have demonstrated the benefits of treating depression in primary care settings, uncertainty remains about the quality of care under real-world conditions (53). Adherence to mental health clinical practice guidelines falters without specific intervention, typically multifaceted and resource-intensive (54). The most recent data from the National Comorbidity Survey found that only about 22% of persons with depression in the United States reported treatment that was adequate in relation to treatment guidelines (31). Currently in North America, routine screening of adults for depression is not recommended without systems in place that assure accurate diagnosis, effective treatment, and follow-up (55).

Much of the care for depression takes place in the primary care sector and consists of pharmacotherapy and supportive counseling. A trend of less psychotherapy and increased pharmacotherapy for depression has been reported in the United States that is thought to have arisen from a greater awareness of depression, marketing of antidepressants, and managed care strategies that limit contact with specialty providers (56). Related to this trend, a large drop in visits to nonmedical providers was observed for those with mood disorders, but this drop was not offset by conjoint care (57).

A fear is that these trends may be responsible for the suboptimal detection and treatment of depression in the primary care sector for women. Much of sub-threshold or minor depression may represent women who remain in care because they have not yet recovered from their initial episode. Less advantaged women may not persist in treatment given insurance and medication costs. While more advantaged women may not fully benefit, less advantaged women may not receive any benefit if they cannot afford treatment. In the absence of alternatives, their illness may become severe with patterns of use of services resembling those of men. However, when men access care, their depression may be detected and treated more aggressively for fear of suicide (58). Men may also be more able to afford specialty services. A disturbing consequence would be if women end up having to prove they cannot work so that they can go on long-term disability insurance in order to pay for treatment.

Cross-sectional data do not capture these processes well. Nevertheless, payers may apply cross-sectional data to justify curtailing use of mental health services for conditions that are not considered severe. From the perspective of third-party payers, managing fewer people with more severe illness may cut costs and boost profits. From a societal perspective, the hidden costs of impaired functioning in social roles from a less severely ill but larger proportion of the population may be immense. In the absence of alternatives, some women would become severely ill, and their use of services might then follow that of less advantaged women.

Effective cheaper treatment alternatives for women whose illness is not severe are worth pursuing. Indeed, the large increase in antidepressant prescription rates, associated costs (59), and potential for adverse events behooves researchers and policy makers to examine alternatives. To the extent that depression is an illness that falls along a severity continuum in the population, bolstering universal interventions that traditionally fall outside of the health care sector, such as affordable child care, may aid both more socially advantaged and disadvantaged women. However, greater coordination between health and social service agencies would be necessary to ensure that policies are integrated before implementation.

Offering promise for women clearly suffering from depression are insurance coverage parity and reforms to primary care (e.g., shared care models and changes in the mix or supply of providers). Currently, for many women treatment may consist of pharmacotherapy or supportive counseling or a combination. Notwithstanding the costs, once the severity of the depression has abated, women may wish to discontinue antidepressants because of side effects such as weight gain or inability to achieve sexual climax. There may also be issues of safety to consider, such as suicidality in younger women. Women who are pregnant or lactating may not wish to take antidepressants. In these instances, evidence-based psychotherapies may be effective first lines of treatment. Combining pharmacotherapy and psychotherapy initially or in phases may help women to recover fully from depression (34). For women who are not responding to treatment, stepped care models that increase the range and intensity of interventions may be necessary. Consultation with specialty providers is recommended when symptoms include suicidality or are psychotic in nature or when concurrent disorders are complicating treatment response (35). Currently, there is a shortage of a skilled workforce trained in evidence-based psychotherapies (24,34). Personnel would need to be trained and recruited for this work.

New treatment models may be designed better, specifically to triage populations of concern. Few clinical trials of acute depression have included ethnic minorities. Ongoing research suggests that Black and Latina women also benefit from antidepressants and psychotherapy (34). Access to care for socially disadvantaged women may need to be carefully tailored to their needs because they face greater barriers to care such as less flexible work hours and access to transportation and child care (60). Women with young children, including those who are pregnant, may not be able to participate in treatment without child care. Women with concurrent substance abuse, pregnant or not, may not disclose substance use for fear of stigma, loss of financial stability, and loss of custody of their children. Depending upon the nature and severity of the substance abuse, brief interventions may prevent substance dependence and associated physical health problems. Women may avoid seeking help for substance use disorders in traditional mixed-sex specialty care settings. Research on whether women with substance abuse problems do better in settings that serve women only and with female providers is limited and conflicting. Lesbians or women with histories of physical or sexual abuse may prefer treatment from same-sex providers (61,62).

In conclusion, it is not known whether women with less severe conditions are accessing primary care to their overall benefit or detriment. Because these women make up a larger proportion of the population (whether in care or not) interventions in the form of withdrawing or reallocating resources demand research and careful planning across health and social service agencies. For women who are clearly suffering from depression, primary care reform and parity of insurance coverage provide hope in improving the detection and treatment of depression. Nevertheless, reforms will require substantial investment and realignment of professional roles (63). To assure reforms are succeeding, longitudinal studies of the full population will be vital in assessing improvements over time in treatment uptake and response without increasing existing disparities. This information can be used to shape where reforms are necessary and to establish a baseline from which to evaluate reforms. The information can also be used as an accountability mechanism for citizens, communities, and governments. Stigma, shame, and the symptoms of depression may prevent women from advocating for a critical discourse on the dominant paradigms, related therapies, practices, and resource allocation. Historically, women have been underrepresented in medicine and economic political structures that govern health care delivery expenditures. More and more women are making their individual and collective health needs and priorities known (64).[a]

REFERENCES

1. Mechanic D. Is the prevalence of mental disorders a good measure of the need for services? Health Affairs 2003;22:8–20.
2. Regier DA. Mental disorder diagnostic theory and practical reality: an evolutionary perspective. Health Affairs 2003;22:21–27.

[a]*Dr. Rhodes is supported by a Career Scientist Award from the Ontario Ministry of Health and Long-Term Care. The opinions, results, and conclusions are those of the author and no endorsement by the Ministry is intended or should be inferred.*

3. Andrews G. Unmet Need in Psychiatry. Cambridge, UK: University Press, 2000.
4. Mechanic D. Policy challenges in improving mental health services: some lessons from the past. Psychiatric Services 2003;54:1227–1232.
5. Blehar M. Public health context of women's mental health research. Psychiatr Clin North Am 2003;26:781–789.
6. Wells KB, Stewart A, Hays R. The functioning and well-being of depressed patients: results from the Medical Outcomes Study. JAMA 1989;262:914–919.
7. Conti D, Burton W. The economic burden of depression in a workplace. J Occup Med 1994;36:983–988.
8. Simon GE, Barber C, Birnbaum H, et al. Depression and work productivity: the comparative costs of treatment versus nontreatment. J Occup Environ Med 2001;43:2–9.
9. Murray C, Lopez A. The Global Burden of Disease: A Comprehensive Assessment of Mortality and Disability from Diseases, Injuries, and Risk Factors in 1990 and Projected to 2020. Cambridge, MA: Harvard University Press, 1996.
10. Sanderson K, Andrews G, Corry J, et al. Reducing the burden of affective disorders: is evidence-based health care affordable? J Affect Dis 2003;77:109–125.
11. Remick R. Diagnosis and management of depression in primary care: a clinical update and review. Can Med Assoc J 2002;167:1253–1260.
12. Bostwick J, Pankratz V. Affective disorders and suicide risk: a reexamination. Am J Psychiatry 2000;157:1925–1932.
13. American Psychiatric Association. Diagnostic and Statistical Manual of Mental Disorders. 4th Ed. Washington, DC, 1994.
14. Murphy J. Diagnostic schedule and rating scales in adult psychiatry. In: Tsuang M, Tohen M, Zahner G, eds. Textbook in Psychiatric Epidemiology. Toronto: Wiley, 1995.
15. Judd L, Paulus M, Wells K, et al. Socieconomic burden of subsyndromal depressive symptoms and major depression in a sample of the general population. Am J Psychiatry 1996;153:1411–1417.
16. Pincus H, Davis W, McQueen L. "Subthreshold" mental disorders: a review and synthesis of studies on minor depression and other "brand names." Br J Psychiatry 1999;174:288–296.
17. Horwath E, Johnson J, Klerman G, et al. Depressive symptoms as relative and attributable risk factors for first-onset major depression. Arch Gen Psychiatry 1992;49:817–823.
18. Kessler RC. Epidemiology of women and depression. J Affect Dis 2003;74:5–13.
19. Ustun T. Cross-national epidemiology of depression and gender. J Gend Specific Med 2000;3:54–58.
20. Rhodes A, Goering P, To T, et al. Gender and outpatient mental health service use. Soc Sci Med 2002;54:1–10.
21. Simonds V, Whiffen V. Are gender differences in depression explained by gender differences in co-morbid anxiety? J Affect Dis 2003;77:197–202.
22. Sinha R, Rounsaville B. Sex differences in depressed substance abusers. J Clin Psychiatry 2002;63:616–627.
23. Cooper-Patrick L, Crum R, Ford D. Characteristics of patients with major depression who received care in general medical and specialty mental health settings. Med Care 1994;32:15–24.
24. CANMAT. Canadian Network for Mood and Anxiety Treatments: Guidelines for Diagnosis and Pharmacologic Treatment of Depression. Toronto, 1999.
25. APA. The American Psychiatric Association Practice Guidelines for the Treatment of Patients with Major Depressive Disorder (Revision). Am J Psychiatry 2000;Suppl 157:1–45.
26. Persons J, Thase M, Crits-Christoph P. The role of psychotherapy in the treatment of depression: review of two practice guidelines. Arch Gen Psychiatry 1996;53:283–290.
27. Ustun T, Kessler R. Global burden of depressive disorders: the issue of duration. Br J Psychiatry 2002;181:181–183.
28. Young A, Klap R, Sherbourne C, et al. The quality of care for depressive and anxiety disorders in the United States. Arch Gen Psychiatry 2001;58:55–61.
29. Diverty B, Beaudet M. Depression and undertreated disorder? Health Rep 1997;8:9–18.
30. Wang P, Berglund P, Kessler RC. Recent care of common mental disorders in the United States. J Gen Intern Med 2000;15:284–292.
31. Kessler RC, Berglund P, Demler O, et al. The epidemiology of major depressive disorder: results from the National Comorbidity Survey Replication (NCS-R). JAMA 2003;289:3095–3105.
32. Sloan D, Kornstein S. Gender differences in depression and response to antidepressant treatment. Psychiatr Clin North Am 2003;26:581–594.
33. Huttner R, Shepherd J. Gonadal steroids, selective serotonin reuptake inhibitors, and mood disorders in women. Med Clin North Am 2003;87:1–8.
34. Segal Z, Pearson J, Thase M. Challenges in preventing relapse in major depression: report of the NIMH workshop on state of the science of relapse prevention in major depression. J Affect Dis 2003;77:97–108.
35. Whooley M, Simon G. Managing depression in medical outpatients. N Engl J Med 2000;343:1942–1950.

36. Hawton K, Arensman E, Townsend E, et al. Deliberate self harm: systematic review of efficacy of psychosocial and pharmacologic treatments in preventing repetition. Br Med J 1998;317: 441–447.

37. Rhodes A, Links P. Suicide and suicidal behaviours: implications for mental health services. Can J Psychiatry 1998;43:785–791.

38. Townsend E, Hawton K, Altman DC, et al. The efficacy of problem-solving treatments after deliberate self-harm: meta-analysis of randomized controlled trials with respect to depression, hopelessness and improvement in problems. Psychol Med 2001;31:979–988.

39. American Psychiatric Association. Practice Guideline for the Assessment and Treatment of Patients with Suicidal Behaviors. 2003. Available at: http://www.psych.org.

40. Moynihan R. FDA Advisory panel calls for suicide warnings over new antidepressants. Br Med J 2004;328(7435):303.

41. Cohen L. Gender-specific considerations in the treatment of mood disorders in women across the life cycle. J Clin Psychiatry 2003;64(S15):18–29.

42. Bijl R, de Graff R, Hiripi E, et al. The prevalence of treated and untreated mental disorders in five countries. Health Affairs 2003;22:122–133.

43. Rhodes A. Gender, type of mental disorder and use of outpatient mental health services. PhD Dissertation, Epidemiology, Graduate Department of Public Health Sciences, University of Toronto, 1999.

44. Canino G, Bird H, Shrout P, et al. The prevalence of specific psychiatric disorders in Puerto Rico. Arch Gen Psychiatry 1987;44:727–735.

45. Leaf P, Livingston Bruce M. Gender differences in the use of mental health-related services: a re-examination. J Health Soc Behav 1987;28:171–183.

46. Albizu-Garcia C, Alegria M, Freeman D, et al. Gender and health services use for a mental health problem. Soc Sci Med 2001;53:865–878.

47. Gallo JJ, Marino S, Ford D, et al. Filters on the pathway to mental health care, II. Sociodemographic factors. Psychol Med 1995;25:1149–1160.

48. Rhodes AE, Jaakkimainen L, Bondy S, et al. Depression and Mental Health Visits to Physicians—A Prospective Records-Based Study (Under review 2005).

49. Rhodes A, Lin E, Mustard C. Self-reported use of mental health services versus administrative records: should we care? Int J Methods Psychiatr Res 2002;11:125–133.

50. Rhodes AE, Fung K. Self-reported use of mental health services versus administrative records: care to recall? Int J Methods Psychiatr Res 2004;13:165–175.

51. Brown C, Schulberg H. Diagnosis and treatment of depression in primary medical care practice: the application of research findings to clinical practice. J Clin Psychol 1998;54:303–314.

52. Peveler R, Kendrick T. Treatment delivery and guidelines in primary care. Br Med J 2001;57:193–206.

53. Schoenbaum M, Unutzer J, McCaffrey D, et al. The effects of primary care depression treatment on patients' clinical status and employment. Health Services Res 2002;37:1145–1158.

54. Bauer M. A review of quantitative studies of adherence to mental health clinical practice guidelines. Harvard Rev Psychiatry 2002;10:138–153.

55. U.S. Preventive Services Task Force. Screening for depression: recommendations and rationale. Ann Intern Med 2002;136:760–776.

56. Olfson M, Marcus S, Druss B, et al. National trends in the outpatient treatment of depression. JAMA 2002;287:203–209.

57. Druss B, Marcus S, Olfson M, et al. Trends in care by nonphysician clinicians in the United States. N Engl J Med 2003;348:130–137.

58. Mechanic D, Angel R, Davies L. Risk and selection processes between the general and the specialty mental health sectors. J Health Soc Behav 1991;32:49–64.

59. Hemels M, Koren G, Einarson T. Increased use of antidepressants in Canada: 1981–2000. Ann Pharmacother 2002;36:1375–1379.

60. Mechanic D. Disadvantage, inequality and social policy. Health Affairs 2002;21:48–59.

61. Brienza R, Stein M. Alcohol use disorders in primary care: do gender-specific differences exist? Gen Intern Med 2002;17:387–397.

62. Copeland J, Wayne H, Didcott P, et al. A comparison of specialist women's alcohol and other drug treatment service with two traditional mixed-sex services: client characteristics and treatment outcome. Drug Alcohol Dependence 1993;32:81–92.

63. Gilbody S, Whitty P, Grimshaw J, et al. Educational and organizational interventions to improve the management of depression in primary care: a systematic review. JAMA 2003;289:3145–3151.

64. Morgan KP. Contested bodies, contested knowledge: Women, health and the politics of medicalization. In: The Politics of Women's Health, S. Sherwin, ed. Philadelphia: Temple University Press, 1998:83–121.

CHAPTER 27

Women's Mental Health: From Hysteria to Human Rights

Jill A. Astbury

The womb is an animal which longs to generate children. When it remains barren too long after puberty, it is distressed and sorely disturbed, and straying about in the body and cutting off the passages of the breath, it impedes respiration and brings the sufferer into the extremest anguish and provokes all manner of diseases besides. (1)

From the ancient Greeks onward, the nature, forms, and causes of women's emotional distress have intrigued philosophers, priests, and scientists. How women's emotional distress has been named over time reflects beliefs about its underlying causes, sets limits on the social and psychological terrain scientists believe is relevant to investigation, and dictates who is entitled to professional "ownership" of the distress. As the quote above from Plato illustrates, the first and longest lasting explanation of women's distress was that it was caused by female reproductive difficulties. The archetypal female malady was called "hysteria" by ancient Greek philosophers and physicians, after the word "hysterus" meaning uterus.

All manner of psychological problems were believed to be caused by the movement of the uterus around the body. Dangers from the "wandering womb" were heightened whenever women did not fulfill their biologic destiny to bear children. Treatments took the form of foul or sweet-smelling potions to coax the vagrant womb back into its correct position. Right up to the early twentieth century, strong-smelling herbs like asafetida, in the form of aromatics, sedatives, and antispasmodics, were still being recommended in pharmacologic textbooks as specific antihystericals

The construction of "hysteria" as a peculiarly feminine disorder shackled women's mental disorders to their supposedly flawed biology for more than 3,000 years. Women's distress, by virtue of its basis in female difference and faulty female anatomy, was deemed an illness; ownership of it was assumed by biologic science and the medical profession.

The prejudicial linking of women's mental health to reproductive functioning meant that sources of distress emanating from outside women's bodies, including social origins, aroused little scientific curiosity. Indeed, the possibility that factors external to and separate from the woman, including the violation of her human rights, could affect her mental well-being remained a neglected space in the psychiatric imagination until very late in the twentieth century.

Interestingly, when human rights are discussed in the context of mental health, it is usually in relation to the rights of the mentally ill not to be stigmatized or discriminated against on account of their mental illness, rather than the other way around: that stigma and discrimination contribute to mental illness. At least one study has shown that stigma can be a determinant of emotional distress (2). In this study, women whose families thought a positive HIV status was shameful were much more likely than others to experience high levels of emotional distress. Such women had the highest levels of HIV-related worry of all HIV-positive women and were the least likely to disclose their HIV status, thus losing the opportunity to extend avenues for psychologically beneficial forms of social support.

Before sex differences were conceptually distinguished from gender differences, research into disparities in rates of psychiatric disorders between men and women were driven by attempts to identify a biologic determinant. For example, a great deal of biologically based research into the approximately 2:1 ratio of depression in women compared with men has looked to genetic, neurotransmitter, and endocrinologic sex differences (3).

Assumptions that scientific research and scientists themselves were necessarily objective and value neutral did nothing to foster a more critical approach to this narrow biologic model of women's emotional distress. As a result, other possible variables of interest, such as the role of childhood abuse, were slow to be recognized, and systematic gender bias in much psychological research was ignored (4). From the 1970s onward and coincident with the rise of second wave feminism, the importance of gender, women's social position, and violence toward women have been recognized as increasingly critical determinants of women's mental health. Interestingly, this recognition has occurred in parallel with an upsurge of research into the social origins of depression and other common mental disorders (5).

In this chapter it is argued that, in order to provide a comprehensive explanation of women's higher rates of depression, post-traumatic stress disorder, and other related comorbid disorders, a model of women's mental health is required that moves beyond brain chemistry and biologic factors. At the very least, it is necessary to include events and experiences that themselves alter brain chemistry and activate biologic stress mechanisms that, in turn, potentiate poor mental health and damage self-esteem (6). Three concepts are needed to inform this expanded model, namely gender, social position, and human rights. Evidence will be reviewed to illustrate the importance of all three and their interrelationships.

The chapter begins with a brief discussion of the right to health as a fundamental human right followed by a summary of gender as a mental health risk factor illustrated by the known pattern of gender disparities in mental health. Research is then reviewed showing the importance of social position in determining mental health status and underlining how gender, as a critical, cross-cutting determinant of health, has implications for both social position and mental health. Finally, gender-based violence and its known impact on women's mental health is used as an example of the interrelationships among gender, social position, and human rights.

HEALTH AS A HUMAN RIGHT

The notion of health as a fundamental human right was articulated as far back as 1946 in the Constitution of the World Health Organization: "The enjoyment of the highest attainable standard of health is one of the fundamental rights of every human being without distinction of race, religion, political belief, economic or social condition."

Despite this early recognition of the importance of the link between health and human rights, the right to health has been neglected in comparison with other rights, even though it has the same international legal status as freedom of religion or the right to a fair trial. As a result of this neglect, the right to health is not as widely recognized as civil and political rights even though it is cited in numerous conventions. These include the Universal Declaration of Human Rights (1948), the International Covenant on Economic, Social and Cultural Rights (1976), the Convention on the Rights of the Child (1989), the Convention on the Elimination of All Forms of Discrimination against Women (CEDAW) (1979), and the International Convention on the Elimination of All Forms of Racial Discrimination (1965).

The claims of human beings on society and government arise from their inalienable rights as human beings and not because of any special favor or privilege that may be conferred or withheld on the grounds of "race, colour, sex, language, religion, political or other opinion, national or social origin, property, birth or other status," in the words of Article 2 of the Universal Declaration of Human Rights.

Proclaimed by the United Nations General Assembly in 1948, the Universal Declaration of Human Rights states that "all people are born equal in dignity and rights" and governments are expected to respect, promote, and protect the human rights of all citizens regardless of their differences. Statements of principle are one thing, and the implementation and protection of rights another. For example, while human rights theoretically cannot be conferred or withheld on the grounds of sex, there is overwhelming evidence that they are. Women continue to occupy a subordinate social position globally, and their status as full human beings from a rights perspective has not yet been realized (7). The need to redress this situation and to articulate gender-specific rights more fully inspired the development of CEDAW.

Many human rights frameworks respond with difficulty to issues of concern for women because they focus on the behavior of government actors rather than private parties. Some of the most critical violations of women's rights occur within the private sphere of the home. The more recent Declaration on the Elimination of Violence against Women (1993) overcomes this difficulty by including as a rights violation violence that occurs within the family, in addition to that which occurs in the community or that which is perpetrated or condoned by the State.

A clear overlap exists between the objectives of human rights and health (8). The linkage between health and human rights derives from "the deep complementarity of the public health goal to ensure the conditions in which people can be healthy and the human right goal of identifying, promoting, and protecting the societal determinants of human well-being" (8, p. 179).

For this reason, public health policies, programs, and practices are uniquely placed to promote and protect people's human rights in the context of their health. Conversely, health policies, programs, and practices can, through the exercise of deliberate or inadvertent discrimination, place an additional burden on the health of the public—especially those segments of the population that are marginalized and vulnerable. These are the groups who may be "overlooked" in the framing of health policies for the general population unless care is taken to include them. Human rights violations can have direct and immediate as well as long-term negative effects on human health, as illustrated by the health impacts of torture on human health. While the violation of any right can be conceived as exerting measurable impacts on physical, mental, and social well-being, it has been suggested that the health effects arising from human rights violations remain "in large part, to be discovered and documented" (9, p. 445).

It can equally well be asserted that there is already a considerable body of evidence regarding the impact of human rights violations on women's mental health, even though this evidence was not collected with the explicit goal of identifying or documenting the mental health effects of human rights violations. Human rights offer a societal level framework for identifying and responding to the underlying societal determinants of health. As such, a rights perspective is a valuable addition to existing conceptions of the social model of health and to the measurement of social position.

GENDER AND GENDER DISPARITIES IN MENTAL HEALTH

To elucidate gender disparities in mental health, an understanding of gender as a social construct and analytic category is obviously essential. Gender has the analytical power to identify and explain differences between men's and women's susceptibility and exposure to specific risks to mental health. Gender is crucially related to the differential power men and women have to control their lives. It also impinges powerfully on the ability to respond and to cope with health risks. Access to health care can also be constrained on gender grounds. The rise of "user pays" medical care ensures that the cost burden falls most heavily on the most economically disadvantaged, namely women. Without the concept of gender, it is not possible to begin to ask questions about how the social categories occupied by women and men differentially affect how they see, experience, and understand the society in which they live and how they are likely to be regarded and treated within that society.

The Global Burden of Disease reveals that 5 of the 10 leading causes of disability worldwide are neuropsychiatric disorders (10). Depression, besides being the most prevalent psychiatric condition, makes an increasingly heavy contribution to the global disease burden. Depression is the most frequently encountered women's mental health problem and accounts for more than 1 in 10 years of life lived with disability. By 2020, depression is predicted to be the second leading cause of disease burden and the leading cause of disability burden.

As noted, earlier attempts to explain the gender difference in depression proceeded largely as if it is a sex difference and exhaustively investigated possible biologic reasons for the difference. The dominant place given to biologic factors resulted in hasty and erroneous interpretation of epidemiologic evidence.

Data from national surveys can be used to compare population-based rates of depression over the life span. The gender difference in depression first emerges in early puberty (11) and declines from midlife onward (12). These changes in rates of depression over the female life cycle were taken as strong evidence that corresponding changes in female sex hormones were responsible. However, while the gender difference in depression is most marked during the reproductive years, strenuous research efforts have not succeeded in tying this difference to changes in sex hormones related to pregnancy, the use of oral contraceptives, or the use of hormone replacement therapy in menopause or natural hormonal changes during menopause (12). Other factors in women's lives also change over time and have proved to be important in explaining depression. For example, some of the methodologically strongest research on depression and menopause has reported that multiple interacting factors best explain why some women experience depression at this time and others do not. Research undertaken by Kuh and colleagues (13) to consider the complex range of factors that impinge on mental health in midlife is reported here in some detail. Factors from childhood, adolescence, and adult life were all examined in relation to psychological distress among women in midlife. Participants in this research on midlife health and menopause were part of the larger Medical Research Council National Survey of Health and Development (MRCNSHD), a prospective cohort study of a representative sample of the British population born in 1946 and subsequently followed. The psychological symptoms on which data were collected when participants were aged between 47 and 52 years included anxiety and depression, irritability, tearfulness, and feelings of panic and a composite psychological symptom score. A very large number of risk factors across the life course were included. Risk factors belonged to six clusters: family background, characteristics of the child, adult health, adult socioeconomic circumstances, social support and life style, and current life stress. The study investigated the nature of links between mental health in midlife and experiences in childhood or in adolescence and early adult life. Pathways through which such risk factors as cumulative losses, social adversity, negative events, and experiences over the course of women's lives influenced their psychological health in midlife were carefully evaluated.

Importantly, no variation in psychological symptoms in midlife was found according to menopausal stage, a finding that is in keeping with the results of the majority of other studies. However, past psychological distress was predictive of current distress, and many of the classical social determinants of depression and poor mental health were found to play a highly significant role in women's mental health in midlife. These included social position in childhood and adult life (lower social class, having lived in council housing, lower educational qualifications, parents who had divorced), negative life events, behavioral risk factors (smoking and being overweight), and marital status, with divorced or separated women having higher symptom scores than those who were married or single (13). A graded relationship was reported between the number of adverse changes in participants' family and work life each year between 47 and 52 years of age and systematic increases in symptom scores over the same time span. Higher social support, including emotional support, good social networks, and access to help in a crisis, positively mediated the likelihood of psychological symptoms. This research underlines the importance of taking a life course approach to women's mental health and employing methodologies capable of eliciting markedly different life course trajectories.

WHY GENDER?

Women are overrepresented among those diagnosed with three or more comorbid disorders, and increased rates of depression among women are accompanied by higher rates of somatization disorder, panic disorder, and certain personality disorders compared with men. High rates of comorbidity are linked with increased use of services, greater severity of mental illness, and higher levels of disability (14). Rates of depression are significantly higher among those living in poverty and experiencing the greatest socioeconomic disadvantage. Once again women are overrepresented among those living in such circumstances (15,16).

These findings have not usually been considered from the perspective of gender and rights, but it is useful to do so, and such an analysis can suggest different approaches to mental health promotion and the prevention and treatment of women's mental health problems.

SOCIAL POSITION AND MENTAL HEALTH

The critical importance of social environment and social position for health has been demonstrated repeatedly. Variations in both mortality and morbidity rates by social class are a consistent finding of epidemiology (17). Adverse mental health outcomes such as depression are 2 to 2.5 times higher among those experiencing the greatest social disadvantage compared with those experiencing the least. Women experiencing such disadvantage have the highest rates of all (12,15,18).

Studies in countries of different income levels have confirmed the existence of what has come to be called the social gradient in health—significant differences in both mortality and morbidity extend from the top to the bottom of the social hierarchy (15,17,19). So strong is the relationship between socioeconomic status (SES) measured by such indicators as income, education, and employment status and a wide range of poor health outcomes that SES is typically accorded the status of a research control variable in order to facilitate the evaluation of other risk factors to health. As a result, little detailed research into socioeconomic status as an etiologic factor in its own right has occurred (19).

Mann (9) asserts that the biomedical foundation of public health, with its concepts and language borrowed from notions of disease, is ill suited to understanding societal level determinants of health and detracts from analyzing and responding to the underlying social conditions responsible for poor health. He is also critical of researchers, program administrators, and policy makers who ostensibly seek to improve public health but attempt to do so by designing behavioral risk reduction programs that assume high-risk health behaviors such as drinking, smoking, and unhealthful dietary choices are under the complete control of the persons who engage in them. Ironically, such programs tend to ignore differences in the social contexts that help to explain variations in rates of these same behaviors.

There is abundant evidence that poverty and material disadvantage are critical predictors of poor mental health. Other dimensions of social position that are important include environmental stressors such as adverse life events and chronic psychosocial difficulties that are more common among people living in poverty and are significantly associated with the lower socioeconomic class predominance for nonpsychotic psychiatric disorders like depression and anxiety. Less access to supportive social networks, at both an immediate personal, contextual level and a broader, societal level, has also been linked with higher levels of morbidity, including higher rates of depression and anxiety (5).

Until now, public health research into the social gradient in health has paid little detailed attention to the gendering of social position or to the contribution that human rights violations might make to the negative mental health outcomes described by the social gradient and disproportionately experienced by women. This omission is even more surprising given that women are so overrepresented among those living in the greatest socioeconomic disadvantage. Traditional indicators of social position such as household income are not ideal for capturing women's social position. Many studies lack substantive data on women's income, and this further reduces the predictive value of income as an indicator of women's social position (20). Additional data are needed on whether women are able to access and exercise control over the expenditure of household income. Assumptions of shared access to household income remain to be tested. Notions of social disadvantage and inequalities in health need to be rethought by considering an alternative causal pathway, namely that disadvantage and inequality are effects of the violation of one or more critical human rights.

Material disadvantage as a cause of differences in mental health status fails to convince when differences in health status exist between groups toward the top of the social hierarchy, where poverty is no longer a relevant variable. Neither does material disadvantage explain different rates of mental illness among women who experience equal levels of material disadvantage.

The time for the integration of a gender and rights perspective into research on social position and health is long overdue. Researchers cannot continue to ignore the fact that "no society treats its women as well as it treats its men" (7) in their models of explanation regarding the relationship between the social environment and health. This ill treatment, like social position itself, has both a material dimension and a symbolic dimension. Status and relative position in a social hierarchy and latitude in decision making are strongly related to physical and mental well-being and self-esteem (6,21). Stansfield and colleagues (17), in their longitudinal study of Whitehall civil servants in Great Britain, found that rank or grade of employment was significantly related to well-being. Work characteristics, especially skill discretion and decision authority, were closely related to employment grade and made the largest contribution to explaining differences in well-being and depression. Those in the highest employment grades had the highest levels of well-being and the least depression, while those in the lowest grades had the highest levels of depression. Furthermore, those in the lowest employment grades experienced a higher prevalence of negative life events and chronic stressors and relatively less social support. Not surprisingly, women were overrepresented among those occupying the lowest grade and had the lowest status jobs and the least discretion in decision making.

Knowledge is accumulating steadily on the defining social variables and critical characteristics of situations and experiences that trigger depression. Depression is most likely to occur when a person experiences feelings of loss and defeat, especially in situations involving an intimate tie and situations that engender feelings of entrapment and humiliation denoting devaluation and marginalization (22). Evidence from research into social rank theory confirms the importance of the depressogenic effect of perceiving the self as inferior or in an unwanted subordinate position, lacking self-confidence and behaving in submissive or nonassertive ways, having a sense of defeat in relation to important battles, and at the same time wanting to escape but being trapped (21). All these factors appear to be predictable subjective responses to the lower rank, lower paid, and less powerful positions that define women's occupational status and extend to their intimate relationships. Inequality outside the home in terms of poorer paid, lower status, and less satisfying jobs can act as a fulcrum that reinforces inequality inside the home.

Research by Brown, Harris, and Hepworth (22) reveals that humiliation is a defining characteristic of the negative life events experienced by women who became depressed. These researchers observe that the meaning attached to an event, its symbolism, is significant in triggering depression and that humiliating events are fitted into understandings that women carry of their position and worth in the larger society: "Probably equally significant to being humiliated and devalued is what is symbolized by such atypical events in terms of the woman's life as a whole—in particular, the experience of being confirmed as marginal and unwanted" (22, p. 19).

This study found that humiliation and devaluation severely undermine women's sense of worth as human beings and hence may be considered to violate the fundamental human right for all people to live equal in dignity and rights. Currently, measures or indicators of dignity and humiliation are not used in research on depression in women despite their obvious relevance. Autonomy and control, the obverse of entrapment and humiliation, *have* been measured and appear to play an important role in lessening the risk of depression occurring in the context of what might otherwise be considered a serious loss such as the loss of an important relationship with a partner. When separation was initiated by the woman, only about 10% of women in the study whose relationships ended in separation subsequently developed depression. When the separation was almost entirely initiated by the woman's partner, around half the women developed depression. The rate of depression increased again if infidelity was discovered and *not* followed by separation (22).

According to Marmot (6), gaining appropriate reward for efforts expended and having control over life circumstances are critically linked to self-esteem and gaining respect. In this regard, gender functions as a socially sanctioned conduit for the granting or withholding of reward for effort and control over life circumstances. Systemic denial of effort-based rewards to women constitutes a structural impediment to self-esteem and violates women's right to self-determination. This right is summarized in Article 1 of the International Covenant on Civil and Political Rights (1976): "All peoples have the right to self-determination. By virtue of that right they freely determine their political status and freely pursue their economic, social and cultural development."

Discrimination on the basis of female gender resulting in inequality in occupational status, reduced autonomy, and lower rates of pay that is described in research on occupational health (17) results in gendered inequalities in health status, especially mental health status. Identifying the particular hazards or risk factors to which women's social position exposes them and ascertaining their effect on emotional well-being are important in themselves and for providing evidence on which to base more meaningful approaches to mental health promotion and treatment for women. To do this, additional indicators of women's social position taken from a human rights framework need to be developed.

One of the most important indicators of gendered social position is the high prevalence of gender-based violence, referred to by Lisa Andermann in Chapter 2 of this book. Unfortunately, most research using a social determinants model of health to give an account of differences in rates of depression across the social gradient does not include gender-based violence as a salient indicator (16). Without examining the role of gender-based violence and other gender-specific risk factors, a coherent account of why differences in rates of depression occur would seem to be out of the question.

A further advantage of a rights-based approach is that it is especially sensitive to individuals and groups who are variously called "vulnerable," "disadvantaged," or "marginalized." It is precisely these groups that human rights analysis identifies and includes, in contrast to traditional public health programs, which exclude or increase the health burden on such groups through inadvertent discrimination (9). A rights-based approach is capable of determining whether different types of health inequalities are causally related to specific rights violations and how these in turn are connected with other characteristics of vulnerable groups, including gender, race, and disability.

GENDER-BASED VIOLENCE: MENTAL HEALTH, GENDERED SOCIAL POSITION, AND RIGHTS

Gender-based violence (GBV) is arguably the most emblematic violation of women's human rights. The Declaration on the Elimination of Violence against Women (1993) recognized that such violence violates, impairs, or nullifies women's enjoyment of their human rights and fundamental freedoms. Such violence encapsulates all three features identified by research into the negative life events and adverse social circumstances most strongly associated with depression, namely humiliation, inferior social ranking, and entrapment. Gender-based violence forces submission at an individual level, and, by engendering fear, defeat, humiliation, and a sense of blocked escape or entrapment, it reinforces women's inferior social ranking and subordination in the wider society.

By definition, gender-based violence expresses contempt for the notion that women are full human beings "born free and equal in dignity and rights" with their male perpetrators (Article 1 of the Universal Declaration of Human Rights). Gender-based violence can result in death, thus violating the absolute right to life; it necessarily destroys a woman's right to liberty and security of person (Article 3). When it involves entrapment and total coercive control over every aspect of a woman's life, it violates Article 5, that no one shall be held in slavery or servitude. When it encompasses repetitive, escalating, humiliating physical, sexual, and emotional abuse, it violates the absolute right of every human being to live in freedom from torture and cruel, inhuman, or degrading treatment. It also violates Articles 12, 13, 16, 18, and 19, the right to privacy, freedom of movement, equality in marriage, and freedom of thought, opinion, and expression.

The multiple negative health outcomes associated with violence provide the strongest evidence of the causal relationship between health and human rights. It goes without saying that being subjected to violence is utterly incompatible with the enjoyment of the highest attainable standard of physical and mental health. Perhaps the most defining characteristic of gender-based violence is that it is most likely to be perpetrated by someone known and often known intimately to the woman. This characteristic deserves special attention when seeking to explain the psychological impact of violence on women's mental health. If the idea of having a home encompasses living in a place that affords physical and psychological safety and security, then a woman experiencing violence at home is in a very real sense, homeless. Such a woman may have shelter, but she does not have a place where she can safely let her defenses down as such violence tends to be repetitive and to escalate in severity over time.

Gender-based violence in childhood and adult life, including physical, sexual, and emotional violence and abuse, is associated with threefold to fourfold increases in the risk of depression and is also linked with marked increases in psychiatric comorbidity, including increased rates of anxiety, post-traumatic stress disorder, suicidality, substance abuse disorders, somatization, panic disorders, eating disorders, and certain personality disorders such as borderline personality disorder (23–25). Of all these outcomes, the finding of an increased risk of depression is the most thoroughly investigated and reported (16). Evidence indicates that the link between gender-based violence and depression is likely to be causal.

Large-scale, population-based surveys in a number of countries (25,26) have found that women who report a history of victimization have significantly increased rates of depression and anxiety compared with those who do not. Even stronger evidence for a causal relationship comes from prospective longitudinal studies of women who continue to be subjected to violence compared with those who are no longer exposed to violence. Studies have found that levels of depression and anxiety remain unchanged or increase among women still being subjected to violence, while they decrease significantly in women who are no longer experiencing violence. This relationship continues to be significant after previous levels of psychological and physical health have been statistically controlled (27).

More recent research that separates out the different forms of violence and its link with depression has reported that the effect of violence ceasing is related to the kind of violence a woman has experienced. For women who have experienced only psychological abuse, the cessation of violence was followed by an insignificant reduction in the likelihood of depression. For women with a history of physical or sexual abuse and psychological abuse, the cessation of violence resulted in a 27% decline in the likelihood of depression; this increased to a 35% decline in women who experienced multiple forms of abuse (28).

A dose–duration relationship has been revealed between the severity of violence and its duration and the number and the severity of subsequent psychological disorders. Not only do women who have "ever" experienced violence differ significantly in their rates of psychological disorder from those never abused, but women who have been doubly or multiply abused have significantly higher rates (29). Women who experienced repeated childhood sexual abuse not only have lower self-esteem than those who experienced few abusive events (30), but they are more likely to develop psychiatric disorders as adults and to be admitted to a psychiatric unit or hospital at some time in their lives (31).

POST-TRAUMATIC STRESS

Women's risk of developing post-traumatic stress disorder (PTSD) following exposure to trauma has been found to be approximately twofold higher than men's. Interestingly, this parallels the gender difference found for depression, and the duration of PTSD has been found to be longer in women than in men (32). In an epidemiologic study of trauma and PTSD, Breslau found that PTSD persisted longer in women than in men and that assaultive violence including rape and sexual assault was associated with the highest risk of PTSD (33). While physical symptoms following rape tend to decrease over the next 12 months, psychological symptoms remain significantly elevated (33).

Women who have experienced domestic violence and sexual assault are at very high risk of PTSD (34). In the US nationwide study on rape, 31% of women who reported being raped subsequently developed PTSD compared with 5% who had never experienced rape (35). There is also a complex interaction between exposure to trauma and the subsequent development of both PTSD and borderline personality disorder. In an analysis of data from the collaborative longitudinal personality disorders study, Yen et al. (36) reported that the severity and number of traumatic events especially of an assaultive and personal nature and an early onset predicted the severity of subsequent personality disorder. Borderline personality disorder participants reported the highest rate of exposure to trauma, especially sexual trauma including childhood sexual abuse.

COMORBIDITY AND THE BURDEN OF VIOLENCE

Depression may be the most common mental health effect of GBV, just as it is the most common psychiatric disorder in the general community, but it typically co-occurs with anxiety, post-traumatic stress, and a range of other psychiatric disorders (37). Indeed, Kessler et al. (18), reporting on the U.S. National Comorbidity Survey, noted that women had higher prevalences than men of both lifetime and 12-month comorbidity of three or more disorders and were more exposed to violence from an intimate. In other words, psychiatric comorbidity, with depression as a common factor, is a characteristic finding of research on the impact of violence on women's mental health (29,37).

To complicate the matter further, psychiatric comorbidity can and frequently does co-occur with physical comorbidity. Just as the form that violence itself takes can be physical, sexual, or psychological, so too, the health outcomes of violence can be manifested in physical, sexual, and psychological disorders. For example, children exposed to sexual, physical, and emotional abuse are at greater risk of subsequent revictimization and increased rates of multiple adverse health outcomes in the long term (38). Although the contribution of a single form of violence, such as childhood sexual abuse, to mental health in adult life can be established by statistically controlling for the effects of other childhood risk factors, it is important to identify all forms of violence as well as other forms of adversity in childhood in order to gain a comprehensive understanding of the relationship between adverse childhood experiences and health in adult life.

Felitti and colleagues (39) demonstrated the importance to adult health of exposure in childhood to multiple adverse experiences, which included psychological, physical, or sexual abuse; violence against the mother and living with household members who were substance abusers, mentally ill, or suicidal or had ever been imprisoned. It is clear that most of these experiences constitute violations of the rights of the child. A strong graded relationship was found between the number of adverse experiences to which the child had been exposed and the number and kinds of poor health experienced in adult life. Importantly, adverse experiences in childhood were strongly interrelated. Poor health included health risk behaviors (smoking, alcohol and drug abuse, physical inactivity, and multiple sexual partners) as well as many of the leading causes of death in adult life. Those who had experienced four or more categories of childhood exposure compared to those who had experienced none had a 12-fold increased health risk for alcoholism, drug abuse, depression, or suicide attempts (39).

Evidence suggests there is a high degree of comorbid psychopathology and multisomatization associated with violence. Studies that have been designed to measure all forms of violence and to measure multiple health outcomes have found complex relationships between the type of violence perpetrated and the consequent health outcomes. For example, analysis of data from the U.S. population–based National Violence Against Women Survey (NVAWS) (40) revealed that higher scores on psychological forms of partner violence were more strongly associated with a range of adverse health outcomes than physical violence scores. These health outcomes included current poor health, depressive symptoms, substance use, chronic disease, chronic mental illness and injury (26). Nevertheless, the majority of studies so far have concentrated on either psychological or physical comorbidity but not both (23,25,29).

Resnick and colleagues (23) have argued that the most critical task facing researchers and clinicians is to elucidate the important causative and mediating factors involved in the complex web of interrelatedness among the many negative health effects of violence and to identify the determinants of specific negative outcomes. Many of the risk factors for violence that have been identified as independent risk factors for depression can also be considered to reflect rights violations. These include unemployment in both the victim and the perpetrator, inadequate income, history of violence in childhood, and adult life. Moreover, these risk factors and rights violations facilitate and reinforce the perpetration of gender-based violence and engender its associated pernicious effects on women's mental health. Acknowledging the existence of GBV and its profound impact on women's mental health demands significant revisions to the models of public health and mental health. GBV suggests the need to integrate a gender and human rights perspective into public health research, policy, and programs.

Not only is there a heavily gendered social gradient for depression, but this in turn is mediated by the occurrence of violence. A large, prospective longitudinal study has found that women experience an increased risk for victimization when their income is below the poverty level and when they are newly divorced. In addition, victimization appears to increase women's risk for unemployment, taking time off work, reduced income, and divorce (41). In other words, violence can further weaken women's social and material position while increasing their psychological vulnerability to depression and other disorders. Conversely, the presence of social support, developing positive subsequent relationships, forging achievements in some sphere of life, and gaining employment can positively mediate the risk of adverse psychological health outcomes developing after violence has occurred (25,26,30).

The same combination of adverse social factors and violence has been reported to predict high rates of psychiatric morbidity in low-income countries (15) including Arab countries. Maziak et al. (42) investigated predictors of mental distress among low-income women in Aleppo, Syria. The most important predictors of psychological distress were physical abuse, low education (including illiteracy), polygamy, residence, age, and age of marriage. Education was a significant modifier of poor psychological outcome because higher education meant women were significantly less likely to marry young, enter polygamous marriages, or be physically abused. Illiteracy not only indicates a denial of the right to education but increases the likelihood of other rights violations related to age at marriage, "choice" of marriage partner, and type of marriage entered into, which in turn increases the risk of women being exposed to subsequent physical violence. Together, these violations are risk factors for significant levels of psychological distress. From a psychiatric perspective it would be accurate to call this distress "depression," but other terms might also be accurate.

CONCLUSION

Terminology is always important. As noted at the beginning of this chapter, how a phenomenon is named reflects beliefs about its underlying causes, determines which etiologic factors are included in research and which are excluded, and underpins policies, programs, and practices designed to ameliorate the phenomenon in question. If what is currently named "depression," treated as a psychiatric disorder, and believed to have a biologic basis amenable to psychopharmacologic rectification were to be renamed "demoralization" and believed to have a basis in rights violations, then the possibilities for treating and responding meaningfully to this new disorder would expand.

Interventions would have to address the source or sources of demoralization, seek to redress the rights violations that had occurred, and look to ways and means of protecting and improving women's enjoyment of their human rights. Naming is an essential first step and logically precedes measurement. Before childhood sexual abuse and gender-based violence were named, they could not become visible as meaningful social, public health, or human rights issues, nor could the prevalence or the severity of their mental health effects be ascertained. Increased attention and questioning on an issue drives the search for evidence, not the other way around (4).

As Marmot (6) notes, autonomy, self-esteem, and health are linked together and reflect much more than natural endowment. They are also dependent on life chances, opportunities, and achievements. Life chances and opportunities are enabling factors for self-esteem, respect, and good health, including good mental health. Globally, women's life chances are lower than men's, and even in high-income countries, the level of gender development lags behind human development (16).

Changing the psychosocial context that determines women's life chances, opportunities, and treatment is necessary for any meaningful attempt to be made in reducing the current burden of ill health associated with depression and other common mental health problems that disproportionately impact on women. Some of the most pressing changes that need to be made if women's right to good mental health is to be realized include reducing the unacceptably high level of gender-based violence, increasing women's status as human beings, eliminating the gender gap in rates of pay, and equalizing the double shift of paid and unpaid work.

It is argued that such changes are essential to change depressed women's mood and will be more effective in the long term than psychotropic medication in maintaining good psychological health and preventing relapse. This is not to say that psychotropic drugs do not change mood; clearly they can be extremely efficacious in doing so. Nor is it to argue that psychiatry and psychotherapy are not valuable in assisting women with mental health problems. What is argued is that an approach based on rights, with a focus on human dignity, is needed to complement traditional clinical approaches to mental health. It is also asserted that psychotropic drugs or psychotherapy alone can do nothing to change the psychosocial context or the conditions that are currently not conducive to supporting women's right to mental health. A large body of evidence on gender-specific risk factors for mental health that has been reviewed here leaves no doubt that current social arrangements and their widespread facilitation of rights violations against women are instrumental in triggering and maintaining women's high rates of mental disorders. Identifying and analyzing rights violations in relation to health contributes a new perspective to the socioeconomic and structural factors usually considered within a social model of health. Evidence on the mechanisms through which gender and rights violations link to poor mental health in women is sparse. Mann (9) suggests that an exploration of the meanings of dignity and the forms of its violation and how this in turn affects physical, mental, and social well-being may uncover "a new universe of human suffering" (9, p. 449). Such an exploration could represent the first step in identifying and understanding how to reduce gender-specific risk factors for poor mental health.

Certainly, women's understandings of what constitutes dignity for themselves have not previously received attention from public health researchers interested in mental health at the level of the population. Experiences of self-worth, autonomy, adequate income, and safety are some of the likely ingredients of a sense of dignity that are systematically denied, along with the rights that these experiences represent. In a number of countries, women's equal right to dignity and right to life, liberty, and security of person have been subordinated to notions of family honor. In practice, this is synonymous with men's honor because women have not had the power to assert alternative notions of honor that work in their interest. The result is not only that "honor" killings have occurred but that those who perpetrated them did so with impunity.

A gendered rights-based approach signals a shift away from the biologically reductionist and tautological propositions that women have mental health problems because they are women and have a biologically based proneness to such problems. Research that confines its attention to socioeconomic indicators of risk typically ignores the normative orders that inform those indicators. The use of a gendered rights-based approach offers a means of analyzing those normative orders with regard to the impediments they create for women in accessing their right to mental health.

REFERENCES

1. Archer-Hind RD. The Timaeus of Plato. London: Macmillan, 1888.
2. Bennetts A, Shaffer N, Manopaiboon C, et al. Determinants of depression and HIV-related worry among HIV-positive women who have recently given birth, Bangkok, Thailand. Soc Sci Med 1999;49:737–749.
3. Blehar MC, Oren DA. Women's increased vulnerability to mood disorders: integrating psychobiology and epidemiology. Depression 1995;3:3–12.

4. Astbury J. Crazy for You: The Making of Women's Madness. Melbourne: Oxford University Press, 1996.
5. Brown GW. Genetic and population perspectives on life events and depression. Soc Psychiatry Psychiatr Epidemiol 1998;33:363–372.
6. Marmot M. Self esteem and health. Br Med J 2003;327:574–575.
7. World Health Organization. The world health report. Geneva: World Health Organization, 1998.
8. Mann JM, Gostin L, Gruskin S, et al. Health and human rights. In: Mann JM, Gruskin S, Grodin MA, et al., eds. Health and Human Rights. New York: Routledge, 1999:7–20.
9. Mann JM. Medicine and public health. In: Mann JM, Gruskin S, Grodin MA, et al., eds. Health and Human Rights. New York: Routledge, 1999:439–452.
10. Murray JL, Lopez AD. The global burden of disease. Boston: Harvard School of Public Health and World Health Organization, 1996.
11. Wade TJ, Cairney J, Pevalin DJ. Emergence of gender differences in depression during adolescence: national panel results from three countries. J Am Acad Child Adolesc Psychiatry 2002;41:190–198.
12. Kessler RC. Epidemiology of women and depression. J Affect Disord 2003;74:5–13.
13. Kuh D, Hardy R, Rodgers B, et al. Lifetime risk factors for women's psychological distress in midlife. Soc Sci Med 2002;55:1957–1973.
14. Kessler RC, Sonnega A, Bromet E, et al. Posttraumatic stress disorder in the National Comorbidity Survey. Arch Gen Psychiatry 1995;52:1048–1060.
15. Patel V, Araya R, de Lima M, et al. Women, poverty and common mental disorders in four restructuring societies. Soc Sci Med 1999;49:1461–1471.
16. Astbury J, Cabral M. Women's mental health: an evidence based review. Geneva: World Health Organization, 2000.
17. Stansfield SA, Head J, Marmot MG. Explaining social class differentials in depression and well-being. Soc Psychiatry Psychiatr Epidemiol 1998:1–9.
18. Kessler RC, McGonagle KA, Zhao S, et al. Lifetime and 12-month prevalence of DSM-III-R psychiatric disorders in the United States: results from the National Comorbidity Survey. Arch Gen Psychiatry 1994;51:8–19.
19. Adler N, Boyce T, Chesney MA, et al. Socioeconomic status and health: the challenge of the gradient. Am Psychol 1994;49:15–24.
20. Macran S, Clarke L, Joshi H. Women's health: dimensions and differentials. Soc Sci Med 1996;42:1203–1216.
21. Gilbert P, Allan S. The role of defeat and entrapment (arrested flight) in depression: an exploration of an evolutionary view. Psychol Med 1998;28:585–598.
22. Brown GW, Harris TO, Hepworth C. Loss, humiliation and entrapment among women developing depression: a patient and non-patient comparison. Psychol Med 1995;25:7–21.
23. Resnick HS, Acierno R, Kilpatrick DG. Health impact of interpersonal violence. 2: Medical and mental health outcomes. Behav Med 1997;23:65–78.
24. Astbury J. Gender disparities in mental health. In: Mental health: a call for action by world health ministers. Geneva: World Health Organization, 2001:73–92.
25. Campbell JC. Health consequences of intimate partner violence. Lancet 2002;359:1331–1336.
26. Coker AL, Davis KE, Arias I, et al. Physical and mental health effects of intimate partner violence for men and women. Am J Prev Med 2002;23:260–268.
27. Sutherland C, Bybee D, Sutherland C. The long-term effects of battering on women's health. Women's Health 1998;4:41–70.
28. Kernie MA, Holt VL, Stoner JA, et al. Resolution of depression among victims of intimate partner violence: is cessation of violence enough? Violence Vict 2003;18:115–129.
29. Roberts GL, Lawrence JM, William GM, et al. The impact of domestic violence on women's mental health. Aust NZ J Pub Health 1998;22:796–801.
30. Romans SE, Martin JL, Anderson JC, et al. Factors that mediate between child sexual abuse and adult psychological outcomes. Psychol Med 1995;25:127–142.
31. Mullen PE, Martin JL, Anderson JC, et al. Childhood sexual abuse and mental health in adult life. Br J Psychiatry 1993;163:721–732.
32. Breslau N. Gender differences in trauma and posttraumatic stress disorder. J Gend Specif Med 2002;5:34–40.
33. Kimerling R, Calhoun KS. Somatic symptoms, social support, and treatment seeking among sexual assault victims. J Cons Clin Psychol 1994;62:333–340.
34. Kubany ES, McKenzie WF, Owens JA, et al. PTSD among women survivors of domestic violence in Hawaii. Hawaii Med J 1996;55:164–165.
35. Kilpatrick DG, Edmunds CS, Seymour AK. Rape in America: a report to the nation. Arlington, VA: National Victim Center and Medical University of South Carolina, 1992.
36. Yen S, Shea MT, Battle CL, et al. Traumatic exposure and posttraumatic stress disorder in borderline, schizotypal, avoidant, and obsessive-compulsive personality disorders: findings from the collaborative longitudinal personality disorders study. J Nerv Ment Dis 2002;190:510–518.

37. Danielson KK, Moffitt TE, Caspi A, et al. Comorbidity between abuse of an adult and DSM-III-R mental disorders: evidence from an epidemiological study. Am J Psychiatry 1998;155:131–133.
38. Coid J, Petruckevitch A, Feder G, et al. Relation between childhood sexual and physical abuse and risk of revictimisation in women: a cross-sectional survey. Lancet 2001;358:450–454.
39. Felitti VJ, Anda RF, Nordenberg D, et al. Relationship of childhood abuse and household dysfunction to many of the leading causes of death in adults. The Adverse Childhood Experiences (ACE) Study. Am J Prev Med 1998;14:245–258.
40. Tjaden P, Thoennes N. The role of stalking in domestic violence crime reports generated by the Colorado Springs Police Department. Violence Vict 2000;15:427–441.
41. Byrne CA, Resnick HS, Kilpatrick DG, et al. The socioeconomic impact of interpersonal violence on women. J Cons Clin Psych 1999;67:362–366.
42. Maziak W, Asfar T, Mzayek F, et al. Socio-demographic correlates of psychiatric morbidity among low-income women in Aleppo, Syria. Soc Sci Med 2002;54(9):1419–1427.

Mental Health Services for Women in Third World Countries and Immigrant Women

Nalini Pandalangat

"The ones doing the looking are giving themselves the power to define" (1). This statement by Merata Mita, though drawn from a parallel context, resonates with meaning when one looks at how women's health is defined and addressed the world over. This assumes greater significance in "Third World countries" or "developing nations," where sociocultural, economic, and political factors further color the "looking" and the "defining."

Access to mental health services for women in Third World countries is a multifaceted issue, shrouded by blankets of marginalization. Marginalized by gender, the nature of the health issue, and the socioeconomic conditions of Third World countries, access to health and health services is particularly challenging (2). The cultural context in many of the Third World nations has its share of enablers and underminers that influence women's health status.

This chapter focuses on interface between many complex factors that affect access to services for women in Third World countries. It dwells on challenges and opportunities and the innovations that address some of the challenges. Finally it looks at service access for immigrant women in Canada. The understanding, gleaned from the initial section, of factors that influence service access in immigrant women's home countries is employed to look critically at how service delivery in the host country needs to be sensitive and based on a similar understanding.

UNDERSTANDING THIRD WORLD COUNTRIES AND THEIR HEALTH RESOURCES

So-called Third World countries are widely defined as countries that are poorer than a certain wealth threshold. Countries above the threshold are called First World countries. "Developing nations," "less developed nations," "nonindustrialized nations," and "the Global South" are some terms used interchangeably with the term "Third World countries" (3).

The World Health Report of 2001 (4) reiterates the fact that mental illness is associated with poverty and disadvantage the world over. By this yardstick, it is arguable that mental health in developing nations warrants closer attention. However, due to severe resource constraints, again attributable to the socioeconomic conditions of the countries in question, that attention is not accorded.

Statistics show that in low-income countries the median numbers of psychiatrists and psychiatric nurses are 0.06 and 0.1 per 100,000, whereas in high-income countries the numbers are 9 and 33.5 per 100,000 (4). The stark inequities are illustrated by a case in point: Africa. The African region, with a population of 620 million people, is served by 1,200 psychiatrists and 12,000 psychiatric nurses. In the European region, which includes countries of the former Soviet Union, a population of 870 million is served by 86,000 psychiatrists and 280,000 psychiatric nurses.

The dearth of resources impedes national and policy-level commitment to mental health (5). Of the 10 African nations, four that comprise 60% of the population of the African continent have no national mental health policy. One third (33%) have no relevant action program, and 25% have no legislation regarding mental health (4,6). About one third of the world's population lives in nations that invest less than 1% of their respective total health budgets in mental health. Looking at regional disparities, four fifths (78.9%) of the countries in the African region spend less than 1% of their health budgets on mental health. Two thirds (62.5%) of countries in Southeast Asia spend less than 1% of their health budgets on mental health. In contrast, in the European region, more than 54% of the countries spend more than 5% of their health budgets on mental health. In terms of income, of the low-income countries, 61.5% spend less than 1% on mental health (7). Again, this figure is dismal given that, in many countries with poor economies, the gross domestic product is small (8).

It is in this highly "lacking" context that we need to juxtapose our discourse of mental health services for women. It is not surprising that not much literature is available on the status of mental health services for women in Third World countries when one considers the reality that health services in general and mental health services specifically are themselves challenged entities in many of the Third World countries.

"DEFINING" WOMEN'S HEALTH

Tunnel vision is common in viewing women's health issues. Gender role expectations have significantly influenced the defining and addressing of women's health needs. A woman is seen primarily as a "reproducer" and "caregiver." This is more so in developing countries, where women are defined primarily as "wives" and "mothers" (9). In participatory action research on South Asian women who had immigrated to Canada, a very important theme that emerged was placing family needs before self (10). Given this context, often the basic focus among health-care professionals and policy makers has been on reproductive, maternal, and child health issues (9,11). Even in those areas, issues arise around the locus of control. In many countries, men continue to be the decision makers and still control women's reproductive and sexual health decisions (12). This lack of autonomy in itself could lead to stress and mental health difficulties. A growing recognition of the need for empowerment of women in reproductive health matters and related policy making has resulted in targeted action (13–15). Men's involvement in reproductive health matters is now being addressed within the framework of women's emancipation. Men's involvement is seen as being imperative to encourage responsible and shared decision making in sexuality and reproduction as well as to promote gender equity. Empathy to women's needs, revision of all forms of negative behavior that adversely impact women's physical and mental well-being, and support of women in the exercise of their rights are important aspects of male involvement (13,16).

WOMEN'S MENTAL HEALTH

THE ROLE OF PSYCHOSOCIAL STRESSORS

This focus on stressors for women in Third World countries does not make it a problem exclusive to the developing nations. Any assumption of such a dichotomy is artificial and merely serves to reiterate colonial views of the Third World nations. What is significant is that world over, poverty, lower levels of education, and gender inequalities affect the mental health of the population. Because the challenges of poverty and educational attainment are greater in developing nations, gender inequities become more pronounced and warrant closer consideration there. Leyla Gulcur (17) draws attention to the fact that the existing human rights treaties and consensus documents address the right to mental health only in very general terms. They do not address the specific ways in which cultural, social, and economic conditions interact with gender inequalities to produce gender differentials in mental health. Marginalization, powerlessness, poverty, overwork, stress, and the increasing incidence of domestic violence have been linked to mental disorders (18). Research has consistently shown that poverty, economic dependence, lower educational levels, lack of decision-making power, and high levels of domestic and child care responsibilities are negatively correlated with mental health (19).

A review of evidence shows that in the developed world, around 28% of all women report at least one episode of physical abuse, whereas in developing countries, studies indicate a prevalence ranging from 18% to 67% (20). While this is concerning, we have to exercise caution in drawing inferences regarding these disparities because the methods employed by studies to collect information might have been very different. The aforementioned review of evidence (20) also looked closely at six studies that examined the issue of violence against pregnant women in developing countries by reviewing six different studies undertaken in India, China, Pakistan, and Ethiopia. It concluded that the prevalence of violence against pregnant women in developing countries ranges from 4% to 29%. The main risk factors identified were low socioeconomic status, low education in both partners, and unplanned pregnancy.

A statistical profile of women in Bangladesh shows that life expectancy is lower for women than for men. The average age at marriage is around 18 years for women, while it is 25 years for men. The maternal mortality rate was 600 per 100,000 live births. Literacy rates for men and women in 1991 were 45.5% and 24.2%, respectively. Women generally work more hours in a day than men, largely doing unpaid family work. They are largely employed in the agricultural and related industrial sectors and the garment industry. Spousal abuse in Bangladeshi homes was related to issues of dowry, finances, custody of children, and suspected adultery (21).

In explaining the source of their psychosocial health problems, like "thinking too much," "worrying too much," tiredness, insomnia, and multiple somatic complaints, participants of a study conducted in Ghana, West Africa, identified a number of primary contributing factors: gender division of labor, heavy workloads, the "compulsory" nature of their work, financial insecurity, and the considerable financial responsibility they assumed for their children (9). It is significant that reproductive health problems did not figure prominently among the problems outlined by the women. The authors of the study underscore two important facts. One is that the psychosocial symptoms described do not find place in the discussions of the burden of disease in the developing world. This is because the women themselves are not involved in health-care decisions relevant to them. The second fact is that women in developing countries have too long been defined as childbearers, and their role as workers and the stresses related to the nature and proportion of work have been neglected. Studies of women in developing countries have shown that a higher risk for depression is partly accounted for by negative attitudes toward women, lack of acknowledgment of their work, fewer opportunities for them in education and employment, and a greater risk of domestic violence (22). However Gulcar (17) suggests that disparities between developed and developing nations are not acute. She draws in on the findings of WHO's Global Burden of Disease and states that, for women of reproductive age, of the 10 leading causes of disease burden, depression has currently become the major leading cause in both developing and industrialized regions.

A country's social and political climate also determines the stresses and the discrimination to which women are subjected. Gender apartheid was practiced in Afghanistan from 1996, during the Taliban regime. Gender apartheid refers to the gender-based segregation policies that severely restricted women's ability to function in society. Women were not allowed to work outside the home, except to a limited capacity in health care. Education was denied to them. Their mobility was severely restricted; they could travel only when accompanied by a male relative. This resulted in very restricted access to health and other essential services (23). It is little wonder that a survey by the Physicians for Human Rights showed a marked decrease in mental health of Afghanistani women under Taliban rule. Almost all Afghanistani women studied (97%) were diagnosed with depression, and 42% were diagnosed with post-traumatic stress disorder. This can well be attributed to the then ongoing war as well as the deteriorating conditions for women in Afghanistan (24). Worldwide, it is estimated that 80% of the 50 million people affected by war are women and children (25). In a large-scale survey (26) of the Sri Lankan Tamil community in Toronto, members of which had experienced a decades-long war and ethnic conflict in their home country, it was found that one third of the respondents reported traumatic events such as witnessing combat or experiencing physical assault or rape. Rates were higher for women (36.8%) than for men (30.7%).

CULTURAL FACTORS AND MENTAL HEALTH

Collectivistic or primarily non-Western cultures require a high level of related-ness and moderate levels of autonomy to maintain mental health (27). Many de-veloping nations have collectivistic cultures, which have greater connectedness than Western cultures and extensive social networks. Hence in social contexts where there is a moderate level of autonomy, a woman's degree of social and emotional connectedness, by virtue of her gender role as a caregiver, mother, and nurturer might actually enhance her mental well-being. In a study comparing the prevalence of alexithymia in rural India among women with functional somatic symptoms and those without, women without functional somatic symptoms showed coping such as talking to family members and seeking help and emo-tional support (28). However when the cultural context in developing countries or within communities stresses the caregiving and the homemaker roles while de-valuing the contributions of women and disempowering them, then this is a ready formula for mental health problems.

Murthy (29) states that mental health programs in developing countries should be implemented in ways that strengthen the positive aspects of rural life, which generally symbolize a collectivistic culture. The availability of community sup-port for patients, increased cohesion in patients' families, and simple ways of life that more easily accommodate a patient's rehabilitation and community reinte-gration are the strong points of a rural culture. Developing countries may present avenues for prevention of mental disorders because their traditional lifestyles often emphasize the importance of social supports in crisis (30). Research has shown better prognoses for people with psychiatric disabilities in developing na-tions than in Western countries. The emphasis on interdependence, the external-ized locus of control, and family involvement are significant factors in caring for people with psychiatric disabilities (31). However, further research is needed to assess whether this cultural advantage is retained for women in particular when there is a shift from women as caregivers to women as care recipients when fac-ing a mental health challenge.

ACCESS TO HEALTH AND HEALTH-CARE SERVICES

A review of the literature highlights the role of sociocultural, socioeconomic, and sociopolitical factors in influencing the mental health of women (see Chapters 26 and 27 in this volume). It reveals that the health of women is challenged by the existing social conditions. So unless the importance of the social determinants of health is acknowledged and pervasive action is undertaken, no health-care sys-tem, however evolved, will be able to address the mental health challenges for women in the developing world. Moreover, the paucity of resources in the mental health-care system of developing nations almost forces definitive social action as a viable mechanism.

According to a United Nations Development Program (UNDP) report in 1997 (32), of the 146 countries surveyed, none had a Gender Development Index (GDI) greater than its Human Development Index (HDI). Around 39 countries had a GDI of less than 0.500, indicating that the women in these countries did not reach even half the level of human development as assessed through the three indicators: life expectancy, educational achievement, and income. This meant that women were well behind their male counterparts in the ability to access opportunities for development. However it is heartening that many developing countries are realizing the need for gender empowerment to balance the equation. Some developing countries are surpassing developed nations in achieving gender empowerment in political, economic, and professional activities. For example Barbados, Guatemala, and Guyana have UNDP Gender Empowerment Measure (GEM) rankings in the top third of all countries.

It is in the light of gender empowerment and improving social circumstances as a means to access mental health services and promotion of better mental health that the role of grassroots organizations and community mental health initiatives gains significance. As Farmer (33) very succinctly observes when talking about behavioral change for better health, "Throughout the world, those least likely to comply are those least able to comply."

In the account of the Ghanaian women (9), although the study did not dwell on access issues, it could be safely surmised that the "compulsory" nature of work of Ghanaian women coupled with the magnitude of the workload might adversely affect the women's capacity to take the time to live healthily. It might also hinder access to services because the women might not be able to cut down on workload or share it with their male counterparts.

In the Taliban regime, where women were disempowered, male doctors were not allowed to see or touch a female patient during examination. This made diagnosis and treatment almost impossible. Also, male doctors could examine women only when a close male relative was present. Female health professionals were very scarce. All this restricted women's access to health-care services (34,35).

India, a nation with great diversity, is mixed in its responses to women's health and access issues. While some regions are making major strides in the empowerment of women, others are still in a deep slumber. Health services are concentrated in urban centers, and women and children are particularly at risk. Gender inequalities are particularly pronounced in the northern states. The inequalities have hindered access to education and health services (36). Good (11) notes that the attitudes of the health-care provider make it difficult for the woman to disclose psychological distress or the consequences of sexual violence, which is very often stigmatized. Communication among health workers, physicians, and women patients tends to be highly authoritarian in many places in the world regardless of the sex of the physician or the health worker.

Studies of women's mental health (25) show that up to 20% of those attending primary health care in developing countries suffer from anxiety or depressive disorders. In most cases, these needs are not recognized and hence not treated.

Worldwide, the Atlas project evaluated the availability of essential drugs to treat mental and neurologic disorders and concluded that more than 25% of the countries do not have the most common prescriptions of antipsychotic, antidepressant, and antiepilepsy drugs at the primary care level (37). Also, basic drugs are relatively less affordable in low-income countries, where 40% of the costs of mental health care are paid by the consumers (6). These factors will definitely infringe further on women's access to essential medication in societies with gender inequalities and marked socioeconomic challenges.

Another important factor influencing access to care is the differences in explanatory factors attributed to a condition, which are largely determined by cultural factors. Kleinman (38) states that perceptions of illness differ across cultures. Many cultures blend the natural with the supernatural in determining explanatory models of illness, and this definitely affects the kind of help sought (see Chapter 2 in this volume). Kakar (39) elaborates on the different sources of help that people in India seek to alleviate their psychic distress dependent on their predominant systems of belief.

Those who believe in possession by spirits seek relief from shamans; those who believe that psychic distress is the result of "karma" (the sum effect of one's deeds/misdeeds in one's previous lives) seek help from mystics, priests, and sadhus; and those who believe in the medical nature (physical or psychological) of illness seek help from physicians and psychiatrists. Much of the world outside North America and Europe regards the conditions or illnesses defined by *Diagnostic and Statistical Manual of Mental Disorders* as products either of fate or of weak character (40). These assumptions might lend themselves to shifting the locus of control and to escalating stigma, respectively, thus affecting help-seeking behavior. Another important factor is that often the mental health consequences of rape are not addressed because of cultural beliefs that equate a woman's worth with her virginity (41). It is important to consider how these belief systems affect help-seeking behavior in women who live in disadvantaged circumstances where they have less access to education, health information, and rights education than their male counterparts.

INNOVATIONS: TOWARD BETTER HEALTH

Recognition of the need to look at women's mental health has been increasing in recent years as the spotlight has turned to social origins of psychological distress for women. Addressing the health concerns of women is therefore happening at two intersecting levels: addressing the social origins of many problems through grassroots empowerment initiatives as well as enhancing sensitivity and access within the "socialized" health-care system to make it more responsive.

Legal reforms and major educational campaigns addressing domestic violence have been initiated in developing countries like Ecuador, India, and Mexico as a result of concerted activity of nongovernmental organizations (NGOs). In Brazil, feminist action has resulted in all-female police stations to assist victims of violence (42). Qualitative evaluations in African and Asian settings have found that interventions like the Stepping Stones program that focus on strengthening intimate relationships through parent training, mentoring, and marriage counseling have helped men communicate and show new respect for women. Given the linkages between domestic violence and mental disorders, such initiatives will definitely have a positive impact on mental well-being of women (22).

Adult literacy programs and programs to resist oppression are helping to reshape community mental health programs throughout the world's local communities (43). It is heartening that NGOs in the mental health sector are active in around 86% of the low-income countries and are often the pioneers of mental health service reform (44). In the area of reproductive health, as mentioned earlier in the chapter, organizations are working toward increasing the decision-making power of the childbearer in reproductive health issues, encouraging male involvement within the paradigm of female emancipation, and improving access to education and information. An example of this is "Suraksha," a community-based NGO in South India that focuses on women's reproductive rights as well as their rights to overall well-being (16).

Community mental health initiatives are gaining ground in developing countries as a way to address the lack of specialized mental health resources and personnel. Although they are not focused exclusively on women, these initiatives have many elements that promote a more gender-sensitive attitude and increased consumer participation.

A mental health program was drafted in Iran and received approval in 1986. This program's basic tenet was the integration of mental health into the primary care system through strategizing services, training, and administration. It is noteworthy that this program identified the special needs of vulnerable groups like adolescents, children, pregnant women, and the elderly (45). Although this is definitely a step forward, it is interesting to note that this program confines vulnerability among women to pregnant women and is thus another instance of women's health being seen through a reproductive lens.

A study in rural India took a community-based approach to combating alcoholism and promoting mental health of families through a participatory action research model. This gave an opportunity to young people and women to be involved in the community movement called "Liberation from Liquor," which included action against drunken men and advocacy to politicians to limit the sale and distribution of alcohol. This led to a 60% decrease in alcohol consumption and a reduction in domestic violence (46).

Several developing countries in Asia, Africa, and South America are now involved in the integration of mental health and primary care (29). The canvas has spread beyond the formal health system and encompasses the work of NGOs and citizens using a variety of community-oriented care programs. In Colombia, ancillary nurses are providing care for persons with nonpsychotic conditions. This could mean that conditions like "anxiety" and "nerves," which go undetected in the female population, now have better chances of being identified and treated. As identified by the World Health Organization document "Nations for Health: A Focus on Women" (41), gender-sensitive training with regard to the identification and management of mental health problems affecting women is essential. This includes developing sensitivity and heightened awareness toward psychosocial and sociocultural factors that impact mental health. In recent years, pilot integrated programs have been started in Bangladesh, Egypt, Nepal, Pakistan, and Indonesia. All this will increase access to care for previously underserved segments of the population, including women.

In a nutshell, it can be surmised that women in Third World countries face challenges both in attaining good health and in accessing health-care services. Contributing to these challenges are gender inequities, psychosocial stressors, socioeconomic disadvantages, and the paucity of resources of the Third World countries as well as their political climate, prescribed gender roles, and elements of culture. However, the picture is not all bleak. Gender empowerment, elements of culture, increasing participation in community health initiatives, and the work of grassroots NGOs are all helping to promote mental health and well-being of women in developing nations. It is important to realize that different countries and different regions within a country are at different phases of this journey. Hence, while looking at access issues for immigrant women from these countries, an appreciation of this diversity and unique personal circumstances is essential to develop population-specific strategies for health promotion and intervention.

IMMIGRANT WOMEN: ACCESS TO HEALTH AND HEALTH CARE

A perusal of the preceding section helps us readily identify factors impinging on access that accompany the woman in her migration and hence assume relevance in the host country as well. Some of the factors thus identified are lower levels of education, gender role identities that focus on caregiving and nurturing, cultural explanations to mental health, inhibitions to disclosing violence, and the like.

When there is a shift from the traditional, collectivist context to the individualistic, egalitarian context, the woman brings with her a family-oriented psyche without the support network that might have been an integral part of her life in her home country. Add to this the effects of forced migration (in some cases), financial strain, the need to take on an additional role (as wage earner), the need to balance family and outside work, incompatible social skills, and inadequate language skills. These demands leave the woman with little or no time, will, or agency to take care of herself or her health-related needs.

Studies of Asian women in North America have shown that they continue to maintain their gender role identities as immigrants (10). In a study of 118 caregivers for the elderly in South Asian families, 60% of the caregivers were found to be women. Among female caregivers, 20% were daughters and 38% were daughters-in-law, while the reminder were other female caregivers. Of the 40% male caregivers, 34% were sons and only 4% were sons-in-law (47). This finding is interesting from a sociocultural perspective. While women are expected to be responsible for the care of their husband's family, there is no similar expectation of men. This could be hypothesized as the patriarchal system feeding into gender inequities.

Another challenge for women who immigrate to North America is exposure to freedoms and opportunities that were unavailable to them earlier. These opportunities might conflict with the sex role socialization and the expectations of other family members, leading to intrapsychic and interpersonal stress as women try to preserve the norms of their home country and live up to family expectations while dealing with the aspirations generated in a new cultural context (48,49). An inquiry into changes in family dynamics, conflicting expectations, and levels of acculturation becomes important in this context.

Immigrant women face multiple disadvantages in the country of resettlement. Loss of social networks, financial instability, functional illiteracy, marginalization, and racial discrimination are some confounders (50). Because their families survive on shoestring budgets, immigrant women who are not fluent in the English language might not have the luxury of affording child care to attend English language classes (50). Immigrant and refugee women are also known to have average incomes that are much lower than their English-speaking counterparts, even if they have comparable education and experience (51,52). All of these factors detract not only from mental well-being but also from the woman's ability to access health care. Inadequate fluency in English makes the navigation of the health system difficult; a low-paying job might not allow the flexibility to meet the requirements of illness management like taking time off for a doctor's or clinic appointment. So here again, as in the immigrant's home country, there arises a need to address the social circumstances that influence health and health care. A summary of recommendations for health promoters recognizes this need and recommends focusing on reducing informational, cultural, linguistic, economic, and systemic barriers to care, using an empowerment philosophy, and involving the community in planning, design, and delivery of interventions. It also recommends that this be a dynamic process as attitudes, beliefs, and behaviors change as a consequence of acculturation (53). The settlement services in Canada are geared toward facilitating the integration of immigrants and newcomers and helping them address some of the challenges of resettlement. A number of settlement services are geared toward addressing the issues that immigrant and refugee women face in the host country. These organizations also play a significant role in advocating for these women.

Studies or findings focused on factors influencing access and the responsiveness of the health-care system yield interesting insights. In a study of the Sri Lankan Tamil community in Toronto (26), it was found that seniors and women were particularly likely to encounter linguistic barriers while negotiating the health-care system. It also found that whether a condition is perceived as "physical" or as "psychological" greatly influences the propensity to seek help. The cultural explanations of illness might be an important factor in this case. So understanding what attributions are made to psychological symptoms is imperative in such situations. This would help in reaching out to different clients in a culturally competent manner and addressing issues without deriding their belief systems.

A case study (54) of a female Puerto Rican migrant brings to light the necessity of cultural understanding and cultural competence in addressing mental health issues. The misdiagnosis of the client, leading to unwarranted medication and a poor outcome, is followed by her referral to a Latino clinic, where her condition is reassessed and a diagnosis is arrived at based on a cultural understanding of the client's behavior and cultural information of normative expressions of distress in the Puerto Rican population. Appropriate treatment and sustained improvement results. This finding draws attention to the fact that people who are defining mental illness may not be familiar with cultural expressions of distress. This inference finds support in accounts of mental distress in Ghanaian women as well as in other studies (9,55,56).

Western psychiatry demarcates "mental functioning" as related to different parts of the mind rather than to the person as a whole. Expressions of mental distress are seen as being manifested exclusively through the cognitive and affective domains, which comprise the mind. It is because of this segregatory approach that the Western world sees other populations as "somatising" their emotional disorders (57). This symptom description itself suggests an inherent racism because the assumption that emotional disorders are manifested through a particular symptom profile, which then assumes universal coinage, is based on Western culture from which Western psychiatry derives. Hence expression of distress through "bodily symptoms" is seen as "different" rather than a natural expression of the disorder that goes beyond the domains of the "mind."

A study of health-care utilization patterns among Russian-speaking immigrant women showed that a greater understanding of immigrant population's cultural patterns or orientations toward health-care utilization is needed to improve access and delivery of health-care services to these populations (58). Findings show a consistent reliance of these women on their physicians to refer them to services including prevention and health teaching on topics that will help them stay healthy. The women's unfamiliarity with a health-care system that puts them in charge of their health-care choices is challenging to them. Similarly, a woman from Afghanistan who had been conditioned to the extremely restrictive environment of gender apartheid might not be proactive in help seeking because the sociopolitical environment she came from actively discouraged and even punished such behavior. Health-care providers must be sensitive to such dispositions, which result either from mechanisms of natural socialization or from forced conditioning.

Finally, extreme sensitivity is required in dealing with immigrant and refugee women who are from war-torn countries or countries where they have been exposed to disaster, extreme trauma, and continued gender oppression. A study undertaken in Saskatchewan, Canada, with women who identified themselves as suffering from post-traumatic stress disorder found that while there seemed to be a strong theoretical knowledge of PTSD based on the DSM among service providers, this knowledge did not appear to be translated into practice. Physicians and psychiatrists were not identifying symptoms of the disorder among immigrant, refugee, and visible minority women clients (59). This leads us back to the discussion of cultural sensitivity required in identifying expressions of distress. Because the immigrant and refugee women from areas of disaster are a highly needy group, overlooking their needs is likely to result in serious mental health implications.

Any discussion on women's access to health care should cut through the boundaries of a formal health-care system and move beyond to an approach that looks at the social fabric of the macro system, thus working on improving the social determinants of health, encouraging female participation and empowerment, and building a more responsive system of care and service delivery.

REFERENCES

1. Mita M. "Merata Mita on …" New Zealand Listener, October 14, 1989:30.
2. SDC-Health: Access to health services. Swiss Agency for Development and Co-operation, 2003.
3. Haney D. Third world women. Available at: www.arches.uga.edu. Accessed Jan. 17, 2001.
4. World Health Organization. World Health Report. Mental health: new understanding, new hope. Geneva, 2001.
5. Murthy RS. Mental Health Policy: India—towards community mental health care. 2003. In Mental Illness: Global Challenges, Global Responses—Editorial Staff, Psychiatr Times 2004;20:11.
6. Thornicroft G, Maingay S. Editorial: the global response to mental illness. Br Med J 2002;325:608.
7. World Health Organization. Atlas: country profiles on mental health resources. Geneva, 2001.
8. Goldberg D, Thornicroft G. Overview and emerging themes. In: Goldberg D, Thornicroft G, eds. Mental Health in Our Future Cities. London: Psychology Press, 1998.
9. Avotri JY, Walters V. "You just look at our work and see if you have any freedom on earth": Ghanaian women's accounts of their work and health. Soc Sci Med 1999;48:1123–1133.
10. Choudry UK, Jandu S, Mahal J, et al. Health promotion and participatory action research with South Asian Women. J Nurs Scholarship 2002;34:75–81.
11. Good MJDV, Ware N. "Women." In: Desjarlais R, Eisenberg L, Good B, et al., eds. World Mental Health: Problems and Priorities in Low-Income Countries. New York: Oxford University Press, 1995:ch. 8.
12. Laudari C. Gender equity in reproductive and sexual health. Paper presented at UNFPA workshop on male involvement in reproductive health programs and services. Rome, November 1998.
13. Datta B, Misra G. Advocacy for reproductive health and women's empowerment in India. A Ford Foundation Report, 1997.
14. Karkal M. Family planning and reproductive rights of women. In: Lingam L, ed. Understanding Women's Health Issues: A Reader. New Delhi: Kali, 1998.
15. Sciortino R. The challenge of addressing gender in reproductive health programs: examples from Indonesia. Reprod Health Matters 1998;11:33–43.
16. Salgame L. Toward better reproductive health care in India. Changemakers J. Online journal available at: www.changemakers.net/journal/01june/salgame.cfm. Accessed June 1, 2001.
17. Gulcar L. Evaluating the role of gender inequalities and rights violations in women's mental health. Health Hum Rights 2000;5(1):47–66.
18. Beijing Declaration and Platform for Action of the Fourth World Conference on Women. UN document. A/CONF.177/20, para 100, 1995.

19. Dennerstein L, Astbury J, Morse C. Psychosocial and mental health aspects of women's health. Geneva: World Health Organization, 1993.

20. Nasir K, Hyder AA. Violence against pregnant women in developing countries: review of evidence. Eur J Public Health 2003,13:105 107,

21. Rianon NJ, Shelton AJ. Perception of spousal abuse expressed by married Bangladeshi immigrant women in Houston, Texas, U.S.A. J Immigr Health 2003;5(1):37–44.

22. World Health Organization. Women's mental health: an evidence based review. Geneva: WHO/MSD/MHP/00.1, 2000.

23. Third world women's health: gender apartheid. Available at: http://www.arches.uga.edu/~haneydaw/twwh/apartheid.html. Accessed August 5, 2004.

24. Rasekh Z, Bauer HM, Manos MM, et al. Women's health and human rights in Afghanistan. JAMA 1998;280:449–455.

25. World Health Organization. Gender and women's mental health: gender disparities and mental health: the facts. A WHO document. Available at: http://www.who.int/mental_health/prevention/genderwomen/en/print.html. Accessed August 5, 2004.

26. Beiser M, Simich L, Pandalangat N. Community in distress: mental health needs and help-seeking in the Tamil community in Toronto. Int Migration 2003;41(5):233–245.

27. Sato T, Shippensburg U. Autonomy and relatedness in psychopathology and treatment: a cross-cultural formulation. Genetic Soc Gen Psychol Monographs 2001;127(1):89–127.

28. Geetha PR, Sekar K. Alexithymia in rural health care. NIMHANS J 1995;13(1):53–57.

29. Murthy RS. Rural psychiatry in developing countries. Psychiatr Serv 1998;49:967–969.

30. Prevention of mental, neurological and psychological disorders. Geneva: World Health Organization, 1986.

31. Stanhope V. Culture, control and family involvement: a comparison of psycho-social rehabilitation in India and the US. Psychiatr Rehab J 2002;25(3):273–280.

32. United Nations Development Program. Human Development Report. New York: Oxford University Press, 1997.

33. Farmer P. Social scientists and the new tuberculosis. Soc Sci Med 1997;44:353.

34. U.S. Department of State, Bureau of Democracy, Human Rights, and Labour. Afghanistan country report on human rights practices for 1998. Washington, DC, 1999.

35. Feminist Majority Foundation Stop gender apartheid in Afghanistan: fact sheet. 1999.

36. Country profile: India. A VSO report. Available at: http://www.vso.org.uk/about/cprofiles/india.asp. Accessed October 10, 2004.

37. Current issues and forthcoming events. J Adv Nurs 2001;35(3):311–316.

38. Kleinman A. Major conceptual and research issues for cultural psychiatry. Cult Med Psychiatry 1980;4:3–13.

39. Kakar S. Shamans, Mystics and Doctors: A Psychological Inquiry into India and Its Healing Traditions. New York: Knopf, 1982.

40. Pang KYC. Understanding depression among elderly Korean immigrants through their folk illnesses. Med Anthropol Q 1994;8(2):209–216.

41. Gomel MK. Nations for mental health: a focus on women. Geneva: World Health Organization, Division of Mental Health and Prevention of Substance Abuse, 1997.

42. Heise LL, Pitanguy J, Germain A. Violence against women: the hidden health burden. World Discussion Papers. Washington, DC: The World Bank, 1994.

43. Davis DL, Low SM, eds. Gender, Health and Illness: The Case of Nerves. New York: Hemisphere Publishing, 1989.

44. Friedli L, Parker C, Jenkins R, et al. Developing a National Mental Health Policy. Hove: Psychology Press, 2002.

45. Mohit A. Mental health in Tehran in the context of the national mental health programme of Iran. In: Goldberg D, Thornicroft G. eds. Mental Health in Our Future Cities. London: Psychology Press, 1998.

46. Bang A, Bang R. Action against alcoholism. Health Action 1995;11(2).

47. Guptha R. Consideration of nursing home care placement for the elderly in South Asian families. J Immigr Health 2002;4(1):47–56.

48. Ahmed SM, Lemkau JP. Cultural issues in the primary care of South Asians. J Immigr Health 2000;2(2):89–96.

49. Morrison L, Guruge S, Snarr K. Sri Lankan Tamil immigrants in Toronto. In: Kelson GA, Delaet DL, eds. Gender and Immigration. London: Macmillan, 1999:144–162.

50. Guruge S, Donner GJ, Morrison L. The impact of Canadian health care reform on recent women immigrants and refugees. In: Gustafson DL, ed. Care and Consequences: The Impact of Health Care Reform. Halifax, Nova Scotia: Fernwood Publishing, 2000.

51. Waxler-Morrison N. Introduction. In: Waxler-Morrison N, Anderson JM, Richardson E, eds. Cross-Cultural Caring: A Handbook for Health Professionals in Western Canada. Vancouver: University of British Columbia Press, 1990:3–10.

52. Lee R. Passage from the homeland. Can Nurse 1994;October:27–32.

53. Hyman I, Guruge S. A review of theory and health promotion strategies for new immigrant women. Can J Pub Health 2002;93(3):183–187.

54. Fernandez RL. Cultural formulation of psychiatric diagnosis: diagnosis and treatment of *nervios* and *ataques* in a female Puerto Rican migrant. Cult Med Psychiatry 1996;20:155–163.
55. Escobar JI. Cross cultural aspects of the somatization trait. Hosp Comm Psychiatry 1987;38: 174–180.
56. Canino IA, Rubio Stipec M, Canio G, et al. Functional and somatic symptoms: a cross ethnic comparison. Am J Ortho Psychiatry 1992;62:605–612.
57. Rack P. Race, Culture and Mental Disorder. London: Tavistock, 1982.
58. Ivanov LL, Buck K. Health care utilization patterns of Russian speaking immigrant women across age groups. J Immigr Health 2002;4(1):17–27.
59. White J, Tutt S, Rude D, et al. Post traumatic stress disorder: the lived experience of immigrant, refugee and visible minority women: a research conducted under the auspices of Immigrant, Refugee and Visible Minority Women of Saskatchewan, Inc. 2001.

Index